Isaac D. Johnson

**Johnson's therapeutic key**

Isaac D. Johnson

**Johnson's therapeutic key**

ISBN/EAN: 9783742821164

Manufactured in Europe, USA, Canada, Australia, Japa

Cover: Foto ©Lupo / pixelio.de

Manufactured and distributed by brebook publishing software
(www.brebook.com)

Isaac D. Johnson

# Johnson's therapeutic key

# ГHERAPEUTIC KEY.

BY

I. D. JOHNSON, M.D.,

NORARY MEMBER OF THE AMERICAN INSTITUTE OF HOMŒOPATHY,
AND AUTHOR OF "A GUIDE TO HOMŒOPATHIC PRACTICE,"
"COUNSEL TO PARENTS," ETC.

**Sixteenth Edition.**

*REVISED, IMPROVED AND ENLARGED.*

---

PHILADELPHIA:
HAHNEMANN PUBLISHING HOUSE.
1899.

# PREFACE.

THE demand which has exhausted so large an edition of this little volume in so short a time has prompted the author to again bring out a new edition. And to gratify the wishes of a large number of our professional friends we have reproduced the MATERIA MEDICA—which was left out of the last edition—and given further indications for the use of the remedies, besides presenting other important matter not found in the original text.

The symptoms of each remedy throughout the work are marked according to their estimated value. The asterisk [ * ] represents *characteristic* symptoms, or "*Key-notes.*" Those in *italics* represent similar symptoms, but of a less prominent character; while those left without a sign correspond to a third degree of distinction.

We are indebted to the following gentlemen, whose works have furnished valuable hints in the preparaton of this edition: Drs. Raue, Hering, Guernsey, Lilienthal, Jahr, Hughes, Hale, Hartman, Hempel, Lippe, Gatchel, Arndt, Helmuth, and especially to Prof. A. R. Thomas, for valuable material culled from his excellent work on Post-Mortem Examinations.

The work is submitted to the Profession with the belief that it registers the furthest advance made in Therapeutics, and represents the condensed experience of the leading physicians of our School.

I. D. JOHNSON.

KENNETT SQUARE, PA., January, 1889.

# ABBREVIATIONS.

**āā.**—Ana, *Of each.*
**Ad.**—*To, up to.*
**Ad lib.**—Ad libitum, *At pleasure.*
**Aq. bull.**—Aqua bulliens, *Boiling water.*
**Aq. dest.**—Aqua destillata, *Distilled water.*
**Aq. ferv.**—Aqua fervens, *Hot water.*
**Aq. font.**—Aqua fontana, *Spring water.*
**C.**—Congius, *A gallon.*
**Cerat.**—Ceratum, *A cerate.*
**Comp.**—Compositus, *Compound.*
**D.**—Dosis, *A dose.*
**Dec.**—Decanta, *Pour off.*
**Decoct.**—Decoctum, *A decoction.*
**Dil.**—Dilutus, *Dilute.*
**Enem.**—Enema, *A clyster.*
**Esp.**—*Especially.*
**Ext.**—*Externally.*
**Extr.**—Extractum, *An extract.*
**Fl.**—Fluidus, *Fluid.*
**Ft.**—Fiat, *Let be made.*
**Gr.**—Granum, grana, *A grain, grains.*
**Gtt.**—Gutta, guttæ, *A drop, drops.*
**Inf.**—Infusum, *An infusion.*
**Int.**—*Internally.*
**Lb.**—Libra, *A pound.*
**Liq.**—Liquor, *A solution.*
**M.**—Misce, *Mix.*
**Mist.**—Mistura, *A mixture.*
**Mucil.**—Mucilago, *A mucilage.*
**No.**—Numero, *In number.*
**O.**—Octarius, *A pint.*
**Ov.**—Ovum, *An egg.*
**Pot.**—Potio, *A potion.*
**Proph.**—*Prophylactic.*
**Pulv.**—Pulveris, *A powder.*
**Q.S.**—Quantum sufficit, *Sufficient quantity.*
**℞.**—Recipe, *Take.*
**Ss.**—Semi, *One-half.*
**S., Sig.**—Signa, *Write.*
**Solv.**—Solve, *Dissolve.*
**Sol.**—Solutio, *A solution.*
**Spt.**—Spiritus, *A spirit.*
**St.**—Stet, *Let stand.*
**Sum.**—Sumat, *Let him take.*
**Suppos.**—Suppositoria, *A suppository.*
**Syr.**—Syrupus, *A syrup.*
**Tablesp.**—*A tablespoonful.*
**Teasp.**—*A teaspoonful.*
**Ter dle.**—Ter in die, *Thrice daily.*
**Tr.**—Tinctura, *A tincture.*
**Trit.**—Trituratus, *A trituration.*
**Ung.**—Unguentum, *An ointment.*
**Vin.**—Vinum, *A wine.*
**Vs.**—Venœsectio, *Venesection.*

# WEIGHTS AND MEASURES.

## APOTHECARIES' or TROY WEIGHT.

| Pound. | | Ounces. | | Drachms. | | Scruples. | | Grains. |
|---|---|---|---|---|---|---|---|---|
| ℔. | | ℥. | | ʒ. | | ℈. | | gr. |
| 1 | = | 12 | = | 96 | = | 288 | = | 5760 |
| | | 1 | = | 8 | = | 24 | = | 480 |
| | | | | 1 | = | 3 | = | 60 |
| | | | | | | 1 | = | 20 |

## APOTHECARIES' or WINE MEASURE.

| Gallon. | | Pints. | | Fluid ounces. | | Fluid drachms. | | Minims. |
|---|---|---|---|---|---|---|---|---|
| C. | | O. | | f℥. | | fʒ. | | ♏. |
| 1 | = | 8 | = | 128 | = | 1024 | = | 61440 |
| | | 1 | = | 16 | = | 128 | = | 7680 |
| | | | | 1 | = | 8 | = | 480 |
| | | | | | | 1 | = | 60 |

# PART I.

# DIAGNOSTIC AND THERAPEUTIC HINTS.

## DIAGNOSIS.

EVERY case of disease presents two grand problems to be solved; 1st, to discover its nature, and 2d, to devise its cure. And as it is a matter of vital importance to the physician to be familiar with the most approved methods of diagnosis, in order to take advantage of every possible circumstance that will aid in the cure of disease, a few suggestions, that will facilitate investigation and refresh the memory, will be acceptable to the clinical student who may not have time or opportunity to consult larger works on the subject.

## THE TONGUE.

The tongue and characters of its coating furnish important diagnostic signs in disease.

A *tremulous* tongue is, in all *acute* diseases, of evil import, but has no particular significance in chronic nervous disorders.

*Immobility* and *trembling* of tongue, indicates *torpor of the brain.*

If the tongue is protruded very *slowly*, or left exposed after being shown, it is a sign of great exhaustion, or congestion, or other pressure on brain.

When the tongue is thrust continually to *one* side it indicates hemiplegia of the organ.

A thick and flabby tongue, showing indentations from pressure of teeth, indicates *gastric* and *nervous irritation.*

A *sharp* and *pointed* tongue is often observed in *irritation* and *inflammation of the brain.*

A *bright red* tongue indicates *inflammation* of gastric or intestinal mucous membrane.

A *clean red* tongue, with papilla prominent, or a white coated tongue, with papilla projecting through the fur, indicate *scarlatina.*

**Coating of Tongue.**—Coating on root of tongue does not mean much, most persons have it even in best of health.

A *patchy* or "*map tongue*" denotes irritation or partial inflammation of the stomach.

A thick and *yellow fur* covering the tongue indicates *biliary derangement.*

A dark brown coating on tongue indicates *malignant fever.*

A *dry, blackish*, furred, and tremulous tongue indicates *abdominal* or *putrid typhus.*

A tongue *red on edges* and *tip*, or having a *red, dry streak*, in centre, is typical of *typhoid* and *gastric fevers.*

A *thick, white* coating on tongue indicates gastric derangements.

A *lead-colored* tongue is found in *cholera* and *mortification* of *lungs* and *stomach.*

A *lead-colored* tongue, with thrush, denotes death under all circumstances.—RAUE.

A *bluish tongue* denotes impeded circulation.

A *black coating*, in dysentery, indicates exhaustion, mortification, death. In *jaundice* it denotes organic disease of liver. In *small-pox* it is an unfavorable sign.

---

## THE PULSE.

The pulse of a healthy adult male at middle life beats from 70 to 75 times per minute; but this is not an invariable rule, for some persons enjoy good health with a pulse at 50, and even lower, while others are as well with a pulse at 90. Again, it varies at different periods of life, and according to sex, position of body, etc., thus:—

| | |
|---|---|
| In embryo, its average per minute is . . | 150 |
| At birth, . . . . . . . | 140 to 130 |
| During the *first* year, . . . . | 130 to 115 |
| During the *second* year, . . . | 115 to 100 |
| During the third year, . . . . | 100 to 90 |
| About the seventh year, . . . | 90 to 85 |
| About the *fourteenth* year, . . . | 85 to 80 |
| In the middle period of life, . . . | 75 to 70 |
| In old age, . . . . . . | 65 to 50 |

The pulse of *women* is more frequent by 10 or 15 beats per minute than those of men.

The pulse is more frequent by 10 or 12 beats in the *standing* than in the sitting posture.

Muscular exertion, as dancing, for example, will raise the pulse from 75 to 125, and even higher. And *eating* or *drinking* will likewise increase the heart's action; on the contrary, during sleep the pulse is less frequent.

### OF THE PULSE IN DISEASE.

*Acceleration* of the pulse is a common symptom of all febrile disorders; it augments with their increase and subsides with their decline.

The pulse of an adult rarely exceeds 150 per minute, even in *acute inflammatory* affections; when it runs above 170 per minute, it portends a fatal issue.

A *quick, hard* pulse is very characteristic of *diphtheria* and *scarlatina.*

A *quick, full, bounding* pulse indicates *inflammation*, or fever of an *acute inflammatory* character.

A *sluggish, full* pulse evinces a want of *nervous energy.*

Unusual *slowness* of pulse is chiefly met with in *chronic softening* and in *tuberculous* affections of the brain. It is also a common symptom in diseases attended with *coma* resulting from *concussion*, or compression of the brain.

A *changeable* pulse indicates *nervous* derangement, and sometimes *organic disease of heart.*

A *fine, scarcely perceptible* pulse denotes great *exhaustion* and approaching death.

An *intermittent* pulse is not inconsistent with health; nevertheless, it is more commonly an indication of disease of the heart.

---

## CLINICAL THERMOMETRY.

The temperature of the body in a state of health ranges between 98° and 100° F. It is slightly increased by eating, exercising, and external heat; on the contrary, it is reduced about 1½° during sleep.

To ascertain the temperature of the body, place the bulb of a thermometer under the tongue or in the axilla, carefully protecting it from the air, and after the space of five minutes, the temperature will be expressed by the ascent of the mercury in the instrument.

In *disease*, the temperature of the body deviates several degrees above and below the average of health. When it moves upward, it is far less dangerous than when it moves downward, particularly in children. Even in adults, one degree below the standard of health represents more danger than 2½° above, and 2° below more than 4° above, and so on.

In facial erysipelas, acute meningitis, pneumonia, scarlatina, typhus, small-pox, and intermittent fever it sometimes rises as high as 106° or 107° F. In other febrile diseases it rarely reaches 104°.

A temperature of 105° to 106°, if it continues uninterruptedly for some weeks, leads *certainly* to *death.*

The temperature *rises higher* the *nearer the disease draws to a fatal issue.*

The *lowest* extreme of temperature is sometimes found in the cold stage of cholera, when the mercury rises only 90° or 91° F. It also falls suddenly in some cases of puerperal fever, pneumonia, and abdominal typhus, after a preceding high temperature.

In general, for every degree of the thermometer, the pulse rises 10 beats per minute; but the rise of temperature to 99½° gives more evidence of disease than the rising of the pulse from 70 to 80 beats per minute.

A *decrease* of heat in morning is favorable; an increase from night to morning the *reverse*.

If the temperature remains *above* the *normal* after general symptoms denote convalescence, the patient is in danger of relapse, or the supervention of some other affection.

A *slow* and gradual increase of temperature indicates typhoid fever.

In the course of typhoid fever, a *sudden* notable *fall* of temperature indicates *intestinal hemorrhage.*

The range of the increase of heat in different febrile diseases extends to 110° F., and as a rule, the amount of increase is a criterion of the intensity of the disease. For example:—

| | | | | |
|---|---|---|---|---|
| A temperature | of | 108·6° | indicates | almost certain death. |
| " | " | 107° | " | generally fatal except in intermittent. |
| " | " | 106° | " | intense fever. |
| " | " | 105° | " | high fever; dangerous. |
| " | " | 104° | " | severe fever. |
| " | " | 102° | " | moderate fever. |
| " | " | 101° | " | slight fever. |
| | | 98·6° | " | normal. |
| " | " | 98° | " | sub-normal. |
| " | " | 96·6° | " | collapse. |
| " | " | 94° | " | algid collapse. |
| " | " | 93° | " | fatal collapse, except in cholera. |

## RESPIRATION.

In the healthy condition, respiration is easy, gentle, regular, and without noise. It varies according to age, sex, and individuality, so that the normal number of respirations will average during repose:—

| | | | |
|---|---|---|---|
| 1st year | about | 35 | per minute. |
| 2d year | " | 25 " | " |
| 15th year | " | 20 " | " |
| 25th year | " | 18 " | " |

Respiration is rendered more frequent by exercise, emotions, the process of digestion, etc. In disease it may be preternaturally frequent or slow, rising to 60 or 80, or falling to 8 or 10 per minute. Frequent respiration is common in all *febrile* and *inflammatory* diseases, especially in children. As a general rule, rapid breathing is a sign of thoracic disease. As mental emotions quicken the respiration, so do certain nervous diseases. In *hysteria*, patient often breathes 60 or 70 times a minute.

*Slow* respiration is seldom, if ever, an attendant upon pulmonary disease, but is the result of some structural or functional derangement of the nervous system. It is observed in apoplexy, in effusion of serum within the cranium, in softening of the brain, and in most of the circumstances which occasion coma.

*Abdominal* respiration is where the diaphragm chiefly exerts itself, while the walls of the chest are nearly at rest. This usually occurs in *acute pleurisy*, rheumatism of chest, pericarditis, fracture of ribs, etc.

*Thoracic* or *high* respiration is where the abdomen does not move, respiration being performed entirely by expansion of the chest. This is observed where the peritoneum, diaphragm or its pleural cavity is inflamed.

---

## ALVINE DISCHARGES.

**Signs from Defecation.**—Diarrhœa and constipation are two of the most uniform accompaniments of disease. Even in healthy subjects the character and frequency of the evacuations vary greatly. Infants have from 3 to 6 passages daily, adults usually one, and the aged even less. Persons leading a sedentary life and using stimulating food, often go for a week without a fæcal discharge.

The existence of *Constipation*, except where it leads to an accumulation of fæces in bowels, has but little influence upon prognosis.

In *diarrhœa* the stools vary from 2 or 3 to 40 or 50 in 24 hours.

*Diarrhœa* occurring in the commencement of an acute attack of disease seated elsewhere than in abdomen, is of *unfavorable* significance. If it occurs later in the disease, followed by alleviation of symptoms, it is sometimes critical. Dropsies have been cured by spontaneous diarrhœa.

*Involuntary* stools, without consciousness or without patient being able to prevent it, indicates fatal result.

**Consistency of Fæces.**—Children at the breast pass fæces of pap-like consistence; with the advance of years they grow progressively harder.

In *disease*, the excrements may be as hard as dry clay, or as thin as serum.

In *mania*, melancholy, and lead-colic, fæces are extremely compact. When long retained they will be globular, resembling sheep's dung.

In *stricture* of rectum, fæces assume shape and size of aperture, may be flattened, indented, or long and slender.

*Color* of fæces varies. In children at the breast they are habitually light-yellow. During first dentition, and in summer complaint, they often resemble hashed spinach.

In *cholera*, stools contain little flakes of fibrin, giving them appearance of rice-water.

A *deficiency* of *bile* makes stools grayish-white like potter's clay.

An *excess* of *bile* makes the stools brown or dark colored.

*Redness* of the stools, is due to the presence of blood, seen in dysentery, congestion of liver, spleen, and in hæmorrhoids, typhus, scurvy and purpura.

---

## THE URINE.

### PHYSICAL EXAMINATION OF.

A healthy adult person passes from 30 to 40 fluidounces of urine in 24 hours; the quantity in summer varying from 30 to 35 ounces. Certain articles of food, drink, and drugs change its quantity and quality. Fruits, as apples, peaches, melons, etc., increase its quantity; while *madder* imparts to it a deep *orange-color; logwood, raspberries, mulberries,* and *blackberries*, increase its REDNESS; *indigo* makes it *blue*, *rhubarb* and *angusturia* YELLOW; *carbolic acid* and preparations of iron *blacken* it, and *tannin* renders it colorless. *Turpentine* gives to it an odor of *violets; cubebs* its characteristic smell, and *asparagus* a *fetid* odor.

Color. Healthy urine is light amber or straw colored, but it may be colorless as water. It exhales a peculiar aromatic odor, which it loses on cooling. About 93 parts in 100 of such urine are pure water; the remainder are chiefly *urea*, saline and organic matters.

### DIAGNOSTIC HINTS.

A *smoky* tint is diagnostic of the presence of blood.

*Red urine* generally indicates an excess of acid.

*Deep yellow* urine indicates the presence of bile.

*Dark brown* or *black* urine occurs during many malignant diseases, and are due to rapid morbid changes in the tissues and to decomposition of the blood.

*Turbid* urine indicates the presence of mucus or pus.

*Pale* urine contains an excess of water, urea, or sugar.

*Colorless* urine is seen in *hysteria*, and after eating certain fruits.

The *froth* on normal urine readily disappears, but if it be permanent, the presence of albumen or the constituents of bile may be suspected.

### CHEMICAL ANALYSIS OF THE URINE.

Before commencing the examination of the urine, the clinical student should provide himself with the following apparatus and reagents:—

Two Cylindrical Urine Glasses capable of holding from 4 to 6 ounces each.

A Urinometer, the stem graduated from 1000 to 1060.
Blue and Red Litmus and Turmeric Paper.
A Test Tube.
A Spirit Lamp.
Nitric and Acetic Acid.
Liquor Potassæ or Liquor Soda.
Ferrocyanide of Potassium.
A Glass Funnel and some Filtering Paper.

## SPECIFIC GRAVITY.

The specific gravity of urine varies in health from 1010 to 1025; a fair average is about 1020. The simplest way of testing its density is by means of the Urinometer.

The urine to be examined should be a portion of the *whole quantity passed in 24 hours.* Put about 4 ounces into a cylindrical glass, care being taken to remove all froth. The Urinometer is then introduced, and allowed to float freely without contact with the glass. To obtain a correct reading, place the eye on a level with the surface of the fluid, and look through the glass at the scale on the stem of the instrument.

*Sugar* in the urine is the most common cause of a high specific gravity; if this substance be not present, *uric acid* will be the most probable cause.

A low specific gravity is often noticed in chronic Bright's disease, in hysteria, in anæmic conditions, and in diuresis from any cause.

## REACTION.

Healthy urine is generally acid, as may be proven by test-paper (turning *blue* litmus-paper red).

A very acid, high-colored urine favors the occurrence of *calculus* and *gravel.*

*Alkaline urine* is rarely observed; when it is, it will be found to turn red litmus-paper blue. *Acid* urine sometimes becomes alkaline by standing long.

## EXAMINATION FOR ALBUMEN.

Urine not distinctly *acid* should be rendered so before testing it for albumen, by adding a few drops *Acetic Acid.* If *permanently turbid,* it should be *filtered* before boiling.

**Test.**—Place half an ounce of urine in a *clean* test-tube, heat slowly to boiling point; if a whitish cloud forms, add a few drops of *Nitric Acid,* and if the cloudiness *remains,* it is due to albumen; but it disappears if due to the earthy phosphates.

**Dr. Smith's Test.**—To a little urine in a test-tube add one-third its bulk of *Acetic Acid*, and afterwards a few drops of a solution of *Ferrocyanide of Potassium;* if albumen be present, a distinct whitish precipitate will occur.

**Renal Casts.**—The search for *renal casts* should always follow the detection of albumen, as this substance alone does not indicate kidney disease unless tube-casts are found. Allow the urine to settle in a tall glass, then pour off the top, and use last few drops, which place under microscope for examination.

## EXAMINATION FOR SUGAR.

Sugar in the urine is the most common cause of a high specific gravity; if it rises above 1030, sugar may be suspected.

**Moore's Test.**—Equal parts of urine and liquor potassæ or liquor sodæ are poured into a test-tube, and the upper layer of this mixture heated to boiling over a spirit-lamp. The heated portion becomes *brown-red*, *dark-brown*, or *black*, according to the amount of sugar present. If the mixture does not perceptibly darken on boiling, it may be assumed to be free from a hurtful quantity of sugar.

**Cautions.**—High-colored urines, and urines containing excess of phosphates, darken perceptibly on boiling with caustic alkalies, and if the urine be albuminous, the color will be greatly deepened, though no sugar be present. Before applying the tests, therefore, to albuminous urine, the albumen must be removed by filtration after boiling with a few drops of *Acetic Acid.*

**Trommer's Test.**—Put about a drachm of the urine into a test-tube, and add about half the quantity of liquor potassæ or sodæ. A weak solution of *sulphate of copper* (10 grains to fluidounce) is now dropped into the mixture. The precipitate first formed is redissolved on shaking the test-tube. The copper should be carefully dropped in, and the test-tube shaken after each drop is added, so long as the precipitate is easily redissolved. The solution will now be a blue transparent liquid. The mixture is next heated to boiling, when, if sugar be present, an *orange-red* precipitate will first be thrown down, which, after standing, becomes reddish-brown.

**Quantity of Sugar in the Urine.**—To estimate the amount of sugar in the urine, put about 4 fluidounces into a 12-ounce bottle with a piece of German yeast the size of a chestnut; set it in a warm place, *lightly* covered, and by its side place another bottle of the same urine without any yeast, and tightly corked. After a period of 24 hours, the fermented urine is poured into a wineglass, and the specific gravity taken. The specific gravity of the unfermented urine is also taken, and the number of "degrees of density lost" in the *fermented* urine will give the number of grains of sugar contained in a fluidounce.

**Observations.**—Modern research has shown that a healthy man excretes daily through the kidneys about 15 grains of sugar; therefore, unless the tests show a much greater quantity than this, it is of little value in a diagnostic or therapeutic sense. It has also been ascertained that the excretion of sugar in diabetes is far greater during the night than during the day.

### PUS IN THE URINE.

*Pus* is frequently present in the urine, and produces a thick sediment at the bottom of urine-glass. It rarely becomes *alkaline*, and readily decomposes after being passed. It is permanently turbid; that is, the turbidity is unaffected by heat.

The deposit from urine containing *pus* is rendered *viscid* and *gelatinous* by the addition of about half its quantity of liquor potassæ. Urine containing *mucus*, on the other hand, becomes more *fluid* and *limpid* by the addition of liquor potassæ.

### URINARY DEPOSITS.

The microscope affords the best means of determining the character of urinary sediments.

A *light*, flocculent, cloudy deposit is commonly mucus, epithelial cells or spermatozoa.

A *yellow*, orange, or pinkish deposit, dissolving when heated—urine acid—is due to *urates*.

A *dense*, *abundant white* deposit, dissolving when *Acetic Acid* is added—urine alkaline—consists of phosphates.

A granular or crystalline reddish deposit, is uric acid.

A *dark*, *sooty* and *dingy-red* deposit, is usually *blood*.

Bodies *resembling earth-worms*, are sometimes passed from the bladder; they are *coagula of blood*, moulded in the ureters.

---

## THE SICK-ROOM.

The room to be occupied by the sick should be large and airy, on the upper floor of house, exposed to direct rays of sun and as retired as possible. The *temperature* in winter should not exceed 70° F.

**Ventilation.**—*A constant supply of pure atmospheric air is an absolute necessity in the sick-room.* Remove all perfumery, camphor and quack nostrums; open the windows and doors, and let in the pure fresh air of heaven. Observe the strictest regard to cleanliness, and exclude all persons *not absolutely* needed, as they tend to vitiate the atmosphere.

**Furniture.**—The *bed* should be a *hair mattress*, covered with a gum blanket or oilcloth to prevent its being soiled; over this place the under sheet and then the upper coverings. Use *hair* pillows, and where special support is needed [as in case of bed-sores] *air cushions.* Where *contagious* diseases are rife, have as little furniture in room as possible, especially upholstered, and no carpets, curtains or rugs.

**Disinfection.**—No disinfectant can take the place of free ventilation and cleanliness. Volatile chemical agents, such as *Carbolic Acid*, *Chlorine*, *Bromine*, *Iodine* and *Sulphurous Acid*, when used in sufficient quantities to destroy *disease germs*, will also destroy the patient; therefore, it is found impractical to disinfect an *occupied* room by such means. Bad *odors* may be neutralized, but this is not disinfection; better turn *foul air* out the window or up the chimney, than attempt to purify it.

*Pulverized Charcoal* put in dishes and set about the room is an excellent purifier of vitiated air. *Cold fresh* water, put in a wide tub and placed under the bed, is a good absorber of gases. It should be renewed two or three times a day.

**Disinfection of Excreta.**—Receive all alvine and other discharges in a *porcelain vessel* containing a solution *Chloride Lime* [4 ounces to gallon], let stand ten minutes, then remove and bury. If impracticable to bury discharges, empty into water-closet, and frequently throw down a solution *Sulphate of Iron* [1 lb. to gal.].

Another powerful disinfectant is: ℞. *Corrosive Sublimate* and Permanganate of Potash, āā ℥ii, water Cj: dissolve and use same as *Chloride Lime*. Being odorless, it has this advantage. It is *very poisonous*, and will injure leaden pipes and metallic vessels if allowed to remain in them long.

**Disinfection of Clothing.**—All soiled clothing should be immersed in *Chloride of Lime* water [2 ounces to gal.] for two hours before being sent to the wash. Clothing and bedding which cannot be washed should be exposed to a temperature of 230° for three hours, and where this cannot be properly done, they should be burned.

**Sputa.**—All matters or secretions expectorated by patients suffering with *scarlatina*, *diphtheria*, *small-pox*, *typhus*, *phthisis*, etc., should be disinfected by being discharged in a cup half full of Chloride of Lime Water [4 oz. to gal.].

**Fetid Odors.**—Offensive odors arising from morbid secretions, exhalations, etc., may be deodorized as follows: Dissolve an ounce of *Chlorate Potassæ* in a gallon of water, saturate cloths in the solution and hang them about the room.

**Fumigation.**—After scarlatina, small-pox, diphtheria, typhus and yellow fever, fumigation should be resorted to. Take three lbs. of *Sulphur* [for every 1000 cubic feet of air space in room], put it in an earthen pan, set it on a brick in a tub part full of water, place this in the room and set it on fire with live coals. All heavy clothing should be opened out and fully exposed, and all *metallic* substances removed. Keep the room *tightly closed* for twenty-four hours, then open and air thoroughly.

**Privy Vaults, Cess-Pools, etc.**—For the disinfection of privy vaults, cess-pools, etc., dissolve two pounds of Sulphate of Iron in two gallons of water and throw into pit or drain. This should be repeated from time to time as occasion may require.

---

## DIETETIC PREPARATIONS.

**BEEF TEA (Liebig's Receipt).**—Take half a pound of fresh beef, finely minced, one pint soft water, four drops *Muriatic acid*, and a little salt. Dissolve the salt and acid in three-fourths of the water and add to it the meat. Let stand *an hour*, then strain through a sieve or cheese-cloth, and wash the residue with the extra quarter of a pint water, and mix the two liquids together.

To *warm up* beef tea put it in a teacup and set the cup in a vessel of *hot* water.

**BEEF TEA (Gatchel's Receipt).**—Take a pound of fresh beef cut fine, soak over night in third of a quart cold water. Now put the meat in two-thirds of a quart water and *simmer* two hours, adding a little water occasionally to replace what is lost by evaporation. When done pour the *broth* into the liquor in which the meat was soaked, squeezing meat dry as possible. Put meat on plate in oven, and when perfectly dry, powder in a mortar and mix it with the liquor. Add a little salt, 20 drops *Muriatic ac.*, and 3 grs. *Pepsin.*

This preparation contains all the elements of the meat in a liquid form. It makes an excellent *nutrient* enema.

**BEEF TEA [No. 2].**—Take a pound of lean beef, pound thoroughly, put it in a pint of cold water, place over a slow fire and let it come to a boil, then remove it from the fire, skim off the top and season with a little salt.

**BEEF JUICE.**—Take a slice of fresh juicy beef without any fat, broil it just enough to heat it well through, score it on both sides and press out the juice with a lemon-squeezer into a *hot* bowl, and serve it warm.

**CHICKEN BROTH.**—To a pound and a half of chicken, cut in small pieces and bones broken, add three pints cold water and a teaspoonful of rice. Bring slowly to a boil and let simmer two hours closely covered. When done pass it through a sieve into a *hot* bowl pressing through the rice. Let stand a few moments, skim off the fat and season with salt.

**MUTTON BROTH.**—Put a pound of mutton cut in pieces in a quart of cold water, bring it slowly to a boil, and let simmer for two hours; when done pour through a sieve, skim off the fat, and season with salt and a *very* little red-pepper. A little fresh, well boiled rice may be added.

**OYSTER SOUP.**—Put one pint of oysters in a saucepan, add a teacupful of water; place on the fire, and when it comes to a boil, remove it and pour off the liquor into a *hot* bowl, and the *oysters* in another vessel. Return the pan to the fire and put into it a lump of butter the size of a walnut, and when it begins to bubble stir in a spoonful of finely powdered cracker, then add the juice of the oysters and half a teacupful of cream. Let cook a few minutes, then add the oysters, and when thoroughly hot, season with salt and serve immediately.

**BARLEY GRUEL.**—Mix gradually a tablespoonful of *barley flour* with an ounce of *cold* water, then add two ounces of boiling water and a pinch of salt. Cook for a few minutes and then add three tablespoonfuls of milk; let it again come to a boil and sweeten with a little sugar.

**GRAHAM-FLOUR GRUEL.**—Take two heaped tablespoonfuls of Graham flour; one pint of water salted. Rub up the flour in half a teacupful of cold water; put the pint of water in a *water bath* (or farina-kettle) over the fire, and when it boils, stir in the flour and cook three-quarters of an hour. When done, strain through a thin cloth, add a tablespoonful of sweet cream, and serve warm. This is an *excellent* article of diet for children or persons with delicate stomachs.

**RICE GRUEL.**—Take one tablespoonful of ground rice, one pint of water, and a pinch of salt. Rub up the rice in a little cold water; put the pint of water in a saucepan over the fire, and when it boils, stir in the rice and cook twenty minutes. If a *richer* gruel is desired, use *milk* instead of water.

**GRAHAM BREAD.**—Take one cupful bread sponge; half a cupful warm water; three cupfuls Graham flour; lard the size of an egg; half teaspoonful salt. Mix ingredients together and put in a deep pan and set in a warm place. When well raised, bake immediately.

**TOAST.**—Use *stale* bread; cut slices thin and even; place on a thin platter in an open oven, and dry it through; then place in a toaster and turn from one side to the other until it receives a deep yellow and uniform color. If to be served *dry*, place on a hot plate, butter and salt slightly.

To make WATER TOAST, prepare the bread in the same manner as described above, then pour over it a cupful of boiling water, cover with a dish, and set in a hot oven for a few minutes.

**CREAM TOAST.**—Prepare the bread as described above; pour over it boiling water, and after standing a moment, drain it off; butter and salt it slightly, then pour over it a little fresh cream. Set in a hot oven for a few minutes, then serve it immediately.

**GRAPE JUICE.**—To one quart of grapes add a pint of water; let simmer from five to ten minutes; then strain through a cloth and sweeten to taste.

**APPLE WATER.**—Take a juicy apple; pare, core, and cut in slices; boil in a closely covered vessel till thoroughly cooked; then strain and sweeten to taste.

**LIME WATER.**—Take a lump of *unslacked* lime, size of small hen's egg; pour over it a quart of *hot* water; when slacked, stir thoroughly and let stand over night; then pour off the clear liquid and bottle.

**TO KEEP ICE.**—Tie a flannel cloth over the mouth of a deep vessel; let the cloth hang down loosely in the vessel; put the ice in this and cover with another flannel. Ice will keep in this way many hours in warm weather.

---

## ARTIFICIAL DIGESTION.

Pepsin and Pancreatin are extensively used at present for the purpose of digesting food artificially. *Pepsin* is usually prescribed in ten-grain doses immediately before or after each meal to assist digestion. It should be mixed with arrowroot and given in sweetened water. If administered while fresh or in an active condition, it will be found very *useful* in some forms of chronic dyspepsia, and in convalescence after acute exhausting diseases.

*Pancreatin* is mixed with the alimentary substances, such as milk, gruel, beef-tea, etc., and the food allowed to undergo *partial digestion* before being taken into the stomach. Food treated in this way has been found especially useful in that form of indigestion sometimes called "intestinal dyspepsia."

**To Peptonize Milk.**—Dissolve 5 grs. *Ext. Pancreatis* and 15 grs. Bicarbonate Soda in 4 ounces of water. Pour this into a quart bottle and add to it a pint of fresh milk. Place the bottle in a temperature of 100° F. to keep it warm; let stand from 30 to 60 minutes, according to the degree of fermentation desired. When the milk turns grayish yellow and tastes bitter, it is thoroughly *peptonized.* The process of fermentation may be arrested at any point by heating the food to the boiling point, or putting it in a refrigerator and keeping it *cold.*

---

## RECTAL ALIMENTATION.

When it becomes necessary to nourish a patient, where food cannot be taken by the mouth or retained by the stomach, nutrient injections have been resorted to for the purpose of sustaining life.

Milk, beef-tea, broths, gruels, etc., are employed for this purpose. *Peptonized* foods used in this manner have been found very valuable.

The rectum should be well emptied and washed out by *warm* water injections before giving the food. The temperature of food should be about 98° F. Inject about *two ounces* at a time, at intervals of two hours. Use syringe with long tube; inject slowly and as high up as possible.

**Nutrient Suppositories** are largely used in cases requiring food in this way. They are manufactured and for sale at most drug stores.

---

## DIET OF INFANTS.

The question of *Diet for Infants* "reared by hand," is one of great importance to the clinical student. On account of the difficulty experienced in obtaining a suitable substitute for mother's milk, various articles and compounds have been introduced to meet the wants of the infant.

**WET-NURSE.**—The mother's milk, where she is healthy, is undoubtedly the best food for child; but where this cannot be obtained, a proper substitute must be furnished. Breast-milk being the natural food for infant, a *wet-nurse* should be procured. Before engaging one, however, her physical condition should be closely scrutinized. She should have a robust constitution, be free from all eruptions, herpes, ulcers, leucorrhœa, syphilis; in a word, she should be healthy and free from all vices and pernicious habits.

**COW'S MILK.**—Cow's milk is perhaps the best food for infants where the mother's milk is out of the question, or a suitable *wet-nurse* cannot be obtained. But there are many points to be considered in its selection. It is important that the milk be taken from *one cow*, and not from a mixture of several. For a *new-born infant*, the cow should be fresh or nearly so, and the milk *first drawn* used, as it is weaker and will not require the admixture of water. If the milk be *rich*, add one-third warm water and sweeten with *Sugar of Milk*. As child grows older, add less water. The milk should not be boiled, but heated in a *water-bath*, or given fresh from the cow. When cow's milk disagrees, a *little salt* added will often be of great advantage.

Cow's milk is slightly *alkaline*, but sometimes when the animal has been milking several months, it becomes slightly acid, in which case some physicians advise adding a little *lime-water*. To test the acidity, dip a strip of *blue* litmus-paper in the milk, and if paper turns *red*, milk is acid and unfit for a young infant. Good cow's milk will turn *red* litmus-paper blue.

**SUGAR OF MILK.**—Where the mother has a deficiency of milk, and the child requires additional food, dissolve a large teaspoonful of *Sugar of Milk* in half a teacupful of boiling water, and add an equal quantity of *fresh unskimmed milk*, and give in proper quantities to the child. In using this preparation, if the milk or caseum is thrown up or passed from the bowels undigested, add a little pulverized *gum arabic* to the mixture.—DR. MOORE.

**WHEAT GRUEL.**—Boil a handful of *unbolted* wheat flour in a quart of water for three-quarters of an hour; strain through a cloth, slightly season with salt and sugar, and thin so as to pass through the nursing-tube. A little cream added will make it more nourishing, or if *marasmus* threaten, pulverized hard-boiled yolk of egg may be added. This is an excellent article of diet for young children. As they grow older, get their teeth, and are of an age to wean, it should be prepared in the form of mush, and eaten with a little sugar and cream.

**GELATINE.**—Take a piece of sheet gelatine about the size of silver dollar, soak half hour in water. Then put it in a pint of fresh water and boil till dissolved. Rub three tea-spoonfuls of Bermuda arrowroot in a little milk, stir it into the gelatine-water, boil six or eight minutes and add a pinch of salt. Now add six tablespoonfuls of new milk and boil. After removing from the fire, add four tablespoonfuls of cream and a little sugar. If the child be constipated do not boil the milk.

**WHEAT FLOUR.**—Tie some flour in a cloth, boil for several hours until it becomes hard, when dry grate it down, and add a little milk or cream, with sugar. This is a very suitable diet for children after weaning, and does well for a change.

**WHEY.**—Sweet whey prepared by separating the whey from the curd by rennet, is especially indicated when the child suffers from imperfect digestion.

**BEEF TEA.**—Put one pound of fresh, lean beef in two quarts of water, and boil down to a pint; to a spoonful of this add one of water and one of milk. Advised where there is great *prostration.*

**BRAN TEA.**—To a teacupful of wheat bran add a quart of water, and boil several minutes; add a little milk, and sweeten to suit. Advised in *constipation.*

---

## WATER, IMPURITIES IN.

The taste and odor of a water are not to be relied upon in any degree. Water of delicious taste, clear and sparkling. may contain deadly impurities, while that tasting and smelling badly may be innocuous.

**Organic Matter.**—Evaporate a quart of the water from a porcelain dish and note the residue, which should not be great. It may be due to excess of mineral matter not especially harmful. Put residue into iron spoon and heat over a lamp. If it turns black, organic matter is present. The odor given off while heating, will help to determine nature of impurity.

**Test.**—To a given quantity of water add enough *Permanganate Potash* to give it a pinkish hue; cover carefully to exclude air; if organic matter is present a brownish color will develop in a few hours.

**Fermentation Test.**—To given specimen of water add a *Syrup of Sugar*, and keep warm enough for fermentation to take place. If organic matter be present, gas bubbles will be seen rising. Such impurities may be removed by filtration through sand, gravel, or charcoal.

**Chlorides.**—To half pint of the water add a drop of *Nitric Acid*, then a few drops of a solution *Nitrate Silver*. If a white precipitate is formed which turns black on exposure to sunlight, *chlorides* are present, and if in large amount these waters should be avoided.

**Lead.**—Water is often impregnated with a salt of lead from being kept in cisterns or pipes formed of this metal. Among the *tests*, none are so efficacious as *Sulphuretted hydrogen;* it reveals a *brown-black* precipitate where less than the 100,000th part of the salt is present.

*Again*, to a glass of water add two or three drops of a solution *Sulphide of soda*. If the water becomes dark-colored, add two or three drops *Hydrochloric acid;* if the color does not disappear, lead is present; if it does, first discoloration is due to iron.

**Carbonate of Lime.**—Water containing *lime* is usually termed "hard water." The degree of hardness is exhibited by its power to curdle soap. When it can be removed by boiling or evaporation, it depends upon the presence of *Carbonate of lime*, and when irremovable by this treatment, *Sulphate of lime* is usually present. Such water is unfit to use in the preparation of medicine. It may be detected by adding to the specimen a portion of *lime-water*. The lime unites with the carbonic acid, which holds the carbonate of lime in solution, and the latter is set free in the form of a white powder.

**Sulphate of Lime.**—Add to the water a few drops of *Nitrate of Baryta*, and if sulphate of lime be present, a white insoluble precipitate will be thrown down.

**Sulphate of Copper.**—*Sulphuretted hydrogen* gives a deep chocolate-brown precipitate; or, if the copper be in small quantity, merely a brown color. A slip of *polished iron* (a common needle), suspended by a thread in the water, is speedily coated with a layer of copper.

**Sulphate of Iron.**—*Ferrocyanide of Potassium* added to the liquid gives a greenish-blue precipitate, becoming deep blue on exposure to the air. *Hydrosulphuret of Ammonia* gives a black precipitate.

**Oxide of Zinc.**—*Ammonia*, or *Sesquicarbonate of Ammonia*, throws down a white precipitate.

# WATER AS A CURATIVE AGENT.

As a hygienic and curative agent, water has been employed from time immemorial. That it possesses great palliative and curative powers has been well attested, both in public and private practice. It is an important auxiliary in the treatment of disease when employed in conformity with the homœopathic law of similars.

**Bathing.**—Every bath should be taken while the body is *warm.*

No bath should be taken on a *full stomach*, or soon after a meal.

Being in a perspiration is no objection to taking a bath.

Delicate persons should not remain long in a bath. Should *leave* the water feeling vigorated.

**THE SPONGE BATH.**—Apply the water by means of a sponge or crash towel, then rub briskly and thoroughly dry. Any invalid may take this bath with benefit. The water may be *warm* [90° to 100° F.] or cold [50° to 60°] to suit the patient.

**THE WARM BATH.**—The patient should lie in the bath and be rubbed by the nurse. If a bath-tub is not at hand, use a large wash-tub, which the patient may sit in, while the nurse dashes the water rapidly over the neck and shoulders for three or four minutes, then wraps him in a *clean dry* sheet, places him in bed, and allows him to dry *without being rubbed.*

In cases attended with *high* fever, *restlessness* and inability to *sleep*, this form of bath will have a salutary effect.

**WET SHEET PACK.**—Remove all clothing from mattress, place a pillow at the head, over this and the mattress spread two comforts, then a blanket; next take a sheet previously wet in cold water and well wrung out, spread this over the blanket. Now, the patient *unclothed*, lies down on his back in middle of sheet, head on pillow and arms raised; the nurse now brings one side of sheet over the patient and tucks it under him; the arms are now dropped and the other side of sheet turned over opposite side and tucked in *closely* about the neck, shoulders, and body; the blanket is next turned over, first one side, then the other, and *snugly* tucked in; then in like manner the comforts are wrapped over by successive manipulations until the packing is complete.

The patient may remain in pack half an hour or longer, according to circumstances, after which he should be sponged off, a *dry sheet* thrown over him like a cloak, and in this and with this rubbed thoroughly dry.

Valuable in *rheumatism*, and all fevers, to lower the temperature, and in *scarlatina* and *measles* it helps to bring out the rash, while in some *chronic* skin diseases it is an important remedy.

**THE SITZ BATH.**—Take an ordinary wash-tub, prop it on edge, place in it enough water to rise to patient's navel when he sits down in it. The temperature of bath must be regulated to suit the occasion; in some cases it should be as *hot* as can be borne.

Valuable in *amenorrhœa*, menstrual *colic*, *nephralgia*, *piles*, constipation, etc.

**THE FOOT BATH.**—Immerse feet and legs in *warm* water to the *knees;* add gradually from time to time *hot* water to *raise* the temperature. In this way temperature of bath may be raised to 150° without endangering the skin. The nurse, however, must be the thermometer, as patient's limbs should be constantly rubbed during the bath.

Valuable in *croup*, bronchial catarrh, congestion of lungs, brain, spasmodic asthma, etc.

**HOT AIR BATH.**—Seat patient *unclothed* on a chair with wood-bottom; place around him, including the chair, a blanket, tucking it in closely about the neck; over this place a thick comfort in like manner, securing it in place with pins. Now put two ounces of *Alcohol* in a saucer, and set it in a deep plate, half filled with water [to guard against accident], place this on the floor, under the chair upon which the patient is seated, and set fire to the *Alcohol*. Soon the patient will perspire freely, and after doing so for five or ten minutes he should be sponged off and dried in a sheet, as advised after taking "WET SHEET PACK."

---

## POULTICES.

**LINSEED POULTICE.**—Stir in boiling water ground flaxseed enough to make a thick pap. Spread evenly on muslin and smear the surface with a little olive oil or fresh lard before applying it. Cover outside with oiled silk and several folds of flannel, to retain moisture and heat. Should be applied hot and frequently changed.

Useful emollient to *inflamed* and *painful* parts.

**OATMEAL POULTICES.**—May be prepared and used in the same way.

**BREAD POULTICE.**—Put bread crumbs into milk and simmer over a gentle fire till reduced to proper consistence. Beat smooth with a spoon, then spread on muslin and apply hot as can be borne.

Indicated for the same conditions as the *Flaxseed Poultice.*

**SLIPPERY ELM POULTICE.**—This is made by adding boiling water to powdered bark of *Ulmus Fulva*, stirring it constantly. It is a light, bland, unirritating cataplasm.

**CHARCOAL AND YEAST POULTICE.**—To a sufficient quantity of brewer's yeast, stir in as much powdered *Charcoal* as it will bear, and apply to the diseased part.

Used as a stimulant and *disinfectant* application to *gangrenous* and *phagedenic* sores.

**MUSTARD POULTICE.**—Add warm water to equal parts of ground *Mustard* and wheaten or rye flour, stirring until a thick paste is formed. This is spread on linen or muslin, then covered with gauze and applied to the skin.

Where a speedy effect is desired, the mustard may be mixed with a little water and the white of egg to form a thick paste. Spread on muslin and apply directly to skin.

Used in almost every form of local pain, such as *neuralgia, rheumatism, pneumonia, colic*, etc.

**HOT FOMENTATION.**—This is a folded cloth wrung out of *hot water*, applied to the painful part, and covered with oiled silk and dry flannel to prevent evaporation. Their utility may be increased by impregnating the water with the *indicated remedy* chosen in conformity with the law of similars.

Useful in *acute rheumatism, gout, peritonitis*, muscular spasm, etc.

**SPONGIO-PILINE.**—This is a thick fabric composed of sponge and wool, coated on one side with rubber. The sponge-surface is wet in *hot water*, wrung out and applied to the diseased parts. This is a very convenient and efficient means of applying fomentations, which may be medicated as suggested above.

**COLD FOMENTATION.**—This is a folded cloth wet in *cold water*, applied to the affected part, and left *uncovered* to favor evaporation. In mechanical and other injuries, *cold compresses* can only do good when used in *early stage*. When congestion or inflammation has occurred, *hot* compresses should be employed.

Used to prevent congestion, and in the treatment of *burns, scalds*, and frost-bites when applied promptly after the injury and kept in constant operation.

**HOT SALT PADS.**—Flannel bags half filled with *hot salt* or *hot sand*, and applied to the affected parts, are excellent palliatives in many forms of local pain.

*A rubber bag* filled with *hot water* is also a very convenient method of applying dry heat, and will be found far preferable to moist fomentations in many cases.

---

## ENEMATA.

This is a well-known method of conveying water and other medicinal agents into the intestinal and vaginal canals. The best instrument for the purpose is the "Fountain Syringe." The temperature of the enema may range from 50° to 110° F., and the patient lying on *left side*, with hips well raised, should receive the injection and retain it long as possible. The quantity used must vary according to age and circumstances. For an infant, *one ounce* will suffice; for child two years, *two* to *four ounces;* for one five to ten years, *six* to *eight ounces;* and for an adult, *one* to *two pints.* In some cases it will be necessary to repeat the clyster several times in order to obtain the desired effect.

**WATER ENEMA.**—Water, at a temperature of 80° to 90° F., forms a simple injection for all ordinary cases of constipation.

**GRUEL ENEMA.**—To a pint of thin gruel or soap-suds, add a lump of lard size of hen's egg, or half ounce castor oil; mix well and administer hot. Useful in obstinate *constipation* and in *flatulent* and *spasmodic colic.*

**MUCILAGE ENEMA.**—Warm *slippery-elm* or *flaxseed tea* makes a bland and suitable injection for infants.

**STARCH ENEMA.**—Take of *clear starch* sufficient quantity, add boiling water to make the consistence of cream. Useful in cholera infantum and dysentery attended with *colic* and *tenesmus.* Should be given in small doses [one to two ounces].

---

## VAGINAL INJECTIONS.

In the treatment of dysmenorrhœa, leucorrhœa, prolapsus, and other diseases of the genital organs, vaginal injections are highly important. The *internal indicated remedy* mingled with the menstruum, may be used with the happiest results.

**WARM WATER ENEMA.**—Injections of *warm water* (100° F.) will often recall the flow in *suppression* of the *menses* and *lochia.* In *post partum hemorrhage,* copious injections into the uterus of *hot water* (110°) have been very successful.

---

## ANÆSTHETICS.

**Test for Chloroform.**—If equal parts Chloroform and Sulphuric acid be shaken together in a glass-stoppered vial, no color should be imparted to either liquid after standing 24 hours. Again, pure Chloroform poured on blotting-paper and evaporated, ought to leave no rancid odor behind.

**Caution.**—Never give Chloroform or Ether to patient with heart disease, phthisis pulmonalis, tumors or abscess of brain. Unfavorable subjects are old drunkards, persons with enlarged tonsils, swollen epiglottis, and epileptic patients. Make provision for plenty fresh air; have dressing forceps ready to grasp tongue, and *Ammonia* to use if necessary.

**Administration of Chloroform.**—Many advise a mixture of one part *Alcohol,* two parts *Chloroform,* three parts *Ether,* used same as chloroform. Have patient in recumbent position, *clothes loose, stomach nearly empty.* Fold napkin into a cone, place small sponge in apex containing 15 drops Chloroform, hold about two inches from face; instruct patient to breathe through open mouth slowly and deeply. Administer slowly at first, allowing *plenty of air.* If any choking, remove napkin a little further. When first 15 drops are exhausted, repeat same quantity, and continue to do this till requisite degree of narcotism is produced. Watch the pulse and respiration; if either stop, remove napkin and proceed at once

**To Resuscitate Patient.**—*Lower* the head. Pull tongue forwards. Open windows. Loosen clothing. Dash cold water on face. Shake chest vigorously. Hold *Ammonia* to nostrils. These failing, apply battery—one pole to inner surface of cheek and other over pit of stomach. Institute artificial respiration, about 18 per minute.

**SULPHURIC ETHER.**—This agent may be administered the same as *Chloroform.* It is regarded as safer, but not so pleasant for patient. Commence with two drachms at first, push vigorously, especially in stage of excitement. Keep napkin close to face, and *exclude air* in giving this drug, whereas in administering *Chloroform* allow *plenty of air.*

*Precautions* the same as taken to guard against accidents from Chloroform.

---

## LOCAL ANÆSTHETICS.

**COCAINE.**—This local anæsthetic has been used for most part in ophthalmic surgery. It is especially adapted to mucous tissues whose sensitive nerves lie near the surface, as those of the eye, ear, nose, larynx, etc.

A few drops of a *four per cent.* solution may be applied to the parts to be acted upon, and repeated at short intervals until the parts become insensible to contact.

**INTENSE COLD.**—Take a lump of ice, put in a canvas bag and crush finely by pounding. Add to this one-half its weight common salt and mix quickly. Place in a thin gauze bag and lay over the part to be benumbed. Watch the effect and do not freeze the parts.

**ETHER SPRAY.**—Use in minor operations, in opening abscesses, extracting foreign bodies, small tumors, etc. It is applied by projecting a stream of atomized pure ether upon the parts until they are benumbed.

**COMPOUND ETHER.**—To one part *Hydride of Amyl* add four parts of *Ether.* This is applied by means of an atomizer, and will induce perfect insensibility in from ten to twenty seconds.

**RHIGOLENE.**—This volatile fluid is more speedy and certain in its action than ether, is comparatively odorless and inexpensive. Used same as ether.

## HYPODERMIC MEDICATION.

The hypodermic use of *morphia* has been greatly perverted by its injudicious employment. Indeed, it is questionable whether its discovery has not been a curse instead of a blessing to mankind. Its value, however, as a means of relieving pain, cannot be denied, and it is the duty of the physician to make use of all means in his power to relieve the suffering patient.

The *dose* of different substances may be as follows:—

| | |
|---|---|
| Muriate of Morphine, . . | $\frac{1}{8}$ to $\frac{1}{2}$ of a grain. |
| Sulphate of Morphine, . . | $\frac{1}{8}$ to $\frac{1}{2}$ of a grain. |
| Sulphate of Atropine, . . | $\frac{1}{100}$ to $\frac{1}{30}$ of a grain. |
| Sulphate of Soda, . . . . . | grs. ii. |
| Sulphate of Quinine, . . | grs. ii to grs. iv. |
| Tinct. Hyoscyamus, . . . | gtt. x to xx. |
| Tinct. Cannabis, . . . . | gtt. x to xx. |

If the remedy is soluble in water, it will be better to use that as a vehicle for the injection.

*Operation.*—Having loaded the syringe, pinch up a fold of integument between the thumb and forefinger, insert the needle well beneath the skin and inject slowly.

---

## THE ASPIRATOR.

This is an instrument constructed on the principle of the exhausting syringe, and is used for the purpose of withdrawing pus and other fluids from internal cavities. The needles are hollow and of various sizes to suit requirements. It may be used in abscess of the liver, retention of urine, ovarian cysts, hydrocephalus, strangulated hernia, hydrothorax, etc.

---

## SIGNS OF DEATH.

In all cases of apparent death occurring suddenly or from external violence, and whenever there is any doubt in the matter, extraordinary precautions should be taken in order to settle the question. The cessation of respiration and circulation (so far as can be observed) does not determine the matter, and even the absence of animal heat is not conclusive, for life may exist, and recovery take place where this is not an attendant. In all doubtful cases the following tests should be applied:—

1st. Apply the *Stethoscope* to determine if the heart is acting.

2d. Put the body in a *dark* room, place the hand (with fingers close together) between the eye and a lighted candle; if life is *not extinct*, hand will show *transparent* redness as in life.

3d. Tie a cord tightly around a finger; if the end becomes *swollen* and *red*, life is *not extinct*.

4th. Inject a few drops of *Aqua Ammonia* under the skin: if life still exists a red or purple spot will form.

5th. Insert a bright steel needle into the flesh, allow it to remain half an hour; if life is extinct it will *tarnish* by oxidation.

6th. Place the surface of a cold mirror over the mouth; if moisture condenses on its surface, *respiration* has not ceased.

7th. In from 12 to 18 hours after death, eye-balls become soft, inelastic, feel flaccid.

8th. In from 8 to 12 hours after death, *hypostasis* or congestion of blood in capillaries begins to form in all *depending* parts of body.

9th. *Putrefaction* is positive proof of death, and unless this takes place by the end of *third* day, *interment should be postponed until it does.*

---

## ARTIFICIAL RESPIRATION.

Turn patient on abdomen, one arm under forehead; raise body to empty stomach and air-passages of water or mucus.

Remove all clothing from chest; lay patient on his back; place a bundle of clothing [a man's body will do] under his back, to raise stomach and lower the head; pull tongue forward and secure it by tying string over it and under the jaw; stand astride or kneel at patient's head; grasp his arms below the elbows, and draw them outwards, upwards and backwards till they meet over the head; keep in this position two seconds, then carry them down to sides of chest again till elbows nearly meet over stomach, and press firmly for two seconds; repeat these manœuvres at the rate of 16 to 18 per minute.

Persevere in these efforts for hours, or until breathing has become restored; then promote the circulation by friction, artificial heat, etc. Soon as patient can swallow, give some hot milk, beef-tea or coffee to drink.

# PART II.

# PRACTICAL GUIDE IN THE TREATMENT OF DISEASE.

## ABSCESS.

**THERAPEUTICS.** The best remedies are

For **ACUTE** abscesses: **Acon. Ars. Asa. Bell. Bry. Hep. Lach. Led. Merc. Mez. Puls. Rhus. Sil. Sulph.**

For **CHRONIC: Aur. Cal. c. Con. Hep. Iod. Lyc. Merc. Nit. ac. Phos. Sil. Sulph.**

In **BONES: Asaf. Aur. *Cal. c. *Cal. phos. Hep. Merc. Nit. ac. Phos. *Sil. Sulph.**

In **HEPATIC** abscesses: **Bell. Chin. Hep. Kali. c. Lach. *Merc. *Phyto. Podo. Ruta. Sil.**

In **SCROFULOUS** abscesses: ***Bary. c. Bell. *Cal. c. Cal. phos. Con. Dul. Hep. Kali. c. Lyc. Merc. Nit. ac. Phos. Rhus. t. Sil. Staph. *Sulph.**

**ACUTE ABSCESS.** This is a collection of pus in a cavity the result of a morbid process. It usually commences with the ordinary signs of acute inflammation, such as fever, throbbing pain, redness and swelling, ending in suppuration.

*Internal* abscesses generally require the same remedies as external.

**TREATMENT.** *Leading indications.*

**ACONITE.** The tumor is swollen, red, and shining. Violent cutting pains; parts burn, as from hot coals, [**Ars.**] Great nervous and vascular excitement. *Gets desperate about pain. *Great fear and anxiety of mind. Aggravation in evening, and during night.

**ARSENICUM.** The abscess threatens to become gangrenous, and is accompanied with *great debility*. *Violent burning pains; the parts burn like fire, [**Acon.**] Restless tossing about. *Great thirst, but can drink but little. Aggravation during rest; better by motion.

**ASAFŒTIDA.** The abscess discharges a thin, fetid pus; is very painful to contact, especially the surrounding parts. *Pains, with numbness of affected parts. Nervous, hysterical, scrofulous individuals.

**BELLADONNA.** Tumor much swollen, hard, and of an erysipelatous appearance. Pressing, burning, stinging or throbbing pains, [**Hep.**] *Pains which appear suddenly and leave as suddenly. *The parts have a hot, dry sensation, with much throbbing; gets worse about 3 P. M. Mammary abscess.

**BRYONIA.** Mostly in beginning, when abscess is hard, swollen, and *feels heavy*, [**Bell.**] The tumor alternates in color, is either very red or very pale. *Stitching pains, aggravated by the slightest motion. *Hard, dry stools, as if burnt.

**HEPAR SULPH.** *Where suppuration is inevitable, [**Lach Merc. Sil.**] Throbbing pains, frequently preceded by a chill; the tumor *hard, hot*, and swollen. Scrofulous persons, and after the abuse of mercury.

**LACHESIS.** Where pus has already formed, or where the inflamed portion assumes a *purplish hue*, or becomes gangrenous, [**Ars.**] *Symptoms all worse after sleep. If caused by introduction of poisonous matter into the system.

**LEDUM.** In the early stage, when abscess is distended and hard. *Stinging and tearing pains, aggravated by heat. *Tensive, hard swelling*, with tearing pains. If caused by external hurts, splinters, etc.

**MERCURIUS.** In commencement, often prevents suppuration; or *after suppuration has taken place*, promotes discharge, [**Lach.**] *Glandular abscesses;* particularly when not inflamed, or with *intense, shining redness, beating and stinging*, [**Bell.**] Where disease extends to sheaths of tendons and ligaments of joints, [see **Mez.**]

**MEZEREUM.** Abscesses that occur in fibrous and tendinous structures, or where they arise from abuse of mercury. Stinging and throbbing pains, worse at night and from contact or motion.

**PHOSPHORUS.** Incipient stage, to prevent formation of pus. Especially in *mammary abscesses* [**Bel.** ***Bry.** ***Phyto.**] it facilitates the suppurative process, and guards against cicatrices.

**PULSATILLA.** Abscess bleeds easily, with stinging or cutting pains, [**Apis.**] Violent itching, burning, and stinging in periphery of abscess. Pus copious and yellow. After violent and long-continued inflammations. *Mild, tearful persons; they weep at everything.

**RHUS TOX.** Especially abscesses of axillary or parotid glands. Stinging or gnawing pains in tumor, which is very painful to touch. Discharge of a bloody-serous matter. *Pain worse during rest, relieved by moving the affected parts, [**Ars.**]

**SILICEA.** Where suppuration is imminent [**Hep. Lach. Merc.**], or where discharge becomes fetid, thin, and watery. Fistulous openings form, which are very slow to heal.

**SULPHUR.** Inveterate cases, when there is a profuse discharge of matter, with emaciation, hectic fever, etc. Constant tendency to a return of the disease, [**Hep.**] Scrofulous persons who are frequently troubled with boils. *Psoric diathesis. *Lean persons who walk stooping.

**LOCAL MEASURES.** *Poultices* relax the parts, soothe the pain and promote formation of pus. They should be large, light and soft. *Linseed-meal* or bread and milk generally used; they should be covered with oiled silk to prevent getting dry. Hot water dressings are good substitutes for poultices. Soon as pus forms, use local *anæsthetic* and open at most *dependent point.* Support strength by a good *nourishing diet,* rare beef, beef-tea, milk, etc.

---

## AFTER-PAINS.

*After-Pains,* as a general rule, should not be interfered with, at least for several hours after delivery, as they are caused by uterine contractions in efforts to expel portions of membrane or coagula which should come away.

**TREATMENT.** *Leading indications.*

**ARNICA.** *Sore feeling all through the patient as if from a bruise.* The pains are not very violent, but there is a bruised, sore feeling, with pressure on the bladder and retention of urine. *After difficult labor.*

**BELLADONNA.** *Severe bearing-down pains, as if everything would protrude, [Nit. ac. *Sep.] Pains come on suddenly and leave as suddenly. Fullness and great tenderness of abdomen; *every jar hurts her.* Sleepiness, but cannot sleep.

**GELSEMIUM.** *Uterus as if squeezed by a hand. Numbness of extremities, uterine cramps extending upwards and backwards.

**CAULOPHYLLUM.** After *protracted and exhausting labor;* pains spasmodic, across the lower abdomen, extending into groin.

**CHAMOMILLA.** Great nervous excitement, with restless tossing about. The *pains are very distressing,* and she becomes almost furious. *Very impatient, can hardly answer one civilly. Dark lochial discharge.

**CIMICIFUGA.** After-pains worse in groins; over-sensitiveness, [Cham.] She feels the pains very acutely, and they make her sleepless, restless and low spirited.

**COFFEA.** Great sensitiveness, with general excitability. *Violent pains, driving her almost to despair [becomes desperate, Acon. Cham.] Extreme wakefulness.

**CUPRUM ACET.** *Terrible cramping pains, often accompanied with cramps in extremities. Spasms, with nausea and vomiting.

**IGNATIA.** The pains are cramp-like and pressing, resembling labor pains, [*Cham.] *Sadness and sighing, with empty feeling in stomach.

**NUX VOMICA.** When pains are aching and more like colic; fainting after every pain. Violent contractive pains in uterus, [**Sec.**] *Every pain causes an inclination to go to stool. Much pain in small of back, worse by turning in bed.

**PULSATILLA.** Severe colicky pains extending to back. The pains grow worse towards evening: are too long and too violent, [**Sec.**] Bad taste in mouth, with desire to vomit. *Persons of a mild, tearful disposition.

**SECALE COR.** Excessive uterine contractions, which are long continued. *In thin, feeble, scrawny females, or women who have borne many children; *feels cold, but does not wish to be covered.* Thin, offensive lochial discharge.

---

## AMENORRHŒA.

(*Suppression of the Menses.*)

**TREATMENT.** *Leading indications.*

**ACONITE.** If the result of direct application of cold. Congestion of head or chest, with flushed face. Shooting and beating pains in head, with delirium or stupefaction. *Vertigo with faintness on rising from recumbent position. Age of *puberty*, [**Kali. c. Puls.**] Young *plethoric* girls. If caused by *fright* or anxiety of mind.

**APIS MEL.** Suppression, with congestion of the head. *Chlorosis, with puffy, bloated, waxy appearance of face; œdematous swelling of eyelids and feet. Very busy and restless; constantly changing from one thing to another; very awkward, often breaking things. Aching pain, especially in right ovary.

**ARSENICUM.** Pale, waxen color of face. Great prostration of strength. Loss of appetite; sadness and melancholy. Fear of death and being alone. Much chilliness; wants more clothes on, or to be near fire. *Intense thirst, but drinks little. *Sufferings all worse after midnight.

**BELLADONNA.** Throbbing headache at approach of each menstrual period. Red face, with determination of blood to head when stooping. *Bearing-down pain in hypogastrium as if menses would appear, [see **Cham.**] *She cannot bear light or noise.

**BRYONIA.** Swimming in head, with painful pressure in temples. *Bleeding of nose*, when menses should appear, [**Bell Puls.**] Drawing pains in lower part of abdomen. *Hard, dry stools. *Symptoms all worse from motion.

**CALCARIA CARB.** Scrofulous subjects. The menstrual period is preceded by swelling and soreness of breasts, headache, colic, shiverings and leucorrhœa. *Cold, damp feet, and swelling at pit of stomach. *Dizziness on going up-stairs.

**CAUSTICUM.** Yellow, discolored complexion. Weakly, scrofulous subjects with glandular swellings. Melancholy moods; she looks on dark side of everything. Hysterical spasms and pinching pain in sacrum. *Leucorrhœa only at night, [**Amb. g.**]

**CHAMOMILLA.** Pressure towards genital organs, like labor-pains. Cutting colic, and drawing in thighs previous to a menstrual period. *She is very irritable, can hardly answer one civilly. *One cheek red, other pale, [**Acon. Nux.**] Passing large quantities of colorless urine.

**CHINA.** Pale, sickly complexion. Weakness of digestion; fullness and distension of abdomen, particularly after eating [**Lyc. Nux.**] *Debility from loss of animal fluids. After chagrin, [**Cham.**]

**COCCULUS.** Leucorrhœa in place of menses. *During menstrual period she is extremely weak. Sometimes a few drops of black blood are discharged. Nervous hysterical subjects.

**COLOCYNTH.** Amenorrhœa from anger and silent grief. *Severe colicky pains which compel one to bend double. Great anguish and restlessness.

**CONIUM.** Much vertigo, particularly when lying down, or when turning over in bed. *At every menstrual effort, the breasts enlarge, become sore and painful. Much difficulty in voiding urine; it intermits in its flow. Great weakness after the least walk.

**CROCUS.** Sensation as if the menses would appear, with colic and dragging down in the direction of the pudendum [see **Bell.**] *Sensation of something alive in abdomen, [**Saba. Sulph.**] Discharge of thick, black, stringy blood from the nose, [see **Bry.**]

**DULCAMARA.** Amenorrhœa from exposure to cold, or from getting wet, [***Puls.**] *At each menstrual period a rash appears on the skin; [violent itching of old tetter eruptions when menses should appear, **Carb. v.**] Every time she takes cold has urticaria or some other eruption on skin.

**GELSEMIUM.** Suppression, with sensation of heaviness in uterine region. Feeling of fullness in hypogastrium; slight uterine pain and aching across sacrum, as if menses would come on. Headache, with great dullness of head and vertigo affecting vision.

**GRAPHITES.** Suppression of menses, with a sense of weight in arms and lower extremities. An occasional show of menses, discharge being very pale and scant. Swelling and coldness of feet. *Eruptions on skin oozing sticky fluid.

**KALI CARB.** Amenorrhœa, with anasarca. Pains in abdomen resembling false labor-pains. Shortness of breath and violent palpitation of heart. *Little sac-like swellings over upper eyelids in morning. Age of puberty, [**Acon.** ***Puls.**]

**LILIUM TIG.** Amenorrhœa, accompanied with cardiac distress or with ovarian pains of a burning or stinging character. Prolapsus or other displacements of womb, [**Merc. Sep. Nux.**] Thin, acrid leucorrhœa, which stains linen brown. Partial amenia, the menses returning occasionally, and then remaining off again.

**LYCOPODIUM.** Chronic suppression of menses; also from fright. *Sour eructations, with nausea and vomiting*, especially in morning. *Great fullness in stomach and bowels.* *Red, sandy sediment in urine.

**NUX MOSCH.** Suppression of menses from exposure to wet, [**Dulc. Rhus.**] with severe pains in abdomen. *Irregular menstruation, blood thick and dark. *Sleepiness and inclination to faint.* *Great dryness of tongue, particularly after sleeping. Pain in back as if broken and bruised. Enormous distension of abdomen after eating.

**PHOSPHORUS.** *Spitting and vomiting blood at menstrual nisus, [see **Bryo.**] Menses *too late* or not appearing, [**Puls. Sulph.**] *Tight feeling in chest, with dry, tight cough. *Long, narrow, hard stools, [**Caust.**] *Tall, slender, phthisical subjects.*

**PULSATILLA.** *Suppression, especially from *getting feet wet*, [**Dulc.**] Aching pains over forehead, with pressure on vertex. Vertigo, with buzzing in ears. Stitching toothache, pains suddenly shifting. Palpitation of heart. Pain in stomach, with nausea and vomiting. *Constant chilliness even in warm room. *Mild, tearful disposition, with tendency to sadness, [**Ign. Sep.**] Symptoms all worse in evening.

**SEPIA.** Frequent paroxysms of hysteric or nervous headache. Toothache, with great sensitiveness of teeth. *Sallow complexion or dingy spots on face. Nervous debility and great disposition to sweat. *Painful sensation of emptiness in stomach, [**Ign.**] *Feeble, delicate* women.

**SULPHUR.** Aching and tensive pain in head, especially from occiput to neck. Rush of blood to head, with whizzing noise in brain. *Constant heat on top of head, [**Graph.**—*Coldness*, **Verat.**] Pale, sickly complexion, blue margins around eyes. Frequent weak, faint spells through day. *She gets very hungry about 11 A. M.

**VERATRUM ALB.** Nervous headache at every menstrual period, with hysterical symptoms. Pale, livid face, and cold sweat on forehead. Coldness on top of head, [**Sep.**—*Heat*, ***Sulph.**] Cold hands, feet and nose. *Great weakness, with frequent spells of fainting.

**AUXILIARY MEASURES.** Hot *sitz baths* will be found valuable in *sudden* suppression of menses from exposure to cold or getting wet, especially when there is fullness in the head, and bearing-down pains in pelvic region. *Hot water* injections will often have a salutary effect in recalling the flow in such cases.

Rubbing, bathing, and proper physical exercise in open air should of necessity enter into the treatment.

---

## ANGINA PECTORIS.

**TREATMENT.** *Leading indications.*

**ACONITE.** *Intense anxiety, with fear of death. Has to sit straight up, can hardly breathe. Pulse thread-like and feeble. Intense pain in all directions, [see **Cimi.**] Suffocative constriction of chest, so distressing that he sweats from agony, [**Ars.**] Flushed face; pain in region of heart, going down left arm. Suitable to *strong plethoric* subjects.

**AMYL NITRITE.** *Sharp pain* in cardiac region. Tumultuous action of heart and quick respiration. Sense of fullness in temples. *Burning of the ears. Bronchial irritation. Some physicians advise inhalations of this remedy. Put six or eight drops on a little cotton in small vial, and inhale during an attack.

**ANGUSTURA.** In lighter forms; chest is in constant motion; *spasmodic breathing;* palpitation of heart. Cutting shocks in sternum and back, and painful shocks in region of heart.

**ARSENICUM.** Indescribable agonizing pain in præcordial region, extending to neck and occiput. Can only breathe very gently with his chest *stooping forwards.* Oppression and stitches in præcordial region, with anxiety and a fainting sort of weakness. Pulse *feeble, irregular,* intermittent, [**Dig.**] *Restlessness, prostration, intense thirst, drinking little and often.

**BRYONIA.** Attacks from mental excitement or fright. Sense of great oppression; it seems as if something should expand but will not. *Cutting pain in right chest;* also a cutting pain *extending down left arm,* [see **Acon.**] *Patient exceedingly irritable.

**CACTUS GR.** *Feeling of *constriction* at heart, as if an *iron band* prevented its normal action. Acute pains in region of heart, with difficulty of breathing. *Palpitation* worse at night or when lying on left side. Attacks of suffocation with fainting.

**CIMICIFUGA.** Intense anxiety about the heart, with pain in left shoulder extending down arm and into back. Where the attack *arises* from *uterine derangements.*

**DIGITALIS.** Sharp stitches, or contractive pains in region of heart, [**Arn. Rhus. Spig.**] Pulse feeble, irregular, spasmodic, slow, intermitting. *Sensation as if the heart would stop beating if he moved. Indescribable deathly anguish, the paroxysms keep coming closer together as the disease progresses.

**GELSEMIUM.** *Sudden hysterical spasms;* nervous chills in very sensitive subjects. Feeling as though heart would stop beating if she did not walk incessantly, with a feeling of impending death, [see **Dig.**]

**HYDROC. ACID.** Heart disease, with *violent palpitations;* long fainting spells, [see **Lach.**] Feeling of suffocation, with torturing pains in chest. Irregular feeble beating of heart

**LACHESIS.** Anxious pain, with beating of the heart. Choking, constriction, or rising in the throat, with organic disease of heart. Cannot lie down, must sit up bent forwards. *Very distressed after sleeping.

**LAUROCERASUS.** Attacks of suffocation, with gasping for breath; feeling as if he was not going to breathe again. Stitches in region of heart. Violent pain in stomach, with loss of speech; cold, moist skin.

**PHYTOLACCA.** *Fatty degeneration of heart;* feeling of lassitude and indisposition to move. Lame feeling in left side of chest, near cardiac region, with much nervous restlessness. *Pain extends to right arm or right side, [*left* arm, **Rhus.**] Rheumatic diathesis, [**Rhus.**]

**RHUS TOX.** Stitches in heart, with painful *lameness* and *stiffness* of whole body and limbs. Pain extending down left arm, [down right arm, **Phyto.**] *Rheumatic diathesis.*

**SPIGELIA.** **Organic disease of heart.* Severe stabbing stitches in heart at every beat; pain rapidly passing around body from left to right. *Palpitation so violent can be seen and heard at a distance, [**Dig. Verat. a.**] Can lie only on right side, with trunk well raised. Worse stooping, bending forward, touching stomach, lifting arms, or from any motion.

**TABACUM.** *Death-like paleness of face, with sick stomach, features pinched. *Icy coldness of legs from knees down.* Violent constriction in throat, with tightness across upper part of chest; cannot speak. *Trembling all over, with palpitation of heart.

**VERAT. ALB.** *Painful spasmodic constriction of chest, [see **Cact.**] Periodical attacks of contractive, crampy pain in left chest, or cutting pain, with excessive agony. Visible palpitation of heart, [**Dig. Spig.**] *Cold sweat, particularly on forehead.

**AUXILIARY MEASURES.** During an attack, place patient's feet in *hot bath*, and have them rubbed briskly. Apply *hot fomentations* or bags of *hot salt* to region of heart, enjoin perfect quiet, and allow an abundance of fresh air.

Persons subject to this complaint should be strictly temperate in their habits, avoid excitement, and all *stimulating food, drinks*, and use of *tobacco*.

## APHTHÆ.—CANCRUM ORIS.

**TREATMENT.** *Leading indications.*

**ACONITE.** Dry, hot skin, with much heat about head. Constant restlessness, cries, frets most of the time, bites its fist, and has green watery diarrhœa. *Excessive sensibility* to least touch.

**ARSENICUM.** The mouth is reddish-blue, and inflamed. Fetid smell from mouth; great restlessness. *Green, watery diarrhœa, attended with great weakness. *Emaciation*, skin hanging in folds.

**BAPTISIA.** Child can swallow only fluids, even a small portion of solid food causes gagging. Long-standing ulcerations of mouth, extending through alimentary canal, with watery discharge. *Sore mouth of nursing infants [of *pregnant* and *nursing* females, Caulo.]

**BORAX.** Red blisters on tongue, as if skin were pulled off. Shriveling up of the mucous membrane. *The child frequently lets go the nipple, and cries as if in pain. Light yellow slimy stools. *Fear of falling from a downward motion.

**CALC. CARB.** Scrofulous children, especially during dentition. *Large, open fontanelles, [**Merc. *Sil. Sulph.**] Much perspiration on head and face, [**Sil.**] Hard, undigested stools of a light color. *Cold, damp feet. *Emaciation* and good appetite.

**CAULOPHYLLUM.** Especially in *pregnant* and *nursing* females; also in children. **Eupa. ar.** is highly spoken of in similar cases.

**CHAMOMILLA.** Child starts and jumps much during sleep. Wants different things and rejects them when presented, [***Bry. Staph.**] *Very uneasy, and must be carried all the time to be quieted.

**MERCURIUS.** Tongue inflamed, swollen and ulcerated on edges. The gums bleed, and incline to ulcerate about teeth, [see **Nit. ac.**] Very fetid breath. *Profuse secretion of saliva in mouth. Dysenteric diarrhœa, with griping and tenesmus.

**NITRIC ACID.** Mouth full of fetid ulcers, with putrid-smelling breath, [**Merc.**] *Ptyalism of a corrosive nature, causing fresh ulcers to break out on lips, chin or cheeks. Bleeding gums, [**Ars. Staph.**] *If syphilitic dyscrasia exists, or patient has taken much *mercury*.

**NUX VOMICA.** If disease assumes the character of stomatitis. Painful swelling of gums, with bloody saliva. Fetid ulcers or blisters in mouth, on gums, palate or tongue. *Constipation, with frequent urging to stool. Irritable mood.

**STAPHISAGRIA.** Spongy excrescence on gums and in mouth. Vesicles under tongue. Mouth and tongue ulcerated and covered with blisters. Sickly complexion, with sunken cheeks, hollow eyes surrounded with blue margins. *The aphthous patches bleed easily, and gums are spongy.

**SULPHUR.** Thick whitish or brownish aphthous coating on tongue. Blisters and aphthæ in mouth, with burning and soreness. Ptyalism or bloody saliva. *Acrid, slimy or greenish diarrhœa excoriating the parts*, [**Cham.** ***Merc.**] *The child does not take its usual long nap, but wakens often.

**SULPHURIC AC.** Mouth appears very painful, and child very weak. Vesicles on inner side of cheeks; ulcers on gums. Profuse flow of tasteless saliva. *Diarrhœa with great debility, and inclination to sweat; *night sweats.*

**HYGIENIC MEASURES.** Cleanliness, daily bathing, washing out mouth frequently with *tepid water*, avoidance of all sugar-teats, keeping breasts and nipples clean, using proper ventilation, taking child into open air and sunlight, are the best preventive means.

Washing out the mouth three or four times a day with a weak solution of Borax [grains ji; water, ℥j] is useful in many cases, but should not be pushed too far.

---

## APOPLEXIA.

**TREATMENT.** *Leading indications.*

**ÆSCULUS HIP.** *Severe vertigo*, with reeling and staggering. Vertigo with nausea, dimness of vision, and confusion of head; thickness of speech; great weakness, with trembling.

**ACONITE.** Head hot, carotids throbbing, redness of face, [**Bell.**] Eyes red, sparkling, and prominent, with dilated pupils; fixed look. Paralysis of tongue, trembling, stammering speech. *Great difficulty in swallowing*, [***Bell. Hyos.**] Pulse full and hard, but not intermittent. *Plethoric habit.*

**ARNICA.** Head hot, while rest of body is cool. Paralysis of limbs, especially left side. Loss of consciousness, with stupefaction and stertorous breathing, [**Opi.**] Staring eyes and contracted pupils. *Sighing, muttering, and involuntary discharge of fæces and urine. Stout, plethoric persons.

**BARYTA CARB.** Apoplexy of aged persons, and those of intemperate habits, [**Nux Opi.**] Paralysis of limbs, right side, [left side, **Lach.**] *Disturbed consciousness, acts childish;* inability to keep body erect.

**BELLADONNA.** Face swollen, bluish and dark red. Veins of head and neck distended. *Visible throbbing of carotid and temporal arteries, [**Acon.**] Drowsiness with loss of consciousness and speech. Paralysis of limbs, right side, [left side, **Lach.**] *Mouth drawn to one side; difficult or impossible deglutition. *Loss of sight, smell, and speech. *Involuntary micturition.*

**COCCULUS.** Paroxysm preceded by a *stupid feeling in head and vertigo.* Convulsive motions of eyes. Paralysis, especially of *lower limbs,* with insensibility. *Head and face hot, feet cold.

**GELSEMIUM.** Threatened or actual apoplexy, with stupor, coma, and nearly general paralysis. Headache, with nausea, tightness of brain; giddiness; tendency to stagger, with dimness of vision, [see **Æsc.**] Vertigo and intense passive congestion to head, with nervous exhaustion.

**HYDROCY. AC.** Features spasmodically distorted; eyes fixed and turned upwards; pupils immovable; breathing stertorous, [**Opi.**] Pulse almost imperceptible. *Paralysis of œsophagus; fluids pass down throat with a gurgling sound.

**HYOSCYAMUS.** *Sudden falling down with a shriek. Loss of consciousness and of speech; foam at mouth. Constriction of throat, and inability to swallow, [**Bell.**] Brown-red, swollen face, and staring distorted eyes, with dilated pupils. Paralysis of bladder and sphincter ani. *Twitching and jerking of all muscles in body.

**LACHESIS.** Attack *preceded by absent-mindedness* or vertigo. Apoplexia with paralysis of left side, and coldness of hands as if dead. *Mouth drawn to one side,* [***Bell.**] *Cannot bear anything to touch his neck. Entire inability to swallow. Climacteric period, [**Puls.**]

**LAUROCERASUS.** Sudden attack of apoplexia where patient falls down without any precursory symptoms. Eyes staring, or lightly closed; *pupils dilated,* or contracted and immovable, [**Hyd. ac.**] Slow, feeble moaning, or rattling breathing.

**NUX VOMICA.** The paroxysm is preceded by vertigo, with headache and buzzing in ears, or nausea with urging to vomit. Stupefaction, with stertorous breathing. *Paralysis of lower jaw, and often lower extremities, which are cold and without sensation. Persons of sedentary or intemperate habits.

**OPIUM.** *The patient lies in a state of sopor and unconsciousness, with half-open eyes and dilated pupils. Redness, bloatedness, and heat of face. *Respiration labored, snoring, and rattling. *Convulsive motions of extremities, or tetanic stiffness of whole body,* [**Nux.**] *Slow pulse, [**Verat. v.**]

**PULSATILLA.** Stupefaction and loss of consciousness. Bloated and bluish-red face. Loss of motion, violent palpitation of heart, and almost complete suppression of pulse. Restless sleep and tossing about. *Amenorrhœa.* *Persons of a mild, tearful disposition.

**VERATRUM V.** *Congestive headache;* he becomes stupid, has ringing in ears, bloodshot eyes, thickness of speech, hot head. Full, slow, *hard* pulse, [see **Opi.**] Convulsions, dimness of vision, with nausea and vomiting.

**AUXILIARY MEASURES.** When an attack occurs, loosen all tight clothing, place patient on side or face to prevent tongue from falling back; have head and shoulders well elevated; allow plenty fresh air. Put feet in warm bath, add *hot water* and make temperature 130°. Apply *hot fomentations* to head. Soon as patient can swallow give indicated remedy. In severe cases, if head and neck are livid, apply *dry* cups to the spine.

**HYGIENIC.** Persons subject to apoplexy should avoid all *stimulating food* and drinks, over-eating, excitement and exposure to hot sun, heated rooms, and excesses of every kind.

---

## APPARENT DEATH.—ASPHYXIA.

**TREATMENT** of apparent death.

**ASPHYXIA FROM NOXIOUS GASES.** If a person has become insensible from inhaling **Carbonic Acid, Carbonic Oxide, Fumes of Burning Charcoal, Chlorine, or Sulphuretted Hydrogen Gas,** expose him at once to fresh air. Bathe face and breast with *vinegar*, and let him inhale the vapor. Give strong *coffee*, apply cold water to head, and warmth to feet. If necessary, have recourse to the method of resuscitation explained under "Apparent Death from *Drowning*," or apply *positive pole of battery* to upper part of spine, and *negative pole* on chest, over diaphragm.

If there is congestion to head, loss of consciousness, throbbing carotids, and red, bloated face, give **Bell.** If face is purplish and swollen, with soporous sleep, stertorous breathing, and vomiting, give **Opi.** If patient is excited, talks much, complains of shooting pains, feels giddy when lying down, give **Coffea.**

**ASPHYXIA FROM CHLOROFORM, ETHER SULPHURIC, ETC.** Place body in a horizontal position, *lower* the head; open windows; loosen clothing; dash cold water on face; shake chest vigorously, and hold **Ammonia** to nostrils. *Introducing a piece of ice into the rectum has proved salutary.* These failing, apply *Galvanic Battery;* one pole on throat, the other over ensiform process, keeping up the current for hours in severe cases. The method of inducing artificial respiration, explained under "Apparent Death from Drowning," should likewise be tried.

After breathing is established, and if patient complains of chilliness, and a sense of intoxication, nausea, vomiting, and quick pulse, give **Nux v.**; if *pulse is slow*, give ***Opium** or **Verat. v.**

**ASPHYXIA FROM COLD.** Always place body in a *cold* room, and rub with snow, or bathe in ice-cold water, until limbs become soft and flexible, then place in a dry bed, and rub briskly with flannel, at same time have recourse to artificial respiration, explained under "Asphyxia from *Drowning*." Soon as there are signs of returning life, give small injections of *coffee* without milk, and if patient can swallow, give him spoonful doses of *coffee*.

For the severe, burning pains which usually follow resuscitation from intense cold, **Acon. Ars. Carb. v.** or **Bry.**, will be found sufficient.

**ASPHYXIA FROM DROWNING.** The length of time that a body may remain under water, and then be restored to life, has been variously estimated. Some say that no recovery has taken place after complete submersion for five minutes. On the contrary, cases are recorded that have been restored after submersion for *half an hour* and longer. Recent experiments have shown that animals bled to death may be restored to life eighteen hours thereafter by the transfusion of blood into the veins, and a resort to artificial respiration.

**TREATMENT.** Place patient on abdomen, one arm under forehead; raise body to empty stomach and air-passages of water or mucus. Remove all clothing from chest. Lay patient on his back, place a bundle of clothing [a man's body will do] under his back to raise stomach and lower the head. Pull tongue forward and secure it by tying string over it and under the jaw. Stand astride or kneel at patient's head; grasp his arms below the elbows, and draw them outwards, upwards and backwards till they meet over the head; keep in this position two seconds; then carry them down to sides of chest again till elbows nearly meet over the stomach and press firmly for two seconds. Repeat these manœuvres at the rate of 16 per minute.

Persevere in these efforts for hours, or until breathing has become restored, then promote the circulation by friction, artificial heat, etc. Soon as patient can swallow, give some hot milk, beef-tea or coffee to drink.

In addition to the mechanical means resorted to, a dose of **Lach.** may be placed upon the tongue, or administered as an injection. **Tart. e.** is also a valuable remedy in these cases.

**ASPHYXIA FROM HANGING, CHOKING, ETC.** Endeavor to induce artificial respiration by same method as recommended for asphyxia from drowning, and give **Opi.** or **Tart. e.** by injection.

**ASPHYXIA FROM LIGHTNING.** *Dash cold water* on head, face, and whole body; pour it on head from a height. If this does not revive, place the naked body in a freshly-made opening in ground, in a half-sitting posture, and cover it all over, except face, with fresh earth. Give **Nux v.** as soon as there are any signs of returning life. For blindness that sometimes follows, give **Phos.**

---

## ARTHRITIS.

**TREATMENT.** *Leading indications.*

**ACONITE.** Synochal fever. The parts affected are swollen, red, shining. Tearing or stitching pains, less when moving the parts, [***Rhus.**] *The pains are intolerable at night, the patient becoming desperate.

**ARNICA.** *Hard, red swelling of big toe joint.* Violent pains as if sprained or contused, with a sensation as if *resting upon something hard*, [**Bapt.**] *Great fear of being struck or touched. Aggravation by moving the parts, [***Bry.**] After *mechanical injuries.*

**ARSENICUM.** Swelling of feet, hot, shining, with burning red spots. *Burning pains—the parts burn like fire, [**Acon.**] Wants to be in warm room. Great anguish, restlessness, and fear of death, [**Acon.**] Intense thirst, but drinks little. Symptoms all worse at night, particularly after midnight, [***Rhus t.**]

**AURUM MUR.** *Continued gnawing-boring pain deep in joints after the inflammatory symptoms have subsided. After abuse of mercury.

**BELLADONNA.** Wide-spreading redness and swelling of the parts, like erysipelas. *Stitching, burning, and throbbing pains, which come on suddenly and leave as suddenly. Throbbing headache. *Sleepiness, but cannot sleep, [**Lach.**] Worse 3 P. M.

**BRYONIA.** Red or pale tensive swelling, particularly of joints. *Stitching, tearing pains, aggravated by motion and relieved by rest, [reverse, **Rhus.**] *Patient wants to remain perfectly quiet. Extremely irritable; everything makes him angry. *Dry, hard stools, as if burnt. *Dry mouth and lips.*

**COLCHICUM.** Little or no swelling of affected part; the skin is rose-colored, and leaves a white spot under pressure of finger. *Paroxysms of tearing, stitching, jerking pains, particularly in finger-joints. *Urine dark and scanty, depositing a whitish sediment. Pains intolerable at night, [**Acon.**]

**FERRUM MET.** The patient has a pale, consumptive look. Several joints are affected at same time; pains violent, stinging and tearing, obliging him to move parts constantly, [**Rhus.**] *The least emotion or pain produces a red, flushed face.

**MERC. VIV.** Red and hot swelling of affected joints. Pains drawing and lacerating, or joints feel as if dislocated;

*worse in cold, damp weather*, and at night, [Rhod.] *Much perspiration, which affords no relief.

**NUX VOMICA.** Pains tensive, *jerking*, or pulling, worse in morning, from mental exertion, from motion and slight contact; *but strong pressure relieves*, [Nat. c.] *Persons of intemperate or sedentary habits, and those who live on rich and highly seasoned food. Constipation, or morning diarrhœa.

**PHOSPHORUS.** Arthritic affections of wrist and finger-joints, [knee-joint, Arn. Rhod.] Pains as if lacerated or sprained, worse early in morning or in evening. *Long, narrow hard stools, very difficult to expel. *Sensation of weakness and emptiness in abdomen. Lean, slender persons, [Nux.]

**PULSATILLA.** Red and hot swelling of parts, particularly of knee joints and feet. The pains are tearing, stitching, burning. *Erratic pains, shifting rapidly from one joint to another. *Worse towards evening*, or at night. *Craves fresh cool air; worse in a warm room, [better, Ars.] *Persons of a mild, tearful disposition.

**RHUS TOX.** Rheumatic gout; the joints are red, shining, and swollen. Stiffness and lameness of affected parts. The pains are tearing, burning, or as if sprained, [Arn.] *Aggravation on first moving limb after rest, or *during rest; relieved by motion.*

**SABINA.** Swelling, redness, and stitches in big toe. Nodosities of joints, [Graph.] Pains tearing and stinging, almost insupportable when limbs hang down; *relief in open air.*

**AUXILIARY MEASURES.** During an attack have limb elevated, and apply *hot water* compresses to the parts. Cloths wrung out a solution of *Arnica*, [10 drops to the ounce,] and applied where this remedy is indicated, will afford great relief. In some instances, warm fomentations of hops will be found very efficacious.

**HYGIENIC.** Diet very important. Food easily digested should be chosen, consisting of vegetables, fruits and farinaceous articles. Milk-cure has done good in some cases. All alcoholic beverages should be strictly prohibited.

Flannel should be worn next the skin throughout the year; the body frequently bathed, and moderate exercise taken daily in the open air.

---

## ASCARIDES.—SEAT-WORMS.

This variety of parasite is a source of great annoyance, especially to children. They inhabit for most part the rectum and folds of mucous membrane at the verge of the anus, and cause intolerable itching, pain and tenesmus. In females they sometimes crawl into the urethra and vagina, develop in large numbers, and cause great irritation and a discharge of mucus.

**TREATMENT.** *Leading indications.*

**ACONITE.** *Intolerable itching and tingling at the anus, throwing child into fever. Urging to stool, with discharge of slime. *Great restlessness.*

**CALC. CARB.** Pale, *bloated face, with swollen abdomen and good appetite.* *Itching of anus, commencing towards bed-time. Scrofulous habit.

**MERCURIUS.** Greediness for food, and still grows weaker. *Fetid breath,* [**Nux.**] *Slimy, bloody stools with tenesmus. *Profuse perspiration.*

**NUX VOM.** Itching of anus, worse when sitting. Worms crawl out on external parts. *Blind or bleeding piles, [**Sulph.**] *Constipation;* sedentary habits; high-livers; *very irritable.*

**SULPHUR.** *Creeping, biting in rectum. Passage of ascarides and tænia. Nausea before meals, and faintness before dinner. *Early morning diarrhœa. *Extremely fretful.*

**TEUCRIUM.** *Terrible itching in the anus from seat-worms, [**Urti. ur.**]

**LOCAL MEASURES.** On account of the intolerable itching and annoyance caused by these intestinal parasites, a variety of local remedies have been used for the purpose of obtaining relief. Injections of cold water, *salt* and water, *vinegar* and water, *lemon* juice, etc., have been found useful in allaying the itching. Injections of *turpentine* [20 to 30 drops in 2 ounces mucilage of starch] will settle the little villains instanter. A solution of *carbolic acid* [gtt. xv. aq. ferv. ℥iv.] injected into the rectum, and the parts well washed with this solution, we have found very efficacious. After this injection rectum should be well washed out with *warm* water. Insert just within the anus a pledget of lint soaked in a solution *chloral* [1 to 50], and repeat daily, is highly commended. Anoint anus and parts around with lard or olive oil to prevent *propagation* of ascarides.

---

## ASCITES.—DROPSY.

**TREATMENT.** For dropsical effusions in

The **ABDOMEN**: *Apis. *Apo. can. Ars. Aspar. Bry. Chin. Dig. Hell. Kali o. Lach. Lyc. Sene. Sulph.

The **CHEST**: Apis. Apo. can. *Ars. Bry. Colch. Dig. Kali o. Lach. Lyc. Spig. Squil. Sulph. Tart. e.

The **JOINTS**: Ant. Ars. *Bry. Cal. c. Con. *Dig. Iod. Kali hy. Merc. Sil. *Sulph.

The **OVARIES**: *Apis. Ars. Bry. Bell. Chin. *Iod. Lach. Lyco. Plat. *Prun. spi. Sep. Staph.

The best remedies for dropsical effusions

After **ANIMAL FLUIDS**, loss of: **Apo. c. *Chin. Ferr. Helon. Lyco. Merc. Sulph.**

After **DIPHTHERIA**: ***Apis. Ars. Ascle. syr. Bell. Cal. chlor. *Merc. iod. Sulph.**

After **ENTERITIS**: **Apis. *Ars. Dig. Dulc. *Chin.**

After **EXANTHEMATA**, suppression of: **Apis. Ars. Bry. Dig. Hell. Rhus. Sulph. Verat. v.**

After **INTERMITTENT** fever: ***Ars. Chimaph. Dull. *Ferr. *Hell. Lach. Merc. *Nux v. Sulph.**

After **MERCURY**, abuse of: **Chin. Dulc. *Hep. *Nit. ac. Phyto. Sulph.**

After **SCARLET FEVER**: **Apoc. *Apis. Ars. Ascl. syr. Bell. Chin. Colch. Dig. *Hell. Helon. Scill. Senc.**

*Leading indications.*

**APIS MEL.** Dropsical effusions, *with waxy paleness of skin.* [**Ars.**] *Dropsy of right ovary, [**Bell.**] Great soreness in abdominal walls, [**Apo. can.**] *Stinging, burning pains in different parts of body. Must sit straight up to get any ease, [**Ars.**] *Urine scanty, dark, like coffee-grounds, [***Hell. Lach.**] Complication with *scarlet fever*, uterine tumors, etc.

**APOCYN. CAN.** General dropsy, with *sinking feeling at pit of stomach. Bruised feeling in abdomen, [see **Apis.**] Irritable condition of stomach; obliged to sit up; lying down produces violent dyspnœa, [**Ars.**]; urine very scanty, thick, yellow and turbid. After scarlatina, [**Apis. Ars.**]

**ARSENICUM.** The skin, particularly that of face, looks *livid*, pale or *greenish.* Dropsical swellings of abdomen and extremities. *Great debility and prostration. Faint feeling from slight motion. Suffocative spells, especially at night. *Great thirst, but drinking but little, [**Apis. Chin.**] *Anxiety, restlessness, and fear of death.* Dropsy *after scarlatina*, and when complicated with heart disease.

**ASPARAGUS.** Countenance pale, wax-like, and bloated. Expression of anxiety and distress. Visible throbbing of heart, especially at night. Great fullness of chest. Urine scanty, straw-colored and offensive. Advised in dropsies as an article of food.

**BRYONIA.** Lower eyelids œdematous, [upper lids **Kali c.**] Lips bluish, dry and cracked. Stitching pains in region of heart. Wants to lie perfectly quiet, [**Bell.**] Great thirst and scanty urine. Very irritable. *Constipation of dry, hard stools.*

**CHINA.** Countenance pale or sallow, sunken and sickly. *General debility.* Organic affections of liver and spleen, [**Ars. Ferr.**] Great thirst, drinking little and often, [**Apis. Ars.**] In old people [**Kali c.**], and where it arises from *loss of animal fluids*, [**Ars. Ferr.**] .

**COLCHICUM.** Face yellow and œdematous. Swelling of feet and legs, [**Ars. Bry.**] Skin dry and cold, or alternating with heat during night. Visible palpitations of heart, [**Ars. Dig.**] Pulse full and hard, or quick and small. *Scanty dark-colored urine.*

**CONVOLVULUS.** *Abdomen filled with water. Urine almost entirely suppressed.* Weakness, with a good appetite; could eat much if there was room for it.

**DIGITALIS.** Doughy swelling, which easily yields to pressure. Paleness of face, blue lips, and swelling of eyelids. Hydrothorax originating in organic disease of heart. *Strong visible pulsations of heart, and irregular pulse, [**Ars. Spig.**] *Dropsy of knee joint and scrotum.*

**HELLEBORUS.** General anasarca, *acute cases.* Throbbing or compressive headache. Oppression at chest and stomach. Cramp-like pains in abdomen. Frequent desire to urinate, with scanty emissions; *after standing the urine looks like coffee-grounds, [**Apis. Lach.**] After scarlet and intermittent fevers.

**KALI CARB.** Dropsy, especially of old people, [**Ars. Chin.**] In complication with liver and heart diseases. *Stitching pains. *Swelling over the eyelids.*

**LACHESIS.** Dropsies complicated with liver, heart and spleen diseases, [**Chin. Kali c.**] *Left ovary swollen, with pressing, stitching pains, [see **Apis.**] *Can bear no pressure upon uterine region. Urine *black* and scanty. Worse after sleeping, [**Apis.**]

**LYCOPODIUM.** Upper portion of body emaciated, while *lower* is greatly swollen. *One foot cold, the other hot, [one *hand* hot, the other cold, **Musch.**] Oozing of water from sores on feet. *Urine scant, with *sandy* sediment, [**Phos. Sep.**] After abuse of alcoholic liquors, [**Nux.**]

**SENECIO.** Abdomen very tense. Feet and legs swollen, [***Ars. Bry. Colch.**] Pain in lumbar region, and in ovaries, [*stinging pains in right ovary, ***Apis. Bell.**] Urine scanty and high-colored, or profuse and watery.

**SULPHUR.** Dropsical, burning swelling of external parts. Bluish spots on skin; it *is dry and husky.* *Greatly exhausted without any apparent cause. After *suppressed itch* and other cutaneous eruptions.

**PARACENTESIS ABDOMINIS.** This operation is frequently called for in advanced stages of dropsy, to palliate patients' sufferings. Permanent relief sometimes follows these tappings.

**Operation.** Patient seated on side of bed or in a chair. Bladder *must be empty.* Mark the spot exactly in *median line* where abdomen is to be pierced. Apply a broad bandage around abdomen, cross ends behind and give into hands of two assistants. Make an opening in centre of band, through which to operate. With a trocar in canula and end of forefinger about two inches from point of instrument, plunge it through *linea alba*, then withdraw trocar, leaving canula in for fluids to escape through. Draw off fluids *slowly*, assistants tightening bandage as fluids escape. Having done, cover wound with adhesive plaster and compress, pin bandage tightly around abdomen.

---

## ASTHMA.

**TREATMENT.** *Leading indications.*

**ACONITE.** Shortness of breath, especially when sleeping. Dyspnœa, with inability to take a deep breath. Spasmodic, rough, croaking cough, with constriction of windpipe *Great fear and anxiety of mind, with nervous excitability. *Fear of death [**Ars.**], predicts the day he will die.

**AMBRA.** It is said that *amber beads* worn around the neck will *prevent* "hay asthma." It has succeeded in many cases. Internally, it is advised for children and old persons.

**ARSENICUM.** Anxious and oppressed shortness of breath, with labored breathing, particularly when ascending an eminence. Attacks of *suffocation, especially at night*, in evening, or when lying down. *Great anguish, extreme restlessness, and fear of death. *Drinks often, but little at a time, [**Apis. Chin.**] *Cannot lie down for fear of suffocation. Wants to be in a warm room. Anæmic persons, [plethoric, **Bell.**]

**BELLADONNA.** Paroxysms mostly in afternoon or evening. *Sensation of dust in lungs, better bending head back, and when holding breath. Face and eyes red, head hot. Dry, spasmodic cough, especially at night. Uneasiness and beating in chest. *Sleepiness, but cannot sleep. Plethoric individuals and young people.

**BROMIUM.** Gasping for breath, with wheezing and rattling in larynx and spasmodic closure of glottis. Sensation as if air-passages were full of smoke; constriction of chest, with difficulty of breathing; *must sit up in bed.* *Asthma of sailors, as soon as they go ashore; affections begin in bronchia and ascend to larynx.

**BRYONIA.** *Patient wants to remain perfectly quiet, *worse* from least exertion. Frequently dry cough, or cough with expectoration of a quantity of mucus. Stitches in chest, especially during an inspiration, or when coughing, [**Acon. Bell.**] *Sitting up in bed causes nausea and faintness. *Dry, hard stools.

**CHAMOMILLA.** Oppression in chest, as from incarcerated flatulence in epigastrium. Hoarseness and cough from rattling mucus in trachea, [**Ipe.**] *Much hot perspiration about face and head, [*cold* perspiration, **Ars. *Verat.**] One cheek red, other pale. *Very impatient, can hardly answer one civilly. Especially adapted to children; they are very cross, and *want to be carried all the time.*

**CHINA.** Suffocative fits, as from mucus in larynx, in evening in bed. Difficult inspiration and quick expiration. *The patient appears as if dying. Cough, with difficult expectoration of clear, tenacious mucus, [Ferr.] Worse at night and after drinking. *Better every other day.

**FERRUM.** Asthma most violent when lying down, obliging one to sit up, [Ars.] Spasmodic cough with expectoration of transparent, tenacious mucus, [Chin.] *With every paroxysm of coughing, face becomes fiery red. Always better when walking slowly.

**IPECAC.** Spasmodic asthma, with violent *contraction in throat and chest.* Contraction of chest with short panting breathing. *Rattling noise in bronchial tubes during inspiration. *Suffocation threatens from constriction in throat and chest; worse from least motion, [Bry.] *Nausea with a feeling of emptiness in stomach.

**KALI CARB.** Difficult wheezing respiration. Spasmodic asthma, worse about 3 A. M., relieved by sitting up and bending forward, resting head on knees. Cough, excited by tickling in throat, with sourish expectoration, or of blood-streaked mucus. *Great aversion to being alone.

**LACHESIS.** Shortness of breath, after every exertion. Tightness in chest, with inclination to vomit. *Can bear nothing to touch larynx, seems as though it would suffocate him, [Apis.] *Aggravation after sleeping, and during rest.

**LOBELIA IN.** The attack is preceded or accompanied by a kind of *prickly sensation through whole system, even to ends of fingers and toes. *Sensation as of a foreign body in throat, impeding breathing and deglutition. *Nausea* and *vomiting,* with a sense of great emptiness in stomach, [Ipe.]

**PHOSPHORUS.** Loud panting respiration. Spasmodic constriction of chest, [Acon. Ars.] *Complete loss of voice. *Sensation of weakness and emptiness in abdomen, [Ipe.] *Long, narrow, hard stools, very difficult to expel. Tall, slender people.

**SAMBUCUS.** Violent dyspnœa, with anguish and danger of suffocation, especially when lying down. *Nightly suffocative paroxysms, with spasmodic constriction of chest, [Phos.] Mucus rattling in chest. Especially adapted to children, [Cham.]

**SILPHIUM LAC.** Wheezing in chest during all inspiration. Scraping, tickling, and irritation in throat; sick, faint feeling in stomach. Moist cough, with copious expectoration of white frothy mucus. Especially in old people, [Ars.]

**SPONGIA.** *Difficult respiration, as if to breathe through a sponge. Wheezing respiration or slow and deep breathing, as if from debility. *Awakens often in a fright, and feels as if suffocating. Hoarse, hollow, wheezing cough. Cannot lie down.

**SULPHUR.** Attack comes on during sleep, or in evening, with tightness across chest, and a sensation as of dust in air-passages. Dry cough with hoarseness, or *loose cough* with soreness and pressure in chest. *Frequent weak, faint spells. *Constant heat on top the head.

**TARTARUS EM.** Anxious oppression, difficulty of breathing and shortness of breath, with desire to sit erect, [***Ars.**] *When patient coughs, it seems as if bronchial tubes were full of phlegm, but none comes up, [***Ipe.**] *Coldness of surface*, with clammy perspiration.

**VERAT. ALB.** Attack mostly occurs in cold, damp weather, and early in morning. Anguish, suffocation, and oppression about heart. Coldness of nose, ears, and lower extremities. *Cold sweat on forehead [*hot* sweat, **Cham.**] with great prostration.

For **HAY ASTHMA: Ailanth. Allium cep. Ars. Arum tri. Euph. Lobe. in. Mosch. Sang. Sili. Sticta.**

**AUXILIARY MEASURES.** Among the various remedies employed to relieve the severity of an attack are: *Stramonium*, *Nitrate of Potash*, Chloroform, Ether, *Amyl Nitrite*, etc. *Stram.* is used by smoking the dried leaves. *Nitrate of Potash* by soaking coarse paper in a saturated solution, drying it thoroughly and inhaling the fumes while the paper is burning. *Chloroform* and *Ether* are administered by inhalation. *Amyl Nitrite* is used by putting 3 or 4 drops on a handkerchief and inhaling it; this often gives prompt relief—should be used cautiously. *Pilocarpin* is strongly recommended; ten drops of a 2 per cent. solution is injected into the arm. *Grindelia robusta* is highly extolled at present in this disease. ℞. Fl. Extr. Grindelia robusta, ℥ji., Glycerine, ℥j., Aq. font. ℥ji. Mix and give a teaspoonful every hour till paroxysm is relieved.

---

## ATROPHY OF CHILDREN.

**TREATMENT.** *Leading indications.*

**ABROTANUM.** *Child cross, depressed, very peevish. Face wrinkled as if old, [**Opi.**] *Ravenous appetite, all the while emaciating. *Distended abdomen.* *Food passes undigested. *Skin flabby, hangs loose.

**ÆTHUSA C.** The child throws up its milk soon after nursing, *with great force, suddenly*—then falls asleep as if from exhaustion, to awaken for a fresh supply. The milk disagrees; *aphthæ in mouth.*

**ARSENICUM.** General emaciation, with dry parchment-like skin. Pale œdematous swelling of face. Sunken eyes with blue margins. *Feverish heat with desire to drink often, but little at a time. Great restlessness, particularly at night. Painful, offensive, undigested stools. *Prostration* and coldness of extremities.

**BARYTA CARB.** *Swelling and induration of glands. Emaciation, bloated face, swollen abdomen, and constant desire to sleep. Indisposed to work or play. *Scrofulous children that do not grow.

**BELLADONNA.** Glandular swellings painful or suppurating. Eyelids inflamed and ulcers on cornea. *Child sleepy, but cannot sleep. *Sudden starting and jumping during sleep. *Precocious* children.

**BRYONIA.** The child throws up its food immediately after taking it, [**Ars.**] Mouth and lips very dry, with thirst for large quantities of water. *Child very irritable and wants to be quiet; feels worse at every *hot spell.* *Dry, hard stools, as if burnt.

**CALC. CARB.** Large *head with open fontanelles,* [**Merc.** ***Sil. Sulph.**] Dry *flabby* skin. Enlargement and hardness of abdomen. *General emaciation with good appetite, [See **Abrot.**] Diarrhœa, with clay-colored stools. *Cold, damp feet. *Much perspiration about head in large drops, [**Merc. Sil.**] Cough, with rattling mucus in bronchia.

**CHINA.** Pale, sickly appearance. Enlargement of liver and spleen. Copious sweats, especially at night; great debility and prostration. *Painless, undigested, offensive stools. *Abdomen distended with flatulence.

**MERCURIUS.** Yellow, earthy color of face. Large head and open fontanelles, [***Cal. c.**] Swelling and suppuration of glands. *Slimy or bloody stools, with much straining. *Profuse night sweats. Child is never so well during wet weather.

**PHOSPHORUS.** Pale and bloated face. Sunken eyes, with blue circles under the same, [**Ars.**] Dry, hacking cough. Diarrhœa, with white, watery, undigested stools. Great debility and oppression after least exercise. *Children of tall, slender stature.

**PULSATILLA.** The child seems to be very changeable; gets better for a time, and then without any apparent cause gets worse. *Diarrhœa, especially at night, no two stools alike, [**Sulph.**] *Worse towards evening; *better in open air.* Pale face, blue eyes.

**RHUS TOX.** Herpetic eruptions on face. Swelling and induration of glands. Diarrhœa, with thin, red mucous stools; great appetite. *The child always gets worse after midnight.

**SARSAPARILLA.** *Fully developed marasmus. Great emaciation; skin hangs in folds; the face is shrivelled; *aphthæ in mouth,* and herpes on the skin.

**STAPHISAGRIA.** Hollow eyes, with weary look. Swelling of submaxillary and cervical glands, [**Bary. c.**] Unhealthy, readily ulcerating skin. *Canine hunger, even when stomach is full of food.

**SULPHUR.** The child frequently awakens from sleep with screams. Great voracity, wants to put everything in mouth. ***Diarrhœa**, excoriating anus, [**Ars. Cham. *Merc.**] ***Copious morning sweats, after waking.** *Unhealthy skin.*

---

## BED-SORES.

Bed-sores are the result of long-continued pressure on prominent parts of the body, as the sacrum, brim of ilium, great trochanter and spine, caused by long confinement in bed. The parts first become red, look rough, then ulcerate, or turn black and mortify.

**TREATMENT.** On the first appearance of the sores, they should be bathed with a weak solution of *Arnica*, and the pressure removed by a change of position or the use of circular *air-cushions.*

If the part becomes ulcerated, a linseed-meal poultice may be applied to hasten separation of the slough, after which it should be dressed with carbolated *Calendula.*

Sponges wet in *hot* and *cold* water applied *alternately* to the sores, are said to be very successful. Each sponge should be allowed to remain on about one minute, and the entire time occupied from 10 to 15 minutes. Should be repeated several times daily.

**GALVANISM.** This is said to be singularly successful. "A thin *silver* plate, not thicker than paper, is cut exact size and shape of sore, a zinc plate about same size is connected with silver plate by a silver or copper wire 6 or 8 inches long; the *silver* is placed in immediate contact with the sore, and the *zinc* plate on sound skin above, piece of chamois skin soaked in vinegar intervening; this must be kept *moist* to insure action of battery." Dr. Hammond states that he has seen bed-sores three to four inches in diameter, half inch deep, heal entirely over in 48 hours under this treatment.

Dr. Hering advises placing an open vessel filled with water under the bed of patient, to prevent bed-sores. In many cases the internal administration of **Arn. Carb. v. Chin. Plumb.** or **Sulph. ac.** will be useful.

---

## BITES AND STINGS OF INSECTS.

When a person has been bitten by a venomous snake, tie a ligature tightly round the limb above the wound, to check circulation, suck the wound thoroughly and inject into it with a hypodermic syringe a solution *Permanganate of Potash* [1 to 100], or cut the bitten part out and suck the wound, or lastly, *cauterize it with Liq. Ammonia, Nitric* or *Carbolic Acid.*

**RATTLESNAKE.** There is every reason to believe that Prof. Bibron's antidote for the bite of a rattlesnake is effectual. It is as follows:—

| ℞. | Potassii iodidi, | . . . . . | 4 grs. |
|---|---|---|---|
| | Hydrarg. chlor, | . . . . . | 2 grs. |
| | Brominii, | . . . . | 4 drachms. |

Give ten drops of this mixture, diluted with a spoonful of wine or brandy, and repeat if necessary.

Another favorite remedy for this species of poisoning, is to make the patient drunk by giving large quantities of alcohol.

**BITES OF SPIDERS, ETC.** The bite of spiders, centipedes, etc., is not usually followed by any bad consequences. One of the best local applications is tincture *Apis Mellifica.* Washing the parts well with hot water, and then applying raw onion, is a good remedy, also *Arnicated Collodion.*

**STINGS OF BEES, ETC.** Examine the parts with magnifying glass, and extract the stings with fine forceps, if visible. *Aqua Ammonia* or *Tr. Arnica,* dilute, among the best applications. *Bicarbonate of Potash,* wood *ashes* and water, moist clay, raw *onion* and tincture of *Camphor,* are also good local remedies.

If the wound cause inflammation and fever, give **Camph.** to smell, and if this be insufficient, give **Aconite.**

If tongue is the seat of injury, give **Aconite,** and if this does not relieve, **Arnica. Bell.** will be required if there is much redness, swelling and tenderness of parts.

For stings in the *eye,* **Acon.** and **Arnica** will be found the best remedies.

---

## BOIL.—FURUNCLE.

A boil is a small phlegmon, which appears in the form of a conical, hard, circumscribed tumor, having its seat in the dermoid texture. At the end of an uncertain period it becomes pointed, white or yellow, and gives exit to pus mixed with blood.

**TREATMENT.** *Special indications.*

**ACONITE.** Boil *highly inflamed,* attended with a good deal of fever, *restlessness* and *anxiety.*

**ARNICA.** *Many small painful boils, very sore. Boils following mechanical injuries. Where there is a tendency to a recurrence, [**Lyc. Phos. Sil. *Sulph.**] Plethoric subjects with red face. Applied locally gives much relief.

**BELLADONNA.** *Fiery-red or erysipelatous appearance. *Swelling of glands* under the arms and in the groins. Fever, hot, dry skin, thirst and headache. Young full-blooded subjects.

**BERBERIS VUL.** *Hastens suppuration*, and removes predisposition to a recurrence.—HELMUTH.

**HEPAR SULPH.** *Hastens suppuration, pain throbbing, [see **Merc.**] Boil very painful to *touch* [**Rhus.**] *Unhealthy skin, slight injuries suppurate.

**MERC. VIV.** *After pus has formed; pain throbbing, stinging, [stinging when touched, **Lyco.**] Axillary *glands swollen;* inclination to sweat, [boils of axillary glands, **Rhus t.**]

**SULPHUR.** Where there is a *strong predisposition* and *frequent return* of the disease, [**Calc. c. Lyc. Phos.**] Glandular swellings, [**Merc.**] Skin *rough, scaly, scabby.*

**LOCAL TREATMENT.** *Hot poultices* or *fomentations*, medicated with the *internal indicated remedy*, will have a salutary effect. Soon as suppuration is established, open with sharp lancet.

---

## BRIGHT'S DISEASE.

(*Parenchymatous Nephritis.*)

Under this head some writers include acute and chronic inflammation of the kidneys, in fact all conditions in which *albumen* is found in the urine. Only where there is *granular* or *fatty* degeneration of the kidneys can we have positive evidence of the existence of so-called *Morbus Brightii.* This can only be determined by a chemical and microscopic examination of the urine. Such examination should be made at short intervals so long as *albumen* is present in renal secretions.

**TREATMENT.** *Leading indications.*

**APIS MEL.** *Impaired memory.* Headache and vertigo. *Pain in hypochondriac region, extending upwards. Renal pains, soreness on pressure or when stooping. *Urine scanty, milky, albuminous, containing uriniferous tubules and epithelium. *Eyelids œdematous, with baglike swelling under the eyes, [over upper lids, **Kali c.**] *Œdema of hands and lower extremities. Especially after scarlatina, [**Kali c. Helon. Sec.**]

**ARGENT. NIT.** *Dullness of the head and mental confusion.* Dizziness with tendency to fall sideways. *Head feels too large, [**Gel. *Nux.**] *Irresistible desire for sugar. *Belching after every meal, stomach as if it would burst.* Acute pain about kidneys, extending down ureters to bladder.

**ARSENICUM.** *Fear of death, restlessness, trembling, prostration. Intense frontal headache. *Œdematous swelling of face, *Edge of tongue red, takes imprint of teeth, [see **Merc.**] Stitches in renal region when breathing or sneezing. *Urine scanty, dark brown, and *albuminous. Great thirst, drinking often and little,* [**Apis.**] Pale, waxy skin. *General dropsy.

**BERBERIS.** Fretful humor, with weariness of life. Beating and fluttering in ears. *Smarting, burning in region of kidneys, [**Tereb.**] Bloody urine, which settles at bottom of vessel in a cake. Transparent, jelly-like mucus passes with urine, followed by *great exhaustion.* **Albuminous urine,* [**Apis. Helon. Tereb.**] Pain in loins and hips. Hard, lumpy stools.

**CANTHARIS.** Whining and complaining, with anxious restlessness. Great thirst, with burning in stomach, [**Ars.**] Cutting, burning pains in region of both kidneys, the parts being sensitive to pressure. *Painful micturition, by drops, of burning, bloody urine. *Albuminous urine containing cylindrical casts, mucus, and shreds ; looks jelly-like.* Great weakness, prostration, faintness.

**HELONIAS.** *Mind dull and inactive,* wants to be let alone. Great languor, [**Berb. Phos. Tereb.**] *Feeling of weakness and weight in region of kidneys. Frequent desire to urinate. *Urine profuse, light-colored, albuminous.* Dropsy, general debility, uterine atony.

**KALMIA.** Anxiety, with *palpitation of heart.* Scanty albuminous urine, with fibrinous casts and epithelial cells [see **Helon.**] Oppression of chest, dyspnœa, vertigo, dullness of head. Persistent pains in lower extremities.

**MERC. COR.** Mind sluggish, with torpid digestion. Œdematous swelling of face, [**Apis. Ars.**] Metallic taste, mouth feels as if scalded. Bloated abdomen, painful to touch. Filaments, flocks or dark flesh-like pieces of mucus in urine. Albumen in urine after diphtheria. Yellowish tint of the skin.

**PHOSPHORUS.** Great indifference, and *lowness of spirits.* Skin on face and forehead feels tense. Puffiness under the eyes. *Feebleness of sight, [**Kalm.**] *Granular and fatty degeneration of the kidneys.* *Albumen and exudation cells in urine. Sensation of weakness or emptiness in stomach. *Constipation, stools *long, slender, and hard* like a dog's, [**Caust.**]

**SARSAPARILLA.** Dull, stupid feeling, cannot keep the mind on his study. Throbbing in top of head, worse from walking. *Dimness of sight, as if looking through a fog,* [***Ars. Merc.**] *Tenesmus of bladder, with discharge of white acrid *pus and mucus.* *Severe pain at *conclusion of urination.* Trembling of hands and feet.

**SECALE.** Anxiety, sadness, melancholy; fear of death. Feeling of lightness in head, [great *heaviness,* **Gel.**] Obscuration of sight. *Morbus Brightii after scarlatina, [see **Apis.**] *Urine pale or bloody, with deposits looking like cheese.* Desire to be uncovered ; *worse in a warm room.*

**TARTAR EMET.** Weariness in every part of body. Numbness of head, with stupefaction. Trembling of head and hands, with great debility, worse when lying and getting warm in bed. *Dimness* of sight, sees things as through a veil, [*white* veil, **Ars.**—*gray*, **Phos.**] Longing for acids and fruits. *Continuous nausea, [***Ipe.**] *Albuminous urine.* Visible palpitation of heart.

**TEREBINTHINA.** Sudden vertigo, with obscuration of sight. Burning and drawing from right kidney to hip. *Urine black, with sediment like coffee grounds. Blood is thoroughly mixed with urine. *Albuminous urine.* If caused by living in damp dwellings.

**HYGIENIC MEASURES.** These are of first importance. Over-taxing of body or mind, exposure to inclement weather, the use of alcoholic stimulants and imprudence in eating, should be interdicted. Frequent bathing with tepid water, and friction to promote healthy action of skin and circulation, clothing to secure uniform warmth, and outdoor exercise to extent of patient's ability, are important measures to be adopted.

**DIETETICS.** A diet exclusively of *skim-milk* is highly commended. Begin with moderate quantity, increase it daily to the exclusion of all other food. Continue this for at least a month, and if no improvement, gradually return to other diet. We have found good *fresh buttermilk* one of the very best articles of diet in this disease, and greatly prefer it to skim-milk.

---

## BRONCHITIS.

**TREATMENT.** *Leading indications.*

**ACONITE.** Mostly in commencement of acute attacks. Chill and synochal fever, dry, hot skin, and great restlessness. Short, dry cough, worse at night, with constant irritation in larnyx. *Great fear and anxiety of mind, with nervous excitability. *After exposure to dry, cold winds, [**Hep.**]

**APIS MEL.** Sensation of soreness in chest as from a bruise. *Cough, particularly after lying down and sleeping, [**Lach.**] A clear, tough, stringy phlegm rises in throat, which causes him to hawk frequently, [**Kali b. Rumex.**] *Œdema glottidis.

**ARSENICUM.** Dry, hacking cough, with soreness in chest, as if raw, or moist cough, with difficult expectoration of blood-streaked mucus. Difficulty of breathing, obliging him to sit up, [**Apis.**] *Dryness and burning in larynx.* Great thirst, but drinks little. *Restlessness, debility, and fear of death.

**BELLADONNA.** Face flushed and eyes red. *Great fullness in head, or splitting headache. Hot skin, with inclination to perspire. Spasmodic cough which does not allow one time to breathe. *Children cry after every coughing spell.* Sleepy, but cannot sleep, [**Opi.**] *Starting and jumping during sleep.

**BRYONIA.** Short, difficult respiration, obliging him to sit erect, [**Ars.**] Dry cough, with stitches in chest. Violent morning cough, with expectoration of quantities of mucus. *Sensation when coughing as if head and chest would fly to pieces. *The patient wants to remain perfectly quiet.

**CARBO VEG.** Obstinate hoarseness, particularly in evening, [in morning, ***Caust. Phos.**] Severe burning in chest as from hot coals. Violent cough, with discharge of a quantity of yellowish pus. Stitching pains between scapula, [burning. **Bry.**] *Patient craves air; wants to be fanned all the time.

**CAUSTICUM.** Hoarseness and roughness of throat, particularly in morning. Short, hacking cough, with rawness in throat. *When coughing, pain over the hip, [**Bell.**] Involuntary emissions of urine, [**Puls.**] Loss of voice, [**Phos.**] *Tightness* of chest.

**CHAMOMILLA.** Hoarseness and cough from rattling mucus in trachea, the place feeling sore from whence the mucus was detached. *Scraping, dry cough from tickling in larynx, *worse at night*, even during sleep; *expectoration only in daytime.* *One cheek red, other pale, [***Acon. Nux.**] *Very impatient, can hardly answer one civilly.

**EUPATOR. PER.** *Rough scraping cough, with soreness in chest. Has to support *chest* when he coughs, [***Nat. s.**—has to support *head*, ***Nice.**]

**HEPAR SULPH.** Dry, hoarse cough, and roughness in throat. *Rattling, choking cough, worse after midnight. Hoarse, anxious, wheezing breathing, with danger of suffocation when lying down. After exposure to cold west winds, [***Acon.**]

**IPECAC.** *Rattling of mucus in bronchia. Suffocative cough, with great difficulty of breathing. Chest seems full of phlegm, but does not yield to coughing, [***Tart. e.**] *Much nausea and vomiting of mucus. Face livid during cough.

**KALI BICHRO.** Burning pain in trachea and bronchia. *Cough, with expectoration of tough, stringy mucus, which can be drawn down to feet, [**Phos.**]

**LACHESIS.** Hoarseness with feeble voice and constriction of throat. Short, hacking cough, caused by a tingling in throat. Difficult yellow expectoration. *Larynx and throat painful when touched; pressure produces violent cough, [**Rumex.**] *Always worse after sleeping.

**MERCURIUS.** *Hoarseness* and *sore throat.* Catarrh of whole mucous membrane. Violent, racking cough, particularly at night, as if it would burst the head and chest, [see **Bry.**] Alternate chilliness and heat, [**Bell.**] *Cough worse when lying on right side, [on *left side*, **Phos.**] *Much perspiration, without relief.

**NUX VOMICA.** Roughness and scraping in larynx, inducing cough, [**Caust.** ***Phos.**] Dry cough from midnight till morning. Cough with headache as if skull would split, [**Bry. Merc.**] Nose stopped up. Fever, but chilliness from slight motion. *Always worse after 4 A. M. *Habitual constipation. After previous use of cough mixtures.

**PHOSPHORUS.** *Complete loss of voice,* [**Caust.**] *Cannot talk, larynx so painful, [**Apis.**] *Tightness across the chest, [**Ars. Puls.**] Cough with expectoration of frothy, pale-red, or rust-colored mucus. Severe and exhausting cough, which the patient dreads and avoids as long as possible. *Sensation of weakness and emptiness in the abdomen.

**PULSATILLA.** Scraping and dryness in throat, [**Nux v.**] *Dry cough at night, going off when sitting up in bed,* [**Hyos. Sang.**] Loose cough, with copious expectoration of yellow or greenish mucus. *Chilliness even in a warm room. *Hot, dry skin, with little or no thirst. Persons of a mild, tearful disposition.

**RHUS TOX.** Cough excited by a tickling under middle of sternum, worse from laughing or loud talking, [**Phos.**] *Rheumatic pains in bones, worse when at rest, [*better, **Bry.**] *Worse at night, particularly after midnight. After getting wet when heated.

**SANGUINARIA.** Dryness of throat, and sensation of swelling in larynx. *Severe cough, *with circumscribed redness of cheeks and pain in breast.* Pain in root of nose. Fluent coryza and thin diarrhœa. Burning in hands and feet at night. *Sweats* at night.

**SPONGIA.** Great dryness in larynx, with hoarse, hollow, wheezing cough, worse in evening. Sawing respiration. *The voice frequently gives out when talking or reading aloud. *Croupy* subjects.

**SULPHUR.** Hoarseness and loss of voice. Sensation as of something creeping in larynx, [**Carb. v.**] Loose cough, with expectoration of thick mucus and soreness in chest. *Stitches in chest extending to back. Pain in left side. *Frequent weak, faint spells. Constant rattling in chest. *Lean persons who walk stooping.

**TARTARUS EM.** Large collection of mucus in bronchia, with difficult breathing. *When patient coughs, it seems as if much would be expectorated, but nothing comes up, [***Ipe.**] *Nausea and vomiting of much mucus. Great oppression and difficulty of breathing.

**VERAT.** Dry, hollow cough as if proceeding from lower parts of chest or abdomen. *Rattling of mucus in chest, but can't get rid of it, [see **Ipe.**] Vomiting, with diarrhœa and great prostration.

---

## BUNION.

This is an enlargement over the metatarsal joint of great toe. It is frequently found in persons of advanced years, causing considerable deformity, and at times much pain.

**TREATMENT.** *Special remedies.*

Remove all pressure caused by tight shoes, and if part is inflamed, apply *linseed-meal* poultice, or hot fomentations medicated with dilute *Arnica.*

**ACONITE.** Red, shining, hot swelling of joint. Violent cutting pains, part burns like fire, [**Ars.**] Nervous, restless, very excitable.

**ARNICA.** If caused from a blow, *pressure* or *constant friction.* *Bluish redness of the part and intense soreness.

**LEDUM.** Indicated for similar symptoms to those found under **Arnica.** *Stinging tearing pains, aggravated by heat.

**GRAPHITES.** Chronic enlargement of the joint, with redness of surrounding parts; swelling and itching of toes. *Unhealthy skin, ulcerates readily.

**Hepar, Merc.** or **Sili.** Where there is a tendency to suppurate.

**IODIDE POTAS.** The most effectual remedy for chronic form of the disease.—Helmuth.

**STICTA PULM.** In the *acute form,* with circumscribed redness of the parts.

---

## BURNS AND SCALDS.

All charred or burnt clothing must first be carefully cut away from burned surface. Then wash parts with solution *Cantharides* or *Urtica Urens,* [ʒi, *warm water* ℥iv], or solution *Creasote* [ʒi, water Oi.] Prick any vesicles with needle, and apply such dressings as will absolutely exclude the air. Thick layers of cotton best protection to the parts. Dress parts soon as possible after injury. Use first remedy at hand, till others can be procured.

**TREATMENT.** *Principal remedies.*

**ALCOHOL.** For burns or scalds, where blisters have not already formed, the external application of this remedy is highly extolled.

**BICARBONATE OF SODA.** Valuable in all superficial burns or scalds, [see **Canth.**] Soon as can be after accident, apply the powdered soda to burnt surface and lay over it a wet cloth. The pain will almost immediately subside and wound readily heal.

**CANTHARIDES.** In superficial burns or scalds, this is one of the best remedies. Put twenty drops of *Tincture* in a gill of water, and keep injured parts constantly wet with rags or lint saturated with the solution. After the acute symptoms have subsided, dress with *simple cerate.*

**CARBOLIZED OIL.** One of the best remedies in deep-seated burns. Mix one drachm **Carbolic Acid** with one pint of olive or linseed oil, and apply with cloths.

**CASTILE SOAP.** Make a thick salve by mixing it with warm water, spread it upon soft linen or muslin, and apply to the injured part, change twice daily.

**FLOUR AND OIL.** A good application and most always at hand. Soon after accident as possible, oil injured surface with sweet or linseed oil, and dust it over with flour from a common dredging-box until thickly covered.

**GLYCERINE.** For burns in mouth, throat or stomach, this is an excellent remedy. Equal parts of glycerine and water may be taken in spoonful doses, and mouth and throat gargled with same. Take *Urtica Urens* internally for burns of this character.

**URTICA URENS.** Valuable in all classes of burns, not only for slight and superficial cases, but in severe and more deeply penetrating injuries of this kind. It may be applied same as directed for use of **Cantharides.**

## INTERNAL TREATMENT.

**ACONITE.** Chills, fever, dry, hot skin and much thirst, following extensive burns. *Great fear and anxiety of mind, with much nervous excitability.

**ARSENICUM.** Dark, watery, offensive diarrhœa. Rapid prostration, with sinking of vital forces. *Extreme thirst, drinking often, but little at a time. Great anguish, restlessness and fear of death.

**CHAMOMILLA.** In *convulsions* arising from severe burns. Becomes furious about the pains, [**Acon.**] *Very impatient, can hardly answer one civilly. Warm sweat about the face and head.

**CHINA.** Extensive suppuration, producing much debility, [**Hepar. Merc.**] Painless diarrhœa of dark, watery stools, particularly at night

**SILICEA.** When the ulcer heals slowly, or proud flesh is disposed to shoot up, and the parts burn.

**SULPHUR.** There is a strong tendency to the production of proud flesh, and there is no appearance of granulations, [**Sili.**] Much itching, burning and inflammation around the ulcers.

**CLINICAL REMARKS.** Be in no hurry in removing first dressings. If injury is extensive, apply dressings so they can be removed without exposing too great surface at once. At each dressing, bathe part well with *carbolized* water, drachm to pint, When suppuration is profuse, and reaction begins, cover parts with carded cotton, and keep wet with *Calendula.* Give same remedy internally.

*Extensive* burns, even of slight severity, are always dangerous.

If *one-half,* or even *one-third,* the surface is burned, death is almost certain to follow.

Burns on the *trunk* more dangerous than those of equal extent on extremities.

**Periods of Danger.** First. Immediately after injury, from *shock.* Second. During third or fourth day, from fever or sympathetic affections of brain or bowels. Third. During period of suppuration, hectic or pyæmia may supervene.

## CARBUNCLE.—ANTHRAX.

This is a species of malignant tumor. It commences as a livid red swelling, attended with a *burning, itching, smarting* pain, which gradually grows worse as the disease progresses. After 5 or 6 days, softening and suppuration take place, and when it bursts, instead of having a central opening as a boil, it is flat on top with several openings which discharge a thin acrid fluid. These openings gradually widen, coalesce, and large pieces of decayed cellular tissue are thrown off by sloughing.

Carbuncles vary in size from that of a chestnut to that of a man's fist, and when occurring about the head are very dangerous.

**TREATMENT.** *Principal remedies.*

**ANTHRACINUM.** Violent burning pains not relieved by **Ars.** Sloughing; abundant discharge of ichorous, terribly smelling pus.—Raue.

**ARSENICUM.** *Intense burning in parts. Sensation as if boiling water was running beneath integuments. *Great restlessness, thirst and debility. Worse at night, better from warm applications.

**BELLADONNA.** Bright redness, of an erysipelatous character. *Throbbing pain, drowsiness and inability to sleep.

**CARBO VEG.** Dark bluish appearance of tumor. *Great foulness of the discharges. Cachectic persons, whose vital powers have become weakened.

**HEPAR SULPH.** If given early will sometimes abort anthrax, later it promotes suppuration. When extensive cavities have formed, discharge profuse and purulent.

**LACHESIS.** Bluish purplish appearance of parts. [See **Carb. v.**] *Impending gangrene. Blood-poisoning.

**MURIATIC AC.** Scorbutic individuals, ulcers on gums, with fetid breath. Feeling of great emptiness in stomach and abdomen.

**RHUS TOX.** The parts have a bluish gangrenous appearance, [see **Lach.**] Itching, burning around the carbuncle. *Great restlessness; patient feels better while moving about.

**SILICEA.** During process of ulceration. *Fistulous openings with offensive discharge; parts around hard, bluish-red. Promotes healthy granulations.

**CLINICAL REMARKS.** Avoid use of "free incisions." Dress sore with solution *hot* **Calendula** [drachm to pint.] Cover compress with oiled silk, and trust to internal medication. If parts become gangrenous, apply poultices of *charcoal and yeast.* Allow nourishing diet and discard all stimulants.

"A commencing carbuncle may be successfully aborted by injecting into its centre several drops of *pure carbolic acid.*" —Gatchell.

## CATARRH.—CORYZA.

**TREATMENT.** *Leading remedies.*

For **DRY CORYZA,** with stoppage of the nose, ***Am. c. Bry Dulc. Nit. ac. Nux v. Phos. *Sep.**

For **FLUENT CORYZA,** with mucus or watery discharges, ***Alli. c. Ars. Arum. t. Bell. Cham. Dul. Euph. Hepar. Kali b. *Merc. Puls. Sulph.**

**LEADING INDICATIONS.**

**ACONITE.** Mostly in first stage; chilliness, with burning heat, especially in head and face. Profuse lachrymation, [**Euph.**] Short, dry cough, from tickling in larynx. *Fear, anxiety, and great restlessness. *From dry, cold winds, [**Hepar**—*cold damp air*, **Gel.**]

**ALLIUM CEPA.** *Profuse discharge from eyes, and burning excoriating water from nose. *Catarrh, with profuse flow of tears; smarting in the eyes, and violent sneezing.* Terrible laryngeal cough, compelling patient to grasp larynx; it seems if cough would tear it. *Feels better* in fresh air.

**AMM. CARB.** *Burning and pain in eyes*, with lachrymation. *Dry coryza*, with stoppage of nose, especially at night, [**Nux.**] Dry, *nightly* cough, and stitches in the chest. Frequent chilliness.

**ARSENICUM.** Frequent sneezing, profuse fluent coryza, stoppage of nose. Burning and soreness of nostrils. Profuse lachrymation and burning in the eyes, [**Acon. Euph.**] Dryness in mouth and loss of taste. Chilliness, particularly after drinking. *Intense thirst, drinking little and often. *Restlessness and prostration.

**ARUM TRIPH.** *Coryza, with discharge of burning, ichorous fluid from nose, excoriating nostrils and upper lip, [**Ars.**] Nose stopped up; can only breathe with mouth open. Hoarseness and sore throat. Dry, feverish heat and hot skin.

**BAPTISIA.** Stiffness of all the joints as if strained. Rheumatic pains, and *soreness all over*, [see **Gel.**] *Tickling in throat, provoking cough, *fauces dark red.* Thick mucus from the nose. Dull frontal headache.

**BELLADONNA.** Sore throat and hoarseness. *Throbbing headache, worse from motion. Dry, hoarse cough; *children cry when coughing.* Alternate chilliness and heat. [**Merc.**] Swelling and stiffness in nape of neck. *Sleepy, but cannot sleep.

**BRYONIA.** Dry coryza, with inflamed, ulcerated nostrils. *Lips parched, dry, and cracked; *splitting headache.* Dry cough, apparently from stomach, worse after drinking. *Constipation of hard, dry stools as if burnt. *Patient wants to keep very still. Exceedingly irritable.

**CARBO VEG.** Beating or pulsating headache, [**Bell.**] Burning in eyes and profuse lachrymation. Stopping of nose, particularly in evening. Fluent coryza, with hoarseness and rawness of chest. *If coryza return in evening.

**CHAMOMILLA.** *Fluent acrid discharge* from nose. Chilliness and feverish heat. *One cheek red and hot, the other pale and cold, [Acon. Nux.] Hoarseness and cough from rattling mucus in bronchia. *Dry cough, worse at night, even during sleep. *Patient very irritable. *Children want to be carried all the time.

**DULCAMARA.** Dry coryza, aggravated in cold air. *The symptoms are aggravated by every cold change, [Gel.] and in wet weather; better when moving about.

**EUPHRASIA.** *Profuse fluent coryza, with burning acrid tears. Cough only during day. Ulceration of margins of eyelids, [*Merc. Sulph.] *Earache.*

**GELSEMIUM.** Liability to take cold from change in any weather, [see Dulc.] Sore throat, with pain on swallowing, shooting up into ear, [Apis.] *Dull aching and muscular soreness in limbs,* [see Bapt.] *Fever without thirst; wants to lie still and rest.

**HEPAR SULPH.** Great liability to take cold, especially after abuse of mercury. Roughness and scraping in throat, [Nux v.] *Stitches in throat as if caused by a splinter, [Arg. n.] *Hoarse croupy cough, phlegm being loose and choking.

**IPECAC.** Aching pain over the eyes. Fluent coryza, stoppage of nose, loss of smell. *Rattling of phlegm in chest, but does not yield to coughing, [Tart. e.] *Nausea and vomiting large quantities of mucus. Oppressed breathing as of asthma. Suitable to *children.*

**KALI B.** Fluent coryza, worse in evening and in open air. Flow of acrid water from nose, excoriating the nostrils, [Ars. Arum. t.] *Cough, with expectoration of tough phlegm, which can be drawn into long strings. Loss of smell, [Ipe. Sep.]

**LACHESIS.** Fluent coryza. Dryness of mouth, with *burning as if from pepper.* Dry cough, shortness of breath, and stitches in chest. *Can bear nothing to touch his throat [Apis.]; it excites a cough and produces a sense of suffocation. *Symptoms worse in afternoon and after sleeping.

**MERCURIUS.** *Catarrhal headache.* Burning in eyes and profuse lachrymation. Pain in jaws and teeth. *Frequent sneezing and profuse fluent coryza. Inflamed and *ulcerated tonsils,* [Bell.] Short, dry, fatiguing cough, worse at night. *After sweating at night, the cold is no better. Feels better in a warm room, [Ars.]

**NUX VOMICA.** Chilliness and feverish heat. Fluent coryza during the day; dry at night. Dry cough with headache as if skull would burst. *Very irritable and wishes to be alone, [Chin.] Constipation, with frequent urging to stool. *Aggravation* in morning.

nose stopped up - alter. fr. side to si

nose stopped up

**PULSATILLA.** Yellowish, green, thick, fetid mucus from nose. Loss of taste and smell, [**Sulph.**] Toothache and otalgia. *Craves fresh, cool air; worse in warm room, [better, ***Ars.**] *Chilliness even in warm room. Loose cough, with expectoration of yellow mucus. *Symptoms all worse towards evening. Mild, tearful disposition.

**SAMBUCUS.** *Stoppage of nose, with thick tenacious mucus. Sudden starting from sleep as if suffocating. Circumscribed redness of the cheeks, [**Sang.**] *Snifles of infants, can't breathe through the nose,* [**Nux.**]

**SEPIA.** Nose swollen and inflamed, with sore ulcerated nostrils. Obstruction of nose, and *violent dry* coryza. Loss of smell. Pain in back and stiffness in nape of neck, [**Bell**] *Cough worse in morning, terminating in an effort to vomit. *Great sense of emptiness in stomach.

**SULPHUR.** Catarrh, with fluent coryza. Soreness and pressure in throat as from a lump. Complete loss of taste and smell, [***Puls.**] Coldness of the extremities and chilliness. *Frequent weak, faint spells. *Great liability to take cold.

---

## CHRONIC NASOPHARYNGEAL CATARRH.

**TREATMENT.** *Leading indications.*

**ÆSCULUS HIP.** Dull frontal headache, fluent coryza, thin watery discharge. Stinging and burning in posterior nares and soft palate, [**Cap.**] *Hawks up ropy mucus of sweetish taste, [**Alum.**]

**AILANTHUS GLAN.** Loss of smell, [see **Hepar.**] *Copious thin, ichorous, bloody discharge from nose, without fetor, [see **Graph.**] Hawking of mucus, constant effort to raise hard lumps of whitish matter, [see **Mag. c.**] Throat dark red and swollen, [see **Arg. n.**]

**ALUMINA.** Chronic nasal catarrh, with scurfy, sore nostrils, [see **Cal. c.**] Discharge of dry, hard, yellow-green mucus from nose. Thick mucus dropping from posterior nares, [**Coral. r. Hydras. Phyto.**] Ulcers in fauces, secreting a yellowish-brown, badly smelling pus.

**ARGENT. NIT.** Violent itching of nose, [of *tip*, ***Sili. Caust.**] Discharge of whitish pus, with clots of blood. *Uvula and fauces dark red, [**Bapt. Bell.**] *Thick tenacious mucus in throat, obliging him to hawk, [**Æscu. hip. Hepar. Hydras. Graph.**] Rawness, soreness and scraping in throat, [**Hepar. Phos.**] *Head feels too large. *Craves sugar.

**AURUM MET.** Sensitive smell; everything smells too strong. Fetid discharge from nose, [see **Nit. ac.**] Frontal headache, [see **Puls.**] *Caries of nasal bones, [**Merc. Nit. ac.**] Tip of nose "knobby" red.

**BARYTA CAR.** Frequent nosebleed, [**Graph. Hepar.**] Formation of scabs in posterior nares, and behind base of uvula. *Liability to quinsy*, [Hepar. Lach. Sulph.] *Chronic induration of tonsils, [Baryta m. Hepar. Ign. Lyc.]

**CALC. CARB.** *Scrofulous habit*, [Baryta o. Ferr. Merc. Sulph.] Unhealthy, ulcerated skin. Great liability to take cold, [Graph. Sili. Sulph.] Nasal discharge thick, pus-like. Sore ulcerated nostrils, [Graph. Nit. ac. Lyc.] General sick feeling. *Cold, damp feet.

**CISTUS CAN.** Eczema of nose. Fauces inflamed and dry. *Tough, gum-like, thick, tasteless mucus brought up by hawking, mostly mornings. *Strips* of tough mucus on back of throat.

**FERRUM.** Anæmic condition, [Chin.] Dropping of fluid from posterior nares or frontal sinuses, [hangs down in strings, Phyto.] Headache, it feels dull and full. *Least emotion or exertion produces a flushed face.

**GRAPHITES.** Burning spot on top of head, [Sulph.] Loss of smell, [Ailan. Puls.] Discharge of thick, yellowish, *fetid* mucus from nose. Dry scabs in nose, with sore, cracked, ulcerated nostrils, [Alum. Puls.] *Roughness and rawness in throat*, [Arg. n. Phos. Puls.] Hawking of phlegm, [see Arg. n.] *Eruption on skin, oozing sticky fluid.

**HEPAR SULPH.** Sense of smell acute, [*obtuse*, Ailan. Arg. n. Cal. c.] Sore pain on dorsum of nose, when touching it. Itching in nose, [see Arg. n.] *Cracking in ear when blowing nose.* Scraping in throat when swallowing. Hawking up mucus, [see Arg. n.] Sensation of plug in throat, [Bary. c. Ign. Lyc.] Unhealthy skin.

**HYDRAS. CAN.** Air feels cold in nose. *Dropping of mucus from posterior nares into throat, [see Alum. Arg. n.] Soreness of cartilaginous septum, bleeding when touched. Ozæna, with bloody purulent discharge, [Aur. m. Nit. ac.] Dull heavy headache over eyes, [see Puls.]

**IODIUM.** Chronic *fetid* discharge from nose. Buzzing in ears, [*crackling*, Bary. c. Kali b. Nit. ac.] Ulcers in throat, with swelling of glands of neck. Scrofulous persons, with low state of system, [see Ferr.] After abuse of *Merc.*

**KALI BI.** Fetid smell from nose. *Discharge of tough green masses, or plugs from nose, [see Mag. c.] Ropy, tough discharge from posterior nares, [see Alum.] *Œdematous uvula. *Ulcers in fauces and pharynx, discharging cheesy lumps, of fetid odor, [see Mag. c.]

**LYCOPO.** Humid scurfs on and behind ears, [Graph.] Catarrh of nose and frontal sinuses, discharge yellow and thick. Frontal headache, aggravated by warmth, [Puls.] Chronic induration of tonsils, [see Bary. c.] Hawking of bloody mucus, or hard greenish-yellow phlegm, [see Mag. c.]

**MAGNE. CAR.** Epistaxis, especially in morning, [Nit. ac.] Vesicular eruptions in nose. Burning in throat and palate, with dryness and roughness as if scraped. *Hawking up soft, fetid tubercles, color of peas, [see Merc. io. r.]

**MERCURIUS VIV.** Fluent corrosive discharge from nose, with much sneezing. Nostrils bleeding, sore and scurfy, [see **Graph.**] *Greenish, fetid pus from nose, nasal bones swollen. Chronic ulcerated sore throat. Glands of neck swollen.

**MERC. IOD. RUB.** *Hawks mucus from posterior nares, which feel raw. Crusty eruption on wings of nose. Sensation of a lump in throat, [see **Hepar.**] Hawks up hard greenish lumps, [see **Mag. c.**]

**NITRIC ACID.** Fetid, yellow, nasal discharge, [see **Merc. v.**] *Syphilitic ozæna, [see **Hydras.**] Dirty, bloody mucus from posterior nares. Green casts from nose every morning. Sore throat, extending up into nose. **Strong-smelling urine.*

**PETROLEUM.** Pain at root of nose, with purulent discharge. *Scurfs around mouth.* Throat feels swollen and raw. Hawking of tough, bad-tasting phlegm, mornings. When swallowing, food enters posterior nares.

**PHOSPHORUS.** Chronic inflammation of nasal membrane, with acuteness or loss of smell. *Rawness* and *scraping* in *pharynx*, worse toward evening, [see **Arg. n.**] Hawking of phlegm, mornings, [see **Pet.**] *Great dryness of throat, it fairly glistens. *Long, *narrow*, tough stools.

**PULSATILLA.** Loss of smell, [**Ailan. Hepar.**] *Green, fetid, nasal discharge, with diminished taste and smell. Frontal headache, [**Hydras. Lyc.**] Ears feel as if stopped. Throat dry mornings, feels as if she would choke. *Mild, tearful disposition.*

**SEPIA.** Fetid smell before the nose. Swollen, inflamed nose; nostrils sore, ulcerated, scabby, [see **Graph.**] *Blows large lumps of yellow-green mucus, or crusts from nose, [see **Kali b.**] Hawking of mucus in morning, [see **Arg. n.**] *Herpes circinatus.

**SILICEA.** Loss of smell, [see **Puls.**] Gnawing and ulcers high up in nose. *Intolerable itching of tip of nose, [see **Arg. n.**] Throat feels if filled up, [**Cimi. Gel.**] *Constipation, stools recede after being partially expelled.

**SULPHUR.** *Dry ulcers or scabs in nose, with chronic obstruction. Excoriation and ulceration of nostrils, [see **Graph.**] Scrofulous or syphilitic taint. Skin *rough, scaly, scabby.*

**THUYA.** Blows out thick, green mucus, mixed with blood; later brown scabs form. Nose sore, red eruptions on alæ. Throat feels raw, dry, or as if constricted. *Watery purulent otorrhœa.

---

## CHOLERA ASIATICA.

**TREATMENT.** *Leading indications.*

**ACONITE.** Forming stage, where there is great vascular excitement. *Violent heat* and *dryness of skin.* *Great fear and anxiety of mind, with nervous excitability. Full and frequent pulse. *Vertigo, particularly on raising the head. *Bitter, greenish vomiting. Stools whitish, with discharge of lumbrici. *Fear of death, predicts the day he will die.

**ARSENICUM.** *Great anguish, extreme restlessness, and fear of death, [**Acon. Verat.**] *Sudden prostration, with sinking of vital forces. Tongue dry, blackish, and cracked. Violent burning pains in stomach. Vomiting watery, slimy, greenish, brownish, or blackish substances; worse after drinking. *Vomiting and purging simultaneously*, [**Ipe. Verat.**] *Great thirst; drinks little and often. Skin cold and covered with clammy sweat, or dry and shriveled, [see **Camph. Verat.**]

**CAMPHOR.** One of *first remedies* to be thought of, especially when there is great anguish and *sudden prostration*, [**Ars. Verat.**] *Pulse small and rapid.* Hands, feet, and skin cold. *Burning pains in stomach and throat. *Cramps* in calves, [**Jatro. cur.**] Painfulness of pit of stomach when touched. *Icy coldness and blueness of face and limbs, even of tongue, [**Verat.**] *Half stupid and senseless; he moans and groans in a hoarse, husky voice.

**CARBO VEG.** Mostly in *last stage*, [in *first* stage, **Ipe. *Phos. ac.**] Complete collapse of pulse, patient lies in a state of asphyxia. The spasms and vomiting have ceased, followed by great debility. Cold breath, cold tongue, or coldness all over, [**Camph.**] *Livid countenance, hoarse voice, and sunken eyes.

**CHINA.** Hippocratic countenance, pointed nose and hollow eyes. Yellowish, blackish, or parched tongue. Violent thirst, with a desire to drink often, but little at a time, [***Ars.**] Spasmodic colic. Painless diarrhœa, stools blackish, bilious or whitish. Prostration even unto fainting. *After loss of animal fluids.

**COLOCYNTH.** Vomiting first food, then a greenish substance. *Violent constrictive pain in abdomen as if intestines were squeezed between stones, *relieved by forcible pressure.* *Terrible, cramp-like pains which draw patient almost double. Thin, greenish, slimy, or watery stools; retention of urine. Worse after eating or drinking.

**CROTON TIG.** Watery discharge from bowels, mixed with whitish flakes. *The discharges always come on after drinking, and are expelled with a sudden gush, [see **Jatro.**] *Vomiting whitish frothy fluids.* Great exhaustion with faintness and vertigo.

**CUPRUM MET.** Violent vomiting, with colic and diarrhœa. Rolling of eyeballs, great restlessness and coldness of face. Spasmodic colicky pains without vomiting, or vomiting preceded by spasmodic constriction of chest, arresting breathing. *Extreme thirst, liquids descend the throat with a gurgling sound. *Violent cramps in the stomach, fingers, and toes, [in *legs* and *feet*, **Jatro. cur.**] The vomiting is relieved by drinking cold water.

**IPECAC.** In early stage, and where *nausea and vomiting* is a prominent symptom. *Vomiting large quantities of green jelly-like mucus, or black pitch-like substances, [**Ars. Verat.**] Griping, pinching in abdomen, as if grasped with a hand; excited by motion. *Grass-green mucous stools, having appearance as if fermented. Cramp in calves, fingers and toes, [**Cup. m.**] Coldness of face and extremities.

**JATROPHA CUR.** Violent vomiting of a whitish, jelly-like substance, like white of egg, [*black* bile, ***Ars. Verat.**] Anxiety and burning in stomach. **Profuse watery stools, gushing out like a torrent.* Cramps in legs and feet [in fingers and toes, ***Cup.**] gurgling noise in abdomen.

**NICOTIN.** *Death-like paleness of face, with nausea and cold clammy sweat, while body is warm, [see **Verat.**] *Coldness in abdomen,* with nausea and hiccough; no vomiting or diarrhœa. Slow, irregular, intermittent pulse.

**PHOS. ACID.** In commencement, before vomitings set in Diarrhœa, with whitish, watery, slimy stools, without pain. *Tenacious viscid mucus in mouth; gluey matter on the tongue.* *Indifferent, not disposed to talk. Quiet delirium and stupefaction.

**SECALE COR.** Face pale and eyes sunken. Dry, thick, yellowish white coating on tongue. *Unquenchable thirst,* [**Verat.**] Heat and *burning in abdomen.* Watery, slimy diarrhœa, or involuntary diarrhœa. The evacuations are preceded by vertigo, anguish, cramps in calves, rumbling in abdomen, and nausea. *Great aversion to heat, or to being covered. *Thin, scrawny persons.*

**VERAT. ALB.** Pale, death-like expression of face. Tongue dry, blackish and cracked. *Unquenchable thirst for cold drinks. *Vomiting and purging simultaneously. Black vomit,* [**Ars.**] *Great weakness after vomiting. Severe cutting pains in abdomen. Violent diarrhœa, with greenish, watery flocculent stools, *followed by rapid prostration.* Cramps in calves. Small, almost imperceptible, pulse. Hoarse, weak voice, cold breath. *Cold sweat over whole body.

**CLINICAL OBSERVATIONS.** At beginning of attack, place patient in bed; if he inclines to coldness, surround him with bottles of *hot water* and cover with blankets. Give no drinks but cold water or ice, unless warm toast-water is preferred. Mutton or chicken broth, or beef tea slightly seasoned with salt may be taken. Keep patient quiet as possible; have him use bed pan to avoid getting up.

Disinfect all discharges and soiled clothing with *Chloride of Lime* or *Corrosive Sublimate* as directed on page 14.

In cramps of muscles, friction with dry hand is the best remedy to remove spasm, restore heat and circulation.

**DIETETICS.** During convalescence, great care must be used in regard to diet. Good fresh milk, simple broths and light puddings may be used. No solid food should be taken while there is any looseness of bowels.

**HYGIENIC PRECAUTIONS.** Observe regular habits in all things. Avoid all indigestible food; use goodly proportion of animal food, good bread and ripe fruits. Take no intoxicating liquors. Boil all water used for drinking or culinary purposes. Treat promptly all cases of diarrhœa at the outset. Give *strict attention to cleanliness.*

---

## CHOLERA MORBUS.

**TREATMENT.** *Leading indications.*

**ANTIMO. CRUD.** *Thick, milky-white coating on tongue. Great thirst for cold water, especially at night. Vomiting and diarrhœa, watery or slimy. Suitable after use of sour wine, [see **Chin.**]

**ARSENICUM.** *Violent attacks, *sudden prostration*, great *restlessness*, extreme thirst, *drinking little* and *often*. Severe burning in stomach. Vomiting, especially after *eating* or *drinking*. Vomiting and purging simultaneously, [**Ipe. Verat.**] Skin dry or cold and bluish. Great anguish and *fear of death.*

**CHAMOMILLA.** Frequent vomiting food or mucus, *sour* or *bitter* substances. Severe cutting pains in abdomen. *Patient very *irritable*, can scarcely answer a civil question. Children must be *carried all the time* to be quieted. If excited by a fit of passion, [**Colo.**]

**CHINA.** Sudden attacks in the night; discharges mostly *painless*, containing undigested food. *Great fermentation in bowels; *abdomen bloated.* Weakly persons who have *lost* much *blood*, or after drinking sour beer, eating fruits, etc.

**COLOCYNTH.** Moderate nausea, vomiting and purging. *Violent cramp-like pains in region of navel, relieved by bending double. *Cramps* in the extremities, [**Diosc. Verat.**] Tongue loaded with yellow fur.

**DIOSCOREA.** Vomiting and purging, stools watery, with painful cramps in the stomach, bowels, and extremities. *Violent twisting colic, occurring in regular paroxysms, with remissions, *relieved* by *walking.*

**EUPHORBIA COR.** Forcible vomiting and diarrhœa of watery fluid, with sinking, anxious feeling at stomach. Painful spasms in the bowels, with cold sweat. *Cramps in the hands and feet,* [see **Verat.**] Death-like sensation, with anxiety of mind.

**IPECAC.** Vomiting most prominent symptom. * *Constant nausea and vomiting food, mucus, bile, or jelly-like substances.* Stools as if *fermented*, green as grass, with colic. After eating unripe sour fruit.

**IRIS VERSICO.** Nausea, with *burning in mouth, fauces and œsophagus.* Vomiting and diarrhœa, with violent pain in pit of stomach, *at or before every fit of vomiting or purging.* Suitable when disease occurs in hot weather, [**Podo.**]

**PODOPHYLLUM.** When the disease occurs in hot weather, [**Iris**] *Gagging or empty retching.* *Painless diarrhœa, stools profuse, watery, and gushing, with cramps in the feet, calves, and thighs. Restless sleep, with half-closed eyes.

**PULSATILLA.** *Chiefly useful where the disease has been induced by eating *fat*, *crude*, *indigestible food* or *fruit.* Vomiting food, bile, or mucus. Stools *greenish, bilious, watery,* worse at night. Wants to be in a cool place, or in the open air.

**VERAT. ALB.** Countenance pale or bluish, with *cold sweat on forehead.* Eyes sunken, nose pointed, mouth and lips dry. *Pulse frequent, very weak,* [**Ars.**] *Intense thirst for cold and acid drinks. *Violent nausea and vomiting, with profuse watery diarrhœa, and *severe pinching colic. Great sinking and empty feeling in abdomen after stool.* Cramps in abdomen and extremities. Great anguish and fear of death, [**Ars.**]

For further treatment, see CHOLERA ASIATICA.

**CLINICAL OBSERVATIONS.** If attack was caused by overeating or partaking of indigestible food, induce patient to vomit by giving tepid water or tickling fauces with a feather or something similar.

In many instances taking copious draughts of water—*hot as can be borne*—will promptly relieve.

If extremities incline to coldness, keep them warm with bottles of *hot water*, hot bricks, or friction with dry hands.

**DIETETICS.** Mucilaginous drinks, as rice-water, barley-water, gum-Arabic water, etc., are preferable. A little mutton, chicken, or beef broth may be taken at regular intervals; but in no case should solid food be allowed until patient has wellnigh recovered.

## CHOLERA INFANTUM.

**PROGNOSIS.** Must be guarded.

**Bad Signs.**—Extreme restlessness; or apathy and stupor; convulsions; incessant vomiting; frequent and copious stools; pinched countenance; extremities cold, blue and shriveled.

**Favorable Signs.**—Cessation of vomiting; stools diminished in quantity and frequency; natural sleep; less thirst; returning appetite.

**TREATMENT.** *Leading indications.*

**ACONITE.** *In the beginning, hot skin, quick pulse, and sleeplessness.* Stools green, watery, or white slimy mucus. *Before* and *during* stool, cutting pain and tenesmus. Nausea and vomiting what has been drunk. *Restlessness, child turns from side to side.

**ÆTHUSA CYN.** In bad cases. Stools light-yellow or greenish liquid. *Before* stool, pinching, cutting pain in abdomen. *Violent vomiting coagulated milk.* *Spasms, with stupor and delirium, clinched thumbs, eyes drawn downward, pupils dilated. *Symptoms of hydrocephaloid,* [**Cal. phos.**]

**ANTIMO. CRUD.** *Tongue coated white.* Violent vomiting slimy mucus or lumps of curd, worse after eating or drinking, [see **Ars.**] Stools watery and profuse. Pain before and during stool. Protrusion of rectum. *The child cannot bear to be looked at. Caused from disordered stomach, [**Puls.**]

**APIS MEL.** Tongue dry and shining. No appetite or thirst. Stools *greenish, yellowish,* slimy mucus. *During stool,* griping and tenesmus. Tenderness of abdomen to pressure. The disease slightly improves for a time, then relapses again, when from anæmia and nervous exhaustion it terminates in hydrocephaloid. *Aggravation in morning.

**ARSENICUM.** Pale, death-like countenance. Skin dry and shriveled. Stools *thick, dark green,* or *dark, watery, offensive.* Cutting pain before and tenesmus during stool. *Vomiting immediately after drinking, [**Verat.**] *Great restlessness, extreme *prostration,* and thirst, *drinking but little.* Aggravation *after midnight,* [**Rhus.**]

**BELLADONNA.** Face pale or flushed. Great dryness of mouth and lips. Tongue coated white in middle, with red edges. Stools thin green mucus, or bloody mucus. *Delirium worse during and just after sleep, with desire to get out of bed.* *Sleepy, but cannot sleep, [**Opi.**] *Child cries out suddenly, and ceases as suddenly. *Sudden starting at noise and during sleep.

**BENZOIC AC.** *Fetid, watery, white stools, very copious* and exhausting, [**Podo.**] *During* stool much pressing or straining. *Strong-smelling urine. mostly dark-colored. Troublesome and dry hacking cough. Tongue coated with white mucus, or ulcerated.

**BORAX.** Pale clay-colored appearance of face. Aphthæ in mouth and on tongue. *Light yellow, slimy mucus,* or greenish, watery stools. *Fear of falling from downward motion, even during sleep. *Easily startled at sudden noise, with anxious screams, [**Bell.**] Loss of appetite, with loathing the breast.

**BRYONIA.** Dry, parched lips and mouth. Thirst for *large quantities* of water at long intervals, [reverse, ***Ars. Chin.**] *Vomiting food soon after taking it, undigested. Stools brown, thin fecal, or undigested. Before stool, child cries out, and cannot bear to be moved. *Gets faint and sick on sitting up. After *cold drinks, fruit,* or getting *overheated.*

**CALC. CARB.** Children with *large heads and open fontanelles, scrofulous,* [***Sil. Sulph.**] Swollen, distended abdomen, with emaciation and good appetite. Skin dry and shriveled

Stools whitish and watery, or *chalk-like; undigested,* [**Podo.**] Vomiting sour substances. *Profuse sweat on head when sleeping, [**Sil.**] *Cold, damp feet.

**CAMPHOR.** Sudden attack. *Great and rapid prostration, [see **Ars.**] *Skin cold, yet child will not remain covered. Vomiting and purging sometimes absent, only *coldness* and *prostration.*

**CALC. PHOS.** *Delayed closure, or reopening of fontanelles.* Point of nose icy cold. *Upper lip swollen, and cold sweat on face.* Vomits often and easy. Craves bacon. *Abdomen sunken.* Stools green, loose, and sometimes slimy. Suffocative attack when lifted up.

**CARB. VEG.** Great paleness or gray-yellow color of the face. Stools *light colored; involuntary; putrid: cadaverous smelling,* [**Sil.**] Mostly in last stage, and where the vital powers are greatly exhausted. Restlessness and anxiety, worse towards evening. *Emission of large quantities of flatus, inodorous, or putrid.

**CHAMOMILLA.** Redness and heat of face, sometimes *one cheek red and the other pale,* [**Acon.**] Tongue coated thick yellow, or white. Vomiting sour food, or slimy substances. *Green, watery, corroding* stools with colic; also mixed *white and yellow mucus,* like chopped eggs, [**Nux m.**] Colic *before* and *during* stool. *Child very fretful; must be carried all the time.

**CHINA.** Tympanitic distension of abdomen. Stools *yellow, watery,* undigested, painless, or blackish and offensive. *Before* stool, colic, relieved by bending double, [**Colo.**] Patient worse *after eating* and at night. *Great weakness and inclination to sweat. *Worse every other day, [**Amb.**]

**CINA.** *Disposition to pick and bore at the nose; troubled with worms. White papescent stools. *White, turbid or jelly-like urine, [**Phos. ac.**] *Restless sleep, frequent changing position,* and *waking with cries.* Grinding of teeth during sleep.

**CROTON TIG.** *Dry, parched lips.* Nausea and vomiting water, mucus and bile, especially after drinking. Yellow watery, dark green or greenish yellow stools, *coming out like a shot,* [**Gum. g.**] *Worse after drinking, while nursing. *Great prostration after stool.*

**DULCAMARA.** Dry heat of skin, and violent thirst. Stools yellowish, green, watery or whitish. Colic before and during stool. *The child gets worse at every cold change in weather, or from exposure to cold air. Suitable after taking cold or getting wet, [getting overheated, **Bry.**]

**GUMM. GUTT.** Loud rumbling and gurgling in bowels. Stools *thin yellow fecal,* or *dark green* and *offensive.* *Sudden expulsion of stool, coming in a gush, [***Jatro.**] Nausea and vomiting after eating or drinking, [**Ars.**] The child seems to crave food, but little satisfies it. Aphthæ in mouth.

**IPECAC.** Pale face, with blue margins around the eyes, [**Jatro. Phos.**] Yellowish or white-coated tongue. **Almost* *constant nausea and vomiting*, [see **Verat.**] The child throws up its food and large quantities of green mucus. Stools *grass-green mucus*, or white, fermented, like yeast, [**Arn.**] *Colic* and sick stomach *before* and *during* stool. *After vomiting, inclination to sleep.

**JATRO. CUR.** *Stools *watery; profuse; gushing out like a torrent*, [**Cro. t. Gum. g.**] Vomiting dark green bile, or *watery albuminous substances*, [milky white, **Æth.**] Liquid gurgling in abdomen, [**Gum. g.**]

**LAUROCERASUS.** Sunken countenance; livid grayish yellow complexion. Eyes staring or lightly closed. Tongue white and dry, with violent thirst. Pulse slow, *irregular* or *imperceptible*, [**Verat.**] Stools green, liquid, mucus, involuntary. Cutting pain before and tenesmus after stool. **Rattling sound of liquids when passing through the œsophagus.*

**MAGNESIA C.** Face dark yellow. No appetite, violent thirst, inclination to vomit. *Stools green and slimy, like the scum of a frog-pond, smelling sour. Before stool, *cutting and pinching* in abdomen; after stool, *tenesmus*. Worse in hot weather and during dentition, [see **Cham.**]

**MERCURIUS.** *Dry lips*, with ulcerated corners of the mouth. Tongue *coated as with fur*. Stools yellow, color of sulphur [**Colo.**], sometimes green, slimy or bloody. *Frequent, scanty excoriating stools.* *Colic before, and *tenesmus during and after* stool. *Great tenderness over stomach and abdomen. Cold, clammy sweats, especially at night.

**NUX MOS.** *Great languor;* cold, dry skin, little thirst. Colic worse after eating or drinking; *relieved by application of moist heat.* Stools *thin, yellow*, like beaten or stirred eggs, [***Cham.**] undigested, watery, slimy. Colic *before* and urging during stool. **Great drowsiness and dullness of sense.* Worse at night, and in cool damp weather, [**Merc.**]

**NUX VOMICA.** Tongue coated thick yellowish white. Swelling of gums, fetid ulcers in mouth. Vomiting sour-smelling mucus. Frequent, small, watery, slimy, *dark-colored mucus stools.* Colic before and *violent straining at stool;* relief after stool. *After gastric medicines, and where changing child's food has caused the trouble. Worse in early morning, [**Sulph.**] Very *irritable.*

**PHOSPHORUS.** Pale, sickly complexion; hollow eyes, surrounded by blue margins, [**Ipe. Jatro.**] *Thirst* for cold drinks, which are thrown up soon as they *become warm in stomach.* *Stools *white, watery*, containing little lumps *like grains of tallow;* undigested. Watery stools, pouring away as from a hydrant. Worse in morning, and from lying on left side.

**PHOS. ACID.** Blue margins around the eyes; violent thirst; loss of appetite; profuse perspiration at night. Stools, *whitish, watery*, light yellow, *painless.* *The disease is not marked by *much debility*, though it may continue a long time, [reverse, ***Ars.** ***Verat.**]

**PODOPHYLLUM.** Moaning during sleep, with half-closed eyes, and rolling head from side to side. *Gagging or empty retching*, [**Cro. t.**] *Stools watery, with meal-like sediment; dark yellow mucus, *smelling like carrion.* *Profuse watery, painless stools, very exhausting. *Prolapsus ani during stool, [**Merc.**] Worse in morning and after eating and drinking.

**PULSATILLA.** Tongue coated with tenacious mucus. *Thirstlessness.* *Stools very changeable, no two alike, worse at night, [see **Sulph.**] Before stool, *rumbling* in bowels, [**Phos.**] During stool, *chilliness*, [**Ars. *Merc. Sulph.**] After use of *greasy food.*

**SECALE COR.** Face pale, eyes sunken and surrounded by blue margins, [**Ipe. Phos.**] Dry, thick, yellowish-white coating on tongue. Easy, painless vomiting, without effort. Stools *watery and slimy, involuntary*, [**Bell. Carb. v.**] Before stool, rumbling in abdomen; great exhaustion after stool. *Great aversion to heat, or to being covered. *Thin, scrawny children, with shriveled skin.

**SILICEA.** *Children with large heads and open fontanelles, [***Cal. c. Sulph.**] *Profuse perspiration on head*, particularly during sleep, [***Cal. c. Merc.**] Stools liquid, slimy, frothy, or bloody mucus. Colic, and distension of abdomen. *Psoric derangement.*

**SULPHUR.** Child drowsy through day and wakeful at night. Stools very changeable, attended with pain or no pain at all; *worse in early morning.* *Stools very excoriating, [***Ars. Cham. *Merc.**] When there are repeated relapses, or the case seems to linger a long while. *Hot palms and soles.*

**THUYA.** Great desire for cold drinks; rapid exhaustion; oppressed breathing; great emaciation. *Stools *pale-yellow, watery*, very copious, and gushing like water from a bung-hole, [see ***Jatro.**] Aggravation in morning, and after vaccination.

**VERAT. ALB.** Cold sweat on forehead. Lips dry and dark-colored. *Vomiting excited by smallest quantity of liquids, [**Ars. Nux v.**] The least motion increases vomiting. Stools *greenish watery, with flakes.* Before stool, severe colic; during stool, *cold sweat on forehead*, [warm sweat, **Merc.**] *Violent thirst for cold water. [Pulse almost imperceptible, [**Laur.**]

**CLINICAL REMARKS.** If child resides in the city, remove it to the country. The room it is to occupy should be large, airy and well lighted. Keep child *cool* and free from excitement, and give it an *abundance* of *fresh air.* It should be bathed frequently in tepid water 85° F, then wrap in clean sheet and allow to dry *without rubbing.* Its clothing should be changed daily. Take it riding or carry it into open air frequently, no matter how sick it may be.

**DIETETICS.** The *diet* is of the greatest importance. The mother's milk—if she be healthy—is the best food for child. Breast-milk, when fresh, has an *alkaline* reaction, and an average s. g. of 10.32. When doubts arise about its healthy quality, it should be tested, and if found wanting, rejected. Breast-milk being out of the question, a substitute must be found in cow's-milk or some one of the many preparations of "infants' food" now commended. Cow's-milk, when fresh, is slightly *alkaline;* if of good quality add one part water, sweeten with *sugar of milk,* and add a *little* salt. See article "**Diet of Infants.**" The milk should not be boiled, only warmed or given *fresh* from the cow. If child be greatly exhausted and emaciated, *beef tea* may be given. Great care must be taken to keep bottle, tubes, etc., *perfectly clean.* Allow no *starchy* food until dentition is well advanced.

---

## CHANGE OF LIFE.

(*Menopausis, Critical Age.*)

The change of life, by which is meant the period when menstruation ceases, embraces a period of several months, or may extend over two or more years. It usually takes place between the age of 40 and 50. While this change is in progress, there is more or less disturbance of the general health which calls for medical treatment.

**REMEDIES.** *Leading indications.*

**LACHESIS.** Burning on vertex at menopause [see **Sulph.**] Pressure on vertex, [**Ign. Sep.**] *Flashes of heat, [see **Sang.**] Frequent uterine hemorrhages. Cannot bear least pressure in uterine region.

**PULSATILLA.** Anguish in region of heart, [**Cocc.**] *Vertigo when rising from sitting posture or looking up. Alternate redness and paleness of face, [**Ign.**] *Epistaxis when menses should appear, [***Bry.**] Disordered stomach. *Better in open air or cold room. Mild, tearful disposition.

**BRYONIA.** *Exceedingly irritable. *Fullness* in *forehead* and *splitting headache.* Rush of blood to head, with bloated face. *Constipation of hard, dry stools.

**COCCULUS.** *Nervous weakness* and fainting fits, [**Con.**] Redness of cheeks and heat in face. Reappearance of menses after being suppressed for a year. Palpitation of heart.

**CONIUM.** Nervous attacks, great *weakness every morning.* *Hysteric fits with chilliness. Burning in eyes and impaired vision. *Prolapsus uteri, with induration, ulceration and leucorrhœa, [see **Sep.**]

**IGNATIA AM.** *Full of suppressed grief, [**Puls.**] Weak. empty feeling in stomach, not relieved by eating, [**Sep.**] Uterine cramps with cutting stitches, [**Cocc.**]

**SEPIA.** Sadness and weeping, [**Puls.**] Whizzing and roaring in ears. *Yellowness of face, particularly across nose, *like a saddle.* *Fetid urine, with clay-colored sediment adhering to chamber. Prolapsus uteri and vagina, with burning in back. *Jerking of limbs at night.

**SANGUINARIA.** Redness of cheeks, with burning of ears. *Periodical sick-headache, begins in morning, increases during day, lasts until evening. Os uteri ulcerated, [**Con. Sep.**] *Flashes of heat, and leucorrhœa, [see **Lach. Puls.**] Burning in palms and soles of feet.

**SULPHUR.** Low-spirited, out of humor, inclines to weep. [see **Puls.**] *Constant heat on top of head, [coldness, **Sep.**] *Sour eructations* and great acidity of stomach. Frequent *flushes of heat,* [see **Sang.**] Leucorrhœa of yellow mucus, corroding, [**Con. Puls.**] Pruritis vulva, [**Sep.**] *Frequent weak faint spells.

**CLINICAL REMARKS.** Much benefit will be derived from proper attention to diet, exercise, clothing, etc. Plain simple food, consisting for most part of vegetables, fruits, fresh beef and mutton, will be found preferable. All stimulating food and beverages should be avoided. Daily exercise in the open air, by walking, riding, etc., will be advantageous. The clothing should be warm and comfortable, and adapted to the season. Frequent ablutions, and friction of the skin will assist greatly in preserving the health.

---

## COLIC.—ENTERALGIA.

**TREATMENT.** The principal remedies are:—

For **COPPER COLIC**: **Bell. *Hepar. Nux v. Merc.**

For **FLATULENT COLIC**: **Bell. *Carb. v. Cham. Chin. Cocc. Colo. Diosc. Tart. e. *Lyc. Nux v. *Puls.**

For **GASTRIC COLIC**, where over-eating, or the use of improper food, is the cause: **Ant. c. Ars. Bry. Carb. v. Chin. Hepar. Ipe. *Nux v. *Puls. Tart. e.**

For **LEAD COLIC**: **Ant. c. Alum. Ars. Bell. Cocc. *Nux v. *Opi. Plat. Podo. Zinc.**

For **SPASMODIC COLIC**: **Bell. Cham. *Cocc. *Colo. Cup. Hyos. Ipe. Nux v. Plumb. Puls.**

### SPECIAL INDICATIONS.

**ACONITE.** Inflammatory colic. Difficult and scanty emissions of urine. Great sensitiveness of abdomen, [**Apis. Bell.**] Intolerable cutting pains in belly, so violent that he screams, tosses about, almost beside himself. *Great fear and anxiety of mind. After taking cold.

**ALOES.** Violent cutting pains in bowels, in region of umbilicus. Dull, heavy headache, with dull pains in liver. *Loud gurgling in abdomen, as of water running out of a bottle, [**Jatro.**] *Large and prominent hemorrhoids.*

**ARSENICUM.** Severe cuttting, or spasmodic, drawing pains, as if *intestines had become twisted*, [*as if tied in knots*, **Verat.**] Violent burning in stomach, [**Nux.** ***Phos.**] Watery or bilious vomiting. *Extreme thirst, drinks little and often. *Great restlessness, anxiety, and fear of death. *Prostration* and cold sweat.

**BELLADONNA.** Pad-shaped protrusion of transverse colon. *Clutching in abdomen, as if seized with claws, [as if grasped with a hand, ***Ipe.**] *Constriction of abdomen around umbilicus, as if a ball would form.* External pressure and bending double relieves, [**Chin.** ***Colo. Nux.**] *Periodical pains, which come suddenly, and cease as suddenly.

**BRYONIA.** Painful twisting around umbilicus, with frequent stitches, compelling him to bend double, [see **Colo.**] *Wants to keep perfectly still, least motion or pressure increases pain. Vomiting bitter bile and water, particularly after drinking. *Hard, dry stools.

**CARBO VEG.** *Flatulent colic*, with great fullness in abdomen, as if it would burst. *Incarcerated flatus*, [***Chin. Lyc.**] Frequent eructations affording no relief. *Constant pressure downwards in abdomen, [pressure *upwards*, **Nux.**] Audible rumbling in bowels, and belching sour, rancid food. *Prostration, hippocratic face, with coldness of extremities, [**Ars. Verat.**]

**CHAMOMILLA.** *Flatulent colic*, abdomen distended like a drum. Continual drawing, tearing pains in abdomen, with a sensation as if bowels were rolled up in a ball, [see **Bell.**] Pressing towards abdominal ring, as if hernia would protrude, [see **Nux.**] *Vomiting sour food* or *slimy substances.* *Very impatient, can hardly answer one civilly. *He becomes almost furious about the pains.

**CHINA.** Flatulent colic, with thirst. Violent cutting, pinching pains about navel, relieved by bending double, [***Colo. Nux.**] *The abdomen feels full and tight, as if stuffed, [if it would burst, **Carb. v. Lyc.**] After eating fruit or drinking new beer.

**COCCULUS.** *Violent spasms in stomach*, with a *griping, lacerating* sensation. Contraction of abdomen, with a downward and outward pressure. Flatulent colic at midnight; belching relieves. *Abdomen distended, and feels as if full of sharp stones when moving.

**COFFEA.** Sensation as if bowels would be cut to pieces; horrible cries and grating of teeth. *The patient becomes desperate on account of pains, [**Acon.**] Cannot bear to be touched, parts are so sensitive. Great excitability.

**COLOCYNTH.** *Violent cutting, constrictive, or spasmodic pains.* *Feeling in abdomen as if *intestines were squeezed between stones, compelling one to bend double*, [relieved by stretching body out, **Diosc.**] Great restlessness, moaning, and lamentation. After violent indignation, or after abuse of *opium*.

**CUPRUM M.** Violent spasms in abdomen and in upper and lower limbs, by spells. Cutting and lacerating in bowels.

*A violent piercing pain, as if a knife were penetrating through from umbilicus to back; *abdomen drawn in*, [see **Plumb.**] *Fearful cries as if he were being killed. Intussusception of bowels*, [**Verat.**]

**DIOSCOREA.** *Flatulent colic*, chiefly in persons of feeble digestion. *Continuous* twisting pains in abdomen, [remitting, **Colo.**] Pains *relieved by stretching body out, or walking about*, [reverse **Colo.**]

**IGNATIA.** *Periodical cramp colic*, especially at night, in sensitive, hysterical persons. *Sadness and sighing, with a weak, empty feeling at pit of stomach.

**IPECAC.** Horrid, indescribable pain and sick feeling in stomach. Cutting and pinching around umbilicus, worse by motion, and better by rest, [see **Bell.**] *Constant nausea, stooping causes him to vomit. *After vomiting, inclination to sleep.* After *unripe sour fruit.*

**LYCOPODIUM.** Colic with *incarcerated* flatulence, [**Carb. v.** ***Chin.**] *Sensation as if abdomen would burst, [see **Chin.**] Cutting pain across the hypogastrium, from right to left, [from left to right, **Ipe.**] Belching without relief, [with relief, **Coco.**]

**NUX VOMICA.** Cramp-like pains in stomach, with pressure towards thorax. *Pressure in stomach as from a stone*, [**Ars.** ***Puls.**] *Lead colic, [see **Opi.**] Flatulent colic, from *indigestion, or use of improper food.* *Frequent urging to stool, without effect, [**Lyc.**] *Malicious, irritable disposition; high livers, and victims of drugs.*

**OPIUM.** *Colic from effects of lead, [***Nux v.**] Bowels seem *absolutely closed*, with constant urging to stool. *Squeezing* pains as if something were being *forced through a narrow space.* *Slow pulse.

**PLUMBUM.** *Violent colic*, with *sunken abdomen.* *Terrible contractive pains, drawing in the abdomen to back; abdomen hard as a stone. Constriction of intestines, the navel and anus are violently drawn in. *Obstinate constipation, fæces lumpy, packed together like sheep's dung.

**PULSATILLA.** *Putrid bitter taste.* Aching, drawing pains in stomach, *must walk about to relieve pain.* Frequent loose stools, very changeable, worse at night. Patient can't bear to be covered, and craves fresh cold air. *After *eating rich, greasy food.* Tearful disposition.

**VERAT. ALB.** Pain here and there in abdomen, as if cut with knives, [**Colo. Cup.**] Terrible cutting pains with *violent nausea and vomiting. Intussusception of bowels.* *Intestines feel as if tied in knots. Anxiety, fear and despair. *Cold sweat over whole body. *Great weakness with feeble pulse.* After fruit or vegetables.

**AUXILIARY MEASURES.** If indigestible food be exciting cause, induce *vomiting* by copious draughts *warm water, tickling* the *throat*, or placing salt or mustard on the tongue.

Large draughts of *hot water* often relieve colic. *Hot fomentations*, bags of *hot salt*, friction with dry hand, all beneficial.

**Warm Baths** and injections of *warm water* often afford great relief. The *enemas* should be large, and the patient, lying on *left side* with hips well raised, should retain them long as possible.

---

## COLIC OF INFANTS.

**TREATMENT.** *Leading indications.*

**ACONITE.** The infant has a dry, hot skin, is sleepless and restless. Child bites its fist; seems to suffer pain, and has a green watery diarrhœa. If sudden joy or fright on part of the mother be exciting cause.

**ANISUM STIL.** One of best remedies in so-called "three months' belly-ache." The colic usually comes on in evening and is attended with *distension* of stomach and *rumbling* in bowels.

**BELLADONNA.** *The infant cries out suddenly and ceases just as suddenly; it startles and moans much during sleep. Stools of *thin green* mucus.

**CALC. CARB.** In children of a scrofulous habit. *Large head, with open fontanelles. *White clay-like stools.* Skin dry and *flabby*. Much perspiration about head. **Cold damp feet.*

**CHAMOMILLA.** Colic, with loosenesss of bowels; stools yellowish green and watery. Writhing pain, constant crying and drawing up of limbs, with coldness of feet. *Very irritable and fretful, must be carried all the time to be quieted. Sleepless; starting and jerking while asleep.

**CHINA.** Colic comes on at a *certain hour* every day, [every *evening*, Puls.] Great hardness and fullness of abdomen. *The child screams, and laughs immediately afterwards. Sometimes stools whitish and curdled.

**CINA.** The child is very cross and troublesome. *It will not sleep unless kept in constant motion, must be rocked, carried or dandled all the time. Abdomen hard and distended, [Chin.]

**COLOCYNTH.** *Child writhes in every direction, doubles itself up and seems in great distress. It *screams terribly*, twists, draws up its legs, etc.

**IGNATIA.** If *grief* and *sadness* on part of nursing mother has caused derangement of child's digestive organs. Excessive flatulence.

**IPECAC.** When the cries of child are sharp, as if pains were of the cutting kind. The stools are *fermented* and of a putrid odor. *Much nausea and vomiting. *Flatulent* colic.

**LYCOPODIUM.** Much *rumbling* and *rattling* in bowels. *The child always cries and screams before passing urine, and is relieved immediately afterwards. *Red sand is found in diapers.

**NUX VOMICA.** Child is troubled with hiccough, *constipation*, and throwing up food. *It cries much, draws up its feet and kicks violently. Suitable where the nursing mother lives on *stimulating food.*

**PULSATILLA.** *Flatulent colic*, accompanied with shiverings and paleness of face. Rumbling of wind through the bowels and coldness of feet. The child always gets *worse towards evening.*

**SENNA.** Child cries terribly, and turns blue during its cries. *Colic from incarcerated flatulence.

**VERAT. ALB.** Terrible colic, which causes a cold sweat to stand upon surface, especially *on forehead.* No discharge of flatus up or down.

**LOCAL MEASURES.** Warm *fomentations*, bags of *hot salt*, or what is still better, gum-bags filled with *warm water* applied to the abdomen will often afford prompt relief. If bowels are constipated, injections of warm water will be found useful.

The nursing mother should make no sudden changes in her diet, avoid all indigestible food and stimulating drinks, and observe regular habits in all things. Never *nurse* child *when overheated.*

---

## CONCUSSION OF THE BRAIN.

This signifies a sudden interruption of the functions of the brain, caused by a blow, fall or other mechanical injuries to the head.

In ordinary cases, the patient lies for a time motionless, unconscious and insensible; after a time he moves his limbs as if in uneasy sleep, vomits and frequently recovers his senses instantly, remaining however, giddy, confused and sleepy for some hours thereafter. In the severer cases, patient is profoundly insensible, the surface pale and cold, features ghastly, breathing slow, pulse feeble and intermittent, followed speedily by death, where there is much contusion of the brain substance.

**TREATMENT.** *Leading indications.*

**ARNICA.** First remedy to be thought of. Patient unconscious, insensible and drowsy. Weak intermitting pulse. Cold skin, with depressed vitality.

**BELLADONNA.** Severe injury. Extreme restlessness and jactitation of muscles, with delirium. Eyes red, pupils dilated, [Cic.] Face red and hot or cold and pale. Breathing irregular, short and hurried.

**CICUTA VIRO.** Complete loss of consciousness, with spasms. *Staring at objects, pupils dilated, [Bell.] Oppression, can scarcely breathe.

**DIGITALIS.** Great *weakness*, with *fainting fits*, and inclination to vomit. Very slow pulse, [**Opi.**]

**GELSEMIUM.** Heavy, half stupid look. *Head feels too big, [**Nux.**—Too *small*, **Coff.**] Sensation of a band around the head. Eyelids heavy, can't keep them open. Feels as if intoxicated.

**HYOSCYAMUS.** Rolling head from side to side. *Complete loss of sense. *Stertorous breathing, hiccough* and *vomiting blood.*

**OPIUM.** *Drowsiness and stertorous breathing. Complete loss of consciousness and sensation. Dark red, bloated face. Slow pulse, [see **Dig.**] *Constipation.

**CLINICAL REMARKS.** Place patient in recumbent posture, head well raised. If he can swallow, give **Arn.** in water, otherwise administer by olfaction. Give *no stimulants*, neither try to arouse him. If in a state of collapse apply friction to surface and *warmth* to feet. Keep patient perfectly quiet, and avoid all excitement. In some cases it may be necessary to resort to *artificial respiration.*

**AUXILIARY MEASURES.** If there is contusion of scalp, apply cloths wrung out of solution **Arnica**, [one drachm to pint *cold water*] and change often. Later if head becomes hot, use *warm* water instead of cold, and cover compress with oiled silk.

---

## CONSTIPATION.

**TREATMENT.** *Leading indications.*

**ÆSCULUS HIP.** Constant urging to stool, with ineffectual efforts, [see **Nux.**] Stools large, hard, dry and dark colored. Prolapsus ani after stool, with backache, [see **Ruta.**] *Rectum feels as if full of small sticks. Throbbing in the abdominal and pelvic cavities. *Hemorrhoids, with constant backache.

**ALUMINA.** Great *inactivity and dryness of rectum.* *Stools very hard, knotty, and scant, [see **Graph.**] Sensation of pricking and excoriation in rectum after stool. *Much pressing and straining to pass even a soft stool. *Ailments from lead.*

**AGARICUS.** Stools *first hard and knotty*, afterwards loose, and finally diarrhœic. Itching and tingling of anus, as from ascarides, [**Nux.**] Gastric derangements, *with sharp stitches in region of liver.* *Itching, burning, and redness of feet and hands. *Hysterical subjects.*

**AMMON. MUR.** Whining, peevish, unsociable mood. Empty eructations, and painful stitches in left hypochondrium, early in morning. *Stools large and hard*, followed by soft stools, [see **Anac.**] *Large, hard stools, crumbling as they pass from anus, [**Mag. m.**] *Fæces covered with glairy tough mucus.*

**ANACARDIUM.** Frequent ineffectual urging to stool. *The rectum feels as if stopped up with a plug, [see **Nux.**] If expulsion does not take place soon, a painful twitching is felt across the abdomen. Stools, first loose, afterwards hard and of a pale color.

**ANTIMO. CRUD.** Hard stool, with very difficult expulsion. Alternate diarrhœa and constipation of aged persons, [**Bry.** ***Phos.**] *Sensation as if a copious stool would take place, when only flatus is expelled; finally, a very hard stool is voided. *Milk-white tongue.*

**APIS MEL.** Pain in eyeballs and forehead. Inability to fix the thoughts on any subject. Tenderness of abdomen to pressure, [**Bry. Nux.**] *Sensation in abdomen as if something would break if much effort was made to void the stool.

**BELLADONNA.** Constipation with tendency of blood to head. When stooping, blood rushes to head, followed by giddiness. *Violent throbbing and stitching pains, particularly in forehead. Plethoric individuals.

**BRYONIA.** Lips dry and parched, with much thirst for large draughts of water. Frequent eructations, especially after a meal; food is vomited immediately after eating. Headache as if skull would split; worse from motion, [**Am. c. Bell.**] *Hard, dry stools, as if burnt. *Irritable mood.*

**CALC. CARB.** *Stools large, hard, and sometimes only partially digested, [**Hepar.**] After stool a gloomy feeling in head. *Cold, damp feet. Women who suffer with *profuse and too frequent menses,* [**Bell.**]

**CAUSTICUM.** Frequent and unsuccessful desire to pass stool, with pain, anxiety, and redness of face. *Stools tough, light-colored, whitish, *shining like grease.* Soft, small stool, size of goose-quill, [see ***Phos.**] Soreness in anus and rectum when walking. *Constipation of children.*

**CHELIDONIUM.** Persons subject to hepatic diseases. Sallow, jaundiced complexion. *Constant pain under lower, inner angle of right shoulder-blade. *Shooting pain from liver to back.* *Stools like sheep's dung, [***Plum. Ruta.**]

**GRAPHITES.** *Stools hard and knotty, the lumps united by mucous threads, [see **Alum.**] Sometimes a large quantity of mucus is expelled with stool. Unhealthy skin, [**Cal. c. Sil.**] *Itching blotches over the body, which emit a glutinous fluid.

**IGNATIA.** Anxious desire for stool, with inactivity of rectum, [**Alum.**] Constipation from taking cold, or riding in a carriage, [see **Plat.**] *After stool, a violent stabbing stitch, from anus upwards into rectum. *Full of grief, with a weak, empty feeling in stomach. Blind piles, prolapse with every stool, [**Rhus. Sep.**]

**IODIUM.** Constipation of scrofulous people, with low cachectic state of the system. *Stools hard, knotty, and dark-colored, [see [**Graph.**] Chronic headache and vertigo, especially in old people. Throbbing in the head at every motion.

**KALI CARB.** *Inactivity of rectum*, [**Alum. Ign.**] The stool is too large, and there is a sensation as if the rectum were too weak to expel it. *Distress, with *stitching* colicky pains an hour or two before stool. Aged persons inclined to be fleshy.

**LYCOPODIUM.** Ineffectual urging, particularly in evening. Stools *very hard, scant, and passed with great difficulty.* Sensation after stool as if much remained behind. Acidity and heart-burn, with *great drowsiness* after dinner, [**Phos.**] Much *fermentation* in abdomen. *Loud rumbling and gurgling in bowels. *Red sand in urine, [**Phos. Sil.**]

**MAGNESIA M.** Frequent and severe pressure on rectum with colic. *Knotty stool, like sheep's dung*, covered with blood and mucus. *Large difficult stools crumbling when passing from the anus, [***Am. m.**] Throbbing in the stomach, with dullness of head.

**NITRIC ACID.** *Painless constipation.* Stools *hard, dry and scant.* Headache; head feels as if surrounded by a tight bandage, [**Merc. Sulph.**] *Sour or bitter taste after eating*; sour eructations, [see **Nux.**] Excessive flatulence. *Fetid, strong-smelling urine, like that of horses, [**Chin. s.**]

**NUX VOMICA.** *Constipation with rush of blood to head.* Stools *large, hard*, and passed with difficulty. *Frequent urging to stool, without effect*, [**Bry. Lyc.**] *Sensation as if anus were closed, or too narrow. Frequent eructations of sour or bitter fluids. *Sensation as if a stone or lump of lead were in stomach. Persons of *sedentary habits* and pregnant women [**Bry. Lyc. Sep.**], *high-livers and victims of drugs. Blind or bleeding piles.*

**OPIUM.** Torpor of the bowels, after chronic diarrhœa, or from abuse of cathartics, [**Nux.**] Costiveness for weeks, with loss of appetite. *Stools nothing but *small, hard black balls*, [see **Plumb.**] *Constipation from fright or fear. *Paralysis* of intestines.

**PHOSPHORUS.** Persons with phthisical constitutions, lean and slender. *Stools long, narrow, and hard, like a dog's; very difficult to expel, [see **Caust.**] Alternate diarrhœa and constipation of old people. *Belching large quantities of wind after eating. Very sleepy after meals, especially after dinner.

**PLATINUM.** Constipation while traveling. Stools very scant; they are like putty, and stick to anus. *Cramp-like pressing in temples from without inwards. *Low-spirited* and very nervous. Suitable after *lead poisoning*, [**Alum. Opi.**]

**PLUMB. MET.** Constipation with violent colic. *Stools composed of little, hard, black-brown balls, resembling sheep's dung, [**Chel. Ruta.**] A sense of constriction in sphincter ani, with ineffectual urging.

**PULSATILLA.** Constipation, consequent upon eating *rich, greasy food.* Alternate diarrhœa and constipation, [**Ant. c.**

Bry. *Phos.] Adapted to females, or persons of a mild, gentle, tearful disposition.

**RUTA GRAV.** Hard, scanty stool, almost like sheep's dung. *Frequent urging to stool, with protrusion of rectum, [**Ign. Nux.**] Great difficulty in voiding the stool on account of protrusion of rectum. Constipation following mechanical injuries, [**Arnica.**]

**SARSAPARILLA.** Obstinate constipation, with urging to urinate. Desire for stool, with contraction of intestines and pressure downwards. *Feeling as if the bowels would be pressed out during stool. Frequent scanty emissions of urine, especially at night.

**SEPIA.** Hard, knotty stools, sometimes mingled with mucus, with cutting pains in rectum, [see **Mag. m.**] *Sense of weight or of a lump in anus, not relieved by stool. Especially suited to pregnant women, or to females suffering from uterine difficulties.

**SILICEA.** Difficult stools as if the *rectum had not power to expel them.* *After much effort and straining, the stool *recedes back into rectum* after having been partially expelled. Constipation of females, particularly *before* and *during menstruation;* also of infants and scrofulous children.

**SULPHUR.** Stools hard, lumpy, mixed with mucus, followed by burning pain in anus and rectum, [**Sep.**] Hard, knotty stools, accompanied by hemorrhoids. The *first effort at stool is often very painful*, compelling one to desist. Flashes of heat and throbbing headache. *Constant heat on top of head, [*coldness*, **Verat.**] *Frequent weak, faint spells.

**SULPHURIC AC.** *Hard knotty stools, streaked with blood, very fetid*, [stools lumpy, covered with mucus, **Hydras.**] Pain during stool as if rectum would be torn. *Much debility, with a tremulous sensation over whole body, without trembling. *Sour eructations.*

**THUYA.** *Violent pain in rectum during stool.* Discharge of large, hard, brown fæces, in balls, streaked with blood, [**Sulph. ac.**] Painful contraction in anus and rectum, followed by tearing pains in bowels, [**Nux.**] *Copious and frequent urination, with burning in urethra.

**VERAT. ALB.** *Chronic constipation*, particularly of infants. Stools large and very hard. Inactivity of rectum; it seems as if paralyzed, [**Alum.**] *Much straining, with cold perspiration on forehead. *Great exhaustion and faintness after stool.

**ZINCUM MET.** *Hard, dry, insufficient stool, with much straining*, and rumbling in bowels. *Trembling of hands, with coldness of extremities. *Chronic sick headache, and great weakness of sight. *Fidgety feeling in feet and legs*, must move them constantly.

**AUXILIARY MEASURES.** Patient should *respond promptly* to the call of nature. At a certain hour *daily*, [say after breakfast] retire to water-closet and solicit an evacuation. Kneading abdomen, first over small intestines, then beginning near right groin, pressing gently upwards, following course and direction of colon, will aid materially in expelling delayed contents of bowels.

In some cases it will be necessary to use mechanical means to relieve the bowels. Injections of *warm* water or soap water will generally answer the purpose; they should be large, and patient, lying on *left side* with hips well raised, should retain them long as possible.

When impacted fæces fill the rectum, and cannot be expelled by the natural powers, they must be removed by a scoop, spoonhandle, or some such means, care being taken not to injure the parts.

**DIETETICS.** Corn bread, cracked wheat, oatmeal, bread of unbolted flour, together with juicy fruits, as apples, figs, pears, peaches, prunes, grapes, cherries, melons and vegetables generally are very useful. A glass of water drank every morning before breakfast is beneficial in habitual constipation. Drinking a cup of *hot water* several times a day will also have a salutary effect.

---

## CONVULSIONS, SPASMS.

**TREATMENT.** *Leading indications.*

**ACONITE.** High fever, dry, hot skin, anxiety, restlessness. *During dentition,* [**Bell. Cham. Coff. Gel.**] If caused from irritation of ascarides, [**Cin.**] Grinding of the teeth and convulsive hiccough.

**ARSENICUM.** Spasms preceded by great restlessness, and burning heat. *Extreme thirst, drinking little and often. Patient lies motionless, as if dead; finally, mouth is drawn first to one side and then to other; a violent jerk appears to pass through whole body.

**BELLADONNA.** Heat of head, flushed face, red eyes, and dilated pupils, [**Opi.**] *Starting, jumping during sleep. Drowsiness, with inability to sleep. Convulsive motion of mouth, facial muscles, and eyes. Foam at mouth, grating of teeth. *Drowsiness after spasm. *Precocious* children.

**CAUSTICUM.** Convulsive motions of extremities, grinding of teeth, laughing or weeping. Feverish heat of body, with coldness of hands and feet. Cold water brings on spasms again.

**CHAMOMILLA.** Stretching of limbs, with convulsions of extremities, eyes, eyelids, and tongue. Jerking and twitching during sleep, [**Bell.**] *Redness of face, or one cheek red and other pale. *The child is very cross and fretful. must be carried all the time to be quieted. Hot sweat on forehead and hairy scalp. Constant moaning and craving for drink.

**CICUTA.** Spasmodic rigidity of the body, with head bent either backward or forward. *Without any premonitory signs, child becomes suddenly stiff, with fixed eyes. After spasm, much prostration. If caused by worms, [**Cin.**]

**CINA.** Spasms of the chest, followed by rigidity of the limbs or of the whole body. Especially suited to children troubled with worms. *Constantly picking and boring at nose, [**Phos. ac.**] Frequent swallowing, as if something were in the throat. Dry, hacking cough. *Urine turns milky after standing.

**CUPRUM.** Shrill cries during attack. Drowsy and stupid during intervals, with nausea and vomiting phlegm. *After convulsions, child screams, turns and twists in all directions. If caused from retrocession of scarlatina eruption, [**Bell. Ipe.**]

**GELSEMIUM.** Spasms during dentition, with sudden loud outcries, [violent screaming, **Cicu.**] Nervous, excitable persons who are very sensitive.

**HYOSCYAMUS.** Convulsions with twitching and jerking of all the muscles, especially those about face and eyes. *Convulsions trembling and foam at mouth. After sudden fright, [**Opi.**] *Cough worse when lying down, relieved by sitting up, [**Puls.**]

**IGNATIA.** Sudden starting from a light sleep, with loud screaming and trembling. *Single parts seem to be convulsed, or single muscles here and there. *The spasms return every day at same hour.

**IPECAC.** *Much nausea and vomiting accompanies spasms. Especially if caused by eating indigestible food, or when during an exanthematic fever eruption suddenly strikes in. *Green* diarrhœic stools.

**OPIUM.** Trembling over whole body, and tossing about of limbs. *Loud screaming before or during spasm, [**Cicu.**] The child lies unconscious, as if stunned, with difficult breathing. *Convulsions from fright, [**Acon. Gel.**] *Deep sleep after spasm.*

**SECALE.** Twitching of single muscles, [see **Ign.**] Twisting of head to and fro. Contortions of hands and feet. Labored and anxious respiration. *Thin, scrawny children, with shriveled skin.

**SILICEA.** *Spasms which return at change of moon. Much perspiration about the head. *Constipation, the stool recedes after having been partially expelled. Convulsions *after vaccination.*

**STRAMONIUM.** Convulsions from fright, with tossing of limbs and involuntary evacuations of fæces and urine, [see **Opi.**] *Awakens with a shrinking look, as if afraid of first object seen. If caused by suppressed or delayed eruptions, [**Sulph.**]

**SULPHUR.** *After suppressed eruptions.* *Comes out of spasm very happy, and at termination of paroxysm passes much colorless urine. *Morning diarrhœa. *Scrofulous children.*

**ZINCUM.** *The child cries out during sleep, seems frightened when getting awake, rolls its head from side to side, [**Bell.**] Twitching and jerking of different muscles, more on right side than on left. Cross and irritable. Frequent passages of urine.

**AUXILIARY MEASURES.** If convulsions are caused by indigestible food or overloading the stomach, excite vomiting by tickling the throat, or placing a pinch of salt or mustard on the tongue. If caused by constipation, relieve by injections. If caused by *teething*, lance gums if *swollen* and painful.

During the *spasm*, place lower extremities in *warm* water to the knees and add *hot* water frequently to raise the temperature, or wrap child in *blankets* wrung out of *hot* water, and apply cold water compresses to the head. Put two or three drops *Amyl Nitrite* on a napkin and let patient inhale. This will often cut short the spasm. The inhalation of a few drops of *Camphor* will sometimes relieve. *Chloroform* is sometimes given with the best of results in infantile convulsions.

---

## COUGH.—TUSSIS.

**TREATMENT.** *Leading indications.*

**ACONITE.** *Short, dry cough*, arising from constant tickling in larynx, excited by smoking or drinking; worse *at night.* Stitches in chest, hindering respiration. Cannot breathe freely, the lungs feel as if they would not expand. *Persons of a plethoric habit, [**Bell.**] Induced by a cold west wind, [**Hepar.**]

**ARNICA.** *Dry, short, and tickling* cough, particularly in *morning after rising.* Also for a cough with expectoration of mucus and coagulated blood. *Stitching pain in side of chest,* increased by coughing, [**Bry.**] *The chest and abdomen feel as if bruised.

**ARSENICUM.** Dry cough at night, as if caused by smoke of sulphur, with a sense of suffocation, [see **Chin.**] Cough with scanty, difficult expectoration, sometimes streaked with blood. Anxious and oppressive shortness of breath, particularly when going up-stairs. *Anxiety, restlessness; thirst, drinks little and often.

**ARUM TRI.** *Loose cough*, particularly in children and aged persons, where there is inability to expectorate the mucus, [**Ipe.**] Hoarseness; sore throat of *clergymen and singers,* throat feels as if excoriated. *Discharge of gleety fluid from nose, *excoriating* the parts.

**BELLADONNA.** Dry spasmodic cough, worse at night, *wakes from sleep.* *Soreness in chest, children cry when coughing, [**Cham.**] Sensation as if *down or dust were in throat,* *causing a constant tickling*, with irresistible desire to cough. *Redness and heat of face, with throbbing headache.

**BRYONIA.** *Dry cough*, preceded by tickling or creeping in stomach, and vomiting food, [**Nux. Puls.**] *Cough at night in bed, compelling one to sit up, [and hold the chest, **Nat. s.**] Stitches in chest, when coughing or breathing deep, [***Acon. Bell.**] Sensation, when coughing, as if head and chest would fly to pieces. *Dry, hard stools. Exceedingly irritable.

**CALC. CARB.** *Dry* cough, especially in evening and after midnight, with palpitation of heart. Also cough *early in morning, with yellow expectoration*, [see **Puls.**] *Obstinate, painless hoarseness.* Tightness in chest, as if there was not room to breathe, [see **Acon.**] *When going up-stairs out of breath, has to sit down, [**Ars.**] *Cold, damp feet.

**CAPSICUM.** *Dry cough*, worse in evening and during night. *Throat red, sore, burning.* Headache and inclination to vomit during cough. Throbbing pain in chest. *Shuddering and chilliness in back.

**CAUSTICUM.** *Short, dry cough*, caused by tickling in throat. *Worse in evening until midnight, relieved by drinking cold water, [worse from **Squil.**] *Cough with involuntary emissions of urine, [**Puls. Verat.**] Soreness of chest when coughing. Hoarseness, particularly in morning.

**CHAMOMILLA.** *Dry, tickling cough*, worse at night, even during sleep, especially in children. *Hoarseness and rattling in trachea.* *One cheek red and the other pale, [**Acon. Nux v.**] Patient very irritable. *Children very cross and want to be carried all the time.

**CHINA.** Dry, hacking cough, as if caused by vapor of sulphur, [**Ars. Ign.**] Cough excited by laughing, talking, drinking, or deep inspiration, [**Dros. Phos.**] Also cough *with expectoration of clear tenacious mucus*, or blood-streaked mucus. *After hemorrhage from lungs, and other debilitating losses.

**CINA.** *Dry, spasmodic cough* in children *troubled with worms.* The child starts suddenly, gasps for breath, coughs and gags as if something in throat, [see **Ipe.**] *Continually picking and boring at nose, [**Phos. ac.**] *The urine turns milky.

**DROSERA.** *Loose cough*, with expectoration of yellowish mucus; hoarse bass voice. *Spasmodic, nervous and sympathetic cough. Pain in chest and under ribs when coughing, obliging patient to hold painful part with the hands, [see **Bry.**] Worse at night when lying in bed, after singing or laughing, [**Phos.**]

**HEPAR SULPH.** *Croupy cough*, with loose rattling phlegm in windpipe, [**Sam.**] *Rattling, choking cough, worse after midnight. Also, for *dry, hoarse cough*, worse in morning. *Cannot bear to be uncovered, the least exposure to cold excites cough, [**Rumex.**] Anxious, hoarse, wheezing respiration.

**HYOSCYAMUS.** **Dry spasmodic cough*, especially at night and when *lying down*, relieved by sitting up, [**Puls. Rhus.**] Hysterical females and young girls, [pregnant females, **Con. Nux m. Sabi.**]

**IGNATIA.** *Dry, spasmodic cough*, as if caused by vapor of sulphur or dust, [see **Chin.**] Constant hacking cough in evening in bed. *Full of grief, with weak empty feeling in stomach. *Stitches in hemorrhoidal tumors during every cough.

**IPECAC.** *Dry cough*, caused by tickling in upper part of larynx, [tickling in chest, **Phos.**] Suffocative cough, *with rattling mucus in bronchial tubes when breathing*, [**Sam.**] Children when coughing almost suffocate, and become purple in face. *Much nausea and vomiting phlegm, [***Tart. e.**] *The chest seems *full of phlegm*, but does not yield to coughing, [***Tart. e.**]

**KALI BICHRO.** *Loose cough*, with rattling in chest. Cough with thick, heavy expectoration of bluish, lumpy mucus. *Cough, with expectoration of *tough, stringy mucus* [**Phos.**] During cough, pain in sternum, darting through between shoulders.

**LACHESIS.** *Short, dry cough*, caused by tickling in throat. *The slightest pressure on larynx causes a violent cough and a sense of suffocation, [**Rumex.**] Larynx and throat painful to touch; *cannot bear anything on neck.* Worse during day and *after sleeping.*

**LYCOPODIUM.** Cough, with gray, salt expectoration and great weakness of stomach. Morning cough with *green expectoration* and violent pain in the side. *Fan-like motion of alæ nasi. *Red sand in urine, [**Phos.**] Worse from 4 to 8 P. M.

**MERCURIUS.** *Dry cough*, which sounds as if whole inside of chest were dry. Cough with expectoration of yellowish mucus; sometimes attended with spitting of blood. *Sweat without relief. Worse at night and in damp, rainy weather, [**Dulc. Rhus.**]

**NATRUM CARB.** Hoarseness, with roughness of chest, coryza, chilliness, and scraping painful cough. *Violent dry cough when entering a warm room from the cold air. Short cough with rattling in chest. Chilliness on left side of thorax.

**NATRUM SULPH.** *Dry cough at night, with soreness in chest and roughness in throat, [**Merc.**] Has to sit up and hold the chest with both hands, [hold the head, ***Nicc.**] Stitches in the side.

**NUX VOMICA.** *Dry cough*, caused by a rough, scraping sensation in throat, [**Hepar. Phos. *Puls.**] Cough, with pain in head, as if skull would burst, or a sensation as if bruised in region of stomach. *Constipation, large, hard, difficult stools, [**Lyc.**] After cough mixtures.

**PHOSPHORUS.** Mostly a *dry cough*, arising from tickling in throat and chest, excited by reading aloud, talking, laughing or drinking, [**Bry. Dros. Puls.**] *Dry tickling cough in evening, with *tightness across chest*, [**Puls. Sulph.**] *Long, narrow, hard, difficult stools. Tall, slender persons, with phthisical constitutions.

**PHOS. ACID.** Cough, with expectoration of yellow phlegm, only in morning. Cough with purulent, very offensive expectoration. Headache when coughing, with nausea and vomiting food, or with involuntary emissions of urine, [see **Caust.**]

**PULSATILLA.** *Dry cough* during night, *going off when sitting up in bed*, [***Hyos.**—Worse sitting up, **Kali c.** ***Zinc.**] *Dry cough at night and loose by day*, [**Cham. Nux. Sulph.**] Also, a loose cough, with yellowish, greenish, or bitter expectoration. *Morning cough, with much yellow, salty, bitter, disgusting expectoration; sometimes attended with vomiting. Stitches in chest, particularly when lying down. *All worse toward evening.

**SAMBUCUS.** Profuse debilitating sweats. *Nightly suffocative attacks from obstruction in chest, seems as if he would choke. Attacks of suffocative cough in children, with crying. Cough worse at or soon after midnight, [**Rhus.**]

**SILICEA.** *Dry* or *loose* cough, with expectoration of transparent mucus, Dry, hacking cough, with soreness of chest, [see **Nat. s.**] Also cough, with *vomiting purulent matter.* Want of vital heat, [***Ledum. Sep.**] *Constipation, stools *recede after having been partially expelled.*

**STANNUM.** *Loose cough*, with rattling breathing. *Cough, with profuse greenish expectoration of a disagreeable sweetish taste, [**Phos. Sulph.**] Also cough, with yellowish expectoration, having a putrid taste. After every cough, a sore feeling in chest and trachea. Scrofulous or phthisical subjects.

**SULPHUR.** *Dry cough*, with hoarseness and dryness in throat. Also, a *loose cough*, with expectoration of greenish lumps having a sweetish taste. *Much rattling of mucus in lungs, cough worse in morning. Dry, scaly, unhealthy skin. *Lean persons, who walk stooping.

**TARTAR EM.** *Loose cough*, *without* expectoration. *Throat full of phlegm, but does not yield to coughing, [**Ipe.**] *Nausea, and vomiting large quantities of mucus, [**Ipe.**] *Thirst day and night.*

**VERAT. ALB.** *Deep hollow* cough, *tickling low down in bronchial tubes.* Cough with yellow expectoration, and bruised pain in chest after coughing, [see **Nat. s.**] Violent cough, with blueness of face, and involuntary emissions of urine, [**Caust. Puls.**] *Excessive weakness.*

**CLINICAL REMARKS.** Cough, though only a symptom, is ofter a very prominent one, calling for special treatment.

Persons subject to cough will derive much benefit from frequent bathing in cold water and thorough friction of the body. Drinking freely of cold water or *Gum Arabic* water, in which a few drops of lemon juice has been dissolved, will often have a good effect. Strict attention should be given to ventilation, especially in the sleeping apartment, and all places where smoke or dust abound should be avoided.

The *Diet* must be simple, consisting largely of vegetables and fruits; all stimulating food and drinks should be discarded.

---

## CRAMP IN LIMBS, ETC.

This is a sudden involuntary and painful contraction of a muscle or muscles. It is most frequently experienced in the lower extremities; sometimes, however, it affects the whole body. The attacks frequently occur at night and during sleep.

**TREATMENT.** *Leading indications.*

**COLOCYNTH.** Cramps in abdomen, also in calves, [**Nux v.**] Suitable after grief or indignation.

**CAMPHOR.** *Cramps all over, in inner and outward parts. Cold feeling all over.

**CUPRUM. M.** Violent cramps abdomen and lower limbs, causing patient to scream aloud.

**LYCOPO.**, and **SEPIA** for cramps occurring principally when walking, and during pregnacy.

**NUX VOM.** *Cramps in calves and soles, especially at night, must stretch feet out. High livers and drunkards.

**RHUS TOX** *Cramps during the day, especially when sitting still.

**VERAT. ALB.** *Cramps especially in calves.* *Pain in limbs, as after excessive fatigue.

A dose given every night for a week, will often overcome predisposition to this complaint.

**AUXILIARY MEASURES.** Friction and compression of parts will generally give relief during an attack. For cramps in stomach, copious draughts of *hot* water, and *hot fomentations* applied externally will afford speedy relief.

Persons subject to cramp should take cold baths, and make frequent use of flesh-brush.

---

## CROUP—CATARRHAL.

**TREATMENT.** *Leading indications.*

**ACONITE.** *Inflammatory period,* dry, hot skin, and *restlessness.* After exposure to cold wind, [**Hepar.**] On attempting to swallow, child cries if from pain in throat. *Loud breathing during expiration, but not during inspiration. *Every expiration ends in a hoarse, hacking cough.

**AMM. CAUS.** Deep, weak voice; can scarcely utter a word. Cough with copious expectoration of mucus, especially after drinking. *Difficult, labored, rattling breathing.* Spasms of chest and suffocative fits, **[Sam.]**

**BELLADONNA.** Heat of head; *face flushed, eyes red.* Great soreness of larynx, when touched child seems if it would suffocate, **[Lach.]** *Bright redness of fauces.* Dry, barking, spasmodic cough. *Short, anxious inspirations, with *moaning.* *Sleepiness, but cannot sleep, **[Lach.]** *Starting, during sleep. *Full habit.*

**CALC. CARB.** *Leuco-phlegmatic constitution;* profuse sweat on scalp; inspirations hoarse, rough, loud, and difficult, causing child to cry out with pain. Worse after sleeping, **[*Lach.]** *Cold, damp feet.*

**CHAMOMILLA.** Catarrhal croup, with *much hoarseness, wheezing and rattling of mucus in trachea.* Dry, short, croupy cough, worse at night, even during sleep. *The child is very cross, and wants to be carried. *One cheek red and the other pale.

**HEPAR SULPH.** *Loose, rattling, choking cough;* air-passages seem clogged with mucus, **[Tart. e.]** Violent fits of coughing as if child would suffocate or vomit. *The child cannot bear to be uncovered, and coughs whenever any part of body gets cold. Great drowsiness and profuse sweat. Worse *after midnight.*

**LACHESIS.** Advanced cases, threatened paralysis of lungs, **[Tart. e.]** Patches of exudation on fauces. *Larynx very painful to touch, the slightest pressure causes suffocative cough. Tossing, moaning during sleep. **Distressing aggravation after sleeping,* **[Calc. c.]**

**PHOSPHORUS.** Great hoarseness with soreness of larynx. *Cannot talk on account of pain in larynx. *Trembling of whole body while coughing. Shortness of breath, which otherwise has a natural sound. *Hoarseness* after croup, with tendency to relapses.

**SPONGIA.** **Non-membranous croup,* rough, *crowing, barking* cough. *Slow, loud, wheezing,* and *sawing respiration,* or suffocative fits; inability to breathe, except with head thrown back. *The stridulous respiratory sound is heard during *inspiration,* and the cough, which is *dry,* is excited only during the respiratory act.

**TARTAR EM.** Advanced stages, threatened paralysis of pneumogastric nerves. *Face cold, bluish, covered with cold perspiration. *With every cough, a sound as if a large quantity of mucus were dislodged, but none comes up, **[Ipe.]** Respiration very difficult, short, hoarse, shrill or whistling. The chest expands with great difficulty; head thrown back, much *anxiety* and *prostration.*

For further indications, see **Membranous Croup.**

**AUXILIARY MEASURES.** *Warm* foot-baths beneficial. Immerse feet and legs nearly to the knees in *warm* water, and from time to time add *hot* water until the bath is as hot as can be borne. While limbs are in the bath have them well rubbed by an assistant. When taken out, wipe dry and wrap in warm flannel.

*Hot fomentations* to the throat and upper chest very important; cover with oiled-silk and change frequently. Keep patient quiet as possible.

Give injections of *warm water* unless child is very averse to them. See that room is supplied with an *abundance* of fresh air. Keep temperature of room at about 70° F., and the atmosphere moist.

**DIET.** Mucilaginous drinks, as gum-water, slippery-elm water, etc., during the attack; later, beef-tea, broths and milk may be substituted.

---

## CROUP.—PSEUDO-MEMBRANOUS.

*Membranous* croup is a dangerous disease, the death-rate running as high as 75 per cent. There is little hope when severe and continued dyspnœa occurs with frequent suffocative attacks; marked stenosis, stupor and intermittent pulse.

The disease usually lasts from five to eight days, although in some cases it proves fatal in 24 or 48 hours.

**THERAPEUTICS.** *Leading remedies.*

**ACONITE.** *Inflammatory period*, dry, hot skin, *great restlessness*. After exposure to cold west wind, [**Hepar.**] On attempting to swallow, the child cries as if from pain in throat. *Loud breathing during expiration but not during inspiration. *Every expiration ends in a hoarse, hacking cough.

**BROMINE.** Great difficulty of breathing; *child gasping for air. Spasm of larynx causing suffocation.* Dry, hoarse, spasmodic cough, with wheezing, rattling respiration, impeding speech. *Formation of false membrane, [***Iodi. *Kali b.**] Pulse frequent, feeble, and tremulous. Blue eyes, light hair.

**IODIUM.** *Soreness and pain in throat and chest, which child manifests by grasping parts with hand. *Dry, short, barking cough*, with difficult breathing. *Membranous croup, with wheezing, sawing respiration*, [**Kali b.**] *Face pale and cold; voice deep, rough, and hoarse.

**KALI BICHRO.** *True membranous croup.* The disease approaches *gradually;* at first, slight dyspnœa, with hoarse, croupy cough. *The air, in passing through trachea, *sounds if passing through a metallic tube.* Hoarse, dry, barking cough. Tonsils and larynx red, swollen, and covered with pseudo-membrane. Head inclined backwards; *violent wheezing* and rattling in trachea, heard at a distance. [See **Tart. e.**]

**SANGUINARIA.** *Pseudo-membranous croup. Wheezing whistling cough; metallic sounding; stridulous breathing. *Loss of voice*, with swelling of throat. *Circumscribed redness of cheeks.

**AUXILIARY MEASURES.** See "Croup—Catarrhal," on previous page. Inhalations of *steam* with atomizer, beneficial. *Slacking lime* in room and allowing patient to breathe the vapor, is worthy of trial. A few drops *Tr. Iodine* placed on a sponge in a cup and held near the nostrils, will often give relief. Again: one drachm *Bromide of Potassium*, one grain Bromine, one ounce of water, administered by inhalation, has a salutary effect on dyspnœa.

Great success is claimed from placing patient in closed room, keeping the temperature at 80° F., and surcharging atmosphere with moisture by hanging cloths wet with hot water about the room, or by pouring water on *hot* bricks or heated irons to generate moisture. It is said by this process the exudate is softened and thrown off.

**Tracheotomy** has been successful after all other means have failed, it should therefore be resorted to in all critical cases.

---

## CRUSTA LACTEA.

**TREATMENT.** *Leading indications.*

**ARSENICUM.** Eruption *dry and scaly*, with terrible itching at night. The parts are tender to touch, and *bleed easily* when scratched, [see **Lyc.**] The child has an old look, is weak and emaciated. Worse in the cold air, and *better* from external *warmth*.

**BARYTA CARB.** *Scrofulous children*, [see **Calc. c.**] *Glandular swellings on neck and under the jaw. Eruption moist, with falling off of the hair.

**CALC. CARB.** *Moist, scurfy eruption* on cheeks, behind the ears, and on forehead. Thick crusts, moist or dry; *violent itching of whole face.* *Scrofulous children, with pale, flabby bodies. Glandular swellings and imperfect development of osseous system. *Cold, damp feet;* perspires after eating or drinking.

**CLEMATIS.** Dark miliary eruptions, with *violent itching;* a moisture exudes from the parts, which dries into scurfs as the disease spreads. *Worse during the increasing moon and on getting warm.

**GRAPHITES.** Scabby eruption, particularly on chin and aronnd mouth. *The eruption has a raw appearance, and discharges a sticky glutinous fluid. *Rawness in bends of limbs, groins, neck, behind the ears.* Unhealthy skin; every little injury suppurates.

**HEPAR SULPH.** Eruption in face, scurfy, very painful to touch. The eruption spreads by means of new pimples appearing just beyond the main disease. *Unhealthy skin*, every slight injury suppurates, [Graph.] The eruption secretes a purulent matter.

**LYCOPODIUM.** *Thick crusts*, the surface underneath being cracked and the secretion fetid. The parts bleed easily after scratching, [Ars.] Soreness behind the ears,* in the neck, etc. *Red sand in the urine.

**NATRUM MUR.** Raw, inflamed surface, discharging continually a corroding fluid, which eats away the hair. The parts around margin of hair especially affected. After the use of *Nitrate of Silver.*

**RHUS TOX.** Thick, moist crusts, which secrete a fetid, bloody ichor, [see Lyc.] *Confluent vesicles* containing a *milky* or *watery* fluid. *The parts itch violently, particularly at night, and bleed when scratched.

**STAPHISAGRIA.** *Yellow, acrid moisture oozes from under the crusts. If the scabs are rubbed off, new vesicles at once form, and again burst.

**SULPHUR.** The child has a *dry, unhealthy skin*, and the slightest injury inclines to suppurate. The crusts and pimples itch violently, especially at night; easily bleeding, [Ars.] Aversion to water and the open air.

**LOCAL MEASURES.** All external applications, as washes, ointments, etc., should be discarded. Keep the *parts dry* as possible. A little *cold cream* or *vaseline* may be applied to the parts to allay the intense itching.

The child should be kept scrupulously *clean*, live *out doors* much as possible, and sleep in well-ventilated apartments.

---

## CYSTITIS.

**TREATMENT.** *Principal remedies.*

**ACONITE.** Dry, hot skin, thirst, and restlessness. Frequent and violent urging to urinate, with burning in bladder, [Canth.] *Retention of urine, with stitches in kidneys. Painfulness in region of bladder. *Great fear and anxiety of mind, with nervous excitability.

**APIS MEL.** Stinging pains in urethra during micturiton; *urine dark-colored and scanty*, [brown, black, *Colch. Tereb.] *Incontinence of urine, with great irritation of the parts; worse at night and when coughing. *Sensation as if something in abdomen would break.

**ARNICA.** Retention of urine, with tenesmus of the neck of the bladder. Urging, the urine dropping out involuntary. *Brown urine, with brick-red sediment*, [*Phos. Puls.] *Pain in small of the back as if bruised. After mechanical injuries, [Ruta.]

**BELLADONNA.** Region of bladder very *sensitive; urine hot and red;* sometimes depositing a reddish sediment.

*Constant dribbling of urine, involuntary; also enuresis with profuse perspiration. Sensation of a worm in bladder, [of a *ball*, Lach.] *Pains come on suddenly, and cease as suddenly. Back feels as if it would break.

**CAMPHOR.** Burning heat in bladder, [Acon.] Retention of urine, with constant pressure on bladder and desire to urinate. *Red, thick urine* depositing a thick sediment. Burning in urethra during micturition. *Strangury, especially if caused by abuse of cantharides. Coldness of extremities, with cramp in calves.

**CANNABIS IN.** Inflammation of bladder. Painful discharge by drops of *bloody urine*, [Canth.] Darting stitches in posterior portion of urethra. *Violent burning in urethra during and after micturition. Drawing pain from region of kidneys to inguinal glands, with anxious and sick feeling in pit of stomach.

**CANTHARIDES.** Swelling and tenderness in region of bladder, with tensive and burning pain in loins, [Acon.] *Violent pains* and *burning heat in bladder.* Frequent micturition, with burning, cutting pains, so severe patient screams aloud. Constant desire to urinate, with *scanty emissions of dark and bloody urine.*

**DIGITALIS.** Inflammation in neck of bladder. Continual desire to urinate; each time only a few drops emitted. *Frequent, cutting pains in neck of bladder, as if a *straw was being thrust back and forth.* Urine dark-brown and hot. Can retain urine best in a recumbent posture.

**MERCURIUS.** Stinging pains in small of back, with a sensation of weakness. Constant desire to urinate, with scanty emissions of dark-red urine, soon becoming turbid and fetid. The urine looks as if *mixed with blood*, with white flakes, or as if containing pus. *Worse at night, and in damp, rainy weather.

**NUX VOMICA.** *Burning, lacerating pain in neck of bladder* and *urethra*, [Dig.] Painful, ineffectual desire to urinate, with discharge of a few drops of red, bloody, burning urine, [Canth.] Spasmodic stricture of urethra, with retention of urine. *Constipation, with large, hard difficult stools. Sedentary habits; *after abuse of alcoholic spirits.*

**PAREIRA BRAVA.** *Strangury, with violent pains in bladder*, and at times in back. He cries aloud, and can only emit urine when on his knees. Left testicle painfully drawn up. Pain in thighs, shooting down into feet.

**PHOSPHORUS.** Contractive pain in bladder or stitches in neck of bladder. Urine white like curdled milk, soon becoming turbid with *brick-dust sediment.* Also brown urine, with sediment of red sand, [*Lyc.] Smarting, cutting, and jerking in urethra. *Constipation, stools *long, narrow, hard*, very difficult to expel.

**PULSATILLA.** Aching, burning, cutting pains in region of bladder. *Retention of urine, with redness, heat, and soreness of vesical region externally. *Involuntary emissions of urine when sitting, coughing, or walking, [Caust. Ruta.] *After urinating, spasmodic pain in neck of bladder, extending to pelvis and thighs. *Scant, red, brown urine, with reddish, bloody, or mucous sediment,* [Am. c.] Mild, tearful disposition.

**SARSAPARILLA.** Tenesmus of bladder, with discharge of *white pus and mucus.* Urine red, fiery, turbid, containing flakes. *Severe pain at *conclusion of urination.* Urine contains a quantity of pale sand, [*red sand,* Phos. *Lyc.] Children cry before and during micturition. Pain in small of back, extending toward genital organs.

**SULPHUR.** Obstinate cases, urine mixed with mucus or blood; *very fetid.* *Burning in urethra *during micturition,* Incontinence of urine, particularly at night. *Constant heat on top of head. *Lank, lean persons who walk stooping.

**TARANTULA.** Cystitis, with high fever, [Acon.] Gastric derangement, with excruciating pains in bladder. The bladder seems swollen and hard; great tenesmus from spasmodic action, debilitating the patient, who passes only by drops a dark-red, brown, fetid urine, with a gravel-like sediment.

**AUXILIARY MEASURES.** Great benefit will often arise from cloths wrung out of *hot water* and applied to region of bladder. Warm *sitz-baths,* and if the bowels be constipated, injections of warm *slippery-elm or flaxseed tea* should be resorted to.

In **Chronic** cases benefit may be derived from washing out the bladder with small quantities of *tepid* water. Use fountain syringe, with a flexible rubber catheter.

**DIET.** In *acute* cases adopt a mixed vegetable diet. Avoid meats, oysters, eggs, pastry, and all food highly seasoned with salt. Use no *stimulants,* wines, brandy, beer or ale. Let the drink be pure soft water.

---

## DELIRIUM TREMENS.—MANIA-A-POTU.

**TREATMENT.** *Leading indications.*

**ARSENICUM.** Pale, jaundiced complexion. Bloated face and cold, blue skin. Fainting fits, particularly during vomiting. The patient imagines that vermin are crawling about the bed, and ugly animals are staring him in the face. *Great restlessness and fear of death. *Extreme thirst, drinks little and often.

**BELLADONNA.** *Full plethoric habit.* Flushed face and red eyes, with dilated pupils. *Boisterous delirium, with desire to escape. *Frightful figures and images before the eyes, [Opi. *Stram.] Sudden starting and jumping while sleeping.

**BROMIDE of CAMPHOR.** This medicine given in the 2x trit. 5 grs. every 15 or 20 minutes until sleep is secured, is said to have a happy effect in these distressing cases

**CAMPHOR.** Features distorted; eyes sunken, face, hands, and feet icy cold. Confusion of ideas, maniacal delirium, convulsions, frothing at mouth, and insensibility. *Retention of urine, with constant pressure on bladder.

**COFFEA.** Headache as if a nail were driven into brain. *Excessive irritability and wakefulness. Talks in his sleep and wakes with starting.

**HYOSCYAMUS.** Twitching, jerking of muscles, especially those about eyes and face. *Furious delirium, with wild, staring look,* dilated pupils, throbbing carotids, [*Bell.] Convulsive movements; *subsultus tendinum.* *Grasping at imaginary objects, muttering, and *tremor of the hands.*

**LACHESIS.** Where throat is principally affected with difficult deglutition, [**Bell.**] *Cannot bear anything about his neck, not even neck-tie. Talks much, flying from one subject to another. *The attacks are worse in afternoon and after sleeping.

**NUX VOMICA.** Trembling of limbs and spasmodic twitching of muscles, [**Hyos.**] Makes frequent mistakes in talking. Delirium with frightful visions and efforts of escape. *Very irritable, and wishes to be alone, [fear of being alone, ***Ars.**] *Constipation, with *large* difficult stools. *Thinks he will die.*

**OPIUM.** Patient lies in a comatose state, with eyes half open. *Loud stertorous breathing.* *Complete loss of consciousness and sensation. *Delirious talking, with eyes wide open. Pupils widely dilated or contracted. Pulse full and labored, or *slow and feeble.*

**STRAMONIUM.** Disposed to talk continually. *Sings and prays most devoutly.* *Awakens with a shrinking look, as if afraid of first object seen. *Loquacious delirium, with desire to escape. Dilatation of pupils. Staring eyes, [**Opi.**] Grinding of teeth and distortion of mouth.

To overcome the inclination to drink, all alcoholic beverages must be abandoned, *even as medicine.*

A teaspoonful of *Tr. Chincona rubra* taken thrice daily for ten days, then twice a day for ten days longer, and lastly one teaspoonful a day for a fortnight, will in many cases destroy the appetite for strong drink.

Equal parts of *Tr. Capsicum* and *Fl. Ext. Lupulinæ*, taken in teaspoonful doses as occasion may require, is said to be an excellent substitute for alcoholic stimulants.

**AUXILIARY MEASURES.** During an attack, quietude should be enforced, visitors excluded, and the most favorable conditions enjoined to *promote* sleep. Allopathic physicians claim "great success from large doses of *Bromide of Potassium* [20 grs. in water, every two hours until sleep is procured]. *Capsicum* [30 grs. in capsules] cuts short the delirium."

A cup of *strong coffee*, [without sugar or cream] is very beneficial. Cold affusions to head and the shower-bath useful. Soothe and quiet patient by kindness, using as little compulsion as possible. Have windows and doors securely fastened, and help at hand in case of an emergency.

**DIET.** Patient should be encouraged to take nutritious and easily digested food. *Milk*, beef-tea, soft-boiled eggs, broths, oysters, fruits and vegetables.

---

## DENTITION.—TEETHING.

### Temporary Teeth, [20 in number].

The eruption of the *milk teeth* is very irregular; it takes place, approximately, in the following order:—

| | |
|---|---|
| Central incisors, . . . | 6th to 8th month. |
| Lateral incisors, . . . | 7th to 10th month. |
| First molars, . . . . | 12th to 14th month. |
| Canines, . . . . | 15th to 20th month. |
| Second molars, . . . | 20th to 30th month. |

### Permanent Teeth, [32 in number.]

The permanent teeth put in their appearance with great regularity, and constitute an important means of ascertaining the child's age in the early period of life.

| | |
|---|---|
| First molars, . . . . . . | 7th year. |
| Central incisors, . . . . . | 8th year. |
| Lateral incisors, . . . . . | 9th year. |
| First bicuspids, . . . . . . | 10th year. |
| Second bicuspids, . . . . . | 11th year. |
| Canines, . . . . . . . | 12th year. |
| Second molars, . . . . . . | 13th year. |

During the period of *first dentition*, the infant is especially liable to disease, and should receive the greatest care and attention during this period.

**HYGIENIC TREATMENT.** The child should have a *tepid bath* [85° F.] every morning, followed by gentle, brisk rubbing. It is well, however, to accustom it in early life to the use of *cold baths*, as it fortifies the system and lessens the liability to take cold.

In warm and pleasant weather, it should eat, sleep, and play out of doors. No *matter how sick*, if weather is suitable, dress properly and take it out in the open air. In summer, be careful to guard the head from direct rays of the sun. Keep it in cool place, free from noise, loud talking, and excitement of every kind.

The greatest attention should be paid to cleanliness, especially of *bottles*, *tubes*, *teats*, *pans*, *spoons*, etc. Napkins should be removed soon as they become wet or soiled. Never dry the diapers in room where child is or leave them in an adjoining room to vitiate the air, remove them at once to a distant place.

The nursery should be *freely accessible* to *external light*, and the temperature not under 70° for young children; when older, say a year, 65° will suffice.

**DIETETICS.** Of the greatest importance. Where child cannot have its mother's milk, a proper substitute must be furnished. A suitable wet-nurse the most desirable, [*vide* article **Wet Nurse.**] Cow's milk will in most cases agree with the child. For a *new-born* infant, the cow should be *fresh* or nearly so. If the milk be rich, add one-third *warm* water and sweeten with *sugar of milk*. If cow's-milk will not agree with the child, give a gruel made from *unbolted* wheat flour, [*vide* **Diet of Infants**] which will be found an excellent substitute; being rich in earthy materials, it is especially adapted to teething children.

A child should be fed at regular intervals of three hours during the day, but not at night. An infant six months old should not take more than *two ounces* of food at a time; as it grows older, the amount should be gradually increased. Never feed the child during the night; keep it *warm while taking* its food, and always place it in a *semi-erect* position *while feeding*.

## MEDICAL TREATMENT.

**ACONITE.** *Constant restleseness, which no change of position seems to relieve. The child cries, whines, or frets and cannot be quieted. *Dry, hot skin, disturbed sleep, much heat about head, *great thirst*, [see **Bell.**] *Green, watery diarrhœa* or constipation.

**ALUMINA.** *Constipation* of *bottle-fed babies*. Stools hard and knotty. *Even the soft stool voided with difficulty.

**APIS MEL.** Frequent waking at night, or during sleep, with screams, [***Bell. Cham.**] Red spots here and there over the skin. Urine scanty, sometimes profuse. *Green, yellowish, watery diarrhœa*, worse in morning. *Much yawning and uneasiness.

**ARSENICUM.** Child has a pale waxen look, is very weak. It often vomits all fluids soon after taking them, particularly water, [***Verat.**] *Drinks often, but little at a time, [**Apis. Chin.**] *Very restless, tossing from side to side. Fetid, undigested stools; dry and shriveled skin.

**BELLADONNA.** Child moans a great deal; awakens in a fright, with staring eyes. *Starting, jumping during sleep, [**Ars. Hyos.**] Face and eyes red, pupils dilated, head hot. *Convulsions, followed by sound sleep. Gums swollen and inflamed; numerous *small blood-vessels showing on the surface.*

**BORAX.** Child very nervous, starts and jumps at least noise, [**Bell.**] Sometimes it cries out, and holds on to things as if *afraid of falling*, [when carried, fears it will fall, and clutches, **Gel.**] *Cannot bear a downward motion, [**Berb.**] *Aphthæ in mouth, causing child to cry out when nursing,

**BRYONIA.** Mouth and lips very dry. Child wishes to be

very quiet; gets faint and sick when raised up. *The food is thrown up soon after taking it, [*Ars. Nux.] Thirst for large draughts of water. *Hard, dry stools, or morning diarrhœa. *Desire for things which are rejected when offered. Very irritable.

**CALC. CARB.** Large head with open fontanelles—scrofulous, [**Merc.** ***Sil. Sulph.**] *Head sweats* during sleep, [see **Rheum.**] *Child peevish and fretful; very light sleeper.* *Cold, damp feet. *White, chalk-like stools, or thin and whitish. *Vomiting milk in thick curds, [**Æthu.**] Swollen, distended abdomen, with emaciation and good appetite.

**CHAMOMILLA.** Very *irritable, sensitive and nervous.* Starting, uttering sudden cries, and tossing about during sleep, [**Bell.**] *Very cross, wants to be carried all the time. *One cheek red and the other pale, [**Acon.**] Convulsive twitchings of the extremities. *Greenish, yellowish or whitish, mucous stools, smelling like bad eggs,* [**Nux m.**]

**CICUTA.** *Grinding the teeth, with pressing jaws together, like lock-jaw, [see **Stram.**] Convulsions with limbs relaxed, hanging down, or stiff, rigid, and extended. A kind of half-sleep with tossing.

**CINA.** Paleness of face, particularly around nose and mouth. *Picks or rubs the nose.* *Very restless during sleep, must be kept in motion to be quieted. *Very peevish, wants many things, which it rejects immediately,* [**Bry.**] *Urine whitish like milk, [**Phos. ac.**] Grinding the teeth.

**COFFEA.** *The child is very excitable and sleepless. It *frets and worries in a pitiful manner;* cries one moment laughs next. Child feverish, and greatly exhausted for want of sleep.

**CUPRUM MET.** Great uneasiness and tossing about. Convulsions, *beginning with cramps in lower extremities and drawing in of fingers and toes;* frothing at mouth, and choking in throat. Green, painful stools and vomiting mucus.

**DULCAMARA.** Pale face, with circumscribed redness of the cheeks. Dry coryza and frequent sneezing. Diarrhœa, with yellowish, greenish or whitish stools. Nausea or real vomiting. *Symptoms all worse by every damp, cold change in the weather.

**FERRUM.** Dentition advances slowly, and an obstinate diarrhœa results. *Stools of mucus and undigested food. *Painless, exhausting diarrhœa, sometimes excoriating the parts. Vomiting food soon after taking it, [see **Bry.**] *Sudden flushing of face. *Exhausting sweats.*

**GRAPHITES.** *Unhealthy condition of the skin.* Rawness in bends of the limbs, on neck, and behind the ears, [***Hepar.**] *Eruptions over head and face, with discharge of a sticky, glutinous fluid. Constipation of large, knotty stools, very offensive.

**HEPAR SULPH.** Dry, herpetic eruptions on skin, especially in bend of arms, groin, upon the face and scalp, itching violently. *The gums are very tender and painful. Diarrhœa, stools whitish and smelling sour, [Cal. c.] Stomach inclined to be out of order; craves sour or strong-tasting things.

**HYOSCYAMUS.** The child puts its fingers into the mouth, presses its gums together as if chewing on something. *Convulsions, beginning with twitching of facial muscles, especially about the eyes. *Deep sleep, muttering, and picking at bed-clothes, [Opi.] *Yellow, watery, involuntary stools.*

**IGNATIA.** Frequent flushes of heat, with perspiration. The child awakens from sleep with piercing cries, and trembling all over, [*Apis.] Convulsive jerking of single parts. *The child is much distressed, *sighs, sobs*, and cries. Stools bloody mucus, often attended with tenesmus and prolapsus of the rectum.

**IPECAC.** Pale face, with blueness around eyes. *Continual nausea, with vomiting, [Phos. *Verat.] Diarrhœa; stools green as grass, or fermented. Catarrh, with suffocative cough and rattling of mucus in bronchia.

**KREASOTE.** *Very painful dentition.* The protruding gum seems infiltrated with a dark, watery fluid. *The teeth begin to decay soon as through the gums. Constipation, with hard, dry stools, or diarrhœa with dark-brown, watery, *very offensive stools.*

**LACHESIS.** *The child always awakens in distress, worse after sleeping, [Apis.] Convulsions, which usually occur as child goes to sleep. Gums dark-purple and painful to touch. *Difficult deglutition, can't bear throat to be touched.

**LYCOPODIUM.** Child sleeps with eyes partially closed, throwing head from side to side. Just before passing water, child cries and screams as if in pain. *Red sand in urine, [Phos. Sil.] Much rumbling of wind in bowels. Worse 4 P. M., better during night.

**MAGNESIA CARB.** Green, sour-smelling diarrhœa of long duration. *Stools green, watery, resembling the scum of a frog-pond, [like chopped eggs and spinach, *Cham.] Frequent vomiting of sour-smelling substances.

**MAGNESIA PHOS.** Convulsive cases, when *Bell.* is indicated, but does no good. Spasmodic colic, and looseness of bowels.

**MERCURIUS.** *Copious salivation, redness of gums, and sometimes little ulcers on tongue and mouth. Diarrhœa, with greenish, slimy, or bloody stools, with *much straining*, [Bell.] Yellowish and strong-smelling urine. Profuse *sweating*, especially at night.

**NUX MOS.** Exhausting diarrhœa, with thin, yellow stools, like beaten or stirred eggs, [Cham.] *The diarrhœa is accompanied with *great drowsiness.* Symptoms worse at night and in warm weather.

**NUX VOMICA.** Child *very cross and irritable*, [**Cham.**] *Constipation, with large, difficult stools, or small, frequent, lumpy, or brown mucus stools, [**Lyc.**] *Especially suited to children raised on cow's-milk, etc., or whose mothers indulge in highly-seasoned food, wines, etc. Aggravation in early morning.

**PODOPHYLLUM.** Restless sleep, with half-closed eyes; moaning and grinding teeth. Rolling head from side to side, [**Apis.**] Green, watery or whitish, chalk-like stools, very offensive. Frequent *gagging or empty retching*. *Morning diarrhœa, with prolapsus ani during every stool, [**Sulph.**] Aggravation in hot weather, and after eating and drinking.

**RHEUM.** *Constant sweating of hairy scalp, [see **Calc. c.**] *Sour-smelling diarrhœa, colic before and tenesmus after stool.* *Sour smell of whole body, which washing does not remove, [**Mag. c.** ***Robinia.**] Diarrhœa worse by moving about, [**Bry.**] Restless sleep.

**SILICEA.** *Large head with open fontanelles—*scrofulous*, [see **Calc.**] Profuse sour-smelling perspiration on head, [**Calc. c. Merc.**] Hard, hot, distended abdomen. The protruding gum is blistered and very sensitive. *Constipation, the stool *recedes after having been partially expelled.* Aversion to mother's milk.

**SULPHUR.** *Open fontanelles.* *Eruptions on skin, attended with much itching. Diarrhœa with whitish, greenish or bloody mucous stools, excoriating the anus, [**Merc.**] *Early morning diarrhœa. Frequent vomiting of food. *Frequent weak, faint spells.

**SULPHURIC AC.** *Aphthæ of mouth and gums*, with much slavering, [**Merc.**] Child very irritable, cries much of the time. *Diarrhœa, stools like chopped, saffron-yellow mucus. Loss of appetite, *great debility*, [see **Mag. c.**]

**VERAT. ALB.** Vomiting and severe empty retching, aggravated by least motion, [**Zinc.**] *Diarrhœa, each stool followed by prostration and cold sweat on forehead. Cold, damp feeling of extremities. *Very weak, faint pulse. *Violent thirst for cold water.

**AUXILIARY MEASURES.** When the gum is much swollen, tender and tightly drawn over the tooth, lance it. Bathing the gum with a weak solution of the indicated remedy, and at the same time giving it internally, will be found very efficacious.

If convulsions should occur, place the feet and legs to the knees in hot water, and apply cold compresses to the head, or the whole body may be put in a warm bath and briskly rubbed. When the system relaxes, wrap patient in a blanket and let him dry without rubbing. If he cannot swallow, put a drop of indicated remedy on the tongue, [*vide* **Spasms.**] Injections of warm water often afford relief.

## DIABETES MELLITUS.

A disease characterized by an immoderate and morbid secretion of urine, in which *urea* is replaced by sugar or glucose, attended with excessive thirst and progressive emaciation. In some cases the quantity of urine discharged is excessive, amounting to three or four gallons per day, each gallon containing from one to two pounds of sugar.

The pathology of this singular malady seems still to be wrapped in mystery, and the treatment has been in a great measure unsatisfactory.

**TREATMENT.** *Leading indications.*

**ARGENT MET.** *Whirling in head* as if drunken. Emaciation and great weakness. *Urine of a sweetish taste and profuse. Scrotum and feet œdematous. Hectic fever, [**Plumb.**] Legs feel heavy.

**ARSENICUM.** Insatiable *thirst,* restlessness and prostration. *Vomiting immediately after eating or drinking. Frequent urging with profuse discharge of urine. Feet and legs swollen. Watery diarrhœa.

**CARBOLIC ACID.** Hacking cough. Copious flow of limpid urine containing sugar, [**Phos. ac.**] Unusual appetite and thirst for stimulants, [**Ars.**] Languor and prostration.

**CURARE.** Clear and frequent urine, with digging crampy pains in kidneys. Shooting pains in stomach; dryness of mouth, and great thirst, especially at night.

**HELONIAS.** Dull, gloomy and irritable. Feeling of weakness and weight in region of kidneys. Passes large quantities of clear, pale urine of high specific gravity. *Burning in kidneys,* [see **Tereb.**] Pain and lameness in back; numbness in feet, going off by motion.

**PHOS. ACID.** *Perfect indifference, with silent sadness. Craves something refreshing, juicy. Hawks up tough white mucus. *Frequent profuse emissions of watery urine, which forms a white cloud; urine contains sugar, [see **Tereb.**] Pain in back and kidneys, [see **Helon.**] Complete impotence. *Diarrhœa without weakness.

**PLUMBUM.** Great lowness of spirits. Excessive emaciation and good appetite. Sweet taste and sweetish belchings. *Stools hard, lumpy, like sheep's dung. Hectic fever, [**Arg. n.**] Complete impotence.

**TEREBINTHINA.** Inability to concentrate his thoughts. Sickness of stomach after eating, [see **Ars.**] Burning, drawing from kidney to hip. Frequent urination at night, profuse, watery. Sugar in urine, [**Carb. ac. Phos. ac. Uran. nit.**] Rancid or acrid eructations, and burning in stomach.

**URANIUM NITRATE.** General languor, debility and cold feeling. Purulent discharge from eyelids and nostrils. *Excessive thirst, [**Ars.**] Frequent urination; urine has a fishy smell. Stiffness in loins; restless at night. When disease originates from dyspepsia.

**DIETETICS.** Diet is an important factor in the treatment of diabetes mellitus. All food containing *starch* or *sugar* should be avoided. The following is a list of articles allowed:—

**ARTICLES ALLOWED.** Beef, mutton, poultry, game, oysters, clams, butter, cheese, eggs, fish, including lobsters, crabs, sardines, and soups of all kinds without flour, rice, or other starchy substances.

*Vegetables.* Cauliflower, spinach, cabbage, string beans, cucumbers, lettuce, greens, cresses, onions and olives.

*Fruits.* Tart fruits, as cherries, currants, strawberries, gooseberries, and nuts generally.

*Beverages.* Milk, cream, buttermilk, coffee with cream and glycerine. No alcoholic liquors of any kind.

**Bread and Pastry.** Only those made from *wheat-gluten* flour. Oatmeal, cornmeal, hominy, etc., must not be used.

**FRUITS PROHIBITED.** All sweet fruits, as apples, pears, plums, grapes, bananas, melons, pineapples, raspberries, blackberries, etc.

**Vegetables Prohibited.** Potatoes, beets, beans, peas, carrots, turnips, parsnips, rice, sago, tapioca, vermicelli, or others containing sugar or starch.

**HYGIENIC MEASURES.** Exercise in the open air, cool sponge baths, friction with flesh-brush, encouraging patient, and regular habits in all things have a salutary effect.

---

## DIARRHŒA.

**TREATMENT.** The best remedies are:—

For **ACUTE** diarrhœa, with sudden prostration of strength: ***Ars. Camph. Carb. v. *Sec. Thuj. *Verat.**

**ALTERNATING** with *Constipation:* **Ant. c. Bry. Calo. phos. Lach. *Nux v. Opi. Phos. Rhus. Ruta.**

**CHRONIC: *Ars. Calc. c. Chin. Ferr. Graph. *Gum g. Hepar. Iod. Ipe. Kali. b. Lach. Lyc. Natr. sul. Phos. *Phos. ac. *Podo. Rhus. Sulp. Thuj. Verat. a.**

**CHILL,** after a: **Bell. Bry. Cham. Chin. *Dulc. Merc. Puls. Verat. a.**

**COLD,** after taking: ***Acon. Ars. Bell. Bry. Caust. Cham. *Dulc. Merc. Nux. m. Nux. v. Sulph.**

**COLD DRINKS,** caused by: **Ars. Bry. Carb. v. Dulc. Hepar. Nux m. *Puls. Rhus. Sul. ac.**

**DRUGS,** after taking: **Carb. v. Hepar. *Nux v. Puls.**

**FAT FOOD,** after eating: **Carb. v. *Puls. Thuj.**

**FRIGHT,** after: ***Acon. Ant. Coff. *Opi. Verat.**

**FRUIT,** after eating: **Ars. Bry. *Chin. Colo. *Puls.**

**GRIEF,** from: ***Colo. *Gel. Ign. Phos. ac.**

**INDIGNATION**, from: **Cham. *Colo.**

**JOY**, after sudden: ***Coff. Opi.**

**LYING-IN-FEMALES**: **Ant. Dulc. Hyos. Petro.**

**MAGNESIA**, after abuse of: ***Nux Puls. Rheum.**

**MERCURY**, after abuse of: **Chin. *Hepar. Nit. ac**

**MILK**, from drinking: **Ars. *Calc. c. Nat. c. *Sulph.**

**OPIUM**, after abuse of: **Bell. Merc. *Nux v.**

**OVERHEATING**, after: ***Acon. Aloe. Ant. Bry. *Podo.**

**OYSTERS**, from eating: ***Brom. Lyc. Sulph. ac.**

**PAINLESS** diarrhœa: **Apis. Ars. *Chin. Colch. Cro. t. *Ferr. Hepar. *Hyos. Phos. ac. *Podo. Rhus t. Sec.**

**PEARS**, from eating: ***Verat. al.**

**PHTHISICAL** persons: **Calc. c. Chin. Ferr. *Phos.**

**PREGNANCY**, during: **Ant. Dulc. Hyos. Lyc. Phos.**

**VEAL**, from eating: **Kali nitr.**

**WATER**, impure: **Zing.**—Calcareous water: ***Camp.**

**WET**, after getting: **Acon. *Rhus t. Rhod.**

## LEADING INDICATIONS.

**ACONITE.** Stools frequent and scanty, *watery, whitish, or slimy.* Nausea and sweat *before* and *tenesmus during* stool. *Vertigo or fainting on rising up, [***Bry.**] Restlessness and intense thirst. *If caused by checked perspiration, or exposure to a cold, dry wind.

**ALOES.** Stools *yellow fecal, copious and watery.* Is driven out of bed early every morning, [***Sulph.**] *Before* stool, a feeling of weight and fullness in pelvis. *During* stool, tenesmus and heat in rectum and anus. *Loud, gurgling in abdomen as of water running out of a bottle, [**Gum. g.**] *Worse after eating,* [see **Ant. c.**]

**ANTIMONIUM.** Stools *watery* and profuse, with *deranged stomach.* *Tongue coated white. *Violent vomiting, bitter, bilious,* or *slimy mucus; worse after eating or drinking,* [**Colo.**] *After overeating, or use of acids.*

**APIS MEL.** Stools *greenish, yellowish, slimy mucus,* or *yellow watery.* *Sensation in abdomen as if something would break when straining at stool. Tongue dry and shining; little or no thirst, [**Puls.**] Œdema of the feet. Aggravation in morning.

**ARGENT. NIT.** Stools *green, fetid mucus,* passing off with much flatus. *Nausea with loud eructations.* Vomiting glassy, tenacious mucus. Aggravation at night, after midnight, and after eating sweet things.

**ARNICA.** Stools *slimy mucus,* or brown fermented (like yeast [see **Ipc.**].) Bitter or putrid taste in the mouth. Eructations, especially in the morning, with taste of putrid eggs, [see **Sulph.**] *Aversion to food; bad breath.* Diarrhœa following mechanical injuries.

**ARSENICUM.** Stools *thick, dark green mucus, or brown, black, watery.* Involuntary stools, [**Bell. *Carb. v. Ferr. *Hyos. Rhus. *Sec.**] Diarrhœa, *excoriating* the parts,

[Cham. Gum. g. *Merc. Puls.] *Great weakness, fainting, and rapid exhaustion, [*Verat.] *Restlessness, constantly changing from side to side. *Great thirst, but drinking little, [Chin.] *Vomiting after eating or drinking.* Worse after eating anything *cold*, [*better*, Phos.]

**BELLADONNA.** Stools *thin, green mucus*, small and frequent. Clutching pains in abdomen. *Pains come suddenly, and cease as suddenly. *Sleepy, but cannot sleep, [Opi.] *Sudden starting and jumping during sleep. Worse 3 P. M., and after sleeping.

**BENZOIC AC.** Stools *watery or light-colored like soapsuds; copious, very offensive*, [Psor.] *Strong-smelling urine, mostly dark-colored. Feels weak and exhausted.

**BRYONIA.** Diarrhœa in *hot weather*, or when induced by *taking cold drinks*, [Podo.] Stools brown, thin fecal, or undigested, smelling like rotten *cheese* [like *rotten eggs*, *Cham. Psor.] *Nausea and faintness from sitting up. *Thirst for large quantities of water. Aggravation *in morning soon as he moves;* after suppressed exanthemata, [see Sulph.]

**CALC. CARB.** Diarrhœa of scrofulous persons. Swollen, distended abdomen, with emaciation and good appetite. Stools *whitish or watery*, [*Phos. ac.] *Chronic diarrhœa*, with clay-like stools. *Profuse sweat on head when sleeping, [Merc. Sil.] *Sour vomiting* or regurgitation of food. *Feet *cold and damp.*

**CARB. VEG.** Stools *light-colored; involuntary; putrid; cadaverous-smelling.* In the last stage and where the vital powers are greatly exhausted, [Ars.] *Emissions of large quantities of flatus, inodorous or putrid. *Restlessness and anxiety.* Worse 5 to 6 P. M.

**CHAMOMILLA.** Stools *green, watery, corroding with colic.* *Hot diarrhœic stools, smelling like bad eggs, [Psor.] Colic before and during stool; relief after. Bitter taste with bilious vomiting. *Very impatient, can hardly answer one civilly. Children very fretful, and are only stilled by being carried. *One cheek red, the other pale, [Acon.] Worse at night.

**CHINA.** Stools *yellowish, watery, whitish*, or *blackish;* spasmodic colic relieved by bending double. *Painless, undigested*, and watery stools, with distension of the abdomen, [Ars.] *Great weakness and inclination to sweat. *Emissions of large quantities of fetid flatus.* Thirst, drinks little and often, [Apis. Ars.] Aggravation *at night*, after eating, and *every other day.*

**CINA.** *White, papescent stools.* *Disposition to pick and bore at the nose, [Phos. ac.] *White, turbid, or jelly-like urine, [Phos. ac.] *Restless sleep, frequently changing position*, and waking with cries. Grinding of teeth during sleep, [*Podo.] Troubled with worms.

**COLOCYNTH.** Stools *saffron-yellow, frothy, or thin, slimy, and watery*, [Sul. ac.] Before stool, *cutting colic*, great urging. *Feeling in abdomen as if the intestines were being squeezed between stones, relieved by bending double. Bitter taste in mouth. Aggravation after taking the least nourishment.

**CROTON TIG.** Intermittent diarrhœa, *with debility.* *Stools *yellow, watery,* or greenish yellow, *expelled with great force,* [**Gum. g. *Jatro.**] Aggravation after *drinking, while eating,* [**Ars. Ferr. Pod.**] Gagging, with vertigo. Colic and writhing around umbilicus.

**DULCAMARA.** Stools yellowish, greenish, watery or whitish. Colic before and during stool. Griping pain in region of navel, with vomiting mucus. *If caused by taking cold. Aggravated in cold, damp weather, [**Nux m.**] *Dry heat of the skin.*

**FERRUM.** *Painless, watery, undigested stools, at night, or while eating or drinking,* [see **Cro. tig.**] Bowels feel sore as if bruised. Emaciation, debility, good appetite, [**Calc. c. Iod.**] Vomiting food soon after eating, [**Bry.**] *The least emotion or exertion produces a flushed face.

**GELSEMIUM.** Diarrhœa, induced by *sudden depressing emotions, fright, grief, bad news,* [**Opi. Phos. ac.**] Stools the color of tea, dark-yellow. Desire to be quiet.

**GUM. GUTT.** Stools *yellow* or *green, mixed with mucus; very offensive.* Before and during stool, strong urging, with hot, pinching pain. *Loud gurgling as of water in the bowels,* [***Aloe.**] *Feeling of great relief after stool, as if an irritating substance had been removed, [reverse, **Verat. al.**] **Rapid expulsion of the stool.*

**HELLEBORUS.** *White, jelly-like mucous stools, with urging and tenesmus, [***Coloh. Podo.**] In protracted and dangerous cases, during dentition. Hydrocephalus. *Vomiting green or blackish* substances.

**HEPAR SULPH.** Painless or *chronic* diarrhœa. Stools *light yellow, green, slimy, undigested.* *Sour-smelling stools, [see **Rheum.**] Better after eating, [*worse,* ***Ars. Cro. t.**] Hot, sour regurgitation of food. *Feeling of fullness in stomach, with desire to loosen the clothing, [**Chin. Lyc.**] *After the abuse of mercury or quinine.*

**HYOSCYAMUS.** *Painless, yellow, watery, diarrhœa.* *Involuntary stools without consciousness, [**Bell. Carb. v. Rhus t. Sec.**] Diarrhœa during typhoid fever, and in lying-in women. *Worse from least mental excitement.*

**IODINE.** Especially in *chronic* diarrhœa. Stools *watery, foaming, whitish.* Patient feels better after eating, [**Hep. Lyc.**] *Restlessness, continually changing position. Emaciation, with good appetite, [**Calc. c.**]

**IPECAC.** Stools *grass-green, mucous; fermented.* Before and during stool, nausea and colic. *Vomiting yellow, green or jelly-like mucus, [**Verat.**] Paleness of face and coldness of extremities. **Flatulent colic.*

**IRIS VERS.** Painful, green, watery stools, worse at night, about 2 or 3 A. M. *Burning in rectum and anus after stool, [**Aloe. Gum. g.**] Periodical diarrhœa. Vomiting *sour fluid, with burning in mouth and fauces.* Gastric sick-headache. Loss of *taste* and appetite.

**JATRO. CUR.** *Profuse watery diarrhœa, gushing out like a torrent,* [Gum. g.] Noise as of a bottle of water being emptied in abdomen, [*Aloe.] Vomiting bile or watery albuminous substances.

**LEPTANDRIA.** Stools *black, papescent, tar-like, very fetid.* After stool, sharp, cutting pains and distress in umbilical region. Worse P. M. and evening. After exposure to wet, damp weather, [Dulc. Rhus.]

**LYCOPODIUM.** Chronic diarrhœa. Stools thin, brown, pale, fetid, preceded by chilliness in rectum. A feeling of great fullness in stomach after eating but little, [Chin.] Pain and tenderness of stomach, relieved by loosening the clothing. *Red sand in urine, [Phos.] Weak, dyspeptic persons. *Aggravation 4 to 8 P. M.

**MAGNESIA CARB.** *Sour-smelling* diarrhœa of children, [see Rheum.] *Stools resembling the scum of a frog-pond, or green, slimy and watery. Before stool, cutting, pinching pain in abdomen. *Sour vomiting,* [Nux. Puls.] Œdema of feet to the calves.

**MERCURIUS.** Stools *dark green, slimy, frothy* or *bloody;* also stools like *stirred eggs,* [Nux m.] *Frequent urging and *tenesmus* during and *after* stool. Cutting, pinching pain in abdomen, with chilliness, [Ars. Puls.] Violent thirst for cold drinks. Aphthæ and increased flow of saliva. *Sour-smelling night-sweat, particularly about the head, cold on forehead.* Worse at night and in hot weather.

**NUX MOS.** Stools *thin, yellow, like stirred eggs.* Before stool, cutting pain in abdomen. *Loss of appetite and *great drowsiness.* Colic worse after eating or drinking, [Ars.] The *tongue is very dry,* it sticks to the mouth. Worse at night and in cool, damp weather.

**NUX VOM.** Frequent small, *watery, slimy, browish, mucous* stools. Colic and tenesmus before and during stool, with *relief after,* [Merc.] Dysenteric diarrhœa. *Symptoms *worse early in* morning. *Nausea and sour, bitter vomiting. After use of quack nostrums.

**PHOSPHORUS.** Chronic, *painless* diarrhœa, worse in morning, [Podo.] Stools *undigested, watery, with little white flakes* or *lumps like sago.* Gradual loss of strength. *Paralysis of sphincter ani; anus remaining open, [Apis.] *Vomiting what has been drunk soon as it becomes warm in stomach. *Sleepy in daytime, particularly after meals.*

**PHOS. ACID.** *Painless* diarrhœa; stools *whitish-watery,* or yellowish; very offensive. Great rumbling in the bowels. *Diarrhœa, without apparent debility.* *Very indifferent, wants nothing, and cares for nothing. Frequent *emissions* of *pale, watery urine.* Profuse sweats at night.

**PODOPHYLLUM.** *Painless diarrhœa* or colic before and during stool. *Profuse watery stools,* with meal-like sediment;

also yellow mucous stools, *smelling like carrion*. *Before* stool, loud gurgling in bowels as of water, [***Aloe. *Gum. g.**] **During* stool prolapsus ani. Gagging or empty retching, [**Cro. t.**] Cramp in feet, calves, and thighs. *Always *worse in morning*, at night, and in hot weather.

**PULSATILLA.** Stools *greenish, yellowish, like bile.* *Very changeable stools, [**Sulph.**] Before stool, rumbling and cutting pain in bowels. *Diarrhœa, *worse at night*, from eating fruit or ice-cream, [fruit with milk, **Podo.**] Bitter taste after eating. *Craves cool, fresh air, *worse* in a warm room, [*better*, ***Ars. Rhus.**] White-coated tongue; loss of taste.

**RHEUM.** Stools *green, brown, fermented*, [**Ipe.**] *Sour-smelling diarrhœa of children, [***Mag. c. Rheum.**] Colic *before* and *during* stool, and *tenesmus* after, [**Merc.**] *The whole body has a *sour smell*, not removed by washing. Cutting colic, relieved by bending double, [**Colo.**] Worse after eating.

**RHUS TOX.** Stools *reddish* or *yellowish mucus*. Cutting colic *before* and *during* stool, with relief *after*. Involuntary stools at night while sleeping, [**Hyos. Puls.**] *Aggravation at night, particularly after midnight, and during *rest*.

**SECALE COR.** Painless diarrhœa. Stools *brown, watery*, or *slimy; discharged rapidly with great force*. Great exhaustion during and after stool. Vomiting without effort, with great weakness. Great anxiety, and burning at pit of stomach. **Aversion to heat*, or *to being covered up*.

**SULPHUR.** Stools very changeable, *yellow, brown, green, undigested*. **Early morning diarrhœa*, without pain, [**Rumex.**—With pain, **Aloe.**] Before stool, urging and cutting colic. *Constant heat on top of head, [*coldness*, **Verat.**] Sour or bitter vomiting. *Frequent weak, faint spells. Drowsy during the day, and wakeful at night. *After suppressed eruptions*, [**Bry.**]

**SULPHURIC AC.** Painless chronic diarrhœa, *with debility*, [see **Phos. ac.**] Stools *saffron-colored mucus, stringy, green, watery*. Coldness and relaxed feeling in the stomach. Sour eructations. *Sensation of tremor all over without trembling. Aphthæ, [**Ars. Merc.**]

**THUYA.** Copious, *pale-yellow, watery stools, discharged with great force; gurgling like water from a bung-hole*, [see ***Crot. t.**] Rapid exhaustion and *emaciation*. *Diarrhœa after vaccination.* Worse in morning, and after drinking coffee.

**VERAT. ALB.** Stools *profuse, watery, blackish, greenish, Severe pinching colic before* and during stool. *After stool, *great weakness* and empty feeling in abdomen, [**Sul. ac.**] *The suffering causes cold sweat to stand on forehead. Violent vomiting of frothy mucus. *Intense thirst for cold water. *Excessive weakness*, [**Ars.**] *Desire for fruits and acids.*

**HYGIENIC MEASURES.** Persons subject to diarrhœa should observe strict hygienic and dietetic rules. Light exercise in open air, suitable clothing, flannel next the skin, tepid sponge baths, regular habits and mental quietude, the best preventives.

**AUXILIARIES.** During an attack, patient should assume horizontal position and rest mind and body. Remove all discharges at once. Provide for free ventilation. Apply *warm fomentations* to bowels if they are tender and painful.

**DIETETICS.** Eat sparingly—little and often—the better plan. Well-boiled rice, oatmeal gruel, farina, good fresh milk, mutton broth, thickened with flour or rice, fresh crackers broken into milk or made into gruel, barley water, and in some cases beef-tea, will be found the most appropriate diet.

In *chronic cases*, a more generous diet should be allowed. Milk one of the best articles. Tender beef, mutton, chickens, soft boiled eggs, and good ripe fruits may be taken.

---

## DIPHTHERIA.

**TREATMENT.** *Leading indications.*

**ACONITE.** In forming stage, [**Bell.**] Dry, hot skin and very quick pulse. *Dark redness* of fauces, velum palati, and tonsils, [*bright* redness, ***Bell.**] Burning, fine piercing sensation in throat. *Great fear and anxiety of mind, with nervous excitability.

**APIS MELLIFICA.** Great debility from beginning. The membrane assumes at once a dirty-grayish color, [*dark* color, **Phyto.**] Puffiness around the eyes. **Pain in the ears when swallowing,* [**Lach.**] *Stinging pains in the affected parts. Itching, stinging eruption on the skin. Crawling, as if going to sleep in both arms; *lower limbs feel paralyzed, weakness of sight.*

**ARSENICUM.** Great anguish, extreme restlessness, and fear of death. Fetid breath, and viscid, foul discharge from the nostrils. *Constant desire for cold drinks, but can take but little, [**Apis.**] *Great and increasing prostration. All worse about midnight.

**ARUM TRIPH.** Throat raw and sore, as if excoriated. Putrid odor from mouth. *Burning, *ichorous discharge from nose, excoriating nostrils and upper lip,* [see ***Kali b. Nit. ac.**] Lips sore and swollen, skin peels off; patient very restless and fretful. Submaxillary glands swollen.

**BELLADONNA.** *In forming stage.* Great dryness of fauces; tonsil bright red and swollen. *Very restless, feels drowsy, yet cannot sleep. *Starts in his sleep, or jumps suddenly up in bed. Congestion to head, with throbbing of carotids; eyes injected; delirium.

**BROMINE.** The disease commences in larynx and rises into the fauces, [see **Nit. ac.**] In some cases it extends into the larynx, producing a croupy cough and rattling of mucus. *Suffocating cough, with hoarse, whistling, croupy sound, [see **Kali b.**]

**CALC. CHLOR.** Corroding, watery, nasal discharge. Fauces red, sore and covered with membrane. *Foul breath.* Cervical glands swollen, with engorgement of surrounding cellular tissue. Paroxysms of suffocation. Great prostration, [*Prepare fresh.*]

**CANTHARIDES.** Burning and dryness in mouth, extending to throat and pharynx. Extreme prostration, sinking, death-like turns. *Constant desire to urinate, passing but a few drops at a time.

**CAPSICUM.** Burning and soreness in mouth and throat. Congested appearance of mucous membrane. Fauces partially covered with diphtheric deposit. Sensation of *constriction on swallowing.* Heat and throbbing sensation in head. Rapid pulse, vertigo, and bleeding at nose. *Chilliness in back.

**CARBOLIC ACID.** *Low form of fever;* absence of pain. *Great accumulation of deposits, with terrible fetor. Excessive prostration and thready pulse.

**KALI BICHRO.** Fauces inflamed, and more or less covered with a dirty yellow deposit, forming pseudo-membrane. Yellow brown fur on tongue. *Hoarse, croupy cough, with expectoration of *stringy* mucus, *the disease spreading to larynx.* Deep-eating ulcers in fauces. Tough, stringy discharge from nose, [see **Arum t.**] Swelling of parotid glands.

**LACHNANTHES.** *White ulcers on tonsils,* very little fever, slight prostration; able to take nourishment, [similar to **Bell. Lach. Lyc.**] *Very stiff and painful neck, drawn to one side.

**LACHESIS.** The disease mostly appears on *left* side first, [see **Lyc.**] Throat greatly swollen internally and externally. Discharge from nose and mouth of a fetid, excoriating fluid, [**Aru. t.**] *Can bear nothing to touch larynx or throat—it is so painful. *Fauces covered with diphtheric membrane.* *Patient worse after sleeping, [**Apis.**]

**LYCOPODIUM.** * *Worse or beginning* on *right* side. Brownish red appearance of fauces. Stitching pains in throat when swallowing. *Nose stopped up.* *Widely dilated nostrils with every inspiration. Awakens from sleep very cross and irritable. *Red sand in urine. Worse from *warm* and better from *cold* drinks, [**Lach.**]

**MERC. CYANURET.** *Putrid diphtheria, [**Ars. Nit. ac.**] The disease comes on suddenly, extends all over mouth, fauces, pharynx and larynx. Exudation grayish, leathery and putrid. Laryngo-tracheal whistling, [**Kali b.**] Parotid and submaxillary glands swollen, [**Arum t. Merc. io.**] *Incessant salivation;* great prostration.

**MERC. IOD. RUB.** *Pseudo-membranous deposits on tonsils, uvula, velum palati, and pharynx. Tongue coated, thick, yellow, dirty. Tonsils much swollen, with great difficulty in swallowing. *Breath very offensive. *Expector-*

*ation of tough, fetid saliva.* Hoarse breathing. Swelling of parotid and submaxillary glands.

**NITRIC ACID.** Spreading ulcers in mouth and throat. Putrid-smelling breath. Swelling of submaxillary and parotid glands, [**Merc. io.**] Corroding discharge from nose. Dry, barking cough; intermittent pulse. *Strong-smelling urine, like that of horses. *Sore throat, extending into nose, with profuse, thin, purulent discharge.

**PHYTOLACCA.** *Fauces and tonsils highly inflamed, and covered with dark-colored pseudo-membrane. Excessive fetor of breath. *Deglutition almost impossible. Great prostration.* When rising up in bed, gets faint and dizzy, [**Bry.**] *Violent aching in back and limbs.

For *paralysis* following diphtheria, **Gel. Lach. Nux. Phos. Plumb. Rhus. Zinc.**

**HYGIENIC PRECAUTIONS.** Place patient in large upper room, that can be *well ventilated.* Exclude children and all others not absolutely needed. *Disinfect* all sputa, discharges and soiled linen, [see article "**Sick Room.**"] Change patient's clothing and bed-linen frequently. Keep face and hands clean as possible. Temperature of room 70°, and atmosphere moist. Look after drainage about premises.

**LOCAL TREATMENT.** Dilute **Alcohol,** [ ʒji aquæ ℥j] used as a gargle or by spray, one of best applications. **Liq. calcis chlor.** [ ʒj to ℥jii aquæ] as gargle or spray is highly extolled. **Carbolic ac.** [gtt. v. aq. ferv. ℥j] as a gargle [when being used internally] will be found valuable. Where larynx is involved, and in croupal diphtheria, inhaling vapor of **Ammonia**, or tincture **Iodine**, is efficacious in some cases. Inhaling vapor of *slacking* lime, or *lime-water* by atomizer, is worthy of trial. Burning a mixture of *tar* and *turpentine* near the patient's bed, and the vapors inhaled, is highly commended; will soon *detach* the *false membrane,* and relieve the patient. It is also a good *Disinfectant.*

**DIETETICS.** Cold water to allay thirst, or bits of ice to suck is very grateful. If patient has an appetite, indulge it. Beef-tea, mutton or chicken broth may be taken liberally. Good fresh milk is an excellent article of diet in this disease. Ice-cream or water-ice may be taken in moderate quantities at short intervals. No *alcoholic* stimulants whatever should be allowed, as they only *exhaust* the vital forces, and thereby lessen the chances of recovery.

---

## DYSENTERY.

**TREATMENT.** *Leading indications.*

**ACONITE.** Usually in beginning and when the days are *warm* and nights cool, [see **Colch.**] Stools frequent, small, bloody, or slimy. During stool cutting pains and tenesmus.

*Vertigo on rising up. General dry heat and *great restlessness.* *Fear of death, is afraid he will die.

**ALOES.** Stools *bloody, jelly-like mucus,* [white, jelly-like, ***Hell.**] *Before* stool, a sense of fullness and weight in pelvis, and pain around navel. *During* stool, *tenesmus and burning in rectum.* *Loud gurgling in bowels, like water running out of a bottle. *Large and prominent hemorrhoids.*

**ARNICA.** Dysentery caused by mechanical injuries. Stools *clear mucus* or *bloody, with tenesmus.* Bitter or putrid taste in mouth. *Putrid eructations, like bad eggs, [**Podo. Sulph.**] *Offensive breath.*

**ARSENICUM.** Stools *dark or blackish fluid, mixed with blood, of a putrid, foul smell;* involuntary, [see **Carb. v.**] *During* stool *tenesmus* and *burning* in the rectum. *Great anguish, restlessness, and fear of death. *Extreme thirst, drinks often, but little. Rapid prostration and sinking of the vital forces, [**Verat.**] Aggravation at *night* or *after eating* or *drinking.*

**BAPTISIA.** Stools *scant, bloody mucus. Before* and during stool, violent colicky pains in hypogastrium. During stool great tenesmus. *Soreness of the flesh and whole body, with chilliness. *The sweat, urine and stools are all extremely fetid, [**Carb. v.**]

**BELLADONNA.** Stools *greenish, slimy, bloody.* Great *tenesmus during* and *after* stool, [**Merc.**] *Clutching pains in abdomen, which appear suddenly, and cease as suddenly. *Pains relieved by stopping breath and bearing down. Abdomen hot and tender to pressure. *Sudden starting, and jumping during sleep. *Mouth and throat very dry, with little or no thirst.*

**BROMIUM.** *Stools painless, odorless, and like scrapings from intestines, [see **Canth.**] *Blind, painful* hemorrhoids internally, worse during and after stool.

**BRYONIA.** The disease was induced by getting overheated, or from taking cold drinks when the system was very warm, [**Acon.**] *Thin, bloody stools,* preceded by cutting colic. *Sitting up in bed causes nausea and vomiting. *The patient wants to keep very still. Aggravation in morning and from motion.

**CANTHARIDES.** Stools *white, or pale-reddish, like scrapings from intestines;* [see **Brom. Colch. Colo.**] also *bloody* stools. During and after stools, *burning at anus,* [**Aloe. Ars.**] *Frequent urging to urinate, with slight and painful discharge. High fever with burning and dryness of mouth, *burning thirst* or *no thirst at all. Anxious restlessness.*

**CAPSICUM.** Stools *bloody mucus, or mucus streaked with black blood.* *After stool, tenesmus and thirst, with shuddering after drinking. Tenesmus of bladder, [**Merc. cor.**] Distension of abdomen as if it would burst. *Chilliness in back. *Taste as of putrid water.

**CARBO VEG.** Mostly in advanced stages. Stools of *foul*

*blood and mucus; involuntary, smelling terribly.* *Great prostration and cold breath. *The patient wants more air and to be fanned, [**Bapt**.] Heat about the head. and cold perspiration on extremities. *After long-continued or severe acute disease.*

**CHAMOMILLA.** Stools frequent, *small, green,* or *white mucus,* smelling like bad eggs. Colic before and during stool. *Very impatient, can hardly answer one civilly. *Children are very fretful, must be carried. *One cheek red and hot, the other pale and cold, [**Acon. Nux.**] In first stages and during dentition.

**CHINA.** Suitable for weakly persons, and others who have lost much blood, and for dysentery in *marshy districts,* with intermittent symptoms. Stools *chocolate-colored, smelling putrid. Before* stool colic, relieved by bending double, [***Colo.**] Worse at night, and after a meal. Great weakness and inclination to sweat. *Patient worse every other day, [**Amb.**]

**COLCHICUM.** Stools *jelly-like mucus,* or *bloody, mingled with a skinny substance,* with *severe colic and tenesmus.* Also painless bloody stools, [**Ars. Colo. Sulph.**] During stool, spasms of sphincter ani, with shuddering in back. *Autumnal dysentery, when days are warm and nights cool, [**Acon.**] Œdema of feet.

**COLOCYNTH.** Stools *bloody mucus,* or *like scrapings,* [see **Canth.**] *Before* stool, cutting pain and great urging. * *Violent colicky pains, mostly around navel, causing patient to bend double.* Relief after every evacuation. Abdomen distended and painful to contact. Worse *after a meal;* from *fruit; vexation.*

**DIOSCOREA.** Stools like albumen, but lumpy, with straining and burning in rectum, and *sensation as if fæces were hot.* Before and during stool, severe pain in sacral region and bowels. The pains radiate upwards and downwards, until whole body becomes involved with spasms.

**DULCAMARA.** Stools *green mucus or bloody.* If the disease was induced by exposure to cold. *Symptoms all aggravated by every cold change in the weather. Dry heat of the skin, and much thirst.

**HAMAMELIS.** *Copious stools of dark blood, amounting to an actual hemorrhage. Suitable to persons troubled with varices, passive hemorrhages, etc.

**IPECAC.** Stools *bloody,* or *bloody mucus, fermented like frothy molasses.* Great pressing to stool, with griping and pinching about navel. *Much nausea and vomiting. Disgust and loathing of all kinds of food. No thirst, [**Puls.**] If caused by eating unripe, sour fruit.

**KALI BICHRO.** Stools blackish, watery, bloody, or jelly-like. *During* stool, painful urging and tenesmus. Gnawing pain about navel. *Tongue dry, smooth, red, and cracked. Much thirst, desire for acids.

**MAG. CARB.** Stools *bloody mucus,* or *green, frothy, like scum* *on frog-pond. Before* stool, cutting and pinching in abdomen. *During* and *after* stool *tenesmus*, [Merc.] Tongue coated dirty-yellow. Sour vomiting. In children during dentition.

**MERC. COR.** Stools *pure blood*, or *bloody mucus; green bilious*, followed by *slime tinged with blood. During* stool, painful pressing, *straining* and *tenesmus. Severe pains in the rectum*, continuing *after* the discharge. Almost constant cutting pain in abdomen, mostly around umbilicus. **Great tenesmus* of *bladder*, with scanty urine.

**MERC. SOL.** Stools *bloody mucus*, or *green, slimy, excoriating. Before* stool, violent and frequent urging. *During* and *after* stool, *violent tenesmus.* *Wants to remain a long time at chamber. Pinching and cutting colic, with chilliness, [*Bell. *Puls.] Prolapsus ani, [*Podo.] Profuse night sweats, particularly on head. All symptoms worse at night, and in damp, rainy weather.

**NITRIC ACID.** Stools profuse, bloody. *Before* stool, drawing, colicky pain, *During* stool, *tenesmus* and spasmodic contraction of anus, [anus remains *open*, **Phos.**] Long-lasting pains after stool, very exhausting. *Spreading ulcers in mouth, with fetid breath.

**NUX VOMICA.** Stools *thin, bloody mucus*, sometimes mingled with *lumps* of *fæcal matter*, [**Erig.**] *Before* stool, constant urging; backache. *During* stool, violent tenesmus, and cutting pain in hypogastrium, with desire to vomit. *After* stool, relief. *Persons of intemperate habits, or the victims of drugs. *Symptoms worse in morning.* *Patient very irritable, and wants to be alone.

**PHOSPHORUS.** Stools green, slimy or bloody. Painless dysentery, [**Hepar.**] *The anus remains open, as if paralyzed, [**Apis.**] Symptoms *worse in morning, and from lying on left side.* *Thirst for very cold drinks, which are ejected soon as they get warm in stomach.

**PODOPHYLLUM.** Stools *bloody and green mucus*, or *jelly-like mucus*, with little or no pain, [see **Colch.**] *Prolapsus ani* with stool. Children *toss their heads from side to side.* *Gagging or empty retching. Loud rumbling in bowels.

**PULSATILLA.** Stools *blood-streaked* mucus. Before stool, rumbling and cutting colic. During stool, chilliness and pain in the back, [see **Merc.**] Thick, yellow coat on the tongue, bitter taste. *Thirstlessness. *Worse towards evening and at night.

**RHUS TOX.** Stools reddish mucus or jelly-like. *Before* and *during* stool, cutting colic. *Pain which runs in streaks down the limbs with every evacuation. *Remission of the pains after stool, and from moving about.* After getting wet, [after taking cold, **Dulc.**]

**SULPHUR.** Stools green mucus or blood-streaked mucus; changeable, [**Puls.**] *Before* stool, cutting colic. After stool *tenesmus. Painful sensitiveness of abdomen, as if the internal parts were raw and sore.* *Weak, faint spells. After suppressed cutaneous eruptions, [Bry.] *Lean persons, who walk stooping, or who suffer from piles.

**AUXILIARY MEASURES.** Place patient *in bed* and enjoin quietude; have him use bed-pan to avoid getting up. Provide for *free ventilation.* Receive all discharges in porcelain vessel and *disinfect* them. See article **Sick Room.** Change clothing and bed linen daily. *Small* injections of clear starch, gum-water or white of egg beaten up in water, very beneficial. For the distressing *tenesmus* which occurs in some cases, a few drops of *Laudanum,* [3 to 10 drops, according to age of patient] added to the clyster, will afford prompt relief. Injections of *hot water* also beneficial. *Hot fomentations* to abdomen relieve pain and tenderness. Also *warm sitz-baths,* in which patient may remain five or ten minutes.

**DIETETICS.** Cold fresh water frequently excites pain and tenesmus, and should be taken in small quantities; it should be boiled before drinking. Rice-water, barley-water and gum-water most suitable beverages. The white of an egg beaten up in a pint of water and sweetened, is useful. All solid or irritating articles of food should be avoided. Well-cooked milk and flour, or gruel of farina, oatmeal or rice flour are allowable. Mutton broth thickened with rice boiled to a pulp, may be taken in some cases where patient desires it. *Sweet* ripe peaches, plums, grapes, blackberries, and whortleberries, freed of their seeds and hulls, the only fruits considered safe.

---

## DYSMENORRHŒA.

**TREATMENT.** *Leading indications.*

**AMM. CARB.** Menses premature and abundant, preceded by griping colic and loss of appetite. Discharge blackish, in clots, passing off with pains in the abdomen. Paleness of the face, sadness, and toothache.

**APIS MEL.** Discharge of scanty, slimy blood. *Suppressed menses, with congested or inflamed ovaries. Feeling of weight and heaviness in ovarian region. *Inflammation of right ovary, [Bell.—of the left, Lach.]

**BELLADONNA.** The pains precede the flow, with congestion to head and confusion of sight. Frightful visions and screaming. *Disposition to bite and tear things. Redness and bloatedness of face. *Strong *bearing down,* as if everything would escape through vulva, [Plat. *Sep.] *Pains come on suddenly and cease as suddenly. Discharge copious, and of a bright-red color.

**CACTUS.** Menses scanty and cease to flow when lying down. *Terrible pains, causing her to cry aloud and weep, [see Puls.] Pains come on periodically, mostly in evening.

*A feeling as if the heart was constricted. Palpitation worse when lying on left side.

**CALC. CARB.** Preceding the flow, swelling and tenderness of breasts, headache, colic, shiverings, and leucorrhœa. During the flow, cutting pain in abdomen, toothache, bearing down in genitals. *Feet cold and damp. *Scrofulous diathesis.*

**CAULOPHYLLUM.** *Spasmodic bearing-down pains, with scanty flow. Sympathetic cramps and spasms of adjacent organs, as bladder, rectum, bowels. *Membranous dysmenorrhœa, [**Cimi. Collin.**] After *suppressed menses,* [***Puls.**]

**CHAMOMILLA.** Pressure in uterus, resembling *labor-pains.* Discharge *dark-colored,* coagulated, with tearing pains in thighs, [**Cimi.**] Frequent desire to pass urine. Bloated red face, or *one cheek red, the other pale.* Hot perspiration about head. *Very impatient and snappish.

**CIMICIFUGA.** Scanty or profuse flow of coagulated blood. *Severe pains in back, down thighs, and through the hips of a *neuralgic charater.* Labor-like pains, with pressing down, [see **Cham.**] Hysteric spasms, cramps, tenderness of hypogastric region. Low-spirited and very sensitive.

**CONIUM.** Discharge scant, and brown in appearance. Previous to menses, breasts swell, become hard and painful, [**Calc. c.**] Pressing downwards in abdomen and drawing in legs. *Difficulty in voiding urine, it stops and starts repeatedly. *Aching pains about the heart, and vertigo when lying down or turning over in bed.

**GELSEMIUM.** *Dysmenorrhœa preceded* by sick headache, vomiting, red face, bearing down in abdomen and pain in back and limbs. *Sensation* as if *uterus were squeezed* by a hand. *Loss of voice during the menses.

**LILIUM TIG.** Burning, stinging, cutting, grasping in left ovary. *Pain extends across hypogastrium to groin, down leg. Menses dark, thick, smelling like lochia. Severe neuralgic pains in uterus, cannot bear slightest pressure or jar.

**NITRIC ACID.** Menses early, irregular, scanty, and like muddy water. *Cramp-like pains in abdomen, as if it would burst, with cructations.* *Violent pressing down in genitals, as if everything would protrude, [see **Bell.**] *Very *offensive* urine.

**NUX VOM.** Menses return too soon, discharge thick and clotted. Writhing pains, with nausea, or pains in back and loins. *Soreness across pubis as if bruised. Frequent desire to pass urine. Constipation, with frequent urging, hard, difficult stools. After use of drugs and nostrums.

**PHOSPHORUS.** Menses too early and scant. Very sleepy during flow. Stitches in mammæ, sour cructations, and vomiting sour substances. Great fermentation in abdomen.

Cutting in hypogastric région, chilliness, cold hands and feet. *Sensation of weakness and emptiness in abdomen. **Long, narrow*, difficult stools.

**PHYTOLACCA.** *Painful menstruation, especially in barren women, [**Phos.**] *Mammæ hard and painful.*

**PLATINA.** Menses *dark and clotted*, preceded by spasms, much bearing down, desire for stool, backache. *During the flow, pinching in abdomen, excruciating pains in uterus, twitchings, with screams.

**PULSATILLA.** Delayed menses, blood thick and black, flowing by fits and starts, with *chilliness*. Feeling of heaviness, as if from a stone in pelvic cavity. *Pains so violent she tosses about in all directions, with cries and tears, [**Cimi.**] Drawing sensation and numbness, extending down the thighs. *Vertigo on rising up, with chilliness. *Mild, tearful women. *Worse in a warm room.*

**SEPIA.** Menses too early and scant. Colicky pains and *great bearing down, obliging her to cross the limbs*, [see ***Bell.**] Before menses, leucorrhœa, excoriating the parts. *Painful sensation of emptiness in stomach. She weeps and complains, [**Ign.** ***Puls.**] Hard, knotty, difficult stools, with a sensation of *weight in the anus.*

**SULPHUR.** Discharge thick, black, and acrid. Violent pinching in abdomen, with heat, chilliness, and sort of epilepsy. *Constant heat in top of head, [*coldness*, ***Verat.**] *Frequent flashes of heat and weak, faint spells. Chronic eruptions. *Lean persons who walk stooping.*

**VIBUR. OPU.** *Spasmodic dysmenorrhœa. *Cramps in abdomen and legs. Excruciating colicky* pains in womb and lower part of abdomen, coming on suddenly, just preceding the menstrual flow, often lasting for hours. **Cimi.** and **Caul.** are closely allied to this remedy.

**LOCAL TREATMENT.** *Warm sitz-baths*, in which the patient may remain for fifteen or twenty minutes; *warm fomentations* applied to the hypogastric region, and hot bricks to the feet will be found of infinite value in this painful affection. Taking *copious* draughts of water *hot as can be borne*, will also be found very beneficial.

---

## DYSPEPSIA.—GASTRIC CATARRH.

**TREATMENT.** *Leading indications.*

**AMM. MUR.** Bitter eructations or tasting of food, [**Nux. Puls.**] *Regurgitation* of food or of bitter, sour water, [**Phos.** —*sweet water*, **Plumb.**] *Gnawing in stomach as from worms, [see **Puls.**—*gnawing in stomach when empty, relieved by eating*, **Lith. carb.**] Pain in stomach, *immediately after eating.* *Hard crumbling stools, difficult to expel.

**ANACARDIUM.** *Symptoms disappear *while eating*, and return soon after, [better *after* eating, **Hepar.**] Pain as if a *blunt plug* were pressed into the intestines. *Constant desire to eat, which gives temporary ease.

**ANTIMONIUM.** The disease was caused by overloading stomach. Tongue *coated white.* *Eructations tasting of ingesta, [**Chin. *Puls.**] *Stomach weak, very easily disordered.* Watery stools, mingled with hard lumps.

**ARNICA.** *After mechanical injuries, [**Bry. Rhus.**] Sore, bruised feeling in stomach. *Eructations, tasting like bad eggs, [**Sep. Sulph.**] Sense of fullness in pit of stomach. Tongue coated yellow. After meals, inclination to vomit. Bitter or putrid taste.

**ARSENICUM.** Derangement of stomach from ice-cream, fruit, and acid things. *Nausea and vomiting after eating or drinking. Heat or *burning in stomach,* [**Nux. *Phos.**] *Intense thirst, drinking often, but little at a time. *Anxious restlessness.* *Pressure as of a stone in the stomach, [**Bry. *Nux.**] *Exhausting* diarrhœa.

**BOVISTA.** Pressure and fullness in pit of stomach. *Sensation of a lump of ice in stomach, [*coldness,* **Ars. Phos.**] Tension in the temples; mental anxiety.

**BRYONIA.** Dyspepsia in hot weather, or from drinking cold water when overheated. Loathing of food, even smell of it is intolerable. *Soreness of the stomach. *Frequent eructations, especially after a meal.* *Everything tastes *bitter,* [**Puls.**; tastes *sour,* **Chin. Nux.**] Food is thrown up immediately after eating. *Splitting headache.* *Constipation, stools dry and hard. *Is very irritable.

**CALC. CARB.** Pressure as of a weight in stomach. *Cannot bear anything tight around waist, [***Nux. *Lyc.**] Sour taste. Vomiting food, which tastes sour. Aversion to meat and warm food, with desire for dainties. *Dull, stupefying headache.* *Cold, damp feet. *Profuse menstruation.* Cannot sleep after 3 A. M., [***Nux.**] Stools large, hard, and sometimes only partially digested.

**CARBO VEG.** Frequent eructations, affording temporary relief. The most innocent food disagrees. *Sensation as if stomach and abdomen would burst when eating or drinking, [see **Chin.**] Sour, rancid belchings, and burning in stomach. *Excessive flatulence, with tendency to diarrhœa. After debauching, [**Nux.**]

**CHAMOMILLA.** *Painful bloatedness of epigastrium in morning, with a sensation as if the contents were rising to chest. *Aching pain in stomach and under short ribs. Bitter taste, with bilious vomiting. *Very impatient and cross.

**CHELIDONIUM.** Aching, gnawing pain in stomach, aggravated by pressure, but *relieved* by *eating,* [see **Puls.**] *Prefers hot drinks and hot food, [**Ars.**] Very irregular palpitation of the heart. Stools like sheep's dung, [**Ruta.**]

**CHINA.** *Abdomen feels full and tight, as if stuffed, eructations without relief, [see **Arg. n.**] *Aversion to every kind of nourishment. Craves wine or sour things. Eructations tasting of the food, [**Ant.** ***Puls.**] Debility, with desire to lie down *after every meal.* After loss of blood, or exhausting illness. Indisposed to work.

**GELSEMIUM.** Feeling of emptiness and weakness in stomach and bowels. Burning in stomach, extending up to mouth. *Symptoms all worse from sudden emotions, fright, grief, or bad news. *False hunger—a kind of gnawing in stomach, [**Ars. Nux.**]

**HEPAR S.** The stomach is easily disordered, despite the utmost care, [**Carb. v.**] Craving for acids, [**Bry. Chin. Nux.**] Nausea and eructations, without taste or smell. Putrid or metallic taste. *Accumulation of mucus in throat. Hard, difficult stools. Risings in œsophagus, as if he had been eating sour things.

**HYDRASTIS.** *Dull, aching pain in stomach, which causes a very weak, faint feeling. Burning pain in umbilical region. Eructations of *sour fluid*, [setting teeth on edge, ***Robin.** ***Sul. ac.**] *A feeling of goneness in region of stomach, with violent palpitation of heart. *Stools lumpy, covered with mucus.*

**IGNATIA.** *Dyspepsia, with great nervous prostration, caused by mental depression. *Full of grief, with a weak, empty feeling in stomach, [see **Hydras.**] Painful bloating of stomach after every meal, [**Chin. Lyc.**] *Gnawing, cutting pain* in stomach. *Hemorrhoids*, the tumors prolapse with every stool.

**LYCOPODIUM.** Feeling of great fullness and heaviness in stomach after a meal. *After taking a mere swallow of food, feels full up to throat, [see **Chin.**] *Constant sense of fermentation in abdomen, like yeast working, [**Carb. v. Phos.**] *Much rumbling, particularly in left hypochondria.* Distressing pain in back before urinating. *Red sand in the urine. Constipation, stools hard, scant, and passed with great difficulty.

**MERCURIUS.** *Very sensitive about pit of stomach and abdomen, [**Bry. Nux.**] When sitting, the food feels like a stone in stomach. *Pressure in epigastrium*, eructations and heartburn after a meal. Aversion to solid food, meat, warm food, with desire for refreshing things. Much salivation, with saltish, metallic taste.

**NUX VOMICA.** Putrid or bitter taste early in morning, [***Puls.**] **Frequent sour eructations*, [see **Hydras.**] *Region of stomach very sensitive to pressure. *Cramp-like pains in stomach, with pressure, particularly after a meal.* *Waterbrash, especially of drunkards, [see **Puls.**] *Very irritable, and wishes to be alone. Stools *large, hard*, and passed with difficulty. After *rich* or *highly-seasoned food*, drastic medicine, or debauching. Worse *after eating.*

**PHOSPHORUS.** Regurgitation of food, without nausea, comes up in mouthfuls. *Food comes up soon as swallowed. *Water is thrown up soon as it becomes warm in stomach. *Long, narrow, hard stools.

**PULSATILLA.** Tongue *coated white*, or *yellow, with bad taste in morning.* *Eructations after a meal, tasting of food last eaten, [**Chin. Nux. Sulph.**] *Waterbrash.* Gnawing distress in stomach when it is empty, [**Lith. car.**] *Beating in region of stomach,* [**Sep.**] All kinds of fatty food, pork, pastry, ice cream, etc., disagree, [***Ipe.**] *Vertigo when stooping or rising from a sitting posture. Chilliness and flashes of heat. Nightly diarrhœa.

**ROBINIA.** Great *acidity of the stomach;* soon after eating, food turns sour. Constant sense of weight in stomach, [see **Ars.**] *Intensely *sour fluid* rises from stomach, setting teeth on edge, [***Sulph. ac.**] Burning pain in stomach and between the shoulders. Constant frontal headache. Desire for stool, but only flatus is passed.

**RUTA GRAV.** *Dyspepsia from lifting heavy weights. Burning or *gnawing* in stomach, [see **Puls.**] Cannot eat meat, it causes eructations and itching of the skin. *Frequent urging to stool, with protrusion of rectum, [**Ign. Nux.**] Hard, scanty stool, almost like sheep's dung.

**SEPIA.** Pulsations in stomach during a meal. *Great weakness of digestion. Sour or bitter eructations. *Dyspepsia with amenorrhœa, [**Puls.**] Pressure on stomach as of a stone. *Yellowness of face, with a streak across the nose resembling a saddle. *Hard, knotty, difficult stools, with a sense of weight in anus.

**SILICEA.** Bitter taste in the morning. Nausea, especially in morning or after a meal. *Water tastes badly; vomits after drinking. Pains in stomach, with *waterbrash.* Aversion to *warm* cooked food, desires cold things, [reverse, **Ars.**] No appetite, but great thirst. *Constipation, the *stool recedes after having been partly expelled.*

**STAPHISAGRIA.** Sensation as if the stomach were hanging down relaxed, [**Ipe.**—as if balanced up and down, **Phos. ac.**] *Extreme hunger, even when the stomach is full of food. Craves wine, brandy, tobacco.

**SULPHUR.** Sour eructations and much troublesome acidity in stomach. Region of stomach sensitive to contact. *Feels very faint and weak about* 11 A. M.; *must have something to eat. Regurgitation of food and drink,* [see **Puls.**] *Frequent weak, faint spells. *Burning heat on top of head. *Early morning diarrhœa.

**SULPHURIC AC.** Great debility. Constriction of the throat. **Sour risings which set teeth on edge,* [***Robinia.**] Cold, relaxed feeling in the stomach.

For *aching or burning pains in the stomach, with great distension:* **Arn. Ars. Bell. Phos.**

*Sour stomach, with sour belching and taste; heart-burn; gulping up and vomiting sour matter:* ***Calc. c. Carb. v. Chin. Kali c. *Nux v. Phos. Sulph.**

*Sour stomach always after eating:* **Bry. *Calc. c. Chin. Kali c. *Nux m. *Nux v. Phos. Puls. Sep. Sulph.**

*Rancid belching:* **Carb. v. Mag. m. Puls. Sulph.**

*Foul belching:* **Arn. Ars. Chin. Ferr. Merc. Phos. Sep.**

*Bitter taste, bitter belching, bitter vomiting:* **Ars. *Bry. Cham. *Nux. *Puls. Verat.**

*Total loss of appetite:* **Ars. Chin. Nat. m. Nux. Sep.**

*Ravenous hunger:* **Calc. c. Chin. Nat. m. Nux. Phos.**

*Regurgitation of undigested food:* ***Am. m. Bry. Con. Nux v. *Puls. Sulph.**

*Waterbrash:* **Ars. Calc. Natr. m. *Nux v. *Phos. Sep. Sulph.**

**CLINICAL REMARKS.** Prominent among the causes of dyspepsia are, *mental anxiety; irregular habits; overeating;* the use of *tobacco, alcoholic drinks* and *drug medication.* The first prerequisite in the treatment of the disease, therefore, is removal of the primary cause, to accomplish which, will often be found a difficult matter. Kindly advice should enter largely into the treatment, and the patient encouraged in all laudable efforts to better his own condition. He should maintain a cheerful state of mind, and not brood over his sufferings. He should observe regular habits; avoid all excesses; take moderate out-doors exercise; bathe regularly, use the flesh-brush vigorously, and sleep in a cool room with an abundance of fresh air.

**AUXILIARY MEASURES.** In cases where there seems to be a deficiency of gastric juice, and the stomach is unable to digest the simplest food, pure *Pepsin,* [3 to 5 grains] taken half an hour before each meal, will have a salutary effect. If the bowels more especially are the seat of disorder, *Pancreatin* will be found the most appropriate remedy. "Dyspepsia due to sedentary habits and intense thought, a teaspoonful of *Wine of Coca* after each meal will act like magic."—DR. WINSLOW.

**DIETETICS.** The diet is of paramount importance. It should be nutritious, easily digested, and taken in moderate quantities. Food known to *disagree* should not be taken, and the habit of drinking at *meal-time* avoided, but in the mornings and on retiring at night, a glass of *cold* water may be drank. All vinous or fermented liquors should be discarded.

Foods must be tested; what agrees with one will not always agree with others. A milk diet with oat-meal porridge, cracked wheat, and corn-meal mush suit some, while others cannot digest milk. Buttermilk is excellent in most cases of indigestion. Of meats. mutton, beef, chicken, game and fresh eggs the most suitable; while pork, veal, canned or salt meats should be avoided. Of vegetables, baked potatoes mashed, with cream, *fresh* tomatoes well cooked, beans and peas, will be found to give the most desirable results. Of fruits, peaches, grapes, blackberries, strawberries, prunes, oranges and sweet apples, thoroughly ripe, are seldom harmful.

Food should be taken at regular intervals, eaten slowly and *thoroughly masticated*. The patient should engage in some useful employment or pleasurable amusement that will divert his attention and remove the mental causes that produced or tends to perpetuate the affection.

---

## ECZEMA.

(*Vesicular Eruptions.*)

**THERAPEUTICS.** *Leading indications.*

**ANACARDIUM.** *Eruption of little blisters, itching excessively; cannot sleep on account of the itching. Great weakness and loss of memory. Nervous females and old people.

**ANTIMO. CRUD.** The vesicles are surrounded by a red areola, with itching. Eruptions about the nose and eyes, neck and shoulder and back of ears. *Sore, cracked or crusty nostrils. Thick milky-white coating on tongue, [***Bry. Nux.**] *Alternate diarrhœa and constipation.

**ARSENICUM.** **Dry, scaly* eruptions, with *nightly burning* or terrible itching. Eruption on face or extremities, with corrosive discharge, [***Merc. Rhus.**] *Very restless at night. Water disagrees. *Better in a warm room* and from warm applications, [**Sil.**]

**BARYTA CARB.** *Scrofulous children with swollen lymphatics, [***Cal. Merc. *Sulph.**] Eruption *moist*, itching, burning, and pricking. *Enlargement of tonsils, with chronic sore throat. *Falling off of the hair*, [**Rhus. Staph.**] Eyes inflamed; takes cold easily.

**BELLADONNA.** Diffused *redness of the skin*, burning, itching and sensitive to touch. Eruptions during dentition. Sanguine plethoric temperament.

**BOVISTA.** *Moist vesicular eruption, with formation of thick crusts, [**Lyc. *Rhus.**] Eruption appears in warm weather and during full moon, [see **Clem.**] Flabby skin; fetid sweat.

**CALC. CARB.** **Scrofulous diathesis*, [see **Bary.**] Eruption *moist or dry*, with thick crusts, burning and itching. *Unhealthy, ulcerative skin, [**Graph. *Hepar. Sulph.**] Chronic form of the disease, [**Ars. Sulph.**] *Cold feet, as if he had on damp stockings.

**CANTHARIS.** *Watery vesicles* on an inflamed base, with more burning than itching, *Complicated with urinary difficulties.* Perspiration smells like urine.

**CLEMATIS.** *Moist eczema*, itching terribly, [see **Rhus**] The vesicles break and tend to ulceration. Eruption on neck and occiput, [**Petro.**] *The eruption looks inflamed during the increasing and *dry* during the decreasing moon. Worse from washing in cold water.

**CROTON TIG.** *Scarlet redness of the skin, with rash-like vesicles. *Itching followed* by *painful burning.* Irritation and swelling of submaxillary glands.

**DULCAMARA.** Eruption of itching vesicles, ceasing to itch after scratching. The vesicles exude a watery fluid and become covered with a crust. *Scrofulous subjects with glandular enlargements. *Symptoms all worse by a cold change in the weather.

**GRAPHITES.** Eczema, with profuse serous exudations, in blondes inclined to obesity. *The eruption oozes a glutinous *sticky* fluid, [comp., **Nat. m.**] *Rawness in bend of limbs, neck, and behind the ears. *Very dry skin,* never perspires, [**Kali c.**] Great liability to take cold.

**HEPAR S.** Eczema, spreading by means of new pimples appearing just beyond the old parts. *Moist eruption,* burning and itching after scratching; sore to touch. *Unhealthy skin, every little injury suppurates.

**KALI CARB.** Eruption dry at first, but when scratched exudes a moisture. *Dry skin,* [**Graph.**] Aged persons.

**LYCOPO.** Thick crusts, with fetid secretion underneath, [see **Rhus.**] Eruption moist, suppurating, itching violently, and bleeding easily after scratching.

**NATRUM MUR.** Eruption in bend of joints, behind the ears, on back of head, neck, and in border of hair, [see **Graph.**] *Moist eruption, with gluey discharge, [***Graph.**] Great rawness and soreness of skin.

**PETROLEUM.** Moist eruptions, with great itching and much oozing after scratching. Obstinate, dry eruption on genitals and perinæum; chronic form, worse on occiput. Unhealthy skin, every little injury ulcerates.

**RANUNC. BUL.** *Vascular eruption on face in clusters. The parts *smart* as if scalded.

**RHUS TOX.** *Surface raw, excoriated, thick crusts, oozing and offensive. Incessant itching, burning, and tingling of the parts; after scratching, burning. Better from *moving the affected parts* and from *warmth* in general. Worse in wet or damp weather.

**SEPIA.** *Itching pimples in the bends of joints, with soreness, [see **Graph.**] Itching often changes to burning when scratching, [see **Rhus.**] *Scurfy, humid herpes,* with itching and burning. Suitable to pregnant and nursing females.

**STAPHISAGRIA.** Offensive humid vesicles, especially on head and ears of children. Scalp very sensitive. Scratching sometimes changes the locality of the itching. Skin peels off, and hair falls out, [see **Baryt.**]

**SULPHUR.** *Scrofulous subjects.* *Dry, scaly, unhealthy skin. Eruption on head and behind ears, dry, offensive, scabby, with cracks, easily bleeding. *Voluptuous itching, with soreness after scratching. After *suppressed eruptions*, or the *drying up of old sores.*

**THUYA.** Dry, sealy eruptions on head, temples, eyebrows, ears, and neck, with itching, tingling, biting. *Skin sensitive to touch, *burning after scra'ching*, [see **Rhus.**] Dryness of skin, *sweat only on uncovered parts.* Bad effects of vaccination.

**VIOLA TRICO.** *Eczema, especially on face of infants.* *Eruption, the character of humid tetter, discharging a viscid pus. The crusts are of a brownish-yellow color, and the eruption itches violently, scratching gives temporary relief.

**LOCAL MEASURES.** The intense itching may be relieved by mixing five drops *Croton Oil* with one ounce of *Glycerine*, and rubbing it into the parts two or three times a day. The *Tr. Rhus tox.* and *Glycerine* may be used in same way, especially when this remedy is being administered internally at same time. A solution of *Bicarbonate of Soda*, [half an ounce to four ounces of water] applied to the parts is also efficient in allaying the itching.

In *Chronic* cases, bathe the parts well with *warm* water and mild soap, and when dry anoint with *Cosmoline.*

Persons suffering from *eczema* should refrain from all rich or highly seasoned food, and discard all spirituous and malt liquors.

---

## ENTERITIS.

(*Inflammation of the Bowels.*)

**THERAPEUTICS.** *Leading indications.*

**ACONITE.** In early stage, presenting a high *inflammatory* fever, dry, hot skin, and full, frequent pulse. Mouth and tongue dry, with intense thirst. *Abdomen swollen and tender to touch*, [**Bell. Bry.**] *Cutting, burning, tearing pains in umbilical region, aggravated by least pressure. *Great fear and anxiety of mind, with nervous excitability.

**ANTIMO. CRUD.** Enteritis from disordered stomach. *Milky-white tongue, [**Arn. *Bry. Nux.**] Vomiting, followed by great languor, drowsiness, loathing, and desire for cooling things. *Violent cutting pain, as if the bowels would be cut to pieces, with watery diarrhœa.

**ARNICA.** After *mechanical injuries.* Putrid taste, with putrid smell from mouth. Pains come in paroxysms and obstruct respiration. *Sore, aching pains as if from a bruise. *Everything on which he lies feels too hard, [**Bapt.**] Involuntary urination.

**ARSENICUM.** After chilling the stomach by taking cold things. *Burning in abdomen, with cutting pains, *worse after eating or drinking.* **Great prostration, restlessness, and* *intense thirst.* Vomiting immediately after eating or drinking, [Bry.] Usually in last stage.

**BELLADONNA.** Great *heat and tenderness* of abdomen, *can't bear least jar of bed.* *Violent contractive or clutching pains in bowels. *Pains which appear suddenly, and cease as suddenly. Congestion to the head, with throbbing carotids, [Acon.] *Face flushed, eyes red and sparkling. *Great intolerance to noise and light. Starting and jumping during sleep. Sleepiness, but cannot sleep, [Opi.] Almost constant *moaning.*

**BRYONIA.** Enteritis, with hard swelling around umbilicus. *Stitching or cutting in bowels, worse from least motion, [see Bell.] *Lies perfectly still, don't want to move. *Cannot sit up on account of nausea and faintness. *Lips parched, dry, and cracked.* Great thirst for large draughts of water. Vomiting immediately after eating or drinking, [*Ars.] Very *irritable,* everything makes him angry. *Delirium, thinks he is not at home.*

**CANTHARIS.** Heat and burning in abdomen, which is very *sensitive to pressure.* Cutting, burning pains through the bowels, [Acon. Ars.] *Violent, burning thirst, with aversion to all drinks. *Tenesmus of bladder, with ineffectual efforts to urinate. Stools pale-reddish mucus, like scrapings from intestines. *Anxious restlessness.*

**HYOSCYAMUS.** Enteritis, with typhoid symptoms. *Stupor, with incoherent speech. Tongue brown, dry and cracked, [Rhus.] *Unconsciousness, with involuntary stools, and emissions of urine,* [Rhus.] *Desire to uncover and remain naked. *Abdomen distended, with pain when touched.*

**IPECAC.** *Cutting, pinching, around the umbilicus, as if grasped with a hand; worse from motion. **Constant and continual nausea,* [Tart. e. *Verat.] Diarrhœa, stools green, fermented, or like frothy molasses.

**MERCURIUS.** Abdomen swollen, hard and *painful to contact.* Cutting, stabbing pains in bowels, accompanied by chilliness, [Ars.] *Green or bloody mucous stools, with violent tenesmus. *Profuse perspiration affording no relief. Pale, wretched complexion. Foul smell from mouth; vomiting bitter mucus. *Restless sleep, with moaning.*

**VERAT. ALB.** Burning in abdomen as from hot coals, [Ars.] Abdomen distended, very sensitive. *Vomiting, with continuous nausea and great prostration. Vomiting thin, *blackish* or yellowish substances. *Cold sweat, particularly on forehead. *Sudden sinking of strength, with almost imperceptible pulse.*

**AUXILIARY MEASURES.** The patient should occupy a well *ventilated* room, with a uniform temperature of 65°. The bed should be a soft mattress, with light coverings, and the patient kept *quiet* as possible. *Hot fomentations* applied to the tender, painful abdomen, will have a happy effect. They should be large enough to embrace the greater part of the abdomen, covered with oiled silk or dry flannel, and frequently changed. *Linseed poultices*, applied hot, valuable in some cases.

**DIETETICS.** For the intense thirst, small draughts of fresh water may be taken at short intervals. Bits of ice swallowed, will often arrest the vomiting. In first stage of disease, little or no food should be taken except thin gruel, barley-water or mucilaginous drinks. As convalescence advances, mutton or beef-broth, beef-tea, arrowroot, tapioca and other farinaceous articles may be taken. But until all traces of inflammation have subsided no solid food should be allowed.

---

## ENURESIS.

(*Incontinence of Urine.*)

**THERAPEUTICS.** *Leading indications.*

**BELLADONNA.** Women or children with blue eyes, light hair, fine complexion. Starting, restlees sleep. *Involuntary urination, consequent upon paralysis of sphincter muscles.

**CAUSTICUM.** Involuntary passage of urine when coughing or sneezing, [Puls.] *Wetting bed in first sleep, [Sep.] Children with delicate skin.

**CINA.** Involuntary urination, especially at night. *Suitable to children troubled with worms in the intestines. Restless sleep at night.

**CONIUM.** Frequent micturition at night, the urine cannot be retained. Wetting bed at night. Especially suitable to old men. *During micturition, flow intermits.

**NUX VOMICA.** Where the weakness has been caused by use of intoxicating drinks, and intemperate habits. *Paralysis of bladder, urine dribbles.

**PHOS. ACID.** If self-pollution or solitary vice has been the cause of weakness. Involuntary urination. Great indifference to the affairs of life.

**PULSATILLA.** Urine discharged by drops when sitting or walking. *Involuntary urination when coughing and during sleep, [Rhus t.] Mild, tearful disposition.

**RHUS TOX.** Involuntary discharges of urine at night, or while sitting, or when at rest. Gouty or rheumatic subjects.

**SEPIA.** Incontinence of urine at night, especially in first sleep, [see Caust.] *The urine is very offensive, and deposits a clay-colored sediment which adheres to the chamber.

**SULPHUR.** *Wetting bed at night*, copious discharge. Suitable to *persons* of a *scrofulous* habit, and others who suffer from chronic cutaneous eruptions.

**AUXILIARY MEASURES.** Children and others troubled with incontinence of urine at night should be instructed to retain the urine long as possible during the day. They should sleep in a cold room, on a *hard mattress*, with light covering; drink but little in the after part of the day, and always urinate just before getting into bed. All acid fruits, melons, canteloupes and stimulating drinks should be avoided.

A *cold sitz bath*, 65°, for five or ten minutes before retiring will be found very beneficial. Cool sponge-baths, and the vigorous application of the flesh-brush, every night, will have a salutary effect.

---

## EPILEPSY.

This singular malady, whose pathology is still unsettled, is characterized by sudden loss of consciousness, accompanied with convulsions. The paroxysms occur at irregular intervals. After one attack, months may intervene before another, or they may recur in a few days, or several times a day.

**PROGNOSIS.** The prognosis is most unfavorable. In a majority of cases, the disease tends to become confirmed and, as a rule, a more frequent recurrence of the paroxysms.

**THERAPEUTICS.** *Leading remedies.*

**AMYL NITRITE.** This remedy will often ward off a *threatened* attack. Put ten drops in a small phial, on a little cotton, and let patient inhale when an attack is threatened. Inhalations of **Camphor** will have a like effect.

**ARGENT. NITR.** Cerebral epilepsy, [see **Bell.**] Pupils permanently dilated a day or two before the fit. From fright, during the menses, at night, [see **Bufo. Opi.**]

**BELLADONNA.** *Recent cases, with decided brain symptoms. Illusions of sight and hearing. Convulsions commence in upper extremities and extend to mouth, fauces and eyes. *Foam* at *mouth*, [**Hyos. Opi.**] Involuntary micturition and defecation, [**Hydro. ac.**] Young and sanguine subjects.

**BROMIDE OF POTASSIUM.** Has proved curative in many cases. It must be given in large and increasing doses. Fifteen grains twice or thrice daily, for an adult, to begin with. The doses should be increased, if paroxysms continue, and remedy be well borne. The medicine is to be continued for a year or longer. Should the paroxysms fail to recur for several months, the doses may be diminished, and at length suspended, to be resumed, if paroxysms return.

**BUFO.** Epilepsy *following onanism*, [**Nux v.**] Attacks occur mostly at change of the moon, at time of menses, in sleep, [see **Sili.**] Painful weariness of limbs.

**CALCARIA CARB.** Chronic cases, [**Sili.**] *Scrofulous

habit, [Sili.] Sudden attacks of vertigo; loss of *consciousness without convulsions.* Before the attack sense of something running in arm, or from stomach down through abdomen to feet. Nocturnal epilepsy, [Bufo. Opi. Sili.] *Cold damp feet.

**CAMPHOR.** Epileptic fits with stertorous breathing, red and bloated face, coma. Given early will often prevent or modify the spasm.

**CAUSTICUM.** *Recent and slight* cases, [see **Bell.**] Convulsions, especially on right side. During the spasm, copious discharge of urine, involuntary, [see **Bell.**] Idiotic condition before the attack.

**CICUTA VIROSA.** Attacks with swelling of stomach, as from violent spasms of diaphragm. Hiccough, screaming, redness of the face, suddenly becomes stiff and immovable.

**CUPRUM MET.** *Trembling, tottering and falling unconscious without a scream. Froth at mouth, body bent backwards, limbs abducted.

**HYDROCYANIC AC.** Recent cases, [see **Bell.**] Sudden complete loss of consciousness and sensation. Jaws clenched, teeth firmly set, froth at mouth. Involuntary discharge of fæces and urine, [**Bell. Nux.**] Frightful distortion of face and limbs.

**HYOSCYAMUS.** Epilepsy preceded by vertigo, sparks before the eyes, ringing in ears, hungry gnawing. During attack face purple, eyes projecting, shrieks, grinding teeth; urination. After attack, sopor, snoring.

**NUX VOMICA.** Aura epileptica, body bent backwards, with consciousness, [see **Cup.**] Limbs rigid and go to sleep. Fits excited by emotions, anger, indigestion, [see **Opi.**] *Constipation.*

**OPIUM.** *Spasms begin with loud screams, then foam at mouth, trembling of limbs and suffocation. Eyes half open and turned up, pupils dilated and insensible to light. After attack deep sleep, face red and hot.

**SILICEA.** Nocturnal epilepsy, especially about new moon, [see **Bufo.**] *Chronic cases,* [after **Cal. c.**] Attacks preceded by coldness of left side, shaking and twitching of left side.

**AUXILIARY MEASURES.** During attack, loosen all clothing that constringe the neck or chest, place a cork or piece of wood between teeth to protect tongue and lips, and guard patient against personal injury. If unable to swallow, put a few drops of indicated remedy on a handkerchief and allow him to inhale it.

**HYGIENIC.** Epileptics should observe a regular, quiet mode of life, avoid all *excitement* or over-exertion. Out-doors exercise, suitable clothing, frequent ablutions, friction of the skin, regular habits, and mental quietude, the best preventives.

**DIETETICS.** The diet should be plain, simple and of easy digestion, consisting largely of vegetables, very little animal food, fresh ripe fruits, Graham bread, light puddings, oatmeal mush, etc. All stimulating food, *alcoholic* drinks, and the use of *tobacco*, should be discarded.

---

## EPISTAXIS.

(*Hemorrhage from the Nose.*)

**THERAPEUTICS.** *Leading indications.*

**ACONITE.** Adapted to *sanguine, plethoric* persons, [**Arn. *Bell. Bry.**] *Blood bright-red and copious, with fullness of head

**AGARICUS.** Old people with relaxed state of circulatory system. Nosebleed when blowing nose in morning.

**AMMONIUM CARB.** Epitaxis when washing face in cold water.

**ARNICA.** After external injury. *Nosebleed preceded by tingling sensation in nose.

**BELLADONNA.** *Congestion to head, with red face, [**Acon. Bry. *Erig.**] Blood *bright-red, flowing freely.* Worse from motion, noise, bright light. Persons of full habit.

**BRYONIA.** *Bleeding of nose when the menses should appear, [**Ham. *Puls.**] When occurring in morning, or from *overheating.* Irritable mood; *hard, dry stools.*

**CARBO VEG.** Profuse and long-continued nosebleed. Great paleness of face before and after the attack, [reverse, **Bell.**] After straining at stool. Small intermitting pulse.

**CHINA.** Weakly persons who have lost much blood. *Habitual nosebleed, especially morning on rising. *Ringing in ears,* pale face, fainting.

**CROCUS.** The blood is black, thick, stringy, with cold sweat on forehead.

**ERIGERON.** Congestion to head, with red face, [see **Bell.**] Copious bleeding; febrile action.

**HAMAMELIS.** *In combination with hæmoptysis.* *Flow passive, non-coagulable. *Vicarious menstruation.*

**PHOSPHORUS.** *Frequent recurring attacks of profuse bleeding, especially during stool. *Slight wounds bleed much.* *Long, narrow, hard stools.

**PULSATILLA.** Suppressed or scanty menses, [see **Bry.**]

**SECALE COR.** *Anæmic state,* [**Chin.**] Blood dark, runs continuously, with great prostration. After long continued and exhausting disease, [**Chin.**] Blueness of skin.

**AUXILIARY MEASURES.** Place patient in a sitting posture, body bent slightly forward, neck straight. Instruct him to *close the mouth* and *breathe through the nose,* to favor coagulation. Raise arms above the head, and keep in that position some time. Apply *ice-cold* water to root of nose and nape of neck. Pressure on facial arteries, over the superior maxillary bones just before the vessels reach alæ. Sniff tannin

6*

or powdered matico-leaf up the nostrils. Inject into nostrils solution of *alum* or *chloride of iron*.

In dangerous cases, plug posterior nares: Take a cord, say two feet long, tie in the middle a dossil of lint or piece of sponge less than an inch in diameter. Now pass a female catheter or bougie, armed with another cord, through the nostril into pharynx; seize the end with forceps, bring it out through mouth, and tie the two cords together. Now pull it back through the nose and the sponge guided by the finger will cary it into the posterior opening. Plug front opening if necessary. Remove in a day or two by washing out the coagula, then pushing plug back with a catheter or blunt probe, and drawing on the cord in the mouth.

---

## ERYSIPELAS.

**THERAPEUTICS.** *Leading indications.*

**ACONITE.** Chill and synochal fever, with dry, hot skin and full, quick pulse. Great *redness, tingling* and burning in face, [Bell.] *Vertigo from sitting up in bed. *Great fear and anxiety of mind, with nervous excitability. *Cannot bear the pain, nor to be touched or uncovered.

**AMM. CARB.** *Erysipelas of old people, when cerebral symptoms are developed. Tendency to gangrenous destruction. Soreness of the whole body.

**APIS MEL.** Erysipelas of face and scalp, with œdematous swelling of eyelids, [see **Rhus.**] *Burning, stinging pains in affected parts. *Chilliness from least motion, with heat of face and hands. *Dryness of throat, without thirst, [**Puls.**] Urine dark-colored and scanty.

**ARSENICUM.** **Phlegmonous*, parts assume a *blackish hue, with tendency to gangrene*, [**Carb. v.**] *Burning pains, the parts burn like fire, [**Acon.**] *Rapid prostration of strength. *Great anguish, extreme restlessness, and fear of death. *Intense thirst, drinking little and often. Worse, *particularly after midnight*, [**Rhus.**]

**BELLADONNA.** Especially facial erysipelas. *Smooth, red, shining skin, not much swollen, [**Acon.**] *The redness begins in a small spot, and runs in streaks from the centre. *Congestion to head, with delirium. *Throbbing headache*, worse from motion. *Great intolerance of light or noise. Aggravation about 3 P. M.

**BRYONIA.** Erysipelas of joints, [**Puls.**] Hot, red swelling of affected parts. *Pains stitching, burning and stinging; worse from least motion or touch. *Patient wants to remain perfectly quiet. *Cannot sit up from nausea and faintness. *Lips parched, dry and cracked. Splitting headache.* Very irritable. *Dry, hard stools.*

**CANTHARIS.** *Vesicular erysipelas*, [**Cro. tig. Graph. *Rhus. t.**] Active inflammation of skin, with more *burning* than itching, and exudation of serous liquid raising the epidermis in the shape of blisters. *Constant desire to urinate, passing but a few drops at a time.

**CROTON TIG.** *Vesicular erysipelas,* [see **Rhus t.**] *Scarlet redness of the skin, with rash-like vesicles, [**Canth.**] **Intense itching, followed by painful burning,* [more burning than itching, **Canth.**] Erysipelas of *scrotum.*

**GRAPHITES.** Unhealthy skin; the slightest injury inclines to suppurate, [**Hep.**] *Phlegmonous erysipelas, with burning, tingling pains, [**Bell.**] *Vesicular eruptions, discharging a sticky, glutinous fluid. Persons inclined to obesity.

**HEPAR SULPH.** Where the disease inclines to terminate in suppuration, [see **Graph.**] The eruption is very sensitive to touch. Especially after the abuse of mercury. *Empty feeling at the stomach.*

**OPIUM.** Cases which supervene during *pneumonia,* typhoid or other fevers. *Profound coma, with stertorous respiration. Eyes dull and watery, pupils dilated. Face dark red and bloated. Stools composed of hard, black balls, [**Thuy.**] Slow pulse.

**RHUS RAD.** Erysipelas in hot weather. *Œdematous swelling of face, with *itching, burning* and pricking. Phlegmonous erysipelas, [**Bell. Hep. Graph.**] *Joints stiff.*

**RHUS TOX.** *Vesicular erysipelas, [**Canth.** ***Cro. t. Graph.**] **Left side* of face involved first, then goes to *right,* [if it goes to *scrotum,* **Crot. t.**] Burning and redness of surface, which soon swells and becomes covered with *watery vesicles.* **Intolerable burning, itching and tingling* in parts. Eyelids present a bladder-like appearance. Swelling and redness of face, with *partial or entire closing of eyelids.* Bruised feeling in limbs and back.

**SULPHUR.** In cases terminating in ulceration, and where it has assumed a *chronic* form. The parts burn and itch when near fire, or from getting in a heat. *Frequent weak, faint spells. Vesicular eruptions filled with *pus.* *Constant heat on top of head. Early morning diarrhœa. Dry, husky, scaly skin. *Scrofulous diathesis.*

**LOCAL MEASURES.** It is pretty generally admitted by the homœopathic school that local applications in the treatment of erysipelas are productive of more evil than good. In the simple form of the disease, dusting the parts with *powdered starch* or *rye flour* will allay the troublesome itching and burning that annoys patient so much. In *phlegmonous erysipelas,* where the deep-seated tissues are involved, and there is evidence of suppuration, make free incisions through the skin and apply linseed meal poultices. Should *gangrene* supervene, use poultices made of *charcoal* and *brewer's yeast,* and provide for free escape of pus.

**DIETETICS.** The diet should be very simple; thin

gruel made of rice, arrowroot, tapioca, farina or corn-starch, may be taken in the inflammatory stage; later, or in the phlegmonous variety, a more generous diet must be allowed; milk, broths, beef-tea, etc. Cold water, and abundance of fresh air.

---

## FELON.—WHITLOW.

**TREATMENT.** Among the many remedies advised as *preventives* in this painful affection are the following: In the early stage hold finger in *hot turpentine* for ten minutes, three or four times a day. Wrap the part up in *turpentine and salt.* Immerse the affected part in *lye*, hot as can be borne, for half an hour, three or four times a day. Soon as pain and inflammation are perceived, wrap the *skin* of a boiled egg around the parts, and keep it on some time. Apply a compress wet with tincture of *Lobelia*, and renew it every two hours. This is said to be very efficacious.

**LEADING REMEDIES.**

**ALUMINA.** Early stage, pricking, burning, slight swelling and redness. Brittle nails, and tendency to ulceration of finger-tips. *Apply the moistened clay externally.*

**APIS MEL.** *Burning, *stinging* pain; application of cold water relieves. After the abuse of sulphur.

**ARSENICUM.** *Burning in parts like fire. The sore turns black, assuming a gangrenous appearance, [**Lach.**] *Anxious restlessness, prostration.* Worse about midnight.

**BELLADONNA.** Parts *very red*, the inflammation spreads over the whole hand and up the arm. *Throbbing headache.* Persons of full habit.

**GRAPHITES.** Superficial inflammation about root of nail, with burning pain. *Sore does not heal readily, and "proud flesh" springs up, [**Sili.**]

**HEPAR SULPH.** *Suppuration imminent*, [**Merc. Sili.**] *Violent *throbbing* "gathering pain," accelerates suppuration. *Unhealthy skin, every little injury suppurates.

**LEDUM.** If caused by *external injuries, as splinters*, etc. *Gouty nodosities on hands and fingers.

**MERCURIUS.** If the disease extends to the sheaths of tendons, and ligaments of joints, [**Meze.**] *Caries of the bones, [**Sili.**] *Suppurative process slow.*

**PHYTOLACCA.** When the disease is located in *palm of the hand*, pains sharp and darting. Apply the raw bruised root externally,

**SILICEA.** *Deep-seated, terrible pains, swelling unabated. *Suppuration imminent, or in cases where discharge becomes fetid, thin and watery. Fistulous openings form, slow to heal. *Caries of the bones.

**LOCAL TREATMENT.** *Warm poultices*, made of bread and milk, or *linseed meal*, applied to the part and changed often, will be found useful in softening the skin and relieving the pain.

Should *pus* form notwithstanding the above treatment, make a free incision into the tumor down to the bone. Before doing this it will be better to use a *local anæsthetic* [see article **Local Anæsthetics**], and operate quickly. Continue the poulticing, and if *unhealthy granulations* spring up at any time, sprinkle with *burnt alum,* or touch with caustic.

---

## FOREIGN BODIES IN THE EAR.

Extraneous bodies, as gravel, bits of glass, shot, peas, etc., are often put into the ears by children, and may cause inflammation or deafness, if not quickly removed.

**TREATMENT.** Seat patient so that direct rays of sun will fall upon the ear, or if this cannot be done, use a lamp with a reflector; pull auricle outwards and backwards, and introduce *Speculum* well into meatus, and examine carefully. The foreign body can generally be removed by slender forceps, or a hair-pin bent at an obtuse angle, and passed beyond the object, and withdrawn. Hardened wax, dirt, hair and loose flakes of cuticle, may be dislodged by syringing with *warm* water. Insects in ear should be deluged with olive oil, and when they become visible removed with forceps.

If, before effort is made to extract the object, swelling and inflammation have occurred, they must be reduced before poking instruments into the ear. Apply *hot fomentations,* and give *Aconite,* if patient is *anxious, restless, tossing about; ear hot, red, swollen, very painful. Belladonna, if mind is confused; hearing acute; *shooting pains* in ear; parotid gland swollen and red.

---

## FOREIGN BODIES IN THE EYE.

**TREATMENT.** First examine the cornea, then if necessary evert lower lid, and direct patient to look up. If nothing is discovered, turn upper lid inside out, by taking hold of eyelashes and turning the lid up over a probe.

If dust, fine sand, or like substances have entered the eye, syringe out with *tepid* water, or place the eye in a vessel of water and hold it there for a time.

If caustic, sharp acid or salts get into the eye, drop into it sweet oil.

If mineral substances, paint, cantharides, dead insects, etc., drop into the eye white of egg.

If lime, ashes, dye-stuffs or tobacco, deluge the eye with cream or sour milk.

Particles of iron, cinders, etc., in the eye, may be removed with a bent horse-hair placed around the object and under the lid, and then drawn forward, or by picking off with fine forceps. Failing in these, put a few drops of a four per cent. solution of *Cocaine* into the eye, and when it becomes insensible to contact, pass the point of a cataract needle or lancet under the object and lift it out.

If a foreign body has passed within the anterior chamber, it is best to remove it at once; this may be done with instruments used for the extraction of cataract.

---

## FOREIGN BODIES IN THE NOSE.

**TREATMENT.** Children often put beans, peas, grains of corn, and other foreign bodies into the nose. It is best to extract them at once. This may be done with a scoop, bent probe, a bristle probang or slender forceps. Sometimes the object can be expelled by tickling the nostrils with a feather or a little snuff to cause sneezing. If it cannot be brought through the nostrils, it must be pushed back into throat. Take a female catheter, pass it through nostrils with its convexity upwards and point on object, push back through posterior nares. In some cases it may be necessary to use an anæsthetic in the removal of these foreign bodies.

---

## FOREIGN BODIES IN PHARYNX AND ŒSOPHAGUS.

When foreign bodies get fixed in pharynx or œsophagus, they produce a sense of choking and fits of suffocative cough. They may prove fatal by causing suffocation, spasm of glottis, or ulceration of parts.

**TREATMENT.** When pins, small bones, pieces of glass, etc., become lodged in pharynx, seat patient in a bright light, press down tongue, and if the offending object can be seen, extract it with curved forceps. If it has passed into œsophagus, take a smooth whalebone, tie to the end numerous silk-slings or nooses, pass this into the throat below the object, turning it several times, then withdraw it. A whalebone armed with a dry sponge—surface oiled—introduced with rotary motion, the patient given a sup of water and the sponge withdrawn has been successful. If the substance is large and would do no harm in stomach, push it down with probang.

A *fish-hook*, with line attached, has been swallowed. In this case, drill a hole through centre of a leaden or ivory ball, pass the line through this and cause patient to swallow it, then pull both up together.

Children have swallowed needles [head foremost], with thread fastened in the eye. Take a whalebone or a wire with a hole in the end, pass the thread through this, [if thread is short, tie a piece to it] push this with needle into the stomach, then withdraw both together.

As a last resort in these cases, *œsophagotomy.*

---

## FOREIGN BODIES IN LARYNX AND TRACHEA.

When a foreign body enters the *rima glottidis*, it produces violent spasmodic cough and dyspnœa, fixed pain at particular spot, and loss of voice. When it passes into trachea, it may be heard or felt with finger during a fit of coughing. When it enters the bronchia, [generally the right] it causes a whistling or murmuring sound, detected by stethoscope.

**TREATMENT.** If promptly on the spot, *raise patient by the heels*, and slap him upon the back. Search pharynx with finger and extract the substance. Blow snuff into the nose to induce sneezing, or tickle the throat to excite vomiting. Failing in these, recourse must be had to *Tracheotomy.*

**IPECAC.** May be given for suffocative attacks. *Rattling of mucus in brochia. Inclination to vomit.

**TART. EM.** *Much rattling of mucus in trachea. *Suffocative paroxysms. Breathing rapid.

**OPIUM.** Suffocative paroxysms; patient turns purple in face. *Slow pulse.

---

## FRACTURES.

### GENERAL CONSIDERATIONS.

In a case of supposed frature, if any doubt exists as to the *diagnosis*, *etherize* patient and examine carefully. Do not be in too big a *hurry.*

Bones should be *set* as soon after the injury as possible.

If much tumefaction and soreness, cover the limb with *hot compresses* wet with a solution of *Arnica* [ounce to the pint], and give *Arnica* internally.

The indications for treatment are: 1st. To place fragments in their natural position. 2d. To keep them in position until union takes place.

**DRESSINGS.** These consist of: Bandages, Splints, Adhesive strips, Bran, Cotton padding, Fracture-boxes, etc.

**Bandages.** The common roller bandage, made of cotton or linen cloth, cut 3 inches wide and about 4 yards long is generally used. The *many-tailed* bandage, however, is used in most cases of fracture of lower extremities. For particulars see **Wounds.**

**Splints.** A great variety have been introduced, some valuable, others without merit. Those possessing the essential points must be light, firm and easy of application. Thin strips of wood, heavy binder's board, sole-leather and felt answer well in most cases of simple fracture.

**PLASTER OF PARIS SPLINT.** Take two pieces of flannel or cotton cloth suited to length of splint, and wide enough to encircle the limb and overlap slightly in front. Stitch them together from top to bottom in the middle. Place them under the limb with the line of stitching on back of leg. The upper piece is now turned up on each side and pinned smoothly over the shin. Now mix the plaster with about equal bulk of water and spread quickly over the flannel covering the limb. The outer piece is now brought over and a roller applied to make it smooth and regular. The limb must be held firm and straight until the *plaster hardens*, which will be in five or ten minutes.

This splint can be opened or taken off at pleasure by removing the pins when the sides will separate, the line of stitching acting as a hinge. Suitable openings may be made in the sides in case of compound fractures.

**STARCH BANDAGE.** As a permanent dressing this may be applied in *recent* fractures and where no shortening of limb is to be overcome. Prepare some wheat flour paste, cover the limb with corded cotton, and fill up all inequalities of surface and apply over this a *wet* bandage. Now, with the hands smear on the paste, and then retrace the course of the bandage, again apply the paste and again the bandage. Over this run a dry roller and keep limb in proper position until bandage is dry.

**GENERAL TREATMENT.** The first step in the treatment is to *adjust* the fracture. Second, to bind up the part in such a manner as to insure perfect rest.

Union takes place in from four to ten weeks. Younger the subject, more rapid will be the repair.

Care should be taken not to put dressings on too tightly. If fingers or toes become cold, blue or benumbed, *loosen* bandages.

If *much* pain be felt in parts after dressings are applied. it will most likely be due to displaced fragments; look to this.

Open bandages on third or fourth day to see that all is right.

In fractures near joints, remove dressings frequently, [two weeks after injury] and make passive motion to prevent anchylosis.

**Compound Fractures.** The question of *amputation* will frequently arise in these cases. If it is decided to try to save the limb, remove all fragments and splinters of bone. If a sharp end of bone protrude and cannot be returned easily, saw it off

Dress wound *antiseptically*. See article **Antiseptic Dressings.** Provide for free drainage. Have apertures in splints so wound can be dressed without disturbing whole limb.

Build up general health with appropriate nourishment—beef-tea, broths, milk, eggs, etc.

**Extension** will be required in some cases to prevent over-riding of fragments. In all cases of fracture of *femur*, and occasionally of the *humerus*, it will be necessary to provide for extension.

**MEDICAL TREATMENT.** Care should be taken to correct any constitutional disturbance that may arise by appropriate remedies.

**ACONITE.** *Anxiety, restlessness, and tossing about. High temperature, and other febrile symptoms. Threatened erysipelas.

**ARNICA.** *Stupefaction after concussion of brain. Vomiting dark red coagula. *Bruised, sore feeling all over, [**Ruta g.**] Bed feels hard. *Contusions without lacerations.

**CALCARIA PHOS.** Highly commended in *non-union* of fractured bones. *Scrofulous subjects, especially flabby, shrunken, emaciated children.

Prof. Helmuth advises Churchill's hypophosphites of lime and soda to hasten the formative process. Dose: a teaspoonful in a glass of water, taken during a meal.

**SILICEA.** Compound fractures, with malignant and gangrenous inflammation. *Fistulous openings, discharges offensive, parts around hard, swollen, bluish-red.

---

## FROST-BITE.—EFFECTS OF COLD.

Portions of the body, as the feet, hands, nose, ears, etc., may be frozen, and the patient be quite unconscious of it at the time. The first visible effect is a dull red color, the result of imperfect circulation. If the cold be continued, the parts become of a livid, tallowy paleness, insensible, motionless, and reduced in bulk.

**TREATMENT.** Place patient at once in a *cold* room, and rub the frozen parts briskly with *snow* or ice-water until a slight degree of warmth is obtained. After a time cold water may be substituted for the snow or ice. Soon as the circulation is restored, the room may be made warmer, and the parts wrapped in dry flannel.

For the *fever* and burning pain that usually follows the reaction, give *Aconite*, and apply compresses wet with a solution of the same.

**AGARICUS,** is excellent when the *itching* is very *intense*, with burning. This remedy is frequently sufficient to cure the affection.

## GANGRENE.—MORTIFICATION.

Mortification signifies death of any part of the body, the result of disease or injury. The incipient stage, when the parts are still recoverable, is called *gangrene*, and later when vitality is totally destroyed, mortification.

**Dry Gangrene** is a form of the disease mostly found in persons of advanced years, and is the result of deficient arterial circulation. The parts become hard, dry, shriveled, insensible and of a purple hue.

**THERAPEUTICS.** *Leading indications.*

**ARSENICUM.** *Hot, shining, burning red spots and bluish blisters. Hard, red, blue, painful swellings, relieved by external warmth. *Fetid diarrhœa, worse after midnight, with restlessness and prostration. *Intense thirst, drinking little and often.

**CROTALUS.** Dark redness of the swollen parts, which burn like fire, [Ars.] Livid spots with frequent fainting fits and feeble pulse. Swollen part is cold and painful to pressure. Heat and intolerable gnawing of the feet.

**LACHESIS.** Impending gangrene. Gangrenous blisters, bluish or black-looking, burning and itching. .Tingling in the parts with heat and redness. Ichorous offensive discharge, [Ars.] Traumatic gangrene, [Crotal.] *Great tenderness of throat to pressure.

**SECALE COR.** Gangrene, especially of old people [Ars.] The whole skin looks dingy and shriveled. *Dry gangrene of the extremities, the parts are dry, cold, hard and insensible, of uniform black color. *Painless diarrhœa, with great weakness. Numbness, insensibility and coldness of limbs.

**CHINA.** *After repeated hemorrhages.* Humid gangrene, parts turn black. Coldness of the extremities.

**CARBO VEG.** *Dry gangrene,* [*vide* Sec.] Cachectic persons, where vital powers have become weakened. *Great foulness of all the secretions.

For other remedies and treatment of gangrene, see **Wounds.**

**LOCAL MEASURES.** In *humid* gangrene, where *sloughs* are *superficial,* apply poultices of powdered *Charcoal* and *brewer's yeast.* Incise and remove all dead pieces soon as they loosen. Cleanse the parts frequently with solution *Carbolic Acid,* [gtts. v. Aq. ferv, ℥j] using it as hot as can be borne.

In *gangrene* from extreme *heat* or *cold,* apply emollient poultices, use disinfectants, and wait until nature draws the line by which to amputate.

In *dry gangrene,* wrap the parts in lint and cover with oiled silk. If there is much discharge, change the dressings daily; otherwise, leave on for a week.

**DIETETICS.** Sustain patient by a nutritious diet—broths, beef-tea, milk, eggs, tender steak, cream-toast, rice puddings, etc.

---

## GASTRIC DERANGEMENT.

**THERAPEUTICS.** *Leading indications.*

**ACONITE.** Thirst, frequent pulse and great impatience. Vertigo on raising the head. *Burning thirst for beer, [**Bry. Nux. Puls.**] Everything tastes bitter except water, [see **Bry.**] *Pressure in region of liver. Rumbling and fermentation in abdomen, **Lyc.**] *Watery diarrhœa.

**ANTIMO. CRUD.** *Gastric derangement from overloading stomach.* *Milky-white coating of tongue. *Putrid eructations,* smelling like bad eggs, [***Arn. Sep.**] *Persistent vomiting which nothing can stop.* Cramp-like pain in stomach, [**Nux.**] *Stools watery with hard lumps.

**ARGENT. NIT.** *Constant dull headache.* *Head feels much too large, [**Cimi. Gel. Nux.**] Thick, tenacious mucus in throat, obliging him to hawk frequently. *Belching after every meal, stomach feels as if it would burst with wind, [see **Chin.**] Gastralgia after ice-cream, pain radiating in all directions.

**ARSENICUM.** *Debility and exhaustion.* Putrid, fetid taste. *Loss of appetite, with violent thirst, drinking *little and often,* [**Chin.**] *Water-brash,* [**Bry. Nux. Puls.**] *Vomiting immediately after eating or drinking, [***Bry. Nux.**] *Pressure in stomach as from a stone* After the use of *ice-cream, ice-water, sour beer, tobacco.* *Relief from *hot* drinks.

**BRYONIA.** Irritable mood, wishes to be alone [**Nux.**] *The head aches as if skull would burst, [**Acon. Bell.**] Tongue coated *white* or *brown.* Desire for coffee, wine, [**Nux.**] *All food and drink taste bitter, [**Puls**] *Vomiting immediately after eating, [***Ars. Nux. Puls.**] Stomach sensitive to pressure. *Constipation of dry, hard stools.

**CARBO VEG.** Bitter taste before and after eating. *Longing for coffee, acids, sweet and salt things. *Sour, rancid* eructations. *Pyrosis,* great flow of water, [**Chin. Nux. Puls.**] *Bloatedness of abdomen.* After debauching.

**CHAMOMILLA.** *Irritable, impatient mood, [**Bry. Nux.**] Tongue coated white or yellowish. *Bitter,* sour or putrid taste. *Aversion* to coffee, beer, and warm drinks, [**Chin. Ferr. Lyc.**] *Vomiting bile, what has been drunk, slimy matter, or green mucus. · *Wind colic, abdomen distended like a drum;* relieved by applying warm cloths. *Greenish diarrhœic stools.

**CHINA.** *Bitter taste in back part of throat;* bitter taste of everything, [see **Bry.**] Eructations tasting of food last eaten, [**Nux. Phos.** ***Puls. Sulph.**] *Abdomen feels full and tight, as if stuffed, eructations afford no relief, [relief from belching, **Arg. n.**] Weakly persons who have lost much blood.

**HYDRASTIS.** Peppery taste, tongue as if burnt, [**Verat.**] *Dull, aching pain in stomach, causing a faintish, weak, *gone feeling* in epigastric region. Bread or vegetables cause acidity, weakness, indigestion. Constipation, *stools lumpy* and *covered with mucus.*

**IPECAC.** Flat taste, with white, thickly-coated tongue, [**Ant. c.**] **Constant nausea*, with vomiting food, bile, jelly-like mucus, [**Ant. c.**] Stomach feels relaxed, as if hanging down, [**Staph.**] *Diarrhœa, stools as if fermented, green as grass. After eating *sour, acrid things*, unripe fruit, berries, salads, etc.

**IRIS VERSI.** *Gastric sick-headache. Gums and tongue feel as if covered with a greasy substance. *Burning distress in stomach, with vomiting sour fluid. "Grumbling belly-ache," with watery diarrhœa.

**LYCOPODIUM.** Everything tastes sour, [***Chin. Nux.**] *Heart-burn, water-brash*, [**Nux. Puls.**] *Great fullness* in stomach after taking a mere mouthful of food. *Constant sense of fermentation in abdomen, like a pot of yeast working. Constipation, stools scant, hard, and passed with difficulty. *Red sand in urine.

**MERCURIUS.** Dull and stupid feeling, with dizziness. Head feels as if it would burst, with fullness of brain, [see **Bry.**] *Bitter, sweetish, saltish, putrid or slimy taste. Regurgitation or vomiting food, [see **Puls.**] *Stomach burns, is swollen and sensitive to touch, [**Nux. Phos.**] Symptoms all worse at night, and in damp, rainy weather.

**NUX VOMICA.** The patient is *very irritable*, inclines to scold, and *wishes to be alone.* *Headache, with nausea, and vomiting sour, bitter substances, [**Bry. Puls.**] *All food tastes bitter*, [*tastes sour*, ***Chin. Lyc.**] *Sour* or bitter eructations. *Cramp-like pains in stomach, after a meal. *Habitual constipation, with frequent urging to go to stool*, [**Bry. Lyc.**] *Persons of sedentary habits, or after the use of drug-mixtures, alcoholic drinks, etc.

**PHOSPHORUS.** Belching large quantities of wind after eating, [**Arg. n.**] *Very sleepy after meals, especially after dinner, [**Lyc. Nux.**] *Burning in stomach, extending to throat.* *Constipation; stools long, narrow and hard, like a dog's. Cold feet and legs.

**PULSATILLA.** *Mild, gentle, tearful disposition*, [reverse, **Bry. *Cham. Nux.**] No appetite or thirst. *Everything tastes bitter, [see **Nux.**] *Aversion to fat food, pork, meat, bread, milk.* *Eructations tasting and smelling of food, [***Chin. Phos. Sulph.**] Vomiting food, mucus or bitter, sour substances. *Chilliness*, even in a warm room. *Craves cool, fresh, air, worse* in a warm room, or from eating warm food, [reverse, **Ars.**] After eating *pork, pastry*, rancid butter, etc.

**DIETETICS.** At the outset of attack, *abstain from all food.* Bits of ice may be taken to appease thirst. Three or four times a day, patient should drink a cupful of water, *hot as can be borne.* As improvement advances, nourishment must be taken cautiously. Thin gruel, milk, barley and rice-water. Later, beef, mutton and chicken-broths. Return to use of *solid* food very cautiously.

---

## GASTRITIS.

(*Inflammation of the Stomach.*)

**THERAPEUTICS.** *Leading indications.*

**ACONITE.** *Synochal fever*, hot, dry skin, full, quick pulse, and *intense thirst.* Sharp, shooting pains in stomach, with retching and vomiting blood. *Bitter bilious vomiting, with anguish and fear of death. *Great fear and anxiety of mind, with nervous excitability. Shortness of breath; *great restlessness.*

**APIS MEL.** *Great tearfulness, cannot help crying, [***Puls.**] *Tongue dry*, red at tip, swollen. *Intense thirst*, drinks little, but often, [***Ars.**] Vomits food soon as taken, [***Ars. Bry.** ***Verat.**] Burning heat in stomach, with *great soreness*, [**Acon.**] *Greenish, yellowish, watery* stools, worse in morning.

**ARNICA.** *After mechanical injuries.* *Vomiting dark, coagulated blood, [**Ars. Nux.**] *Sore, bruised feeling all through the body; bed feels hard. Belching, with taste of *putrid eggs.*

**ARSENICUM.** Anxious expression of countenance. *Heat or burning in stomach, with sharp, shooting pains, [see **Bell.**] *Vomiting everything eaten or drank, [**Bry.**] Vomiting. *Urgent thirst for cold water, drinks often, but little at a time, [**Apis.**] *Great restlessness and anxiety, with fear of death. *Rapid prostration of strength.*

**BELLADONNA.** Great *heat and tenderness* of whole abdomen, the skin imparts a sensation of *burning* to the hand. Burning, cutting pains in stomach, [**Ars. Bry.**] *Pains come on suddenly and cease as suddenly. *Congestion to the head, with throbbing headache. *Delirium, with desire to escape* from bed. *Great intolerance to light and noise. *Starting and jumping during sleep.

**BRYONIA.** *Tongue dry and brown.* Region of stomach exceedingly sensitive, *cannot bear least pressure on it.* Stitching and darting pains in the parts. *Burning in stomach*, [***Ars.**] *Vomiting immediately after eating or drinking, [***Ars. Verat.**] *Nausea and faintness from sitting up. Delirium, with desire to escape. *Lips parched, dry and cracked.* Thirst for large draughts of cold water. *Wants to remain perfectly quiet.

**CANTHARIS.** Violent pains in stomach; patient tossing about in despair. *Severe burning in stomach*, sometimes extending down into bowels. *Constant desire to urinate, passing but a few drops at a time. Stools like scrapings from intestines. *Burning thirst.* *Vomiting, with violent retching. Anxious restlessness, [**Acon. Ars.**]

**IPECAC.** Where *nausea and vomiting* are the prominent features. Diarrhœa, *with grass-green mucous stools*, and cutting colic. After eating sour, unripe fruit, berries, salads.

**IRIS VERS.** *Great burning distress in epigastric region.* Intense burning in region of pancreas. *Sharp, cutting pains of short duration, and changing often. Distressing nausea and vomiting with pain in the stomach. Aggravation by motion, [**Bry.**]

**NUX VOMICA.** Face red and bloated. Tongue red, clean and tremulous. *Burning pain in stomach*, which is tender to touch, [**Ars. Bell.**] *Contractive, spasmodic pains in stomach. *Vomiting sour-smelling mucus, also blood. Burning in œsophagus up to mouth. Hard, difficult stools, with frequent urging. Victims of drastic medicines and quack nostrums.

**PHOSPHORUS.** Dejected, thinks he will die, [see **Ars.**] Tongue dry, cracked, covered with crusts, [**Apis.**] *Vomiting sourish, offensive fluid, looking like water, ink and coffee grounds. *Burning in stomach, extending to throat and bowels, [see **Nux.**] Griping or cutting pain in region of stomach, coming in paroxysms. *Profuse watery stools, pouring away as from a hydrant.*

**PULSATILLA.** Epigastrium sensitive. Aching and darting pains in stomach. Nausea and vomiting after eating or drinking, [**Ars. Bry.**] *Suffocating and fainting spells; must have fresh, cool air. *Vertigo when rising up, with chilliness. Watery diarrhœa, especially at night. Bitter taste, constant spitting of frothy mucus.

**VERAT. ALB.** *Hippocratic countenance, [**Ars.**] Eyes sunken and glazed. Lips bluish and dry. Great soreness in region of stomach. *Intense thirst for *cold drinks*. Inability to retain anything on stomach. Extremities cold and covered with clammy sweat. *Extreme prostration*, with anguish and fear of death, [***Ars.**] *Pulse almost imperceptible. Exhausting diarrhœa.*

**HYGIENIC MEASURES.** Provide for an abundance of fresh air; keep room light and patient quiet as possible. Apply *hot fomentations* over region of stomach, and change frequently. Give injections of lukewarm water to relieve the bowels if constipation is obstinate.

**DIETETICS.** In the active stage, *total abstinence from all food;* only sips of cold water or bits of ice to appease thirst. Half a teacupful of *hot water* taken frequently will be found very useful in relieving pain and burning of stomach. When improvement sets in, a little *fresh sweet* milk or thin gruel may be taken. Later, beef-tea, animal broths, etc. No solid food should be allowed until all traces of inflammation have subsided. Return to ordinary diet very cautiously.

---

## GONORRHŒA.

**THERAPEUTICS.** *Leading indications.*

**ACONITE.** In early and *inflammatory stage*, [**Can. s. Gel.**] *Burning, smarting in the glans, on urinating.* Painful erections at night, [***Canth. Cap.**] Young plethoric persons,

**AGAVE AMERICANA.** *Extremely painful erections.* Great difficulty in passing urine, accompanied by *heat, pain,* and tenesmus at neck of bladder. Drawing in spermatic cords and testicles, extending to thighs, so violent he wishes to die.

**AGNUS CASTUS.** *Yellow purulent discharge, especially in old sinners.* *Impotence, with want of sexual desire or erections. Testes cold, swollen, hard.

**ARGENT. NIT.** Burning in urethra during micturition, with a feeling as if the urethra were swollen and sore inside. *Swelling* and *induration* of testicles from suppressed gonorrhœa.

**CANNABIS SAT.** Inflammatory stage with painful symptoms, [see **Acon**.] *Great swelling of prepuce, approaching phimosis, [see **Merc.**] Dark redness of glans and prepuce. *Penis sore, as if burnt, painful *when walking.* *Strangury, [**Agave. *Canth.**] *Burning in urethra* during and after micturition; *stream forked,* [**Canth.**]

**CANTHARIS.** When the inflammation has extended to bladder. **Constant desire to urinate,* with scanty emission, [see **Cap.**] *Painful erections* at night, with contraction and sore pain along the urethra.

**CAPSICUM.** *Cream-like, or purulent, yellow discharge from the urethra, [**Agn. cas.**] Burning, cutting or stinging in urethra when urinating; urethra sore to touch. Painful erections at night, [see **Acon.**]

**HYDRASTIS.** Acute or chronic form. *In second stage, thick, yellow discharge, [see **Sene.**] *Gleet, with copious, painless discharge, and debility.* Dragging in right groin to testicles, [**Merc.**] Feeling of debility and faintness after each passage from the bowels, [**Verat.**]

**IODIDE OF SULPH.** *Stricture, with or without *enlarged prostate.* [Should be kept from light, prepared fresh and used in trituration when needed.]

**MERCURIUS.** *Complicated with chancre,* [**Nit. ac.**] *Discharge yellowish-green, purulent, more profuse at night. *Swelling of prepuce,* and *inflammatory redness of its internal surface.* Urine passes in a thin stream, or in drops, sometimes mixed with blood. *Worse at night, and in damp, rainy weather.

**NITRIC ACID.** Gonorrhœa, with chancres and fig-warts. Small blisters on orifice of urethra and inner surface of prepuce. Bloody mucous or purulent discharge, [**Merc.**] *Gleet* [**Agn. c. Merc. Thuy.**] *Urine *very offensive,* and painful in voiding. After abuse of mercury.

**NUX VOMICA.** After use of *copaiva, cubebs,* and other nostrums. Thin discharge, with burning on urinating and urging to stool. Suppressed discharge, with swelling of testicles, [swelling of *prostate,* ***Puls.**] Dull pain in back part of head. **Habitual constipation; blind or bleeding piles.*

**PULSATILLA.** Thick, yellow, or yellow-green discharge, [see **Lith. c.**] Itching, burning on inner and upper side of prepuce. *Suppressed gonorrhœa, with swelling of testicles and prostate gland, [see **Sulph. Thuy.**] Stools flat, small in size. Inflammation of eyes.

**SARSAPARIL.** *Suppressed gonorrhœa, with rheumatism of joints, [**Thuy.**] Herpes on prepuce. *Severe tenesmus* of bladder. *Severe pain at *conclusion* of urination.

**SENECIO.** Advanced stages. Prostate gland enlarged and hard. Dull, heavy pain in left spermatic cord down to testicles. Lascivious dreams, with pollutions.

**SULPHUR.** Gleet, no pain or only slight burning in urethra. Rheumatic pains in different parts. *Chronic inflammation of eyes. Chronic prostatic affections. *Blind or bleeding piles, [**Nux.**] *Dry, scaly, unhealthy skin.*

**THUYA.** *Discharge thin* and *greenish.* Scalding pain when urinating, *urethra* swollen, stream forked, [see **Cann. s.**] *Checked gonorrhœa, causing articular rheumatism, prostatitis, sycosis, and impotence. Nightly painful erections, causing sleeplessness, [see **Acon.**]

**TUSSILAGO.** Acute stage, with fixed, stinging pain in navicular fossa. Also chronic stage, with inflammation of eyes and swelling of testicles, after suppressed discharge. Persons of irregular habits who use rich food, [**Nux v.**]

**AUXILIARY MEASURES.** A large class of homœopathic physicians treat gonorrhœa with *irritating* injections, while others regard these of doubtful utility. They should never be used except in the *early* stage. *Nitrate of Silver* is the favorite remedy; dissolve two grains in an ounce of water, and use as an injection every three hours. In the *fourth* or *chronic* stage, injections of *Sulphate of Zinc,* [two grains to four ounces of water] may be used with benefit. Ablutions and injections of *warm* water, to get rid of any irritating discharges, should be frequently employed.

**DIETETICS.** A carefully regulated diet. Must be *simple,* digestible, and moderate in quantity. Milk, rice, light puddings, farina, corn-starch, sweet fruits, toast, etc. All rich highly seasoned food, tea, coffee and *alcoholic* liquors must be avoided. Water should be the principal drink.

## GUM-BOIL.—ALVEOLAR ABSCESS.

This is a small abscess commencing generally in the socket of a decayed tooth bursting through the gum-tissue and sometimes through the cheek. It is also seen on a large scale as a secondary affection of scurvy. Sometimes it follows the abuse of mercury, phosphorus and other drugs. In neglected cases, extensive exfoliation of the bone may follow.

**TREATMENT.** Proper attention to the mouth and teeth will in most cases prevent the formation of these abscesses. They should be thoroughly washed and brushed *after each* meal. All *tartar* should be removed from time to time, and when a tooth becomes decayed, it should be properly *filled* or removed. The general state of the health must be looked after.

**BELLADONNA.** Tumor *red, hard* and painful. Pain burning, stinging or throbbing, [**Hepar.**] Bleeding of gums.

**CALCARIA CARB.** Gums painful, tender, swollen, bleeding. Swelling of sub-lingual glands. *Scrofulous diathesis.

**HEPAR SULPH.** *Where suppuration is inevitable, [**Merc. Sili.**] Ulcers on gums, [**Merc.**] *Scrofulous* persons, and after the use of *mercury*. Unhealthy skin.

**MERCURIUS.** In *commencement*, often prevents suppuration, [**Hepar. Sili.**] Paleness of the tumor or intense redness, with burning, stinging, beating pain, [**Bell.**] *Ulcerated gums.

**SILICEA.** Painful inflammatory swelling of gum. *Where suppuration is imminent, or in cases where discharge becomes *fetid, thin*, watery. *Fistulous openings form, which are slow to heal.

**LOCAL MEASURES.** Suppuration may be hastened by poulticing. Chew some bread and cheese very finely, place it over the tumor and retain in position by the lips. A *roasted fig* cut in half and applied to the swollen part, makes a good poultice in such cases. Should fluctuation occur, puncture deep with a lancet.

---

## GUMS, BLEEDING OF.

Bleeding of the gums often takes place as a symptom of other diseases, as scurvy, low forms of fever, etc., but the most troublesome hemorrhage from the gums follow the extraction of teeth.

**TREATMENT.** **Aconite, *Arnica and *Phosphorus** are the chief internal remedies. Where these fail, a solution of **Persulphate of Iron, Tannin, Sugar of Lead,** or **Creasote,** will usually succeed. Take a bit of sponge or dossil of lint, saturate with one of the remedies, and introduce into the cavity of the gum.

In some cases it may be necessary to plug the gum. To do this, first remove all coagulæ, then pack the cavity with *dry* wheat flour, and allow it to remain in for some time.

---

## HÆMATEMESIS.—VOMITING BLOOD.

**THERAPEUTICS.** *Leading indications.*

**ACONITE.** *Febrile excitement.* *Sudden excruciating pain, with gagging, retching, and vomiting blood. Cold sweat on forehead, [**Verat.**] Stage of desquamation in scarlatina. Great *fear* and *anxiety* of mind.

**ARNICA.** If caused by *mechanical injuries* or over-exertion. *Vomiting dark-red coagula. *Soreness all over the body, as if from a bruise.

**ARSENICUM.** *Pale, death-colored face.* Great dryness of mouth, and brown, blackish tongue. *Burning thirst, drinking little and often, [**Apis. Chin.**] *Vomiting brownish* or *blackish substances,' or blood and mucus.* *Burning in stomach, [**Canth. Nux. Phos.**] *Prostration, restlessness.*

**BELLADONNA.** *Congestion to head* and stomach. *Hæmatemesis, with ringing in ears, red cheeks, feeling of fullness and warmth in stomach. *Aversion to all food or drink. Flickering before eyes.

**CANTHARIS.** *Vomiting mucus, tinged with bright-red blood. Violent burning in stomach, [**Ars.**] *Constant desire to urinate, passing but a few drops at a time.

**CARBO VEG.** *Hippocratic face*, with icy coldness of extremities. *Vomiting sour, bilious, or bloody masses. Frequent fainting; intermitting, small pulse.

**CHINA.** Hæmatemesis, great loss of blood, weak, pale, cold hands and feet. *Vomits blackish, bloody substances, [see **Ars.**] Stomach feels sore, as if ulcerated.

**ERIGERON.** Violent retching and burning in stomach, with vomiting blood. Stools small, streaked with blood.

**HAMAMELIS.** *Vomiting black blood*, [see **Arn.**] Sensation of trembling in stomach, or fullness and gurgling in abdomen. Feverish by spells. Violent throbbing in stomach. Pain back of stomach along spinal column.

**HYOSCYAMUS.** Vomiting blood, with convulsions. Vomiting bloody mucus, with dark-red blood. Pit of stomach tender to touch. Dull, aching about liver, abdomen bloated. Limbs numb, weak, trembling.

**IPECAC.** *Sudden attacks*, with great paleness and coldness. *Vomiting blood, or a pitch-like substance, [**Ars. Sec. Verat.**] *Indescribable sick feeling in stomach.

**NUX VOM.** Malicious, *irritable* temperament. *Vomiting blood or black substances after suppressed hemorrhoidal flow. Stomach full and distended, sore to touch. *Constipation*, with black stools. *Intemperate habits.*

**PHOSPHORUS.** Oppression and burning in stomach, [see

Ars.] Vomiting sour, offensive fluid, looking like *water*, *ink*, *and coffee grounds.* *Hemorrhage from stomach, better from drinking cold water. *Long, narrow, hard, difficult stools.

**SECALE COR.** Patient lies still, with great weakness, but no pain. Face, lips, tongue, and hands deadly pale, [**Phos.**] *Vomiting brown, *blackish, decomposed* blood. Thin, scrawny, cachectic persons. Desire to be *uncovered.*

**VERAT. ALB.** Restless, wild look, with pale, distorted face. Vomiting *blood, or thin, blackish substances*, [**Ars. Chin.**] *Slow pulse, coldness, fainting fits, and cold sweat. Nausea from raising up, or the least motion.

**AUXILIARY MEASURES.** Place patient in bed with head low, and enjoin perfect quietude. If hemorrhage is severe, give water to drink *hot as can be borne*, half a teacupful every fifteen or twenty minutes until vomiting ceases. *Dry cups* may be applied over the stomach, and a cataplasm of mustard to the lower part of abdomen. These failing, *Gallic acid*, ten grains every hour or two, should be tried. *Monsel's solution* (Persulphate of Iron), a drachm well diluted, is advised as a dernier resort.

**DIETETICS.** During the attack, and for some time after, no food should be taken—let stomach rest. At first, a little warm milk, thin gruel, barley or rice water may be taken. Later, and as improvement advances, beef-tea and broths may be added. No solid food should be allowed until patient is well nigh recovered.

---

## HÆMATURIA.

(*Hemorrhage from the Urinary Organs.*)

**THERAPEUTICS.** *Leading indications.*

**APIS MEL.** Renal pains, soreness on pressure or when stooping. *Urine red, bloody, hot and scanty; after standing, sediment like coffee grounds, [see **Tereb.**] Urine contains *uriniferous tubes and epithelium*, [see **Canth.**]

**ARNICA.** When caused by *mechanical injuries*, as falls, blows, etc., [after straining from *lifting*, **Rhus.**]

**ARSENICUM.** Hemorrhoids of the bladder, urine mixed with pus and blood. Painful micturition, with scanty secretion. *Burning pain in urinary organs. *Extreme thirst, drinking little and often, [**Apis. Chin**] Prostration and restlessness.

**BERBERIS.** *Smarting, burning in region of kidneys, [**Tereb.**] *Bloody urine*, which settles at bottom of chamber in a cake, [**Millef.**] *Transparent, jelly like* mucus, passed with the urine, *followed by great exhaustion.*

**CANTHARIS.** *Constant desire to urinate, passing only a few drops of bloody, burning urine. **Hemorrhage* from the urethra, with tenesmus. Cylindrical exudations in the urine. Drawing pain from region of kidneys to inguinal glands. Pain increased by drinking water.

**HAMAMELIS.** Hæmaturia from passive congestion of kidneys. Dull pain in renal region. *Hemorrhoids of the bladder, [**Ars.**] Urine scanty and high colored.

**IPECAC.** Hæmaturia, with cutting in abdomen and urethra. *Profuse bleeding, with fainting, paleness and sick stomach. Oppression of chest. After suppressed itch.

**LYCOPODIUM.** *Renal colic, pain is felt along ureters to bladder, especially right side. *Hæmaturia*, especially in connection with gravel or chronic catarrh. Urging to urinate, must wait long before it will pass. **Red sand in the urine*, [**Phos. Sep.**] Craves sweet things, [**Arg. n.**]

**MILLEFOLIUM.** Pain in region of left kidney, followed by bloody urine. *Hæmaturia, after standing blood forms a cake in the vessel, [**Berb.**] If connected with gravel or catarrh of bladder, [**Lyc.**] Hemorrhagic diathesis, [**Ham.**] *Bleeding Piles.*

**NITRIC ACID.** **Active hemorrhage*, with urging *after*, and shuddering along the spine *during* micturition. Suitable to persons who have suffered from *gonorrhœa*.

**NUX VOM.** After abuse of drugs and alcoholic stimulants. *Hæmaturia from suppressed hemorrhoidal flow or menses, [**Sulph. Zinc.**] Pain in small of back, so bad he cannot move. *Constipation, frequent urging.

**PHOSPHORUS.** *Hæmaturia from debility after sexual excesses, blood deficient in fibrin, [see **Secale.**] *Constipation, *stools long*, *narrow* and *hard*, very difficult to expel.

**PULSATILLA.** Young girls during the time of puberty, or from suppressed menses. *Hæmaturia, with burning at orifice of urethra and constriction in region of navel. After suppressed gonorrhœal discharges.

**SECALE COR.** *Passive hemorrhage*, [*active* **Ipe. Nit. ac.**] Blood thin and deficient in corpuscles, [see **Phos.**] Painless discharge of thick, black blood in consequence of kidney disease. Great weakness, with coldness of the body.

**TEREBINTH.** *The blood is thoroughly mixed with the urine, forming a dirty reddish-brown or blackish fluid, with coffee-ground-like sediment, [see **Apis.**] Burning, drawing pains in kidneys. Before urination, pressing and straining in bladder when sitting, going off when walking. Burning in bladder, worse during micturition.

**UVA URSI.** Constant urging to urinate and straining, with discharge of blood and slime, or constant straining without any discharge at all, [see **Canth.**] Cutting and burning in urethra, succeeded by a discharge of blood.

**AUXILIARY MEASURES.** Remedies for the immediate arrest of renal hemorrhage seldom required. Our main reliance must be general treatment. If much blood has coagulated in bladder, it may be necessary to dissolve it before it can be passed. "Inject into the bladder two ounces of warm water, containing in solution 5 drops *Hydrochloric acid* and 16 grs. *Pepsin*." GATCHEL.—This is said to dissolve the clots so they can be passed or drawn off in a few hours.

**DIETETICS.** The diet should be plain and unstimulating. Graham bread, vegetables, rice, light puddings, a small amount of animall food, and ripe fruits, the most suitable diet. Mucilaginous drinks, as slippery elm, gum-arabic tea, fresh soft water and milk the only beverages.

---

## HÆMOPTYSIS.

(*Hemorrhage from the Lungs.*)

**THERAPEUTICS.** *Leading indications.*

**ACONITE.** The attack is preceded by fullness of the chest, and burning pain, [**Bell.**] Palpitation of the heart, anguish and restlessness. *Great fear and anxiety of mind, with nervous excitability.

**ARNICA.** After mechanical injury, or bodily exertion. *Expectoration of dark coagulated blood, [**Puls.**] Tickling under sternum, and a sore pain, as if bruised in chest when coughing. *The bed on which he lies feels too hard.

**BELLADONNA.** *Congestion to head and chest. Constant tickling in larynx, with cough and expectoration of bloody mucus. Stitch-like pains in chest, worse by motion. *Vertigo when stooping or rising from a stooping posture, [**Puls.**] Takes cold from every draught of air.

**CHINA.** After loss of blood or animal fluids, [**Ars.**] *Singing in the ears and fainting spells. Periodical attacks, worse every other day. *Debilitating morning* and *night sweats.* Painless, undigested stools.

**DULCAMARA.** Constant tickling in larynx, with desire to cough, [**Bell.**] Expectoration of *bright-red* blood, [dark, coagulated, **Arn. Puls.**] If caused by a cold or a loose cough which existed some time. *Gets worse at every cold change in the weather. *On waking in morning, feels giddy and dizzy, with a sense of trembling and weakness.

**FERRUM.** Hemorrhage, with flying pains in chest, better when walking slowly about, [worse from least motion, **Ipe.**] *Hæmoptysis, with pain between shoulders. Expectoration of *bright-red* blood, [see **Puls.**] Palpitation of heart, with dyspnœa. *The least emotion or exertion produces a flushed face. Slender persons with sallow complexion.

**HAMAMELIS.** **Profuse hemorrhage* of venous blood, coming into mouth without any effort, like a warm current from chest. Mind calm. Sometimes taste of sulphur in mouth. Frequent paroxysms of pain in left ovary, passing down to uterus.

**IPECAC.** *Copious bleeding from lungs, preceded by sensation of bubbling in chest. Taste of blood in mouth. Cough, with *spitting of blood, occasioned by the least effort. Nausea* and debility.

**MILLEFOLIUM.** *Expectoration of light-colored fluid blood, without much coughing, sometimes in consequence of violent exertions.

**PHOSPHORUS.** *Tight feeling in the chest, with a dry, tight cough.* *Vicarious spitting of blood for the menses, [**Ars. Bry. *Puls.**] Occasional attacks of profuse hemorrhage, *pouring out freely, then ceasing for some time,* followed by anæmia and debility. *Tubercular diathesis.*

**PULSATILLA.** Obstinate cases, discharge black and coagulated, [*bright-red,* **Acon. Dulc. Rhus.**] Loose cough. *Very nervous during the night. *Chilliness even in a warm room. Weakness and pain in lower part of chest. Sickish, empty feeling in stomach. *Craves fresh, cool air, worse in a warm room. *Scanty or suppressed menses.

**RHUS TOX.** Dry cough, which seems as if it would tear something out of chest. Discharge of bright-red blood. *Tickling under sternum, exciting cough. After straining, lifting or stretching arms high to reach things.

**AUXILIARY MEASURES.** Place patient on a mattress bed in a half sitting posture. Enjoin perfect quietude. Provide for an *abundance* of *fresh air.* If the case is urgent, and not time to await the action of medicine, apply a ligature about upper part of *left* arm, then one about upper part of *right* thigh; if this does not arrest hemorrhage, bandage *right* arm and *left thigh* in same manner. Soon as bleeding stops, loosen bandages *gradually.*

**DIETETICS.** During an attack patient may swallow *bits* of *ice* frequently. The food at first should be mostly *milk,* gruel, light puddings, then broths, beef-tea, etc. Persons subject to these hemorrhages, should adopt rigid hygienic measures; live with great regularity; exercise freely in open air, eat wholesome, nutritious food; bathe daily and sleep in well ventilated apartments.

---

## HEADACHE.

**THERAPEUTICS.** *Leading indications.*

**ACONITE.** Violent stupefying headache, with great fullness and heaviness in forehead. *Sensation as if the brain would press through the eyes, [**Bell.**] *Vertigo when rising from a sitting posture, [**Puls.**] Bitter bilious vomiting, with anguish and fear of death. *Gets desperate, and declares he cannot bear the pains.

**ARSENICUM.** Periodical headache, [**Bell. Sang. Spig.**] *Great weight in head,* particularly in forehead, [on *vertex,* **Acon. Cact. Ign.**] *Beating pain in forehead,* with inclination to vomit. *Violent vomiting, particularly after eating or drinking. *Extreme thirst, drinking little and often. *Restlessness, prostration, fear of death. Pains worse during rest, better by motion.

**BELLADONNA.** *Sick-headache*, head feels as if it would burst, [**Bry. Nux.**] Congestion to head, with throbbing carotids. *Violent throbbing pain, especially in forehead, obliging one to close the eyes, [**Acon. *Glon.**] *Boring headache in right side of head. *Vertigo, with stupefaction and vanishing of sight. *Nausea, and vomiting bile, mucus or food.* *Cannot bear noise or bright light. [**Acon. Ign.**] Worse about 3 P. M., and from lying down, [better from lying down, **Glon. Ign.**]

**BRYONIA.** Headache sets in on first waking in morning, [**Calc. c. Nux.**] *The head aches as if it would split, worse by stooping or motion, [**Acon. Bell.**] *Wants to keep perfectly still. *Gets faint or sick on sitting up. *Sour or bitter vomiting.* Lips parched, dry, cracked. *Hard, dry stools, as if burnt. Patient very irritable, [**Cham. Nux.**]

**CACTUS G.** Headache from irregular habits or dissipation. Pulsating pain, with a sensation of weight in right side of head. Pressing pain, as if a great *weight lay on the vertex*, [see **Ars.**] Pain commencing in morning and growing worse as day advances, [see **Spig.**] Must lie perfectly quiet, as motion, noise or light makes him worse.

**CALC. CARB.** Chronic headache. Dull, stupefying, oppressive pain in forehead, with cloudiness of intellect, [**Arg.**] Throbbing headache in morning, continuing whole day. *Feeling of coldness in head. *Feet cold, as if they had on damp stockings. *Much dandruff on scalp. Vertigo on going up-stairs. Menses *too soon, too profuse* and *lasting too long.*

**CHAMOMILLA.** If caused from catarrh, or by drinking coffee, [**Ign. Nux.**] Rending or drawing pain in side of head, extending to jaw. Acute shooting or throbbing pains in forehead. *One cheek red, the other pale, [**Acon. Nux.**] *Bitter, bilious vomiting. *Over-sensitive to pain;* gets almost furious. *Very impatient, can hardly answer one civilly. Dysmenorrhœa, with labor-like pains.

**CHINA.** Headache from suppressed coryza. Soreness of the brain, as if bruised, worse from mental exertion, [***Nux. Sulph.**] *Intense throbbing headache after excessive depletion. *Ringing in the ears, and weak, fainting spells. Worse every other day, [**Amb.**]

**CHIONANTHUS VER.** *Habitual sick-headache.* Severe pain, chiefly in forehead and over the eyes. Eyeballs very painful, feel sore and bruised. *Very sick at stomach;* bitter eructations, nausea and retching, with desire for stool. Vomiting green, ropy bile.

**CIMICIFUGA.** *Headache of drunkards and students, [**Lach. *Nux.**] *Nervous, rheumatic menstrual headaches*, [**Bell.**

**Puls.**] Rush of blood to head, brain *feels too large* for cranium. *Top of head feels as if it would fly off, [as if *opening and shutting*, **Cann. in.**] Dull frontal headache, relieved by pressure, worse from motion. *Frequent, thin, dark, offensive stools.

**COCCULUS.** Sick-headache from riding in a carriage, on a boat, etc., [**Bell.**—Better from riding in carriage, **Nit. ac.**] Tearing, throbbing headache, especially in evening. *Violent headache, which compels patient to sit up, aggravated by *talking, laughing, noise, or bright light.* *Vertigo, with nausea and vomiting from motion of a carriage.

**COFFEA.** Patient very excitable. *Headache as if a nail were driven in brain, worse in open air, [vide **Ign.**] Pain in head as if it would fly to pieces, worse from noise or light. *Head feels too small,* [feels too large, **Glon. Nux.**] *Extreme wakefulness. Burning, sour eructations, [**Iris.**]

**GELSEMIUM.** Severe pain in forehead and vertex, dim sight, roaring in ears. Head feels enlarged, [**Arg. n. Glon. Nux.**] *Patient finds himself getting blind before headache comes on. Wild feeling, *alternating with uterine pains.* Adapted to nervous, excitable, hysterical females.

**GLONOIN.** *Congestive, nervous headache,* with no gastric or bilious symptoms. *Headache from recent exposure to sun, [**Acon.** ***Bell.**] *Violent *throbbing, pulsating headache,* with fullness and upward pressure in head, [**Bell.**] *Undulating sensation in head, worse from turning round. *Sick, faint-like feeling at stomach, with nausea.* Head feels too large. Palpitation of heart.

**IGNATIA.** Boring, sticking pain in forehead, relieved by lying down. *Pain as if a nail were driven out through side of head, [as if driven in vertex, **Nux.**] Headache as if something hard pressed upon the surface of brain. *Patient full of suppressed grief, with empty feeling at pit of stomach. Constipation, with prolapsus ani.

**IPECAC.** *If nausea and vomiting is the most prominent feature, [**Verat.**] Headache as if the brain and skull were bruised even to root of tongue. *Stooping causes vomiting. Diarrhœa; grass-green stools.

**IRIS VERSICO.** **Gastric sick-headache,* with vomiting sweetish mucus, [gastric headache from eating rich, greasy food, **Ant. Ipe.** ***Nux.** ***Puls.**] *The headache always begins with a blur before the eyes, [see **Gel.**] Sharp, cutting pains in forehead, eyes, and right side. Worse from rest, [**Ars. Sulph.**] Use low dilution.

**LACHESIS.** Headache with nausea and drowsiness. Throbbing or beating pains in temples, [**Acon. Arn.** ***Bell.**]. Pressing headache early in morning, worse from stooping. *Cannot bear anything tight about the waist. Vertigo, with paleness of face. *Pain in left ovarian region,* [in *right,* **Bell.**] *Larynx and throat very sensitive. Despondent mood. *Aggravation after sleep.*

**NUX VOMICA.** Headache with sour, bitter vomiting. Pressing, *boring* pain, with sensation as if skull would split, [**Bell. Bry.**] *Stupefying headache, especially in morning, aggravated by mental exertion, [**Calc. c. Sulph.**] *Habitual constipation of large, difficult stools, with frequent urging. *Sedentary* or *intemperate* habits; *troubled with piles.*

**PHOSPHORUS.** *Dull, stupefying headache, [**Calc. c.**] *sensation of coldness in cerebellum* [in vertex **Verat.**] *Headache every other day, [every seventh day, **Sang. Sil. Sulph.**] *Belching large quantities of wind after eating. Very sleepy after meals, especially after dinner. *Stools *long, narrow,* hard and very difficult to expel.

**PHOS. ACID.** Dreadful pain on top of head, as though the brain were crushed, after long-continued grief. *Too early and long-continued menstruation, with pain in liver. *Sensation as if stomach were being balanced up and down, [hanging down relaxed, **Arg. n.**] *Painless diarrhœa;* whitish stools.

**PHYTOLACCA.** *Sick-headache, with pain in back, *comes on every week. Headache of syphilitic patients,* [**Merc.**] Dull, heavy headache *in forehead,* [**Calc. c.**] *Sensation as if brain were bruised, when stepping from a high step to ground, [**Chin. Glon.**] Vertigo and dimness of vision.

**PULSATILLA.** Headache consequent upon eating rich, greasy food, [***Ant. Ipe. Nux.**] *Tearing, drawing,* or *stitching pains,* worse towards evening. *Vertigo, especially when stooping or looking up. *Craves cool, fresh air; worse in warm room, [**Phos.**—better in warm room, **Cocc. Sil.**] *Nausea* and vomiting, with repugnance to food. *Menses too late, scanty or suppressed. Chilliness, even in a warm room. She *weeps* and *complains,* [**Ign. Sep.**] Very bad taste in morning.

**SANGUINARIA.** *Sick-headache,* with vomiting bile, begins in morning, increases during the day; worse from motion, stooping, noise or light. *Pains in back part of head, running in rays from neck upwards. Severe pains in head, especially over right eye, with *nausea and vomiting.* *Has to keep in dark room and lie perfectly still.

**SEPIA.** *Beating, stitching* pains, mostly in forehead or temples, [see **Lach.**] Also violent pains, as if head would burst, extorting cries. *Nausea and vomiting, with a feeling of emptiness in stomach. *Dirty yellow appearance of face, especially across the nose. Constipation, with hard knotty stool. Very *fetid urine,* depositing a clay-colored sediment. *Leucorrhœa* between menses.

**SPIGELIA.** Periodical headache, [see **Ars.**] Pains *boring,* pressing, increased by motion, noise, and especially by *stooping,* [**Bry.**] **Nervous headache,* when one or both eyes are involved. *Headache commencing every morning with rising of sun, gets at its height at noon, when it gradually decreases till sun sets, [see **Sang.**] *Severe pressing and sticking pains in eyes, worse during motion.

**SULPHUR.** Pains mostly in forehead and temples, *pressing, throbbing* or *tearing.* *Constant heat on top of head, [*coldness,* **Sep.** ***Verat.**] *Early morning diarrhœa, driving patient out of bed. *Frequent weak, faint spells through the day. *Suppressed eruptions. Hemorrhoids.* *Lean persons who walk stooping.

**VERAT. ALB.** *Nervous headache,* [**Cham. Coff. Ign.**] Violent pains, that almost deprive patient of reason. *Becomes very weak and faint, with cold *sweat on forehead.* *Coldness on top of head, [*heat,* **Graph.** ***Sulph.**] *Vomiting, with exhausting diarrhœa, and cold sweat. Nervous headache at each menstrual period. *Great thirst for cold drinks.*

**DIETETICS.** In all cases of headache particular attention must be given the diet. Avoid the use of tea, coffee, and all vinous and fermented liquors. All rich and highly seasoned food, fresh bread, sweet cakes, pastry, etc. Eat sparingly of meat; let the diet consist chiefly of vegetables, milk, rice, light puddings, ripe fruits, bread made of *unbolted* flour, and drink plentifully of water.

---

## HEART, PALPITATION OF.

**THERAPEUTICS.** *Leading indications.*

**ACONITE.** *Young, plethoric* subjects, [**Arn. Bell.**] After *fright, over-exertion,* or drinking wine, [see **Opi.**] *Heart beats quicker and stronger, with great fear of death. Palpitation, with a feeling as if boiling water was poured into chest,

**ARNICA.** *After "straining the heart" from violent running. Palpitation after exertion; goes off by rest.

**ARSENICUM.** *Palpitation, with anguish, cannot lie on back. *Strong, visible, audible* beats of heart, worse at night and when lying on back. Fainting spells.

**ASAFŒTIDA.** Nervous palpitation from over-exertion or suppression of discharges (in women).

**BELLADONNA.** Great anguish about the heart, with *congestion to head.* *Palpitation when at rest, increasing during motion. *Violent palpitation, reverberating in brain. A kind of bubbling sensation* at heart when going up-stairs.

**CACTUS G.** Palpitation, with vertigo, loss of consciousness, dyspnœa; worse at night, lying on left side, at approach of menses, from exertion. *Sensation of constriction in heart, as if an iron hand prevented its normal action.

**CALC. CARB.** Tremulous pulsation of heart, worse after eating, at night, with anguish. *After suppressed eruptions and pimples on face.

**CHINA.** Palpitation, with rush of blood to face, and cold hands. *Great weakness from loss of vital fluids.

**COCCULUS.** *Tremulous palpitation* from quick motion and mental excitement, with dizziness and faintness

**COFFEA.** After *excessive exaltation.* Palpitation, violent, irregular, with trembling of limbs, [**Puls.**] *Sleeplessness, with agitation of body and mind.

**DIGITALIS.** *Sensation as if heart would stop beating if one moved. *Palpitation excited by talking, motion, or on lying down. Short, hurried breathing.

**FERRUM.** *Anæmic* condition. *Palpitation, better walking slowly about. *Throbbing in all the blood-vessels.* Soft bellows sound at apex of heart.

**KALI CARB.** *Palpitation in spells, taking away his breath.* Stitches about the heart, through to scapula.

**LACHESIS.** Palpitation and choking from the slightest exertion. *Can bear no pressure on throat or chest, must sit up or lie on right side.

**NITRIC ACID.** When caused by least mental excitement. Palpitation and anguish on going up-stairs.

**NUX VOM.** After *coffee, wines, liquors, spices.* Palpitation in frequent short paroxysms, with pulsating throbs in direction of heart. Tired sensation of heart.

**OPIUM.** After alarming events, causing fright, grief, sorrow, [**Acon.**] *Slow, irregular pulse.

**OXALIC ACID.** Immediately after lying down at night, palpitation for half an hour. *Pain in heart like electric flashes.

**PHOSPHORUS.** *Tightness across the chest,* with dyspnœa and great weakness, [**Puls.**] Palpitation, worse after eating or from mental emotion.

**PHOS. ACID.** Palpitation in children and young persons who grow too fast. *After grief or self-abuse.*

**PULSATILLA.** Young girls during time of puberty, or from suppressed menses. *Palpitation in violent paroxysms, often with anguish, obscuration of sight, and trembling of limbs, [see **Coff.**] After chagrin, fright, or joy.

**RHUS TOX.** Trembling sensation of heart. *Palpitation violent when sitting still. *Numbness and lameness of left arm.* Rheumatic subjects.

**RUMEX.** Heart feels as if it suddenly stopped beating, [*would stop, if he moved,* **Dig.**] followed by a heavy throbbing through the chest. Worse when lying, has to sit up.

**SEPIA.** Palpitation after mental emotion. *Wakes up with violent beating of heart. Palpitation, with anxiety about things which happened years ago. Suppression of menses, [see **Puls.**]

**TABACUM.** Palpitation, especially when lying on left side, [see **Cact.**] *Lassitude from muscular relaxation;* cold extremities. Compare PERICORDITIS, RHEUMATISM, ETC.

**GENERAL MEASURES.** Persons subject to attacks of palpitation should avoid over-exertion of body or mind, walking fast, running, ascending long flights of stairs, etc.

When the trouble arises from gastric disturbance, direct the treatment to this affection. When the bowels are found loaded with fecal accumulations, or distended with flatulence, *copious* injections of *warm water* should be given to relieve this condition.

*Hot foot-baths.* Valuable during an attack, especially if excited by uterine disorders or from hysteria.

**DIETETICS.** Plain, simple food; moderate exercise in open air, regular habits, and frequent ablutions. Avoid over-eating, and all *stimulating food* and *drinks*, tea, coffee and *tobacco*.

---

## HEMORRHOIDS.—PILES.

**THERAPEUTICS.** *Leading indications.*

**ACONITE.** Bleeding piles, [Bell. Caso. *Ham. Nit. ac.] Stinging and pressure in the anus. General dryness of the skin. *Constant restlessness, inability to keep still. Persons of a full, plethoric habit.

**ÆSCULUS HIP.** Large protruding *purple* tumors, with slight hemorrhage. **Itching, burning pains*, with a sense of fullness and dryness of anus, [Am. c.] *Severe aching pains in lumbar and sacral region, with stiffness of back, aggravated by walking. *Constant backache, affecting the sacrum and hips. Topical* applications useful.

**ALOES.** *Hemorrhoids protruding like grapes, with constant bearing down in rectum. *Great heat and tenderness of the tumors, relieved by cold water, [Apis.] Violent tenesmus, with bloody or jelly-like mucous stools. *Fistula in ano. Dull, heavy headache, with dull pains in liver. A feeling of faintness during and after stool.

**APIS MEL.** Hemorrhoids, with stinging, burning and smarting pains, relieved by cold water. *Constipation, with a sensation in abdomen as if something tight would break in voiding the stool. *Enlargement of right ovary, and pain in left pectoral region, with cough.

**ARSENICUM.** Blind piles, which *burn like fire*, particularly at night, hindering sleep. During the day, stinging pains, particularly when walking. *Great anguish, restlessness and fear of death. Much thirst, drinks little and often, [Apis.] All worse at night, particularly *after midnight.*

**BELLADONNA.** Bleeding piles, with great tenderness and pain from slightest touch. *Feeling in back as if it would break, hindering motion, [Ham.] *Pains appear suddenly and cease just as suddenly. Congestion of head, with throbbing in temples. *Sleepy, but cannot sleep.

**CALC. CARB.** Varices swollen and protruded, emitting considerable blood. Burning, pricking in rectum, patient cannot remain still. Drawing, cutting pains in rectum, with a feeling of painfulness, particularly after stool. *Menstruation too frequent and too profuse, [Bell.] *Cold, damp feet. Vertigo on going up-stairs.

**CARBO VEG.** Swollen, protruding varices, discharging pure blood. *Acrid, corroding humor oozing from rectum, emitting a *fetid smell*, [see **Sep.**] Tickling, itching and burning of the varices. Stools of *foul, bloody mucus.* *Eructations of sour, rancid food, with *much flatulence* from bowels.

**CAUSTICUM.** Large and painful varices, hindering stool. *Stinging and burning of the tumors when touched, intolerable when walking. Weak, scrofulous persons, with yellow complexion. Pressure and fullness in the abdomen, as if it would burst.

**COLLINSONIA.** Blind or bleeding piles, with sensation as if *gravel or sand had lodged in rectum.* Obstinate and habitual *constipation;* stools lumpy and light-colored, with dull pain in anus. Dysmenorrhœa. Aggravation in evening, and better in morning.

**DIOSCOREA.** Hemorrhoids, like grapes, around the anus, not bleeding, [see **Aloe.**] Involuntary discharge of slimy mucus from anus. Darting pain from old hemorrhoidal tumor to liver. Black, hard, lumpy stools.

**GRAPHITES.** Hemmorrhoids with prolapsus recti. Painful burning cracks between the varices. Burning, itching, and sticking in rectum. *Prolapsus recti, without straining, as if the sphincter were paralyzed. *Chronic constipation of hard, difficult, *knotty stools.* *Unhealthy skin, and eruptions that excrete a sticky fluid. *Fissura ani.*

**HAMAMELIS.** *Profusely bleeding hemorrhoids,* with burning soreness, and at times rawness of anus. *A slight loss of blood causes exhaustion, [**Hydras.**] The back feels as if it would break, [**Bell.**] *Passive hemorrhage from nose, stomach, or bowels.

**HYDRASTIS.** Even a light hemorrhoidal flow exhausts, [**Ham.**] Constipation, stools lumpy, covered with mucus, [**Caso.**] Flatulent colic, accompanid by faintness. *Sinking, gone feeling in stomach.

**IGNATIA.** Hemorrhoids, with violent shooting pains high up in rectum. *The tumors prolapse with every stool, and have to be replaced, [**Rhus. Sep. Sulph.**] Soreness of the parts as if excoriated. *Bleeding and pain worse when the stool is loose. Drawing pain around the pelvis. *Full of suppressed grief, with an empty feeling in the stomach.

**KALI CARB.** Large, painful varices, with considerable protrusion *during micturition.* Large, difficult stools, as if from inactivity of rectum. *The tumors swell and bleed during stool, with pricking and burning. *Constipation, with distress one or two hours before stool, with colicky, stitching pains.

**MURIATIC AC.** Large, protruding piles, with burning and sore pain. *The tumors are bluish, are *extremely sensitive and painful.* *Violent itching of the parts not relieved by scratching. Discharge of blood with the stool. Prolapsus ani during micturition.

**NITRIC AC.** Bleeding piles, protruding after every stool, *blood bright-red, not clotted.* *Sharp, cutting pain in rectum, lasting for hours after an evacuation, and is worse after a loose stool. *Old hemorrhoidal tumors, secreting much slime, and bleeding profusely after stool. *Fissures of the anus,* [**Ars. Graph.**]

**NUX VOM.** *Blind or bleeding piles.* [**Collin.** ***Sulph.**] Burning, pricking pains in tumors. Discharge of light-colored blood after stool. Horrid tearing, pressing pains in small of back and lower bowels. *Frequent and ineffectual urging to stool. *Habitual constipation. Is very irritable, and wishes to be alone. Persons of sedentary or intemperate habits, and victims of drugs, nostrums.

**PHOSPHORUS.** Bleeding piles, with severe lancinating pains. **The blood flows with each stool in a small stream.* Ulceration of rectum, with discharge of blood and pus. *Stools slender, long, tough, and difficult to expel.

**PODOPHYLLUM.** *Hemorrhoids and prolapsus recti during and after confinement. Prolapsus *uteri* with constipation and subinvolution which so frequently protract convalescence from child-bed.

**PULSATILLA.** Mostly *blind* piles, with painful pressure on the tumors. Stinging, itching in rectum, and *soreness of anus.* *Obstinate constipation, with nauseous, bad taste in morning. *Inclination to be chilly. *Disposition to weep and complain,* [**Ign. Sep.**] *Vertigo on rising from a sitting posture. Symptoms all *worse towards evening.*

**RHUS TOX.** Sore blind piles, protruding after every stool. Drawing in back from above downwards; tension and pressing in rectum. *Pain in small of back as if bruised, relieved by motion. Worse from getting wet, or by lifting heavy loads. Rheumatic diathesis.

**SEPIA.** Mostly *bleeding* piles, with protrusion of tumors and rectum during stool. Continual straining pain in rectum, with heat, burning, and swelling of anus. Oozing of moisture from rectum. [*corroding and fetid,* **Carb. v.**] *Sense of weight or of a ball in anus, not relieved by stool.

**SULPHUR.** *Blind or bleeding* piles. Constant urging to stool, which continues after a thin bloody evacuation. *Stinging, burning, and soreness in and about the anus. Prolapsus recti, during stool. Violent stitching pains in back. Burning pains in urethra during micturition. *Weak, faint spells, especially when standing or walking. *Constant heat on top of head.

**AUXILIARY MEASURES.** In *blind* piles, where tumors are highly inflamed and painful, *hot* sitz-baths are the best palliatives. In *profusely bleeding* piles, inject a solution *Tr. Hamamelis,* [ten drops to ounce water] and give same strength of remedy internally. These failing, use injections of *Tannic Acid* or *Persulphate of Iron* [ten grains to ounce water] to check hemorrhage. For *itching* piles, one part finely powdered *Borax* to five parts *Vaseline*, as an ointment will have salutary effect. Where tumors incline to suppurate apply *linseed meal* poultices.

Persons *subject* to piles, should avoid all vigorous exercise, *over-lifting*, resting on soft cushions, and *sedentary* habits.

**DIETETICS.** Bread from *unbolted* flour, fruits and vegetables fresh and ripe, with moderate amount of meat. Dried fruits, as peaches, apples, prunes, etc., will be found the most suitable diet.

---

## HERNIA.—RUPTURE.

Hernia is divided, according to locality, into *umbilical, inguinal, femoral*, scrotal, etc. And again, according to condition, into *reducible, irreducible*, and *strangulated.*

**Reducible** hernia is where the protruded part can readily be replaced.

**Irreducible** is applied to that form which, in consequence of adhesions or thickening, cannot be reduced, although there is no material constriction.

**Strangulated** hernia is where the opening that gives passage to the protruded intestine is constricted in such a way, that the contents of the protruded bowel cannot be propelled onwards, and the venous circulation is impeded.

**TREATMENT.** The first thing to be done is to *reduce* the hernia. In attempting this, the administration of one of the following remedies will afford adequate *assistance.* Repeat the medicine several time before making any extended efforts at reduction.

**ACONITE**. *Inflammation* of parts, with excessive *sensibility* to touch. Bilious vomiting. *Great nervous excitability.

**NUX VOMICA**. *One of principal remedies.* *Strangulated hernia. Bruised pain in bowels as if raw and sore. Frequent protrusion of inguinal hernia. *Nausea, vomiting* and *constipation.*

**OPIUM**. Redness of face, and slowness of pulse. *Vomiting putrid matter, or fæces and urine, [**Plumb.**] Pain in abdomen, as if intestines were cut to pieces.

**PLUMB. MET.** *Incarcerated hernia*, [**Verat. a.**] *Intussusception, with colic and fæcal vomiting, [see **Opi.**] *Violent colic, abdomen drawn in as by a string to spine. Anxiety, cold sweat and fainting.

**VERATR. ALB.** Incarcerated hernia, not inflamed, antiperistaltic action. *Rushes about bent double*, pressing abdomen. *Cold sweat on forehead.

**TAXIS.** Use anæsthetic. Place patient upon back, elevate hips, flex thigh upon abdomen, and rotate limb inwards. Grasp tumor with one hand, and make gentle and *steady* pressure, while with the other hand manipulate neck of tumor back into abdomen. Continue this operation for half an hour or longer, when, if successful, the intestine will return with a gurgling noise.

**Dry Cup.** A *large* dry cup, as a quart measure, or bowl applied to abdomen, has proved successful.

**Inversion.** Hang patient up by the heels. An assistant stooping at bedside, seizes patient's feet, draws them over his shoulders, then rising lifts the sick man with head hanging down, back to back, carries him about with a jolting motion. This method has been very successful, but it too fails at times, when only an operation dividing the stricture will save the patient's life.

**HERNIA OF INFANTS.** Congenital hernia should receive early attention. Soon as discovered, a suitable bandage should be applied over the protruded part and worn constantly, while the appropriate homœopathic remedy should be given to complete the cure.

---

## HEPATITIS.

**THERAPEUTICS.** *Leading indications.*

**ACONITE.** *Violent inflammatory fever*, with stitches in liver. *Intolerable pains driving one to despair. *Great restlessness, anxiety, and fear of death. Vertigo on sitting up. Headache as if everything would press out of forehead. Bitter, bilious vomiting. *Retention of urine, with stitches in kidneys. *Great nervous excitability.*

**ARSENICUM.** Region of liver tender and swollen, with violent burning pains. Vomiting of *brownish* or *blackish* substances, [**Verat.**] Diarrhœa of blackish stools, worse after eating or drinking. *Violent thirst, drinking little and often. Great restlessness, and fear of death, [**Acon.**] *Rapid prostration* of strength. *Better from warm drinks.*

**BELLADONNA.** Acute pain in region of liver, extending to chest and shoulder. Tension in region of stomach, [**Merc.**] *Tenderness of whole abdomen, aggravated by the least jar. *Congestion of head, with throbbing pains in temples. Almost constant moaning, with *starting and jumping during sleep.* *Delirium, with desire to escape. *Cannot bear noise or bright light.* *Urine yellow as gold.

**BRYONIA.** Burning or stitching pains in hypochondria. Pain in right shoulder and arm. Yellow-coated tongue, with *bitter, bilious vomiting.* *Lips cracked, parched and dry. *Splitting headache,* [**Bell. Merc.**] *Sitting up in bed causes *nausea and faintness.* Region of stomach very sensitive. *Exceedingly irritable, everything makes him angry, [see **Nux.**] *Hard, dry stools, as if burnt. *Wants to keep perfectly quiet.

**CHELIDON.** Acute or dull pain, and tenderness in region of liver. *Constant pain under lower inner angle of right shoulder-blade. Sallow, jaundiced complexion,

[***Merc.**] *Stools like sheep's dung, or soft and bright yellow. Urine scanty, deep yellow, sour.

**CHINA.** *Headache, bitter taste, yellow skin.* Pain in hepatic region, as if from subcutaneous ulceration, [**Lach.**] *Swollen, hard liver,* [**Agar.**] *Colic from gall stones, [**Lyc. Merc. Nux.**] *Abdomen feels full and tight, as if stuffed.

**HYDRASTIS.** *Torpor of liver, with pale, scanty stools. Jaundice, with catarrh of stomach and duodenum. **Goneness* and faintness in stomach, general prostration.

**LEPTANDRA.** Aching pains in liver. Yellow-coated tongue. *Black, profuse, papescent, tar-like, very fetid stools, generally in afternoon or evening. Dark-brown urine, [**Bry.**] *Constant dull pain in region of gall-bladder,* [***Phyto.**] *Jaundice.

**MERCURIUS.** *Threatened formation of abscess.* Inability to lie on right side, [**Puls.**] *Inflammation, with great tenderness of liver to contact, and jaundice-like appearance of skin. *When coughing or sneezing, a stitch runs directly through the chest to back. *Much perspiration affording no relief. *Green, bilious,* or frothy stools, with *frequent urgings* and *tenesmus.* Bilious vomiting.

**LACHESIS.** Acute pain in liver, extending towards stomach. Pain as if something had lodged in right side, with stinging. *Cannot bear any pressure about hypochondria. Suitable after *ague, and to drunkards,* [see **Nux.**]

**NUX VOM.** Stitching or throbbing pains in liver, with great tenderness to contact, [**Bell.**] *Sour or bitter taste in mouth, with bilious vomiting. Shortness of breath, and sense of pressure under the ribs. *Splitting headache, [see **Bry.**] Habitual constipation, large, difficult stools. *Cannot sleep *after* 3 A. M., [cannot sleep *before* 3 A. M., **Merc.**] Persons of sedentary or intemperate habits.

**PODOPHYLLUM.** *Torpidity of liver, with fullness and pain, [see **Hydras.**] Nausea and bilious vomiting. *The patient is constantly rubbing and shaking the hypochondriac region. Bitter taste and risings in mouth. *Painless morning diarrhœa, [**Sulph.**]

**PULSATILLA.** Yellow-coated tongue and bitter taste. Frequent attacks of anguish, especially at night. Nausea and desire to vomit. *Green, slimy diarrhœa, usually at night. *Chilliness, even in a warm room, with vertigo when rising from a sitting posture. *Weeps and complains,* [**Ign. Sep.**] Frequent urging to urinate, with cutting pain. Symptoms all worse towards evening.

**SILICEA.** Hardness and distension of region of liver. Throbbing, ulcerative pain, increased by contact and motion. *Formation of abscess, [**Hep.**] *Constipation; stool recedes after having been partially expelled. *Lymphatic swellings, with inclination to suppurate.

**SULPHUR.** Mostly chronic hepatitis. Swelling and hardness of liver, [**Chin.**] Beating, stitching pains and pressure in liver. *Frequent weak, faint spells, with flashes of heat. *Constant heat on top of head. Constipation, or *early morning diarrhœa.* *Drowsy during the day, wakeful at night.

Hepatic **ABSCESS** requires: **Bell. *Bry. *Hep. Lach. *Merc. Phos. Sil. Sulph. Therid.**

For **ENLARGEMENT**, or induration of the liver: **Agar. Ars. Calc. c. *Chin. Nux v. Sulph.**

**AUXILIARY MEASURES.** Use *hot fomentations* or poultices to relieve pain and soreness. Should an abscess form, and the presence of pus be reasonably suspected, it will be advisable to draw it off through the needle of an aspirator.

**DIETETICS.** Light diet, vegetable broths, gruels, rice, oatmeal mush, farina, corn-starch puddings, roasted apples, plenty of water. Abstain from use of meat, fatty and saccharine substances, and all stimulants.

---

## HEPATIC COLIC.—GALL-STONE COLIC.

Hepatic colic is characterized by severe pain in region of liver, chiefly about the gall-bladder occasioned by the passage of a biliary calculus through the cystic and choledoc ducts. The attack usually comes on suddenly, and the pain ceases soon as the stone gets out of the duct.

**THERAPEUTIC AGENTS.**

**BELLADONNA.** Region of liver painful and sore. *Violent pain, goes to shoulder and neck, can tolerate no pressure or jar. *Worse lying on right side.*

**CALCARIA CARB.** Stitches and pressure in hepatic region. *Feeling of great tightness in hypochondria as if laced. This remedy is highly commended by HUGHS and others.

**CHINA.** Never fails to correct the tendency to formation of gall-stones.—THAYER.

**NUX VOMICA.** Throbbing as if from formation of abscess. *Cutting, cramping pains with desire to vomit. Jaundiced condition, fainting turns. One of best remedies to relieve the pain.

**COLOCYNTH.** *Violent cutting, tearing pain, compelling patient to bend double, [has to bend backwards, **Bell.**] If arising from indignation.

**AUXILIARY MEASURES.** *Hot fomentations*, or bags of *hot salt* applied to painful part will often give relief. Placing patient in hot bath (100° to 110°) is also beneficial. The giving of *three* or *four* ounces of warm *Olive-oil* soon as pain appears, recommended by some, is worthy of trial. Failing to relieve the excruciating pain by these means, resource should be had to the inhalation of *Chloroform*, or subcutaneous injections of *Morphia* (one-eighth to one-quarter of a grain) in the arm, every two hours, until relief is obtained.

## HERPES.—TETTER.

**THERAPEUTICS.** *Leading indications.*

For **HERPES** *Circinatus:* **Calc. *Lith. c. Nat. c. *Phyto. *Sep.**

For **HERPES** *Facialis:* **Ars. Calc. Graph. Ledum. Sars.**

For **HERPES** *Genitalium:* ***Dulc. *Petro. *Phos. ac. Rhus t. *Tellu.**

For **HERPES** *Zoster:* **Iris. *Merc. Rhus t. Sili. Thuy.**

**ACONITE.** *Acute cases*, with febrile excitement. Large red itching pimples, filled with acrid fluid. The disease mostly shows itself on the forehead or temples.

**APIS MEL.** Eruptions which usually come out in cold weather. *Small pustules, with *burning, smarting*, stinging, and which form dry, scaly, laminated, brownish scabs. Worse from *warm*, better from *cold* applications.

**ARSENICUM.** *Confluent herpetic eruptions, with *intense burning*, [see **Merc.**] Chronic dry skin. *Cannot sleep after midnight. Worse from *cold*, better from *warmth*, [reverse, **Apis.**] Herpes having a red *unwholesome* appearance.

**BOVISTA.** *Moist* or *dry herpes*, itching on getting warm, continues after scratching. *Red scabby eruption on thighs and bends of knees, appear in hot weather and with full moon. Tetter on back of hands.

**CALC. CARB.** *Herpes circinatus* (ringworm), with moist eruption, itching violently. *Unhealthy, ulcerative skin, [**Graph. Hep. Sulph.**] *Scrofulous diathesis.* *Cold, damp feet.

**CICUTA.** Herpes, especially on face, confluent burning, suppurating, [**Ars.**] *Burning, suppurating eruptions on and around the ears, and hairy scalp.

**CLEMATIS.** *Scaly herpetic eruptions, with yellowish, corrosive ichor. *Chronic, red, humid herpes*, with intolerable itching from warmth of bed, and after washing. *The herpes is red and humid with the *increasing*, but pale and dry with the decreasing moon.

**CROTON TIG.** Vesicular eruption, with burning, stinging, and redness of the skin. *Herpetic eruption on scrotum*, [see **Petro.**] Itching, followed by painful burning.

**DULCAMARA.** *Herpes moist, suppurating*, [**Lyc. Merc. Sep.**] *Thick *crusts* over the whole body, burning, itching. *Tetter oozing watery fluid, [see **Graph.**] Bleeding after scratching.

**GRAPHITES.** *Rawness in bend of limbs, groins, neck, behind ears, especially in children.* *The eruption discharges a *sticky, glutinous fluid*, [see **Petro.**] Unhealthy skin, every little injury suppurates, [**Hep. Sulph.**] Herpes in females, with scanty menses. *Herpes zoster.*

**LEDUM.** **Dry, scaly* tetter in the face, burning in open air. Crusty eruption around mouth and nose, with itching, smarting, and burning. *Want of animal heat.

**MERCURIUS.** Herpetic spots and suppurating pustules,

sometimes running together, forming dry, scaly spots or crusts, with acrid discharge. *Herpes of the genitals, [**Petro. Phos. ac.**] *Zona*, like a girdle, from back around abdomen, itching and tendency to suppurate.

**MEZEREUM.** *Herpes zoster*, with severe neuralgic pains, [**Ran. b. Zinc.**] The vesicles form brownish scabs, and itch violently. Chilly even in warm room.

**NATRUM MUR.** Herpes labialis during fever. *Moist oozing eruptions in bends of arms and knees, [**Graph.**] *Skin of hands, especially *about nails*, dry, cracked.

**PETROLEUM.** *Tetter, especially on *genitals*, moist, oozing, itching, [**Dulc.**] Itching herpes, followed by ulcers. Worse in open air when perspiring, better from warmth.

**PHOSPHORUS.** *Dry tetter*, [**Ars. Bov. Sulph.**] Vesicles confluent and appear in clusters. Brown-colored blisters between the fingers and toes. *Long, slender, hard stools, difficult to expel. Lean, slender persons; very *sensitive to cold.*

**RANUN. BUL.** Vesicular eruptions as if from burns. *Shingles*, with intercostal neuralgia, [see **Mez.**] Blister-like eruptions in palms of hands.

**RHUS TOX.** Confluent vesicles, containing a milky or watery fluid. *Herpetic eruptions, alternating with pains in chest and dysenteric stools. *The eruption is attended with incessant itching, burning, and tingling. *Shingles.*

**SARSAPARILLA.** Herpetic ulcers, extending in a circular form without crusts, red granulated bases, white borders. The eruption discharges a *reddish secretion.*

**SEPIA.** Itching, burning, *humid tetter*, [**Dul. Graph. Merc.**] *Herpes circinnatus, (ringworm). *Humid* places in bends of elbows and knees, [**Graph. Nat. m.**] The itching is made worse by scratching. Females with uterine difficulties.

**SULPHUR.** Herpes, with great itching, burning, and soreness after scratching. *Dry, scabby, scurfy tetter, [see **Phos.**] *Unhealthy skin*, every little injury suppurates. Aversion to *water and cold air.*

**TELLURIUM.** Herpes filled with a watery, excoriating fluid, smelling like fish-brine. *Ringworms all over the body, more distinct on lower limbs.

**THUYA.** *Herpes zoster*, [see **Merc.**] *White, scaly, dry, mealy tetter, [see **Sulph.**] Eruption only on covered parts, burn violently after scratching. Worse from cold water, from heat of bed at night.

**ZINCUM.** *Dry tetter* over the whole body. *Herpes zoster, followed by neuralgia, [see **Mez.**] Violent itching, especially in bends of joints. *Fidgety feet.

**LOCAL MEASURES.** To allay the itching, which is often very annoying, a little *Vaseline*, or equal parts of *Glycerine* and *Rose-water* may be applied to the affected parts.

**DIETETICS.** Persons subject to this affection should

avoid fatty, rich and indigestible food. The diet should consist chiefly of vegetables, a little meat, bread made of *unbolted* flour, milk, plenty of water, ripe fruits, etc. Pay strict attention to cleanliness, bathing, exercise, regular habits, sleep on hard beds, and in well *ventilated* apartments.

---

## HOARSENESS.

**THERAPEUTICS.** *Leading indications.*

**ACONITE.** *After exposure to dry, cold winds,* [**Hepar.**] *Hoarse, croaking voice, like croup, Larynx sensitive to touch, [**Phos.**] Child grasps its throat when it coughs.

**ALUMINA.** Rawness in larynx on awaking. Sudden complete aphonia. *Hoarseness evening and night, especially towards morning. Voice husky, with nasal twang.

**AMM. CARB.** Hoarseness, cannot speak a loud word, [**Phos.**] Great dryness in larynx, [**Bell.**] Hoarseness worse from speaking. Burning in chest, [**Calc. c. Merc.**]

**BELLADONNA.** **Hoarseness with rough voice.* Talking is very difficult; has to speak in a piping voice. Larynx dry and *sensitive to touch.* *Sore throat.

**CALC. CARB.** **Painless hoarseness,* is unable to speak, especially early in morning. *Chronic hoarseness,* [**Carb. v.**] *Cold damp feet. *Scrofulous diathesis.*

**CARBO VEG.** *Long-lasting hoarseness, worse from talking, and in evening, [worse in morning, **Caust. Phos.**] *Hoarseness after measles,* [see **Dros.**] *Chronic hoarseness,* worse from damp evening air.

**CAUSTICUM.** *Hoarseness and *roughness* of throat early in morning. *Burning and roughness* in throat, with hoarseness. Great dryness of the larynx.

**CHAMOMILLA.** **Catarrhal hoarseness* of trachea, with dryness of eyelids, [see **Dulc.**] Hoarseness or loss of voice in children, with rough cough. *Tough mucus in larynx,* which can only be removed by strong hawking.

**DROSERA.** *Deep, hollow, hoarse* voice, requiring great efforts to speak. *Rough, scraping feeling of dryness in fauces. Hoarseness after *measles,* [**Cham. Dulc.**]

**DULCAMARA.** Rough, hoarse voice after taking cold, [**Cham. Merc. Puls.**] *Hoarseness after *measles,* [after *croup,* **Hep. Phos.**] Worse from every *cold change* in weather.

**GELSEMIUM.** *Hoarse in paroxysms,* with dry, rough throat. *Throat feels as if filled up, [**Sili.**] *Catarrh, with rawness of chest.* Croupy cough.

**HEPAR SULPH.** Hoarseness and roughness in throat, [**Caust.**] *Larynx very sensitive to cold air. *Hoarseness after croup,* [**Lyc. Phos.**] *Rough, barking cough.*

**KALI CARB.** Aphonia, with violent sneezing. *Scraping, dryness, and parched feeling in larynx. *Stitching pains* in the chest, left side, with dry cough.

**LYCOPOD.** Hoarseness, with feeble, husky voice. Dryness in windpipe. Hoarseness remaining after croup, [see **Hepar.**] Loose cough by day, suffocative spells at night. *Fanlike motion of alæ nasi.

**MERCURIUS.** *Catarrhal hoarseness*, [see **Cham.**] Burning, rawness in larynx. *Fluent coryza and sore throat. Profuse sweating, without relief.

**NUX VOM.** *Hoarseness, with roughness and scraping in throat, [**Dros.**] Spasmodic constriction of larynx after midnight; suffocating spells, [see **Lyc.**]

**PHOSPHORUS.** Hoarseness, with cough and *rawness in larynx* and bronchiæ, worse in evening. *Hoarseness, with complete loss of voice, [**Bell. Merc. Sulph.**] *Larynx feels as if lined with fur.* Cannot talk on account of pain in larynx.

**PHYTOLACCA.** Hoarseness and aphonia. Dryness of larynx and trachea, worse towards evening. Burning in air-passages, with sensation of contraction of glottis.

**PULSATLLLA.** Hoarseness and roughness of throat, cannot speak aloud, [**Caust. Phos.**] *Loss of smell, with catarrh. Worse *towards evening.*

**RHUS TOX.** *Hoarseness of singers, or from overstraining* voice, [**Arn. Arum t. Phos.**] Throat feels stiff. Roughness in larynx, with roughness and soreness in chest.

**SULPHUR.** Voice rough, hoarse, with mucus on chest. *Aphonia*, [**Bell. Caust. Phos.**] Talking fatigues and excites the pain. Shooting pains through left chest to back.

---

## HOOPING-COUGH.—PERTUSSIS.

**THERAPEUTICS.** *Leading indications.*

**ACONITE.** If a constant febrile condition prevails, and when at the commencement the cough is dry, whistling, with soreness of throat. *The child grasps at its throat with every cough, as if it were in pain. *Great anguish, restlessness and anxiety.

**AMBRA GRIS.** Severe paroxysms of hollow-sounding cough, worse morning and evening and during the night. Oppression and rapid respiration. Expectoration of large quantities of tough, grayish, or yellow mucus, especially in the morning.

**ANACAR.** When fits of anger cause the cough, and when children are very ill-natured, [**Cham.**] Difficulty of breathing accompanies and succeeds the coughing spells. *Children with uncontrollable tempers.

**ARNICA.** Left cheek swollen and red, with heat in the head and coldness of the body. *Every coughing spell is preceded by crying, [**Tart. e.**—cries after couging, **Bell.**] Feels sore all over, as if bruised. Bleeding from the nose, [***Bell.**]

**ARSENICUM.** Suffocative, dry cough, with scanty or

suppressed urine. *Great prostration, with waxy paleness and coldness of skin. *Intense thirst, drinks little and often. *Feels better in a warm room. Aggravation at night, particularly after midnight.

**BELLADONNA.** Frequent paroxysms, worse in night, hard and barking, like croup. *The child gets very red in face with every coughing spell, [gets blue, **Coral. r.** ***Ipe.**] *Eyes swollen, and sclerotica injected with blood. *Bleeding of nose.* In beginning, or when disease has attained a high degree of severity.

**BRYONIA.** Paroxysms set in principally in evening or at night, or after *eating* or *drinking, with vomiting.* *Cough, with expectoration of brownish phlegm, with stitches through chest, [**Acon. Bell.**] *Dry, hard stools, as if burnt. Exceedingly irritable, everything makes him angry. Lips parched, dry, and cracked.

**CHAMOMILLA.** Dry cough, worse at night, or in cold air. *Child very fretful, must be carried all the time. *One cheek red and hot, the other pale and cold, [**Acon.**] Green, watery, corroding stools, smelling like bad eggs. *Warm sweat about the head.

**CINA.** *During paroxysm, child suddenly becomes stiff, [and blue in face, **Ipe.**] After paroxysm, there is a gurgling noise from throat to abdomen. Cough aggravated by running, talking, laughing, etc. *Paleness of face and blueness around mouth and eyes. Spasms, with jerking and twisting of muscles. *Much picking of nose and other worm symptoms.

**COCCUS CACTI.** Nightly, periodical attacks of cough, from tickling in larynx. Every coughing spell ends with expectoration of large quantities of viscid, stringy mucus, [**Kali b.**] *Cough worse on first waking.*

**CORAL. RUB.** Spasms of cough, so violent that child *loses* its *breath* and *turns purple* and *black* in face, [see **Ipe.**] *Takes very little food or drink. Spasmodic, convulsive cough. *Head feels too large.*

**CUPRUM.** Violent and long-continued paroxysms of cough, completely exhausting patient. *During attack child becomes rigid, turns black in face, and seems as if dead, [**Coral. r.**] Vomiting after paroxysm, and rattling of mucus in chest between attacks.

**DROSERA.** The paroxysm is extremely violent, with chills and fever. *Violent spasmodic cough, threatening suffocation, [**Hepar.**] *Worse, particularly after twelve at night. Vomiting food or mucus, and bleeding from the mouth and nose, [**Bry.**]

**HEPAR SULPH.** Dry, spasmodic cough, with soreness of larynx, worse towards morning. *Cough sounds croupy, and it seems as if patient would choke. Rattling, choking cough, worse after midnight. *Cannot bear to be uncovered, coughs when any part of body is exposed.

**IPECAC.** *Suffocative cough; the child becomes *stiff and blue in the face,* [**Coral. r. Cup.**] *The chest seems full of phlegm, but does not yield to coughing, [**Tart. e.**] The cough causes *gagging and vomiting phlegm*

**KALI BICHRO.** Violent rattling cough, lasting some minutes, with an effort to vomit. *Choking cough, with expectoration of viscid mucus, which can be drawn out in long strings. Burning pain in trachea.

**MEPHITIS.** *Spasmodic, hollow or deep cough,* with hoarseness and pain in chest. *Inhalation difficult, exhalation almost impossible. Vomits all food some hours after eating. Worse at night and after lying down.

**MERCURIUS.** Cough only at night, or only by day. *Two paroxysms succeed each other closely, and are separated from next two by an interval of perfect rest. During vomiting patient bleeds at nose and mouth, [see **Nux v.**] *Profuse sweat at night, with nervous agitation.

**NAPHTHALIN.** Violent *spasmodic* cough, the paroxysms *lasting a long time.* This remedy in 3x dec., trit., is regarded by some as almost specific for whooping-cough.

**NUX VOMICA.** Hard, dry cough, worse in morning. *Child has choking spells, becomes blue in face, bleeds at nose and mouth. Gagging, vomiting and constipation. During paroxysm, pain in umbilical region, as if it would be torn to pieces. After nostrums and cough mixtures.

**PULSATILLA.** Cough from beginning, with profuse expectoration. Frequent vomiting mucus or ingesta, [***Ipe.**] Diarrhœa, especially at night. *Chilliness even in a warm room, and vertigo on rising from a seat. Mild, tearful persons, with blue eyes, blonde hair.

**SQUILLA.** During cough child sneezes, waters at nose and eyes. *Constant rubbing of nose, face and eyes during cough. Cough *excited* by *cold drinks and from exertion,* [*relieved* by *cold drinks,* **Cup.**]

**TART. EM.** Cough preceded by crying, or occurs after eating or drinking or when getting warm in bed. *Rattling cough, bronchial tubes seem full of mucus, but none is expectorated, [**Ipe.**] *Nausea and vomiting large quantities of mucus, with cold sweat on forehead.

**VERAT. ALB.** *Convulsive stage;* worse spring and fall. *After every coughing spell child falls over exhausted; cold sweat on forehead. Vomiting tough, thin mucus, and involuntary discharge of urine. Attacks occur on entering a warm room, or from drinking cold water, [see **Squil.**]

**GENERAL MEASURES.** Patients should take moderate exercise in open air; sleep in well ventilated apartments; live on plain, simple food; take frequent tepid baths, and conform to regular habits in all respects.

# HYDROCELE.

Hydrocele is a term applied to a collection of serous fluid in the areola texture of the scrotum or in some of the coverings, either of the testicles or spermatic cords.

The disease may be distinguished from hernia: By *increase* of tumor from *below* upwards; by semi-transparency of tumor; by fluctuation; by smoothness of surface; by absence of cough impulse; absence of pain and history of case.

The disease can, in most cases, be cured by internal medication, if it has not been neglected too long.

## THERAPEUTICS. *Leading remedies.*

**ARNICA.** When caused from *mechanical* injuries or *contusion*, [Con. **Puls.**] *Involuntary urination during sleep. *Sore all over.*

**CALCARIA CARB.** *Scrofulous diathesis, [**Iodi.**] Loss of appetite, debility, emaciation, dryness of skin. *Cold damp feet.

**CONIUM.** Particularly suitable if caused by mechanical injuries or contusion, [see **Arn.**] Bad effects from excessive sexual indulgence.

**DIGITALIS.** *Hydrocele with swelling of testicles. *Irregular heart action.* One of best remedies in this affection.

**GRAPHITES.** *Hydrocele,* [left side] with herpetic eruptions on scrotum. Dropsical swelling of prepuce and scrotum.

**IODINE.** *Scrofulous habit,* glandular swellings, painless swelling of testicles, with offensive sweat.

**RHODODENDRON.** A valuable remedy in hydrocele. Has proved curative in cases of long standing where there was no disease of testes.

**PALLIATIVE TREATMENT.** This consists in evacuating contents of sac, with a trocar. Grasp tumor from behind, [patient in erect posture], and plunge the trocar into sac, pointing the instrument upwards and backwards, to avoid wounding testicle. The trocar being withdrawn, the canula remains for fluid to make its escape through.

**Radical Method.** Evacuate fluid as above described, and then inject into the sac through canula a teaspoonful *Tr. Iodine*, allowing it to remain with a view of establishing adhesions. Others use *Carbolic acid*, [20 to 30 drops] as an injection, and claim for it superior success.

**Treatment by Seton.** Draw off fluid through canula, insert trocar again, and push it up and out through scrotum above. Now withdraw the trocar and pass a ligature through canula; this done, remove canula and make fast the ligature. Let remain in until suppuration takes place.

## HYDROCEPHALUS.

**THERAPEUTICS.** *Leading indications.*

**ACONITE.** In first stage of irritation. *Intolerance of light and noise, [***Bell.**] *Great fear and anxiety, with nervous excitability. *The child is sleepless, restless, cries much, bites its fist, and has a green, watery diarrhœa.

**APIS MEL.** High fever, with delirium. Sleep interrupted by sudden shrill cries. *Boring head into pillow, [**Bell.**] *Squinting, grinding teeth. *Twitching on one side, while other is paralyzed. Profuse perspiration on head, of musk-like odor, [**Sulph.**] Scanty emissions of urine.

**APOCYNUM.** Sutures open, [*fontanelles,* ***Calc. c. Sulph.**] Forehead projecting. Sight of one eye totally lost, the other slightly sensible. Stupor. Constant involuntary motion of one leg and arm, [see **Hell.**] Urine suppressed.

**ARTEMISIA.** Convulsions of right side, and paralysis of left. Body cold all over. Sopor, yet drinking and swallowing eagerly. Face pale, has oldish look, [**Arg. n. Opi.**] Involuntary stools, which are greenish and thin.

**BELLADONNA.** Face flushed, eyes injected, [**Acon.**] *Pupils contracted or dilated,* [**Hell. Hyos. Opi.**] Boring head in pillow, rolling eyes, squinting, [**Apis.**] *Throbbing of carotids. *Sudden starting and jumping during sleep. Involuntary emissions of urine. *Great intolerance of light or noise.*

**BRYONIA.** Manifest *signs of effusion,* [**Dig. Hell.**] Dark, flushed face, *dry and parched lips.* Tongue coated with a dark-yellowish fur. *Frequent motion of the jaws, as if chewing, [**Hell.**] *Cannot sit up on account of nausea and faintness. *Hard, dry stools, as if burnt. *Scanty, hot, red urine.* Exceedingly irritable.

**CALC. CARB.** *Scrofulous diathesis.* *Large head, with open fontanelles, [**Calc. phos. Sulph.**] *Profuse perspiration on head when sleeping. *Emaciation, with good appetite. Painful and difficult urination, urine having a strong, fetid odor.

**CALC. PHOS.** *Hydrocephaloid condition.* *Delayed closure, or reopening of fontanelles, [see **Calc. c.**] Bones of skull soft and thin. Screaming, grasping the head with hands. Cannot hold the head up, it totters. *Squinting,* and distortion of eyeballs, [***Apis.**] Cold sweat on the face.

**CINA.** Child seems frightened, jumps out of bed, sees imaginary objects, screams, trembles, and talks hurriedly. *Cannot bear to be touched or looked at. Turning the head from side to side. *Picking and boring at the nose, [**Hell.**] Twitching and trembling of body.

**CUPRUM MET.** *Metastasis during catarrhal fever, difficult dentition,* or *exanthematic diseases,* [metastasis of measles, ***Puls.**] *Stage of exudation, [**Bry. Hell.**] Eyes red, *balls constantly rotating.* Squinting, [**Apis. Hell.**] Cannot hold the head up. Great irregularity of pulse.

**HELLEBORUS.** After exudation has taken place, [**Bry.**] *Rolling the head*, [**Hyos.**] *Automatic motions of one arm and one leg. *Soporous sleep, with screaming and starting. *Lower jaw sinking down, [**Opi.**] Chewing motion of the mouth. Squinting, pupils dilated, [contracted, **Zinc.**] Forehead drawn in folds, and covered with cold sweat. Vomiting green or blackish substances.

**HYOSCYAMUS.** Cries out suddenly, [**Apis. Bell.**] *Eyes red, starting, rolling about in orbits*, [**Cup.**] Squinting and grinding of teeth, [**Apis.**] Eyes protruding, [**Bell. Calc. phos. Stram.**] Frothing at mouth, impeded deglutition.

**MERCURIUS.** Precocious mental development, [**Bell.**] Large head, sutures open, [see **Calc.**] *Fetid, sour smelling, oily sweat on head. *Scorbutic condition of gums. *Body bathed in sweat.*

**OPIUM.** *Extreme drowsiness, and coma, with stertorous breathing. Face purplish and swollen, [crimson-red, **Bell.**] *Screaming before or during spasm. Dilated pupils, and general symptoms of paralysis of brain, [**Zinc.**]

**STRAMONIUM.** Convulsive motions of head. Sensation of lightness in head, causing patient to frequently raise it up. *Awakens with a shrinking look, as if afraid of first object seen. *Loquacious delirium, with a desire to escape. No thirst, although mouth is very dry. *Light of brilliant objects and contact renew the spasms. *Black fluid stools.*

**SULPHUR.** Heaviness of head, sinking involuntarily backwards. Sweat on head, with musk-like smell, [**Apis.**] Sour smell from mouth. *Drowsiness in daytime, wakefulness at night. Scrofulous diathesis; dry, husky, scaly skin. *After suppressed or dried-up eruptions on head, and other parts.

**ZINCUM.** *Impending paralysis* of brain. Frequent jerking of whole body, and crying out during sleep. When awakened, expresses fear and rolls the head, [see **Hell.**] *Constant trembling of hands, with cold extremities, [**Stram.**] Gagging and vomiting, with a voracious appetite.

**PROPHYLACTIC MEASURES.** In all cases where there is a predisposition to the disease, **Calc. phos.** should be administered and its action kept up for months. The child should be tenderly cared for, and every precaution taken to maintain its general health. It should be kept in the free open air much as possible, all *mental* excitement avoided and due attention paid to the development of its physical strength.

**AUXILIARY MEASURES.** During an attack, cold applications to the head is commended by some. A *sponge cap*, made by sewing thin pieces of sponge together and covering it with oiled silk, is saturated with *cold* water and placed over the head. A *gum bag*, partially filled with pounded ice, and applied to the head, also beneficial. Keep extremities warm by jugs of *hot* water. Drawing off the *water* with *Aspirator* has been successful.

---

## HYSTERIA.

**THERAPEUTICS.** *Leading indications.*

**ACONITE.** *Great and distressing fear of death, [**Ars.**] She *dreads too much activity* about her, and fears to go into crowds. *Anxiety, restlessness and tossing about. Vertigo on raising head after stooping or lying down.

**ANACARDIUM.** * *Great weakness* or loss of memory, [**Arg. n. Calc.**] Sadness, looks on anxious side of everything. *Irresistible desire to curse and swear, [**Lil. tig.**] Feels as if she had two wills, one commanding to do what the other forbids. *Gastric and nervous headache.

**ARSENICUM.** *Hysterical asthma at every little excitement, worse latter part of night. Cannot lie down for fear of suffocation. *Dread of death when alone or on going to bed, [desires death, **Aur. Bell.**] Great anxiety and restlessness. Wants to be in a *warm room.*

**ASAFŒTIDA.** Fits of great joy, with occasional bursts of laughter. Apprehensions of dying. *Hysterical spasms, *œsophagus being chiefly affected.* *Sensation of a ball rising in throat, [**Lach. Mosch. Sene.**] Soreness in œsophagus. *Nervous palpitation, with small pulse. Colic, with rumbling in abdomen.

**AURUM.** *Suicidal mood, with longing for death, [**Lach. Puls.**] Full of fear, a mere noise makes her anxious. Alternately peevish and cheerful. *Fine eruption on lips, face, and forehead. Hysterical spasms, with alternate laughter and crying, [see **Ign.**] *Great nervous weakness.*

**BELLADONNA.** Remembers things long gone by, [reverse, see **Anac.**] *Confusion of head, aggravated by movement. Weary of life, with desire to drown herself, [see **Aur.**] *Moaning at night, even without much sleep. Sleepy, but cannot sleep, [**Lach. Opi.**] Bright sparks before the eyes.

**BROMIUM.** *Great depression of spirits, [**Calc. c. Puls. Sulph.**] Constriction of chest, with anxious feeling about heart. *Trembling all over,* [**Puls.**] Tickling, itching, pricking, and stitches in skin at various places. *Light hair, blue eyes.*

**CACTUS GRAND.** Cries, knows not why; is very sad. *Constriction of throat, exciting a constant desire to swallow. Feeling as of a *cord drawn tightly* around lower part of chest, [**Ars.**] Palpitation of heart, worse when lying on left side, or when walking.

**CALC. CARB.** Sadness and irresistible inclination to weep, [see **Puls.**] *Fears she will lose her reason, or that people will observe her state of mind. Great anxiety and palpitation of heart, worse as evening approaches. Coldness in or on the head, [**Verat.**] *Weak digestion.* *Cold damp feet.

**CAULOPHYL.** Swimming, or sort of vertigo, with dimness of sight. Severe pains by spells in the temples as if they would be crushed together. *Hysterical convulsions during dysmenorrhœa. Dependent upon *uterine derangement.*

**COCCULUS.** Thoughts fixed on one unpleasant subject, is absorbed and observes nothing about her. *Contractive sensation in trachea, as if irritated by smoke, inducing cough. *Nervous palpitation of heart, [see **Asaf.**] *Paralytic immobility of lower limbs.*

**CONIUM.** Easily disturbed by trifles, or moved to tears. Aversion to man, yet averse to being alone, [see **Lyc.**] *Vertigo, worse when lying down or turning in bed. *Globus hystericus,* [**Asaf. Lach. Mosch**] *During micturition the flow intermits.

**GELSEMIUM.** Excessive irritability of mind and body, with vascular excitement. *Hysterical convulsions, with spasms of glottis. *Wild feeling in head,* alternating with uterine pains. Dysmenorrhœa of a neuralgic character.

**HYOSCYAMUS.** She indulges in much silly laughter and many foolish actions. *Jerking and twitching of muscles during spasms. *She is disposed to uncover herself and go naked. *Constriction of throat,* with impeded deglutition, [see **Ign.**] *Nocturnal dry cough.

**IGNATIA.** *Sadness and *sighing,* with an empty feeling at pit of stomach. *Full of grief,* [**Phos. ac. Puls.**] *Choking sensation from stomach up to throat. *Grumbling in abdomen.* *Single startings of limbs when going to sleep.

**LACHESIS.** Talks, sings, whistles, and makes odd motions. Suicidal mood, tired of life, [**Aur.**] Sensation of a lump in throat; on swallowing it descends, but returns at once. *Cannot bear throat to be touched, seems as if it would suffocate her. *Greatly distressed after sleeping.* *Climacteric period, [see **Ther.**]

**MOSCHUS.** Great anxiety, with palpitation of heart. Great *inclination to scold.* *Talks continually of her approaching death.* *Hysterical paroxysms, with *fainting turns,* succeeded by headache. Great dryness of mouth, [**Nux m.**] *Copious colorless urine. Great tendency to involuntary stools.

**NUX MOS.** Laughter, everything seems ludicrous, talks loudly to herself. *Great dryness of mouth and tongue when sleeping. Head feels full and as if expanding. *Enormous distension of abdomen after meals. *Great sleepiness and inclination to faint.

**PALLADIUM.** Great inclination to use strong language and violent expressions, [**Mosch.**] Excited and impatient; thinks she is neglected. Distended abdomen from flatulence. Pain and weakness, as if uterus were sinking down. Stools hard, like chalk, [**Podo.**] Great sleepiness.

**PLATINA.** Feels as if she would lose her senses and die

soon. Spasms alternating with dyspnœa to suffocation. *Twitches of single muscles*, trembling, shivering, worse at dawn, [see **Hyos.**] *Menses in excess, dark, thick.

**PULSATILLA.** *Easily moved to tears or laughter. *Silent mood, disgusted with everything.* *Symptoms ever changing. Fainting fits, with great paleness of face, trembling all over. *Menses too late, scanty, or suppressed. Very *bad taste* in morning, nothing tastes good.

**SEPIA.** *Fits of weeping and laughter*, [**Ign. Puls.**] *Paroxysms of twisting in stomach and rising in throat. Her tongue becomes stiff, she is speechless, body rigid. Sensation of a ball in inner parts, [in bladder, **Bell.**] *Painful sensation of emptiness in stomach, [**Brom. Ign.**] *Urine putrid, depositing a clay-like sediment which *adheres firmly to the vessel.* Cold hands and feet.

**TARANTULA.** *Epileptiform hysteria, [**Gel.**] Crossness, crying, screaming. Anguish and oppression of chest, nearly amounting to suffocation. Uneasiness without cause, changes position every moment. *Burning heat through whole body, alternating with intense coldness, that causes trembling and shaking. Dysmenorrhœa, with gastric derangement, vomiting, etc.

**THERIDION.** Hysterical affections during puberty and climaxis, [see **Lach. Puls.**] Excessive headache, increased by least noise. Anxiety about the heart. Fainting after every exertion. Violent stitches in chest.

**AUXILIARY MEASURES.** During an attack, guard patient against injury, loosen all clothing, give plenty of fresh air, cold douche to head very successful; hold head over a tub and pour cold water on it until convulsion ceases. After this treat hysterical condition.

**HYGIENIC MEASURES.** Persons subject to hysteria should observe a regular *quiet* mode of life, avoid all mental or emotional excitement, over-exertion, errors of diet, overloading the stomach, and abstain from all stimulating food and drinks. Take open-air exercise, rise early, bathe frequently and use the flesh-brush vigorously.

**DIETETICS.** Use but little animal food, chiefly vegetables, fruits, bread made from *unbolted* flour, rice, hominy, oatmeal mush, milk, etc. Avoid tea and coffee and drink plenty of water.

---

## INGROWING TOE-NAILS.

This painful affection arises not so much from deformity of the nail as from the contiguous soft parts becoming swollen and inflamed from constant pressure against the edge of the nail by wearing narrow and tightly fitting shoes. If the inflammation continues, suppuration takes place, and an ulcer is formed, from whence large fungus growths, or "proud flesh," springs up, which are very sensitive and painful.

**TREATMENT.** *Remove all pressure.* Soak the foot well in *warm* water, then introduce under the edge of nail a pledget of lint saturated with *Calendula.* At same time with a sharp-pointed knife scrape a groove lengthwise through centre of nail from root to point. Repeat the scraping from day to day until it nearly reaches the quick. Cut or notch out the centre of nail, and permit the corners to grow. If this does not have desired effects, ℞. *Salycilic acid* ʒji, *Ext. Cannabis ind.* grs. iv, *Collodion* ℥ss. M. and apply to inflamed parts every evening, first removing the dry coating. Will give prompt relief. If "proud flesh" springs up in the ulcer, and is very sore and painful, take a little *Perchloride of iron* in powder, and insinuate it between the free edge of the nail and ulcer; repeat in 24 hours; will have excellent effect.

Failing in the above measures, remove edge of the nail. Etherize patient and pass sharp blade of pair of scissors under the nail, cut it through and tear away offensive portion with forceps.

In addition to the foregoing, one of following remedies given internally will afford great assistance.

**ARSENICUM.** Pain of a burning character, parts have a blackish look and emit a foul odor, [**Carb. v.**]

**PHOSPHORUS.** Parts hard and dry, with pain as if frozen, [**Agar.**] *The parts bleed easily.

**SILICEA.** Ingrowing toe-nail with offensive discharge. "Proud flesh," stinging and burning. *Sweaty feet, with cadaverous smell.

**SULPHUR.** Thin, shining swelling of the toe. *The parts suppurate, and "proud flesh" springs up, which is very tender and painful.

---

## INTERMITTENT FEVER.

**THERAPEUTICS.** *Leading indications.*

**ACONITE.** Recent cases of young persons of full habit. Violent chill, and heat especially about head and face, [**Gel.**] *Cough during fever.* *Great fear and anxiety of mind, with nervous excitability. Palpitation of heart, and pleuritic stitches in chest.

**ANTIMONIUM.** Much gastric disturbance, [**Ipe. Nux v.**] White-coated tongue. *Great sadness and a woeful mood. *Chilliness predominates.* Great desire to sleep; want of thirst, [**Puls.**] Sticky sweat.

**APIS MEL.** Chill about 4 P. M., [***Lyc.**] worse in warm room or near a stove. Renewed chilliness from slightest motion, with heat of face, hands, and particularly abdomen. Sweat, alternating with dryness of skin. During apyrexia, pain under short ribs, worse on left side. *Sensation in abdomen as if something tight would break if effort were made to void a stool.

**ARSENICUM.** Paroxysms imperfectly developed. Before chill, vertigo, headache, yawning, stretching, and general discomfort. Chill frequently intermingled with heat and fever; or there is internal chilliness and external heat, [see **Calc. c.**] *During fever, great anguish, extreme restlessness, and fear of death. After paroxysm, *great prostration.* *Urgent thirst, drinking often, but little, [**Apis. Chin.**]

**BELLADONNA.** *Slight chill,* with *much fever,* or vice versa. Some parts are cold, while others are warm [**Rhus.**] Violent throbbing headache, with stupefaction. *Heat and red face, with throbbing of carotids. Choking sensation in throat, with dry mouth.

**BRYONIA.** The chill predominates. Great thirst during all the stages. *Violent, dry, racking cough, with stitching pains in the side of the chest, [see **Rhus.**] Stitching pain in the region of the liver and abdomen. *Hard, dry stools, as if burnt. Exceedingly irritable; everything makes him angry.

**CALC. CARB.** Persons of a scrofulous diathesis. Thirst during chill. Chills alternating with heat, or external coldness and internal heat, [**Ars.**] Hardness of hearing. *Feet feel as if they had on cold, damp stockings. Patient very weakly in general; vertigo and shortness of breath on going up stairs. Diarrhœa, stools whitish, undigested.

**CAPSICUM.** Chill with thirst, followed by heat without thirst. *The chill commences in back and from thence extends over entire body, [**Eup. pur.**] *Relief by putting hot things to back during chill.* Drowsiness during fever, accompanied by perspiration. Much pain in back and limbs.

**CARBO VEG.** Paroxyms irregular, sometimes commencing with sweat, followed by chill. The attack is preceded or attended by toothache and pain in limbs. *Thirst only during chilly stage, [**Ign.**] Vertigo, redness of face and sick stomach during hot stage. *When eating or drinking, sensation as if the stomach or abdomen would burst.

**CEDRON.** Chills *regular* and very severe, with cramps, and tearing pains in upper and lower extremities. Dry heat, followed by profuse perspiration. *Numb, dead feeling in leg [in fingers, ***Sep.**]; they feel enlarged. *The entire body feels numb.

**CHAMOMILLA.** Chill generally light. Heat and sweat predominate. Much thirst in hot stage, [only in cold stage, **Carb. v. Ign.**] *Face red, or one cheek red and the other pale. *Very impatient, can hardly answer one civilly. Hot perspiration about the head and face. *Pain in the abdomen, with frequent emissions of large quantities of pale urine.

**CHINA.** The paroxysm is preceded by nausea, headache, hunger, anguish, and palpitation of heart. *Thirst before chill, and during sweating stage. Chills alternating with heat, skin cold and blue, [see **Nux.**] Ringing in ears, with dizziness and a feeling as if the head was enlarged. *Pain in region of liver and spleen, when bending or coughing. Sallow complexion. Miasmatic districts.

**CINA.** Vomiting and great hunger before, during, or after paroxysm. Thirst only during chill or heat. Pale face throughout the paroxysm. Frequent tickling in nose, [**Phos. ac.**] Restless at night. *Dilatation of pupils; perfectly clean tongue.

**EUPATO. PER.** Thirst several hours before chill, continuing during chill and heat. Stiffness of fingers during chill. The paroxysm usually occurs about 7 or 9 A. M., [10 A. M., ***Nat. m.**] *During chill severe aching in back and limbs as if the bones were broken. Sweat not very prominent. *Vomiting of bile at conclusion of chill.

**EUPATO. PUR.** *Chill commencing in back, and then spreading over the body, [**Cap.**] *Paroxysms come on at different times of day.* *Violent shaking, with comparatively little coldness. Thirst during the chill and heat. Violent pain in bones during chill and heat. Head feels light, as if it was falling to left side.

**FERRUM.** Chill, with thirst, headache, and swelling of cutaneous veins. Œdema of face, especially around eyes. [***Ars.**] Womiting everything eaten without being digested. *The least emotion or exertion produces a red, flushed face. *Great loss of muscular power.* *In protracted and badly treated cases by quinine, [by *mercury*, **Hep.**] Swelling of feet.

**GELSEMIUM.** Chill mostly in evening, commencing in *hands and feet, or running up and down the spine; it is followed by gradual and moderate sweat, which always gives relief.* The heat is attended with nervous restlessness and mental anxiety. Vertigo, with a sense of intoxication. Sensitive to light or noise, [**Bell.**] Advised as a *prophylactic.*

**IGNATIA.** Thirst *only* during chill. External heat, with partial internal shuddering. * *The chill is relieved by external heat*, [see **Ars. Cap.**] During fever, *nettle-rash* over whole body, [see **Hep. Rhus.**]

**IPECAC.** Much chilliness with little heat, or much heat and little chilliness. Paroxysm sets in with yawning, stretching, and a collection of saliva in mouth. Chill increases by external heat, [relieved by ***Ign.**] No thirst in cold stage, but a great deal in hot. * *Nausea and vomiting* predominate. The *apyrexia* is marked by more or less gastric disturbance.

**LYCOPODIUM.** *The paroxysm comes on about 4 P. M., and terminates about 8 P. M. *Constant sense of fullness in stomach and abdomen, as though they would burst. Obstinate constipation. *Red sediment like sand in urine. Great fear of being left alone, [wishes to be alone, **Chin.** ***Nux.**]

**NATR. MUR.** *Chill commencing at 10 A. M., with great thirst, drinking often and much at a time. During heat violent headache, *relieved by sweating.* *Dry tongue, and ulcerated corners of mouth.

**NUX VOMICA.** Paroxysm usually at night or early in morning. *Long-lasting, hard chill, with bluish, cold face and blue finger-nails. *Great heat, notwithstanding patient wants to be covered up. Both chill and heat are accompanied with gastric and bilious symptoms, [**Ant. Ipe.**] *During chill,* pain in sacrum. *During fever,* headache, vertigo, red face, pain in chest, and vomiting.

**OPIUM.** Drowsiness or heavy sleep, with loud snoring during the cold and hot stages. *Congestive chills.* *Stertorous respiration, with mouth wide open. Congestion of blood to head, with red and puffy appearance of face. Aged persons and children.

**PULSATILLA.** Attack mostly in afternoon or evening. *Chill* and *heat* simultaneous, [**Ars.**] *No thirst* during entire paroxysm, or only in hot stage. Bitter or sour vomiting of mucus or bile. *Thickly coated tongue, and *bad taste in morning.* Slight disorder of stomach induces a relapse. *Much gastric disturbance. Mild, tearful disposition.

**QUININE SULPH.** Chill every *alternate* day, anticipates from one to three hours. *Decided shake, with thirst. Lips and nails blue, [**Nux.**] Face pale, patient *hungry.* *Intense heat, with *excessive* thirst. Profuse sweating with thirst. In many cases this remedy will have to be given in sufficient doses to counteract the influences that produced the disease.

**RHUS TOX.** Paroxysm usually in after part of day. Chill preceded by stretching limbs and yawning. Coldness of some parts of body, and heat in others, [**Bell.**] Perspiration after midnight or towards morning. During hot stage nettle-rash breaks out. *Restlessness, constantly changing position. *Dry, teasing cough before and during chill, [during fever, **Acon.**]

**SAMBUCUS.** *Profuse debilitating sweat, even in apyrexia. Cold creeps over whole body, with fine stitching formication. *Dry, hacking cough during chill and heat.* Icy-cold hands and feet. Burning heat in face, with moderately warm body and cold feet.

**SEPIA.** General cold feeling, with pressure over temples and eyes. *Great coldness of hands, with sensation as if *fingers were dead.* During heat, vertigo, even to insensibility. Sweating over whole body, with anxiety, and dryness of throat. *Perfect absence of thirst, [**Puls.**] Urine brown, fetid.

**SULPHUR.** Attacks mostly in evening or at night, preceded by thirst and lassitude. Chilliness in back, chest, and arms, with coldness of hands, feet, and nose. During heat, thirst, with burning in hands and feet, and a bruised, tired feeling in limbs. *Burning heat on top of head. *Frequent weak, faint spells through the day. *Early morning diarrhœa.

**VERAT. ALB.** Severe chill, with feeling of internal heat, or both together, [see **Puls.**] Great thirst, especially during chill, and sweating. *Profuse sweat, often cold* and long-continued. *Great exhaustion and sinking of strength. Vomiting and diarrhœa. Intermittents during the prevalence of cholera.

**AUXILIARY MEASURES.** During the *cold stage* give patient a *hot foot* bath, or wrap limbs to knees in blankets wrung out of *hot water*, and give *hot water* to drink.

During *hot stage* sponge the surface with *warm* water, and wrap in a clean sheet, and allow patient to dry *without being rubbed.*

In malarial districts patients should avoid *night air*, and sleep in upper story of house.

---

## INTUSSUSCEPTION.

The slipping of one portion of the intestine into another, causing obstruction, is called intussusception or invagination. Generally it is the *upper* part of the intestine, which is *received into the lower.*

The symptoms are: Pain in region of ileo-cœcal valve; great desire to go to stool with passages of blood and mucus; vomiting of ingesta, bile, and feces. After the invagination continues for a time, congestion and inflammation supervene, which sometimes become gangrenous and slough, being passed per anum, and paticut recovers.

**TREATMENT.** When obstruction is suspected from *twist, convolution* or invagination, one of the following remedies should be exhibited, and will often prove curative if given early.

**BELLADONNA.** *Colic as if a spot in the abdomen were seized with nails. *Constriction around* the *umbilicus*, as if a ball would form. *Periodical pains, which come suddenly and cease as suddenly.

**COLOCYNTH.** *Violent cutting, constrictive, spasmodic pains.* *Feeling as if intestines were being squeezed between stones, compelling one to bend double. The pain radiates from a central point, and is aggravated by motion.

**NUX VOMICA.** Violent pains through to the back, extending to the anus, with urging to stool. Stercoraceous vomiting and singultus, [see **Opi.**]

**OPIUM.** Squeezing pains, as if something were forced through a narrow space. *Anti-peristaltic motion, belching and vomiting a fecal-smelling substance, [see **Verat.**] *Slow pulse.

**PLUMBUM.** *Terrible contractive pains, abdomen drawn in to back. Hard swelling in ileo-cœcal region, painful to touch and motion. *Vomiting fecal matter, with colic,* [**Nux Opi.**]

**VERAT. ALB.** *Intestines feel as if tied in knots. Cramping, twisting or cutting pains. *Anti-peristaltic action;* vomiting bile and black blood. *Cold sweat, particularly on forehead.

**SURGICAL TREATMENT.** Place patient on his back, with hips well elevated, pass a *long rubber tube* into the rectum and up the colon as near to seat of stricture as possible, and inject *large quantities* [a gallon, if necessary] of *warm flaxseed-tea* or olive oil. Manipulate abdomen with hands while the injection is being administered and while it is passing away. Repeat operation several times.

Inflating the bowels with air has been successful. Introduce rubber tube as above directed, and with an ordinary-sized bellows, force the air in until abdomen is well distended. Try also inverting patient's body, as directed for strangulated hernia.

If the above measures fail, and the *diagnosis be clear,* have recourse to *abdominal section.* An incision four or five inches long should be made *below* the umbilicus in *linea alba.* Open peritoneum carefully and search for the obstruction. Use antiseptic dressings.

---

## JAUNDICE.

**THERAPEUTICS.** *Leading indications.*

**ACONITE.** Synochal fever, with acute stitches in region of liver. Scanty, *dark* urine. *Great fear and anxiety of mind, with nervous excitability. *Clay-colored stools.*

**ARSENICUM.** Yellowness of sclerotica, [**Cham. Chin.**] Undigested, light-colored, offensive stools. *Great anguish, restlessness, and fear of death. *Urgent thirst, drinks often, but little, [**Chin.**] Irritable mood, alternating with lowness of spirits.

**BRYONIA.** Stitching pains in liver when pressed upon. Pain in right shoulder and arm. Pain in limbs, worse by motion. Yellow-coated tongue; bitter, bilious vomiting. *Lips parched, dry, and cracked. Nausea and faintness on sitting up. *Constipation, stools dry and hard.

**CALC. CARB.** *Scrofulous diathesis,* [**Sulph.**] *Large head and open fontanelles, [**Sil.**] Stitches in liver during or after stooping. Enlargement of liver. Cannot bear tight clothing around waist. *Clay-like stools, scant and knotty. *Fetid, dark-brown* urine, white sediment. *Cold, damp feet. Swollen abdomen; emaciation and good appetite.

**CHAMOMILLA.** Mostly new-born children, or after chagrin, [**Acon. Nux.**] Yellowness of face and whites of eyes. *Green, watery, corroding stools, with colic, [***Merc.**] Bitter taste, with bilious vomiting. *Very impatient, can hardly answer one civilly. *Children are very fretful, and want to be carried.

**CHINA.** Persons who have been weakened by loss of animal fluids. *Yellow color of skin.* Dullness and muddled condition of head. Oppressive, tearing headache. Liver swollen, hard, and tender. *Bitter taste in back part of throat; everything tastes bitter, [**Bry.**] *Abdomen feels full and tight as if stuffed. Yellow, watery, undigested stools, without pain. *Urine turbid, dark. Aggravation every other day.*

**DIGITALIS.** Frequent empty retching, with clean tongue. Soreness and bloatedness of pit of stomach. *Stools almost white, [**Chin.**] Frequent and *painful* emissions of *scanty, brown or blackish urine. Irregular or intermittent pulse.*

**IODINE.** *Yellow, almost dark-brown color of face. Thickly coated tongue. White diarrhœic stools, alternating with constipation. *Dark, yellowish-green, corroding urine.* Nausea and thirst. After mercurial poisoning. *Scrofulous persons,* [**Calc. Sulph.**]

**LEPTANDRA.** Dull aching in the region of gall-bladder, [**Podo.**] Chilliness along the spine. *Constant distress between the umbilicus and epigastrium. *Clay-colored, or black, tarry stools.* Brown urine.

**MANCINELLA.** **Black, or malignant jaundice,* [**Iod. Phos.**] *Jaundice, with dropsy, when skin assumes a dark-greenish tint, or dark-brown appearance.* Œdema of the whole body, the legs greatly swollen and dark-colored. Tired feeling in region of kidneys; *urine brown.* Diarrhœa, with colic and vertigo.

**MERCURIUS.** **Complete jaundice,* with painfulness of region of liver, *skin very yellow.* *Grayish-white fæces, with tenesmus during and after stool. Thickly-coated, flabby tongue. *Bad smell from the mouth, [**Podo.**] Nausea and vomiting. Loathing of food. Urine scanty and dark-red, with a fetid smell.

**NUX VOM.** *Swelling and hardness of liver,* [**Chin. Merc.**] Sour or putrid taste, with aversion to food. Contractive pain in region of liver. Nausea and bilious vomiting. *Constipation with unsuccessful urging. *Cannot sleep after 3 A. M. *Very irritable, and wishes to be alone. Aggravation in morning. *Persons of sedentary or intemperate habits.*

**PODOPHYLLUM,** Icterus consequent upon obstruction of biliary-duct, [see "*Gall-stone.*"] *Pain in region of gall-bladder, attended with excessive nausea. Fullness and soreness in liver, [**Nux v.**] Worse in *hot* weather.

**PULSATILLA.** Yellow coating on tongue, with bitter taste in mouth, [**Cham.**] Nausea and desire to vomit. Frequent attacks of anguish, especially at night. *Chilliness, with vertigo on rising from a sitting posture. *Green, slimy diarrhœa, especially at night. *Thirstlessness. Amenorrhœa.* Aggravation towards evening.

**DIETETICS.** Rice, oatmeal, tapioca, plain puddings, simple toast, vegetables, ripe and cooked fruits should constitute the diet, and water the principal drink. All animal and greasy food, and stimulating beverages should be avoided.

---

## LEUCORRHŒA.

**THERAPEUTICS.** *Leading indications.*

**ÆSCULUS.** *Constant backache affecting the sacrum and hips. *Discharge dark-yellow, thick, and sticky corroding labia.* *Great fatigue from walking ever so little, on account of weakness in back. Large protruding hemorrhoids and constipation.

**ALUMINA.** Leucorrhœa just before or after the menses, [**Kreo.**] *Profuse, purulent, yellowish, corroding discharge, relieved by cold applications. Severe burning in small of back. Great inactivity of the rectum, with much straining at stool.

**AMBRA.** Discharge of bluish-white mucus. *Leucorrhœa only at night. *Stitches in vagina preceding the discharge. Nervous hysterical subjects. During micturition, burning, smarting, itching of vulva.

**AMM. CARB.** *Very acrid, burning, and watery leucorrhœa, [**Alum. Puls.**] Menses too early, too scanty, or too profuse. Unrefreshing sleep; headache after walking in fresh air. Suits sickly, weak, delicate women. [**Ars.**]

**AMM. MUR.** Leucorrhœa, with distension of the abdomen. *Discharge like white of eggs, preceded by pinching pain around the navel. *Brown, slimy leucorrhœa after urinating, [see **Nit. ac.**] Intolerable pain in the small of the back at night. Menses premature, profuse and composed of black clots.

**ARSENICUM.** Acrid, corroding leucorrhœa, making parts sore, [**Alum. Bovis. Con. Ign. *Kreo. Puls.**] *Discharge thick, yellow, dropping out while standing, or when emitting flatus. Great anguish and restlessness at night. Feeble, weakly women.

**BOVISTA.** Especially *after* the catamenia. *Discharge like the white of eggs, coming away while walking, [see **Am. m.**] Also yellowish, green, corrosive leucorrhœa. Menses too often and too profuse, with painful bearing down towards the genitals.

**CALC. CARB.** Milk-like discharge during micturition, or flowing only by spells, [see **Con.**] Too early and profuse menstruation. Very weakly in general, walking produces great fatigue, [see **Æscu.**] *Very sensitive to cold air. *Feet cold and damp.

**CHINA.** Weakly persons who have lost much blood. *Leucorrhœa before the menses, with painful pressing toward the groins and anus. *Bloody leucorrhœa, with occasional discharge of black clots, or fetid purulent matter. Troublesome itching in the inner parts.

**COCCULUS.** Scanty, irregular menses, with leucorrhœa between the periods, [after, **Puls.**] *Leucorrhœa in place of menses.* *Discharge like serum mixed with a purulent, ichorous liquid. *When bending or sitting down the discharge escapes in a gush. Painful menstruation, followed by hemorrhoids.

**CONIUM.** Weakness and lameness in small of back. *Leucorrhœa, smarting and excoriating the parts. Discharge whitish or milk-colored, and painful. *Induration or ulceration of os uteri.* *Vertigo during menses, particularly while lying down. Dysmenorrhœa, with shooting pain in left side of chest.

**CUBEBA.** *Discharge profuse, yellow, greenish, very acrid and offensive. Small burning pimples, ulcers like aphthæ on the vulva, with intense itching. Fissures and bleeding excrescences upon the os tincæ, [see **Con.**] Womb swollen and painful, as if from a tumor.

**GRAPHITES.** Females inclined to obesity; menses too *late* and too *scanty.* **Leucorrhœa profuse* and of a white color, [*milk-like*, **Con. Sep.**] Great weakness in small of back when walking or sitting. *Eruptions on the skin oozing a sticky fluid.

**IGNATIA.** Violent labor-like pains, with pressing in region of womb. *Purulent, corrosive leucorrhœa, with a weak, empty feeling in stomach. *She seems full of suppressed grief. Difficult stools, causing prolapsus ani, [loose stools, with prolapsus ani, **Merc.** ***Podo.**]

**KALI BICHRO.** *Yellow, ropy leucorrhœa, which can be *drawn out in long strings*, [see **Sabi.**] Much pain and weakness across small of back. Menses too soon, with vertigo, nausea, and headache.

**KREOSOT.** Leucorrhœa *before* and after menses. *Putrid, acrid, corrosive leucorrhœa, with great debility, particularly of lower extremities. Menses too early, too profuse, and last too long, [**Bell. Calc. c.**]. *She always feels chilly at menstrual period.

**LACHESIS.** Leucorrhœa before menses, [after, **Puls.**] *Discharge copious, smarting, slimy, stiffening linen and staining it green, [yellow, **Nux v.**] Menses regular, but too short and feeble. *Inability to bear anything tight around waist. Women at *critical age*, [**Sep.**]

**LYCOPO.** *Profuse leucorrhœa at intervals, *accompanied by a cutting pain across hypogastrium* from *right* to *left.* Pale face, with frequent flushes or circumscribed redness of cheeks. *Red, sandy sediment in urine. Menses too long and too profuse. *Sense of great fullness in stomach after eating.

**NITRIC ACID.** *Leucorrhœa of ropy mucus, [**Kali b.**] Also green mucus, or flesh-colored, acrid, brown, offensive.

Excrescence in cervix uteri, [**Cub.**] *Itching, swelling and burning* of *vulva* and *vagina.* *Urine extremely offensive.

**NUX MOS.** *Leucorrhœa in place of menses [**Cocc.**] *Great drowsiness, always awakens with a very *dry mouth and tongue.* Menses too early and too profuse, with discharge of thick, black blood. *Hysterical women.* *Prolapsus uteri et vaginæ, [**Sep.**] *Great tendency to faint.*

**NUX VOM.** Fetid leucorrhœa tingeing the linen yellow with pain in the uterus as if sprained. *Menses irregular, never at the right time. Habitual constipation, with frequent urging to stool. As a consequence of high living, or sedentary life.

**PODOPHYLLUM.** Leucorrhœa, attended with constipation, and bearing down in genital organs. Discharge of thick, transparent mucus. *Prolapsus uteri and ani. *Morning diarrhœa;* stools watery, green.

**PULSATILLA.** Burning, thin, acrid leucorrhœa. *Milky leucorrhœa, with swelling of vulva, particularly after menses. Also leucorrhœa, with thick, white mucus before and during menses. *Vertigo when rising from a sitting posture. *Menses too late and scanty. Mild, tearful* women.

**SABINA.** *Excoriating leucorrhœa, with pruritus. Discharge ropy, glazy, [ropy, yellow, **Kali b.**]

**SEPIA.** Climacteric period, during pregnancy or puberty, [see **Lach.**] Leucorrhœa with stitches in neck of uterus, and itching in vagina. *Prolapsus uteri et vaginæ.* Yellowish, watery, milk-like, or mucous leucorrhœa. *Dirty, yellow spots on face. Very fetid urine, depositing a clay-colored sediment.

**SULPHUR.** Burning, painful leucorrhœa, making vulva sore. Discharge thin, yellowish, preceded by pinching in hypogastrium, [see **Am. m.**] *Burning in vagina. *Frequent weak, faint spells during the day. *Constant heat on top of head. Burning in soles of the feet; puts them out of bed.

**ZINCUM.** *Leucorrhœa of bloody mucus after menses, causing itching of vulva. Uterine ulcers with bloody, acrid, discharge, the ulcers being rather destitute of feeling. Fidgety feeling in feet or lower extremities, must move them constantly. *Chronic sick-headache;* weakness of sight.

**AUXILIARY MEASURES.** Frequent injections of *warm water,* [95° to 100° F.] are very beneficial. Where the discharge is excoriating and the parts sore, injections of a solution *Hydrastis,* [ ʒj. Aq. ferv. Oj.] will be found very useful.

Measures should be taken to improve the general health by suitable diet, out-doors exercise, bathing, regular habits, etc.

## MASTITIS.

*(Inflammation of the Mammæ.)*

**THERAPEUTICS.** *Leading indications.*

**ACONITE.** *If due from exposure to cold, dry, west winds, [Hepar.] Taken at onset of chill, it will often be sufficient to prevent further development.

**ARNICA.** *If caused from a recent injury. Great soreness of the breasts. *The bed on which she lies feels too hard.

**BELLADONNA.** Breast swollen, hard and feels heavy, [Bry.] Sometimes inflammation resembles erysipelas, *with red streaks running in radii.* Burning heat, with throbbing, stitching pain. *Flushed face, throbbing headache.

**BRYONIA.** *In early stage, breast swollen, hard, and feels heavy, but not very red. Severe stitching pains. *Nausea and faintness on sitting up.

**HEPAR SULPH.** *Where suppuration is inevitable, [Sili.] *Throbbing pains,* often preceded by a chill. Scrofulous persons, and after the use of mercury.

**PHYTOLACCA.** "Gathered breasts," with large, fistulous, gaping and angry *ulcers, discharging a watery, fetid pus.*

**SILICEA.** Suppuration imminent. *Fistulous openings form, which are slow to heal, and discharge a fetid, watery pus. Milk suppressed. *Scrofulous diathesis.*

**LOCAL MEASURES.** On first appearance of hardness, give the appropriate remedy and rub with *hot lard* or olive oil, and cover the parts with a piece of flannel wet with the same. Warm fomentations, impregnated with *indicated remedy,* very useful. The *extreme pain* and tenderness may be greatly relieved by a dish of *hot water* held under the breast, and the heated fluid constantly applied with a sponge.

When suppuration is inevitable, apply linseed-meal poultices. In puncturing, have *edge* of lancet looking *towards* the *nipple.*

---

## MEASLES.

**THERAPEUTICS.** *Leading indications.*

**ACONITE.** *At the beginning, when there is dry, hot skin, full, quick pulse, and much thirst.* *Eyes red, watery, and sensitive to light, [Bell.] Catarrhal irritation, with dry, hacking, or hoarse, croupy cough. *Great anxiety and restlessness. Headache, and vertigo on rising up, [nausea and faintness on rising up, *Bry.]

**APIS.** Confluent eruption and *œdematous* swelling of skin. *Cough and soreness in chest, as if bruised. Oppression of chest, with inability to remain in a warm room, [Puls.] Scanty, high-colored urine. *Diarrhœa in morning, stools greenish-yellow.

**ARSENICUM.** Severe cases, when typhoid symptoms are present. *Burning and great dryness and itching of skin. The eruption disappears too suddenly, [***Ipe.**] *Bloatedness of face, and dry, parched lips. *Great anguish, restlessness, and fear of death. *Constant craving for cold water, drinking often, but little. *Rapid prostration.* Worse about midnight.

**BELLADONNA.** Bright-red appearance of throat and tongue, with difficulty of swallowing. *Red and hot face, with throbbing headache. Back feels as if it would break, [as if broken, **Phos.**] Dry, spasmodic cough. Constant drowsiness, and moaning during sleep. *Starting, jumping during sleep, with flushed face, red eyes. If *complicated with scarlet fever.*

**BRYONIA.** The eruption is imperfectly developed. *Congestion of chest, with shooting, stitching pains, increased by deep breathing, [**Phos.**] *Great dyspnœa and quick breathing. Dry, painful cough, with roughness and dryness of the larynx. *Sitting up in bed causes nausea and faintness. Thirst for large draughts of water.

**CAMPHORA.** When there seems to be a depression of vital forces. *Face pale and skin cold, assuming a bluish color. *The eruption does not make its appearance as it should. Great prostration and stiffness of body, [of back and knees, **Bry.**] *Coldness of skin, yet patient cannot bear to be covered.

**IPECAC.** Eruption slow to make its appearance, with oppression of chest, [**Camp.** ***Puls.**] *Constant tickling cough with every breath, and rattling of phlegm in chest. *Much nausea and vomiting. *Suppression of eruption.* Constant sense of nausea.

**MERCURIUS.** The glands of throat swollen, with difficulty in swallowing, [see **Bell.**] *Soreness of throat and *ulceration* of tonsils. Profuse secretion of saliva, and bad breath. *Great sensitiveness of pit of the stomach. Much perspiration without relief. Green, slimy, or bloody stools, with *severe tenesmus.*

**PHOSPHORUS.** If the disease be complicated with pneumonia, or if *typhoid symptoms* set in. *Tightness across chest, with violent and exhausting cough, and *rust-colored* sputa. Sticking pains in chest, aggravated by coughing or breathing, [***Bry.**] *Hoarseness, with loss of voice.

**PULSATILLA.** Generally in beginning, when catarrhal symptoms appear. Eyes red, watery and sensitive to light, [**Acon. Bell.**] Thick, yellow discharge from nose. *Dryness of mouth, without thirst. *The eruption is tardy in coming out. Loose cough, with thick, yellow, mucous expectoration. *Nightly diarrhœa. *Craves cool, fresh air, worse in a warm room.

**SCILLA.** *Diarrhœa during measles, where the stools are dark-brown or black, slimy fluid; in frothy bubbles,

*Discharges painless and very offensive.* For diarrhœa *following* measles, **Chin. Dulc. Merc. Puls. Sulph.**

For **OTITIS** and **OTORRHŒA**, consult **Bell. Cham. Merc. Puls. Sulph.**

**CLINICAL REMARKS.** Keep patient in uniform temperature, 70° F., room well *ventilated*, and darkened if eyes are sensitive. *Warm baths* to bring out tardy eruption, and *hot foot-baths* to relieve oppression of chest. Gum-arabic or slippery-elm tea may be sipped frequently for troublesome cough, and pure, fresh water drank at pleasure.

**DIETETICS.** Plain simple food at first, consisting of milk, light puddings, rice, plain toast, etc. Later, broths, beef-tea, vegetables, fruits, etc.

---

## MENINGITIS.

**THERAPEUTICS.** *Leading indications.*

**ACONITE.** *In the commencement, when there is a high degree of fever.* *Congestion of blood to the head, with red face, and pulsation of carotids, [***Bell.**] *Great anxiety and fear of death; predicts the day he will die. *Sleeplessness, restlessness, tossing from side to side. Vertigo or fainting on rising up.

**APIS MEL.** Meningitis from suppression or spread of erysipelas, or other exanthemata, [see **Cup.**] Congestion to the head and face, [see **Acon.**] *Sopor, with delirium, sudden shrieking cries, squinting, grinding teeth, and boring head in pillow. *Conjunctiva injected, full of dark vessels. Red spots on the skin, like bee-stings, with stinging, burning pains.

**BELLADONNA.** Violent throbbing, stitching pains in head. *Red, sparkling eyes, with furious look. *Face red and bloated,* [**Acon.**] Great heat in head, with violent throbbing of carotids, [**Hyos.**] *Boring with head into pillow,* [see **Apis.**] *Furious delirium, with desire to escape; he tries to strike, bite and injure those around him. *Great aversion to noise and light. Pupils contracted or dilated. *Starting and jumping during sleep.

**BRYONIA.** Pain in head, as if the *skull were being pressed asunder.* Congestion of blood to head, with heat and burning. *Delirious talk at night, with desire to escape, [**Bell.**] Lips dry and parched, with great thirst. *Wants to keep perfectly still, as the least motion makes him worse. Sudden starting up from sleep. *Sitting up in bed causes nausea and fainting. *Dry, hard stools. *Very irritable.*

**CICUTA.** After *concussion* of the brain; eyes sensitive to light, *pupils dilated.* Starting, trembling of the head, worse on moving it. Face bluish, puffed up. Grinding the teeth, [see **Cup.**] Thirst, with inability to swallow. Spasmodic drawing of head backwards.

**GLONOINE.** *Throbbing in temples, vertex, occiput, and whole head, [see **Bell.**] All the blood seems to be *pumped upwards,* the brain feeling too large; holds head with the hands. Redness of eyes, with soreness of eyeballs. Especially suitable after *sunstroke,* [**Acon. Verat. v.**]

**HELLEBORUS.** Usually in last stage, when serous exudation has taken place. *Face pale and puffed. *Soporous sleep, with screaming and starting. *Rolls head* night and day, [see **Hyos.**] *Lower jaw sinking down. *Chewing motions with mouth. *Automatic motions with one arm and one leg. Squinting, pupils dilated.

**HYOSCYAMUS.** Drowsiness and loss of consciousness. *Rolling the head.* *Delirium, with wild, staring look, jerking the limbs, and throbbing of carotids. White-coated tongue; *frothing at the mouth.* *Staring, distorted eyes, with double vision. Starting up suddenly from sleep, [**Bell.**] *Muttering, with picking at bed-clothes. Involuntary stools and urine.

**OPIUM.** Lethargy, with stertorous breathing, eyes half closed. Stupefaction after waking. *Delirious talking, eyes wide open. Face purplish and swollen, [see **Cicu.**] *Acuteness of hearing, [**Verat. v.**] Fearfulness and tendency to start. After grief, fright, or violent mental emotions. *Stools round, hard, black balls.

**STRAMONIUM.** He does not notice objects around him. Stupefaction of the senses. *Loquacious delirium, with desire to escape, [**Bell. Opi.**] *Awakens with a shrinking look, as if afraid of first object seen. *Talks all the time, sings, makes verses.* *Grinding teeth, with shuddering. Lips sore and cracked, and sordes on teeth. *Glistening eyes and staring look.*

**VERAT. VIR.** Congestion to head from high living or abuse of stimulants, [**Nux v.**] *Great fullness in head, throbbing arteries, [see **Bell.**] **A red streak down the centre of tongue.* Increased sensitiveness to sounds. Dimness of vision, with dilated pupils. Slow pulse, [**Opi.**] Meningitis following sunstroke.

**AUXILIARY MEASURES.** Choose cool, airy room, remote from noises. Exclude all persons not needed. Keep room quiet as possible; avoid whispering. Apply *warm fomentations* to head, covering it well and changing often. Keep extremities warm with bottles of hot water. Use little restraint to control patient. For restlessness and inability to sleep, give warm baths and wrap in *dry* sheet, *without rubbing.*

**DIETETICS.** In febrile state, only thin gruel, toast-water, acid-diluted drinks, and pure fresh water. *Later,* beef-tea, broths, milk and light puddings of farina, corn-starch, rice, etc.

## MENORRHAGIA.

(*Profuse Menstruation.*)

**THERAPEUTICS.** *Leading indications.*

**ACONITE.** Adapted to plethoric females and young girls, [*cachectic subjects*, **Chin. Croc. Sec.**] *Profuse menses, with great anxiety and *fear of death.* *Vertigo on rising from a recumbent position. If induced by exposure to dry, cold wind.

**AMMO. CARB.** Premature and profuse menstruation, with spasmodic pain. *Nose bleed when washing face in morning. Discharge *blackish* or *light-colored;* acrid, making the thighs sore. Great sadness, and pain in small of back.

**BELLADONNA.** Too early and profuse, [**Bry.** ***Calc. c. Cimi. Phos.**] Discharge bright-red, *imparting a sense of heat.* *Violent pressing down, as if everything would escape through genitals, [**Nit. ac. Plat.** ***Sep.**] *Throbbing headache, and pain in small of black. Clutching pain in hypogastrium, with screaming, and disposition to bite and tear things.

**BRYONIA.** Too early and profuse. *Discharge dark-red, with lacerating pains in limbs, [see **Cham.**] Pain in back, and headache as if the skull would split. Cannot sit up on account of *nausea and faintness.* *Wants to remain quiet and still, the least motion makes her worse. *Stools hard and dry, as if burnt. Very *irritable*, everything makes her angry.

**CALC. CARB.** Menstruation too soon, too profuse, and lasting too long, [**Croc. Ign. Phos.**] *Profuse menstruation during lactation.* Preceding the flow, there is swelling and sensitiveness of the breasts, headache, colic and shiverings. During the flow, cutting in the abdomen, toothache and bearing down. *Vertigo when stooping, worse on rising or going up-stairs. *Feet feel as if they had on cold, damp stockings. *Sensitive to least cold air.*

**CHAMOMILLA.** *Profuse discharge of dark and clotted blood, flowing at intervals. *Violent labor-like pains in uterus, and tearing in veins of the legs. Very *impatient*, can hardly answer a civil question. Frequent desire to pass urine.

**CIMICIFUGA.** Too early and profuse. Discharge dark and coagulated, [**Cham. Croc.**] *Severe pain in back and down the thighs, [**Bry.**] Aching across the hips, and pressing down in the uterus. Great nervousness, and hysterical spasms. Severe pains in head and eyeballs, increased by least motion.

**COCCUS CACTI.** *Menorrhagia only in evening when lying down, never when stirring about. Sharp pains in lower part of abdomen, first in right side, then in left. She passes enormous black clots from the vagina. Uurging to pass water.

**CROCUS SATI.** Menses regular, but too *profuse* and long-continued. *Discharge dark, clotted, stringy blood. *The least movement increases the flow. Yellowish, earthy color of face, [**Sep.**] *Sensation as of something moving in abdomen, [**Sabi.**] Great debility and palpitation of heart on going up-stairs.

**IGNATIA.** Too frequent, profuse, and long-lasting. *The patient seems full of *suppressed grief.* *Frequent sighing, with a feeling of emptiness in stomach. Difficult stool, causing prolapsus ani. Cold hands and feet; also numbness of feet and legs.

**IODIUM.** Menses premature, copious and violent, with great weakness. Discharge preceded by heat in head and palpitation of heart. *Ovarian region painful, or sensitiveness to pressure. *Emaciation, with a *good appetite.* Hard, knotty, dark-colored stools.

**KREOSOTE.** Menses too early, profuse, and protracted. *The flow intermits; she thinks she is almost well, when the discharge reappears, [**Nux v. Sulph.**] Discharge *black*, in large quantities, very offensive, corrosive itching and smarting of the parts. Climacteric period, [**Puls. Sep. Ustila.**]

**NUX MOS.** Menses too early and too profuse, with discharge of *thick, black blood*, [**Plat**] *Tongue and mouth very dry, particularly after sleeping. Great pressure in back from within outwards during menses. *Drowsiness and inclination to faint. *Pain in sacrum when riding in carriage. Great *distension of abdomen after eating.*

**NUX VOM.** Menses too early and too profuse; discharge dark-colored blood, [**Nux m.**] *The flow, after continuing several days, stops and then returns, [**Sulph.**] Dragging about the loins, with bearing down in pelvis. *Cramp-like pains in abdomen extending down to thighs. *She gets angry and violent without provocation, [**Cham.**] Habitual constipation, with frequent *urging to stool.*

**PHOSPHORUS.** Menses *too soon*, too copious, and lasting *too long*, with pain in small of back and in abdomen. Great weakness, with cold feet and legs. *Sensation of weakness and emptiness in abdomen. *Belching up large quantities of wind after eating. Very sleepy after meals, especially after dinner. *Long, slim, hard, difficult stools. Tall slender people, with fair skin.

**PLATINA.** Too *long and too profuse* menstruation. Discharge *partly fluid and partly in clots*, [***Sabi.**] *Great pressing down in the genitals, [***Bell. *Sep.**]

**SABINA.** *Very profuse* and debilitating menses. Discharge partly pale-red and partly clotted blood. *Labor-like pains drawing down into groin. *Drawing, tearing pains from back through to pubis. *Plethoric women with habitual menorrhagia*, [see **Acon.**] Great liabitity to miscarry.

**SECALE.** Too profuse and too long-continued. Discharge

dark, liquid blood, increased by motion, [Croc.] *All her common ailments worse just before the menses. Suitable to thin, scrawny women.

**SEPIA.** Mostly too early and profuse. Before menses, violent colic. *Painful sensation of emptiness at pit of stomach. *Fetid urine, having a sediment like burnt clay. *Yellow spots on face*, especially across nose. *Prolapsus uteri et vaginæ, [Merc.] *Sensation as if everything would escape through vagina, [*Bell.] *Icy-cold feet and flushes of heat.*

**SULPHUR.** The menses last too long. *She seems to get almost well, and then it returns again and again. Discharge acrid, corroding the thighs, and smelling sour, [offensive, Bell. Kreo.] *Flashes of heat, followed by weak, faint spells. *Constant heat on top of the head.

**TRILLIUM.** Menses lasting too long; discharge at first bright-red, but grows pale, [Bell.] Between the periods, profuse leucorrhœa of a yellowish color and creamy consistence. *Profuse hemorrhages.

**USTILAGO.** Climacteric period, [*Puls. Sep.] Flooding lasting for weeks. *Chronic uterine hemorrhages. *Blood dark-colored*, with many clots, and vertigo. Dull, heavy headache. *Ovarian irritation.*

**AUXILIARY MEASURES.** In urgent cases, place patient on hard mattress in cool room, and elevate the hips. If this does not diminish the flow, apply piece of ice to mouth of uterus. This failing, bandage extremities to impede circulation, as directed under **Post-Partem Hemorrhage**, or plug vagina.

**DIETETICS.** During attack, all food and drink should be taken moderately cold. Avoid all stimulating food and beverages.

---

## METRITIS.

(*Inflammation of the Uterus.*)

**THERAPEUTICS.** *Leading indications.*

**ACONITE.** *Synochal fever. *Great restlessness and fear of death*, [Ars.] Hard, rapid pulse; hot, dry skin; intense thirst. Sharp, shooting pain in whole abdomen, which is tender to touch. *High temperature.*

**APIS MEL.** *Sopor, interrupted by piercing shrieks. Great *tearfulness*, cannot help crying, [Puls.] *Burning or *stinging* pains in region of uterus or ovaries. *Dry mouth, but no thirst.* Urine scanty, dark.

**ARSENICUM.** Great *fear, restlessness*, trembling, cold sweat, *prostration.* *She is sure she will die, [Acon.] *Edge of tongue red, showing imprint of teeth, [see Merc.] *Burning, throbbing, lancinating pains; burning like fire*, [Acon.]

Cold water aggravates her symptoms. She wants to be covered up, is better from warmth.

**BELLADONNA.** Delirium; she is afraid of imaginary things, and tries to escape or hide herself. *Throbbing headache, with heat and red face.* *Clutching or clawing pains, or transient stitches in uterine region, parts sensitive, *cannot bear least jar.* *Pressure towards the genitals, as if everything would issue through vulva. *Menstrual or lochial discharge suppressed or very offensive.* Involuntary flow of urine.

**BRYONIA.** *Very irritable*, wishes to be alone, [**Nux.**] *Head aches as if it would split open, [**Bell. Puls.**] Severe stitching pain in region of ovaries on taking deep inspiration. *Sitting up in bed causes nausea and faintness. *Sufferings all worse from the least motion. Lips parched, mouth dry and great thirst.

**CANTHARIS.** *Dissatisfied* with every one and everthing, says she must die. *Burning sensation in throat, it feels "on fire." Violent pinching pains, with bearing down towards the genitals, [see **Bell.**] Swelling of neck of uterus. *Inflammation of the ovaries*, [**Apis. Bell.**] *Constant desire to urinate, passing only a few drops at a time, sometimes mixed with blood. *Great thirst.*

**COLOCYNTH.** Metritis following violent indignation. *Severe colicky pains, *bends double*, with great restlessness. *Feeling as if the intestines were squeezed between stones. Great distension of bowels.

**HYOSCYAMUS.** *Metritis, typhoid state. *Stupor, unconsciousness*, and silly expression. *Jerking of limbs and twitching of muscles of face. *She throws off the covers, and wishes to be naked.

**MERCURIUS.** Continuous moaning and groaning, [**Bell. Lach.**] *Head feels as if it would burst, with fullness of brain. *Moist, soft tongue, showing imprints of teeth*, [see **Ars.**] *Stitching, aching, or boring pains in uterus, with little heat, but frequent sweats and chills.

**PULSATILLA.** *Mild, gentle, tearful, yielding, timid*, [**Sep.**] Semi-lateral headache, [**Bell. Lach. Nux v.**] Tensive cutting pain in uterus, which is very sensitive to touch. *Suppression of menses or lochial discharge, [**Sec.**] Bad taste in mouth, no thirst, frequent chilliness. *Nightly diarrhœa*, and scanty urination.

**RHUS TOX.** Anxiety, timidity; worse at twilight; *restless change of place, cannot lie still.* Slow fever, with dry tongue having a red tip. *Pains worse at night, especially after midnight. *Metritis, particularly after confinement*, [**Plat. Sabi.**] Milk-leg.

**SECALE.** *Strong tendency to putrescence*, [**Kreo.**] *Discharge from vagina brownish, very offensive. The inflammation seems to be caused by suppression of lochia or menses, [**Puls.**] Burning, hot fever, interrupted by shaking chills. Vomiting decomposed matter. Offensive diarrhœa.

For other remedies and indications, see **Puerperal Peritonitis.**

**AUXILIARY MEASURES.** Absolute rest in horizontal position. *Hot water* injections into vagina several times a day, using fountain syringe, throwing constant stream on cervix for half an hour, very beneficial. In metritis caused by fragments of placenta or retained lochia, intra-uterine injections of *Carbolic acid*, [5 drops to ounce of water] should be used. *Hot* poultices or fomentations to abdomen, valuable in relieving pains.

**DIETETICS.** In acute stage, thin gruel, rice-water and mucilaginous drinks. Later, milk, beef-tea, broths, soft-boiled eggs, toast, etc.

---

## METRORRHAGIA.

(*Uterine Hemorrhage.*)

**THERAPEUTICS.** *Leading indications.*

**ACONITE.** Persons of full habit, especially young girls, [climacteric period, **Puls. Sep. *Ustila.**] *Active hemorrhage, with fear of death. *Very restless and anxious.* So giddy, she cannot sit up in bed.

**BELLADONNA.** *Plethoric women,* [**Acon. Sabi.**] Violent pains in small of back, as if it would break, [as if broken, **Phos.**] *Profuse bright-red blood, which *feels hot* to the parts. Violent *pressure downward,* as if everything would escape through the vulva. The blood sometimes has a bad smell. Palpitation of the heart.

**CHAMOMILLA.** Hemorrhage of dark, coagulated blood, with *labor-like pains,* [**Cimi.**] Tearing pains in legs, [**Cimi. Hyos.**] Frequent discharge of large quantities of colorless urine. *Very impatient, everything seems to go slowly.

**CHINA.** After miscarriage or labor, and in dangerous cases, [***Ipe. Sabi. *Sec.**] *Discharge of dark clots.* *Heaviness of head, ringing in ears, loss of sight, and fainting, Sudden weakness, coldness of extremities, and pale face. *Wants to be fanned, but not too rapidly.* *Debility and other troubles after loss of much blood.

**CROCUS.** After miscarriage or labor, or from over-exertion, [**Chin.**] *Discharge of dark, stringy blood, worse from the least exertion. *Sensation as if something alive in the abdomen, [***Sabi. Sulph.**] Passive hemorrhage in nervous, hysterical women.

**FERRUM.** Weakly persons of hemorrhagic tendency, [**Ham. Sec. Ust.**] *Frequent discharges of partly fluid and partly black-clotted blood, [**Sabi.**] with violent labor-like pains. *The least emotion or exertion produces a red, flushed face. Frequent short shudderings; headache and vertigo.

**HAMAMELIS.** *Protracted uterine hemorrhage, arising from loss of tone in blood-vessels of uterus. *Hemorrhage after abortion or labor, blood dark, having blackish clots mixed with thin, watery blood, [**Sabi.**] The discharge ceases or is better at night.

**HYOSCYAMUS.** Flooding attended with labor-like pains in uterus, drawing in thighs and small of back. Bright-red blood continuing to flow all the time, [**Ipe.**] Trembling over whole body, or numbness of limbs. *Twitching or jerking of a single limb.

**IPECAC.** *Continuous flow of bright-red blood; patient *gasps for breath.* Cutting pains around navel. Great pressure and bearing down. Chills and coldness of body. Great weakness and inclination to vomit. After *parturition or miscarriage,* [***Sabi.** ***Sec.**] Very *impatient.*

**PULSATILLA.** Labor-like pains alternating with hemorrhage. *The discharge is arrested for a little while, then returns with redoubled violence. *There is want of action in the uterus, [***Sec.**] Palpitation of heart; suffocating, fainting spells, and disposition to shed tears.

**SABINA.** Forcing or dragging pains extending to back and loins. Profuse discharge of bright-red blood, [**Bell.**] Feeling of sinking or faintness in abdomen. *Sometimes the discharge is dark, having blackish clots mixed with thin watery blood. Pains extending from back through to pubis.

**SECALE.** *Passive hemorrhage in feeble cachectic females. After parturition or miscarriage. *Want of action in the uterus, [***Puls.**] *Discharge of dark liquid blood, with little or no pain. Coldness of the extremities, pale or sallow face, small feeble pulse. Desire to be uncovered, worse from warmth.

**SEPIA.** Induration of neck of uterus, with spasmodic painful pressure over sexual organs. Chronic metrorrhagia, when it is excited from least cause. Yellow complexion, with spots on face. *Painful sense of emptiness in abdomen. Fetid urine, depositing a clay-colored sediment which adheres to the vessel.

**SULPHUR.** Frequent attacks of hemorrhage; she seems to get almost well, when it occurs again and again, [**Nux v.**] *Constant heat in top of the head, and cold feet. Frequent weak, faint spells and flushes of heat. Gets very hungry about 11 A. M.

**USTILAGO.** *Persistent or continuous hemorrhage of brownish blood, with want of uterine contraction, [**Sec.**] *Chronic metrorrhagia and passive congestion, [**Sep.**]

Consult: **Arn. Caulo. Eriger. Millef. Phos. Plat. Trill.**

**AUXILIARY MEASURES.** Place patient on hard *mattress* in cool room, and enjoin perfect quiet. Lower head and elevate hips. In urgent cases, apply lump of ice to mouth of womb, or *tampon* vagina. Take a soft handkerchief, insert first one corner, then, folding it on itself, introduce the whole, allowing one end to protrude. Remove in ten or twelve hours. This failing, bandage extremities as advised under **Post-Partem Hemorrhage.**

If hemorrhage is due to inefficient uterine contractions, grasp fundus of uterus, and make firm pressure downwards, while with the fingers of other hand in vagina irritate cervix. This failing, inject *hot water,* [110° F.] into the uterus.

---

## MISCARRIAGE, ABORTION.

The expulsion of the fœtus *prior* to the seventh month, is called *miscarriage.* If occurring *after* that period and *before* the ninth month, it is called premature labor. It most frequently occurs between the eighth and twelfth week of gestation. When it has once taken place it is extremely liable to recur in subsequent pregnancies about the same period.

**THERAPEUTICS.** *Leading indications.*

**ACONITE.** Threatened miscarriage in consequence of *fright, the fear still remaining.* *Hemorrhage, with fear of death. Great fear and anxiety of mind, with great nervous excitability. Dizziness on rising from a recumbent position. *Feverish restlessness.*

**ARNICA.** After a *fall, blow* or *concussion,* especially if labor-pains set in, with discharge of blood or serous mucus, [see **Cinn.**] *Sore feeling all through the patient, as if from a bruise, [**Bapt.**] The bed feels too hard.

**BELLADONNA.** Flushed face, red eyes, throbbing headache. Pain in back as if it would break. *Severe bearing down, as if everything would issue through vulva, [**Sep.**] Profuse discharge of bright red blood, [**Cinnamon.**] *Pains come on suddenly and leave as suddenly. *Vertigo when stooping, or when rising from a stooping posture. Great intolerance to light or noise, [**Acon.**]

**CALC. CARB.** Scrofulous diathesis. She has heretofore suffered from too early and too profuse menstruation. Very weakly in general; walking produces great fatigue; she is out of breath when going up-stairs. When standing, a pressing down, as if everything would issue through vulva, [***Bell.**] *Her feet feel cold and damp. *Vertigo when ascending a height.

**CANTHARIS.** *Threatened abortion from congestion or ulceration of the cervix uteri.* Retention of placenta. *Constant desire to urinate.

**CAULOPHYLLUM.** *Threatened miscarriage, with severe pains in back and loins, but uterine contractions feeble; slight flow. *Want of action in the uterus, [**Puls.** ***Sec.**] *Protracted lochia.*

**CHAMOMILLA.** Periodical pains resembling those of *labor,* with discharge of dark-colored or coagulated blood.

*Violent pains in the bowels, extending to the sides, with *frequent urination.* Becomes almost furious about her pains, [**Acon.**] *Very impatient, snappish and cross. Hot perspiration about the head.

**CHINA.** Weak and exhausted persons from loss of animal fluids, [**Phos. ac.**] After miscarriage, when there is hemorrhage unto fainting; giddiness, drowsiness and loss of consciousness. *Heaviness of head, ringing in ears, and coldness of extremities.

**CINNAMON.** Threatened miscarriage after a *false step, or strain in loins,* [**Rhus.**] *The chief symptom is a profuse flow of red blood, [**Bell. Ipc.**] *Itching of nose and nightly restlessness;* she tosses about even during sleep.

**CROCUS SATI.** Especially where the discharge consists of *dark, stringy blood, which is increased by the least exertion.* *Sensation as if something were alive in the abdomen. [**Sabi.**] Mostly after miscarriage.

**FERRUM.** After miscarriage, when there is a discharge of partly fluid and clotted blood, with labor-like pains. *Least emotion or exertion produces a red, flushed face. Hemorrhagic tendency.

**HYOSCYAMUS.** Miscarriage attended with spasms or convulsions of whole body. Discharge of light-red blood, with labor-like pains. *Twitching and jerking of single muscles or limbs, [**Chin.**] Adapted to hysterical subjects, [**Ign. Nux m.**]

**IGNATIA.** Suppressed grief seems to have been exciting cause. *Sadness and sighing, with an empty feeling in stomach. Uterine cramps with cutting stitches. *Difficult stools causing prolapsus ani.

**IPECAC.** *Profuse and continuous discharge of bright-red blood, with pressure downward, [**Bell.**] *Cutting pains around navel.* *Continual nausea, without a moment's relief. Disposition to faint.

**NUX MOS.** Hysterical females, [**Ign.**] Pressure in the abdomen, and drawing down into the legs from the navel; discharge *dark and thick,* [dark liquid, **Sec.**] Great drowsiness and inclination to faint.

**NUX VOM.** *Every pain produces a desire to go to stool, or to urinate. Writhing pains in abdomen, accompanied by nausea, or pains in back and loins as if dislocated. *Very irritable, and wishes to be alone. High livers; sedentary habits.

**PULSATILLA.** Labor-like pains alternating with hemorrhage. *The discharge is arrested for a little while, then returns with redoubled violence. Suffocative spells; she craves fresh air, worse in a close, warm room, [**Sec.**] *Inclination to be chilly, even in a warm room. Retention of after-birth, [**Caul.** ***Sec.**]

**RHUS TOX.** *If a wrench or a strain is the exciting cause, [**Cinnamon.**] Pains worse in the latter part of the night and during rest; has to change position often to get a little temporary relief.

**SABINA.** *Threatened abortion in early months.* Violent forcing or dragging pains extending from *back to pubis.* *Discharge profuse, consisting of bright-red, partly fluid and partly clotted blood, [**Ferr.**] Feeling of sinking or faintness in abdomen. Women who habitually miscary at third month.

**SECALE.** Threatened abortion in *later months.* Especially after miscarriage. *Copious flow of black, liquid blood, worse from slightest motion, [see **Croc.**] *Passive hemorrhage in thin, scrawny, cachectic women. Want of action in uterus, [***Caul.** ***Puls.**] Great debility, feeble, almost extinct pulse.

**AUXILIARY MEASURES.** In threatened abortion, place patient on hard mattress with light covering and enjoin perfect quiet. Keep room cool and well ventilated, and exclude all visitors. Give indicated remedy and watch patient closely. If hemorrhage is profuse, treat as directed under "Metorrhagia." Should miscarriage take place, remove any fragments of *ovum* or *placenta* that might remain behind and cause secondary hemorrhage or septicæmia. With one hand make pressure over the uterus, and with the finger of the other endeavor to extract the offending object. This failing, use placental forceps.

**DIETETICS.** The diet must be of the simplest kind, and taken moderately cool. All stimulating food must be avoided.

---

## MUMPS.—PAROTITIS.

**THERAPEUTICS.** *Leading indications.*

**BELLADONNA.** Redness of face and eyes. *Bright-red swelling of glands, especially on right side, [dark-red swelling of left side, **Rhus.**] Tendency to erysipelatous inflammation of the parts. *Sudden disappearance of swelling, with throbbing headache and delirium. *Sleepiness, but cannot sleep.

**CARBO VEG.** Slow grade of fever; the swelling becomes very hard and will not disperse as it should. *Metastasis to stomach, with burning, pressure, and sensitiveness of epigastrium, After abuse of calomel. *The most innocent food disagrees.

**HYOSCYAMUS.** If the disease be transmitted to brain. Unconscious delirium, red face, wild, staring look, throbbing carotids, [**Bell.**] *Twitching and jerking of limbs, with great nervous excitability. Giddiness, with stupefaction.

**MERCURIUS.** If the disease was induced by a cold. Erethic fever, with *alternate heat and chills.* *Hard swelling of gland, with stiffness of jaws and difficulty of swallowing. *Perspiration, affording no relief. *Profuse secretion of saliva, and very offensive breath. Dark-green or slimy stools with *severe tenesmus.* All worse at night, and in damp weather.

**PULSATILLA**. When there is *metastasis* to female mammæ, [*to testicles*, **Ars. Carb. v.**] *Inflammation and swelling* of *testicles*, with drawing pain extending up spermatic cords. *Vertigo on rising from sitting posture, with chilliness. *Thickly-coated tongue, with bad taste in morning. Mild, tearful disposition.

**RHUS TOX**. If typhoid symptoms set in, or inflammation assumes an erysipelatous character. Lameness and stiffness of limbs, with pain on *first moving them after rest.* *Parotitis after scarlatina, with dropsical symptoms, [**Ars. Chin.**] *Restless at night; must turn often to find a moment's ease.

**AUXILIARY MEASURES.** Where the inflammation and swelling is very considerable, *hot* fomentations to the parts will be found very beneficial. When suppuration is inevitable, poultices made of linseed meal should be applied, and when the abscess points should be opened with a lancet.

Great care should be observed during convalescence to avoid taking cold, as the disease is very liable to be transmitted to the testicles or female mammæ, and seriously complicate the case.

---

## NEPHRALGIA.—COLICA RENALIS.

**THERAPEUTICS.** *Leading indications.*

**BELLADONNA**. Spasmodic, crampy, straining along ureter to bladder. Retention of urine, it passing off only in drops; *when heated deposits a cloud of phosphates.*

**CANTHARIDES**. *Pressing pain* in kidneys, extending along ureters to bladder, [*dragging pain along ureters*, with emissions in drops of burning, bloody urine, **Cann. in.**] *Mucous sediment* in urine, [*purulent*, **Lyc. Nux.**]

**LYCOPO.** Renal colic, right side, [**Bell.**] Frequent urging to urinate, *passing red sand with the urine.* *Pain in back previous to every urination.

**NUX VOM**. Pain, especially in right kidney, extending to genitals and right leg. *Spasmodic contraction of spermatic cords, the testicles being drawn up. Nausea, vomiting, and tenesmus of bladder. *Ineffectual urging to stool, [**Lyc.**]

**OCIMUM CANUM**. *Renal colic, with violent vomiting. Moans, cries, and wrings his hands. After the attack, red urine, with brick-dust sediment, or discharge of blood with the urine.

**OPIUM.** Pressing, squeezing pains, as though something had to force its way through a narrow space. Shooting pains in bladder and testicles. Vomiting slime and bile.

Great anxiety and restlessness. *Slow pulse. *Bed feels too hot.

**PHYTOLACCA.** Dull pain and soreness in region of kidneys, most on right side, [Bell. Lyc.] *Great uneasiness down ureters; chalk-like sediment in urine.

**TABACUM.** Violent colicky pains in region of ureters. *Constant deadly sickness of the stomach and retching, with cold perspiration, [Verat. a.]

**AUXILIARY MEASURES.** *Hot fomentations* to the loins and abdomen; *hot sitz* baths; copious injections of *hot water* into the bowels, valuable. In urgent cases, small injections of clear starch containing 20 or 30 drops of *Laudanum* may be given, and in very urgent cases, where *Opium* is contra-indicated, inhalations of *Chloroform* may be resorted to.

**DIETETICS.** Persons subject to renal calculi should live upon simple digestible food, for most part vegetable. A little meat two or three times a week, may be eaten if necessary to preserve the strength. All highly seasoned food and *alcoholic* drinks must be avoided. Pure *soft water* may be taken *ad libitum.*

---

## NEPHRITIS.

*(Acute inflammation of the Kidneys.)*

**THERAPEUTICS.** *Leading indications.*

**ACONITE.** In early stage, high fever, evinced by hot, dry skin, quick pulse and intense thirst. *Retention of urine, with stitches in kidneys. *Fear and anxiety of mind, with great nervous excitability. *So giddy, cannot sit up.

**BELLADONNA.** Shooting pain from kidneys to bladder. *Pains which appear and disappear suddenly. *Sensation as of a worm in bladder, [of a *ball*, Lach.] Urine scanty, of a bright-red or yellowish color, depositing a whitish, thick sediment, Heat and swelling in region of kidney. *Back feels as if it would break, hindering motion.

**BERBERIS.** **Smarting burning* in region of kidneys, [Tereb.] Bloody urine, which settles at bottom of chamber in a cake, [Mille.] Transparent jelly-like mucus passed with urine, followed by *great exhaustion.* **Albuminous urine*, [Apis. Helon. Ocimum c. Tereb.] Pain in loins and hips.

**CANNABIS.** Inflammation of kidneys, with dragging or shooting pains along ureters to groin, [Berb. Canth. Lyc.] Painful urging to urinate, passing only a few drops of bloody, burning urine, [Canth.] Burning *during* and *after* micturition.

**CANTHARIDES.** Burning heat, with thirst and anxiety. Shooting, cutting or tearing pains in loins and region of kidney. *Constant desire to urinate, passing but a few drops at a time, sometimes mixed with blood, [Merc.] Burning, cutting pains in bladder, with ineffectual efforts to urinate. *Vomiting, with violent retching and severe colic.

**COCCUS CACTI.** *Nephritic colic*, with copious urine and dull pain in urethra. *Sudden acute cutting pains, extending from left renal region along ureters into bladder. Bruised pain in sacro-lumbar region and in groins. Urine deep colored, with sediment color of brick-dust, which adheres to the vessel. The urine also contains mucus in the form of filaments and flocks.

**HEPAR SULPH.** Where suppuration has occurred, or abscess is imminent, [**Lyc. *Merc. Sil.**] *Sensation of throbbing in region of the kidney. Feeling of weight in the loins. Alternate chilliness and heat, followed by profuse perspiration.

**LYCOPO.** *Renal colic, the pain is felt along ureters into bladder, especially right side. *Red, *sandy* sediment in urine, [**Phos. Sep.**] Cutting pain across hypogastrium, from right to left. *Terrific pain in back previous to every urination, with relief as soon as urine begins to flow.

**MERCURIUS.** For a similar train of symptoms as are described under **Hepar.**, and where that remedy does not produce the desired improvement. Urine scanty and red, with *strong smell.* *Much perspiration, affording no relief.

**NUX VOMICA.** Persons of sedentary habits, or where disease arises from suppressed piles. Pain in small of back so bad he cannot move. *Painful desire to urinate, with scanty emissions in drops, with burning pains. Reddish urine, with brick-dust-like sediment, [**Acon. Berb. Nux. *Puls.**] *Constipation of hard, difficult stools, and frequent urging.

**PULSATILLA.** Persons of a mild, tearful disposition, or females with *scanty* or *suppressed menses.* Aching pain in small of back. *Frequent and almost ineffectual urging to urinate, with cutting pain. Pale watery urine, with *jelly-like sediment*, [**Berb. Phos. ac.**] Chilliness even in a warm room. Headache, relieved by compression. *Craves cool fresh air, worse in a warm room. *Bad taste in the morning.* *Vertigo when rising from a seat.

**SULPHUR.** In chronic cases where only partial relief has been obtained by other remedies. *Burning and drawing pain in small of back. Pulsative stitches in region of kidneys. Painful desire to urinate; discharge of drops of bloody urine. **Very fetid urine*, [**Merc. Sep.**] Frequent weak, faint spells. *Constant heat on top of head.

**TEREBINTHINA.** Burning, drawing pains in kidneys. Pressure in bladder, extending up into kidneys when sitting, disappearing when walking about. *Difficult urination, with burning in bladder, [***Cann. *Canth.**] *Blood is thoroughly mixed with urine, like coffee-grounds sediment.

Nephritis arising from abuse of Spanish fly-blister will be relieved by **Camphor** in drop doses.

**AUXILIARY MEASURES.** Absolute rest in recumbent posture. If there is severe pain and inflammation, apply *hot fomentations* or poultices to loins. Gum-bags partly filled with *hot water* or heated salt-bags afford great relief.

**DIETETICS.** During active stage, thin gruels, rice-water and acidulated drinks. Later, milk, broths, toast, light puddings, ripe fruits, etc.

---

## NEURALGIA.

**THERAPEUTICS.** *Leading indications.*

**ACONITE.** Red and hot face, with pain on one side. *Pains so severe patient becomes desperate and declares *something must be done*, [**Cham.**] *Great fear and anxiety, with vertigo on rising from a seat, [**Puls.**] Pains worse at night, with great restlessness.

**ARSENICUM.** Periodical attacks, chiefly around eye and in temples. *Burning, stinging pain, as if pierced with red-hot needles. Pain insupportable, especially at night, [**Acon. Cham. Coff.**] Great fear and anxiety of mind, with extreme restlessness, [**Acon.**] Aggravation about midnight. Temporary relief from external heat, and from moving about.

**BELLADONNA.** Pain most violent under eye, excited by rubbing the part, [by *contact*, **Chin. Colo. Phos.**] *Violent shooting or tearing pains in eye-ball. *Darting pains in cheek-bones, nose, or zygomatic process. Cutting, tearing pains, with stiffness at nape of neck, and clinching of jaws. *Convulsive jerkings in facial muscles. *Great intolerance to *noise* or *light*, [**Acon.**] Aggravation in afternoon.

**CAUSTICUM.** Tensive or beating pains in facial bones, especially under the eye. *Drawing pains on right side, from cheek-bone to temple, [see **Hep.**] Obstinate constipation and hemorrhoids. *Involuntary urination when coughing, [**Puls. Verat.**]

**CEDRON.** *Periodical attacks, [**Ars. Chin. Spig.**] Pains worse during *menstruation, and after coition.* Flying heat in face.

**CHAMOMILLA.** Stitching, jerking pains that seem intolerable, especially at night, [see **Ars.**] *The pain causes hot perspiration about head, and extorts cries. *Very impatient, can hardly answer a civil question. Great sensitiveness to pain, becomes furious.

**CHINA.** *Periodical attacks*, [**Ars. Spig.**] *Darting, tearing pains, aggravated by the *least contact*. *Ringing in ears*, [**Nux.**] Pain mostly in the infra-orbital and maxillary nerves. *Exacerbation every other day. Weakly persons who have lost much blood.

**CIMICIFUGA.** Intense and persistent pains in eye-balls, of a dull, aching, sore nature. Sensation as if top of head would fly off; the cerebrum feels too large for skull, pressing outwards and upwards.

**COLOCYNTH.** Neuralgia chiefly on left side of face, [**Mez. Sep. Spig.**] *Violent rending and darting pains, aggravated by *touch or motion*, [**Chin. Phos. Spig.**] Tearing, screwing pains, together with great restlessness and anxiety. Better from perfect rest, and from warm applications. If caused by anger.

**GELSEMIUM.** *Throbbing pain in medulla* passing through mastoid to forehead and eyes. Great heaviness of eyelids, cannot keep them open, [**Rhus. Sep.**] Dimness of vision, and confusion of mind.

**HEPAR SULPH.** Pains in malar bones, extending to ears and temples, [**Mez.** ***Puls.**] Worse when in open air, and better from wrapping up face. Fluent coryza, with hoarseness and much sweating. After abuse of mercury.

**IRIS VERS.** Neuralgia of head, eyes and temples. *Begins every morning with a stupid, stunning headache.* *Sharp, cutting pains of short duration, with vomiting a sweetish mucus. *Burning distress in epigastrium.* *Profuse flow of saliva. *Aggravation* from rest, [**Rhus.**]

**MERCURIUS.** Tearing pains, worse at night in bed. *Pain starts in a decayed tooth, and involves the whole side of face, [**Staph.**] Profuse ptyalism and lachrymation. *Much perspiration affording no relief, [affords relief, **Verat.**] If caused from cold.

**MEZEREUM.** Chiefly on left side of face, [on *right* side, **Puls. Verat. Zinc.**] The pains extend to eye, temple, ear, neck, and shoulder. *Boring, pressing pains, coming like lightning, leaving parts numb, [**Verbas.**] Aggravated by taking warm food or drink, or from entering a warm room after being in open air.

**NUX VOMICA.** Drawing, tearing, or compressive pains, chiefly in forehead or in the part just above root of nose. *Tearing pain in facial and infra-orbital nerves, [see **Zinc.**] Numbness of affected part. Redness and lachrymation of the eyes. Fluent watery discharge from nose. Constipation, with frequent urging to stool. *Very irritable, and wishes to be alone, [**Chin.**] Aggravation in morning, and from mental exertion.

**PHOSPHORUS.** Drawing and tearing pain in jaws, root of nose, eyes, and temples. Face swollen and pale. Vertigo, and buzzing in ears. *Sensation of weakness and emptiness in abdomen. *Long, narrow, hard stools. difficult to expel, [**Caust.**] Aggravation from chewing, talking, or touching affected parts.

**PLATINA.** Severe spasmodic or boring ain in cheek-bones, with a sensation of crawling in the parts, [**Nux.**] *The attack is preceded by a feeling of coldness and torpor, [**Lyc.**] Anxiety, weeping, and palpitation of heart, [**Puls.**]

Redness of face and lachrymation. Aggravation in evening and during rest.

**PULSATILLA.** Mostly on right side of face and head. *Darting, tearing pains extending from jaw to orbit and temple. *Profuse lachrymation from affected eye, [**Merc. Nux v.**] Chilliness even in a warm room. *Disposition to weep and complain*, [**Ign. Sep.**] Aggravation towards evening and in warm room. Better from cold and worse from warm applications, [reverse, **Ars.**]

**RHUS TOX.** Drawing, burning, tearing pain in malar bones, root of nose and ear. *Pain aggravated by rest, must move continually to get a little relief, [better from rest, **Acon. Bry. Merc.**] Worse at night, particularly after midnight, and in *wet weather.*

**SEPIA.** Drawing or cramp-like pains in facial bones, mostly on left side. Sensation of emptiness in stomach. *Yellowness of face, particularly across bridge of nose, resembling a saddle. *Sense of great weight in anus, not relieved by stool. Especially during period of gestation.

**SPIGELIA.** Periodical, mostly on left side. *Pains darting or burning, especially in cheek-bones, eyeballs, and above the eye, [**Bell.**] *Commences with rising of sun, gets worse until noon, then decreases until sunset. Redness of parts affected. Flow of water from eyes and nose. Palpitation of heart, and difficulty of breathing. *Pains aggravated by least contact or motion.

**STAPHISAGRIA.** The pain starts in a decayed tooth and extends to eye, [**Merc.**] *Drawing*, tearing pains in cheek-bones. Very sensitive to least impression. Cold hands and cold sweat in face. *Pains worse from slight and better from hard pressure, [**Nux.**]

**STRAMONIUM.** Many nervous symptoms. *Feels too tall.* *Pains unbearable, driving patient to despair. Extreme degree of nervous erethism, with convulsive twitching of muscles of face. Jerking through whole body. *Delirious, talking continually; eyes wide open. *Vertigo when walking in dark.

**SULPHUR.** Mostly chronic cases, or where well-chosen remedies have not the desired effect. *After suppressed cutaneous eruptions. Dry, husky, scaly skin; no perspiration. *Constant heat on top of head, [*coldness*, **Sep. Verat.**] Frequent weak, faint spells.

**VERAT. A.** Drawing, tearing pain in right side of face and above the ear. Sunken eyes and coldness of the extremities. *Attacks of pain, with delirium, or driving to madness, [becomes desperate, **Acon. Cham. Stram.**] Trembling and jerking of limbs. *Cold sweat, especially on forehead.

**VERBASCUM.** Violent pain, jerking like lightning, or pressive numbing, [**Mez.**] The pain is excited by pressure, sneezing, talking, chewing, etc. Attacks recur at same hour every day, and are attended with headache, vertigo, belching and a discharge of tough saliva from the mouth.

**ZINCUM.** Burning, quick stitches, and jerking along course of infra-orbital nerve, right side, [**Chin. Nux.**] Bluish color of eyelids and numbness of tongue. Constricted sensation in throat. *Constant trembling of hands, with coldness of extremities. *Fidgety feeling in feet, must move them continually, [**Sticta. Taran.**]

**AUXILIARY MEASURES.** In some cases *hot* fomentations or *hot salt* bags applied to the painful parts relieve the pain, while in other cases *cold* applications answer a better purpose. Bathing parts with *Tr. Aconite* or *Belladonna* is valuable in some cases. Tracing the course of the nerve with oil of *Peppermint* or oil of *Cloves* will sometimes give prompt relief.

---

## OPHTHALMIA.

**THERAPEUTICS.** *Leading indications.*

**ACONITE.** Purulent ophthalmia, where inflammation runs high; dry, hot skin and full, quick pulse. *Intense redness and swelling of the affected parts, attended with acute pain, [**Bell.**] *Great aversion to light.* *Fear, anxiety, and great restlessness. Flushed cheeks.

**APIS MEL.** *Lids dark-red, everted.* *Burning, stinging, shooting pains. *Scalding tears, profuse.* *Conjunctiva injected, full of dark vessels. *Bag-like swelling under the eyes, [*over upper lids*, **Kali c.**]

**ARGENT. NIT.** Photophobia, eyes filled with mucus. Canthi red as blood, caruncula swollen, standing out like a lump of red flesh. *Bright-red granulations on lids. Lids crusty, swollen, thick.

**ARSENICUM.** Inflammation of conjunctiva and sclerotica; *dark redness and congestion of vessels.* *Burning pains; the parts burn like fire, [**Acon.**] Inflammatory swelling of the lids. Specks or ulcers on cornea, [**Calc. c. Euph. Sulph.**] *Nightly agglutination of the lids. *Great anguish and restlessness.* *Intense thirst, drinking little and often.

**BELLADONNA.** Acute ophthalmia, *with great intolerance to light or noise,* [**Acon.**] *Vivid redness of sclerotica, with discharge of hot, salt tears, or great dryness of eyes. Sharp pains in orbits, extending to brain. Pains which appear suddenly, and cease as suddenly. Double vision, [**Hyos. Nit. ac. Stram.**] Throbbing headache, increased by motion.

**CALC. CARB.** *Scrofulous ophthalmia, [**Graph. Lyc. Merc. Sulph.**] *Swelling and redness of eyelids, with nightly agglutination. *Stinging pains, worse from candle-light. Specks and ulcers on cornea. Constant desire to keep the eyes in darkness. Glandular swellings of neck, and eruptions on hairy scalp.

**CHAMOMILLA**. *Ophthalmia of infants*, especially if caused by exposure to cold, damp atmosphere, or if worse by every cold change of weather, [**Dulc. Merc.**] *Eyes agglutinated in morning with purulent mucus. Very irritable, nothing pleases. *Scrofulous ophthalmia during dentition.*

**EUPHRASIA.** Aching pain in eyes and redness of sclerotica. Vesicles, or specks and ulcers on the cornea, [see **Ars.**] *Copious secretion of mucus and tears. Swelling of the eyeballs. *Fluent coryza and headache. Photophobia, flickering of the light.

**GRAPHITES.** *Scrofulous or chronic ophthalmia.* Purulent secretion from balls and lids, with frequent agglutination, [**Calc. c.**] Ulcers on the cornea, [on sclerotica, **Merc.**] *Eyelids much inflamed and painful.* Constant desire to keep eyes covered. *Unhealthy skin, with eruptions oozing a *sticky, glutinous fluid*, [*watery* fluid, **Dulc.**] Eruptions *behind ears.*

**LYCOPO.** Agglutination of lids at night, [**Ars. Calc. c. Puls.**] *Burning and smarting in eyes, [as from sand, **Euph. Graph. Merc. Sulph.**] Scrofulous or catarrhal ophthalmia. Aptness to take cold. *Red sediment like sand in urine. Obstinate constipation. *Constant sensation of satiety, feels full up to throat.

**MERCURIUS.** *Gonorrhœal*, or *scrofulous* ophthalmia. Violent inflammation and readness of eyes. *Cutting, burning pains, or pressure in eyes as if from sand. Great sensitiveness of eyes to glare of fire, or light, [**Acon. Bell.**] *Vesicles and pimples on sclerotica, with purulent discharge. Pustules and scurfs around eyes and on margins of lids.

**NITRIC AC.** and **HEPAR.** are the best remedies for the removal of mercurial ophthalmia, following the abuse of this drug in syphilis and other diseases.

**PULSATILLA.** Catarrhal or rheumatic ophthalmia. After *suppressed gonorrhœal discharge*, [**Merc. Nit. ac. Tart. e.**] Redness and swelling of conjunctiva and lids. Burning and corrosive lachrymation. Itching burning of the eyes, with disposition to rub them. *Evening aggravation. Mild, tearful disposition.

**RHUS TOX.** *Iritis in rheumatic or gouty subjects*, [**Acon. Bry.**] Conjunctiva red, with yellow purulent discharge; lids agglutinated in morning. Lids much swollen and inflamed. *Eyelids œdematous, or erysipelatous, with scattered, watery vesicles. Aggravation *during rest, after midnight, before a storm.*

**SULPHUR.** *Scrofulous ophthalmia.* *Itching, burning in eyes and eyelids, worse by moving or exposing them to light. *Edges of lids thickened and ulcerated.* *Feeling as if sand were in eyes. Specks and ulcers on cornea, [see **Ars.**] *Flashes of heat, and weak, faint spells. *Burning on top of head. After suppressed cutaneous eruptions.

**AUXILIARY MEASURES.** Keep patient in a darkened room, and free from all mental or emotional excitement.

Apply *hot fomentations* medicated with indicated remedy. In gonorrhœal ophthalmia, and also in severe forms of catarrhal ophthalmia, Dr. Dudgeon and others advise a local solution of *Nitrate of Silver*, [grs. ji, aqua dest. ℥j.] a small quantity introduced beneath the lids with a camel's-hair brush once a day, every two or three days.

**DIETETICS.** Light puddings, farina, corn-starch, tapioca, ripe fruits, vegetables, etc. All stimulating food and drinks should be strictly avoided

---

## OTALGIA.—EARACHE.

**THERAPEUTICS.** *Leading remedies.*

**ACONITE.** External ear *hot*, *swollen*, *red*, painfully sensitive, [Puls.] *Acute pain, caused by exposure to *cold wind*, or sudden stoppage of a chronic discharge from ear.

**BELLADONNA.** *Shooting pains* in the ears, with hardness of hearing. *Great sensitiveness to noise and light. *Roaring* and *humming* in the ears. Pain in the head and eyes, with heat and fullness in head. Right parotid gland swollen and red.

**CHAMOMILLA.** Stitches in ear, especially when stooping. *Earache by spells, with tearing pain, extorting cries. Patient becomes almost furious about the pains; worse in open air and at night. *Children very fretful, must be carried all the time.

**DULCAMARA.** *Earache, with nausea, buzzing in ear, worse at night and when still. Earache after measles, [Puls.] Worse from every *cold* change.

**MERCURIUS.** Boils in external canal. *Suppuration imminent, [Hepar.] Ear *inflamed*, with stinging, tearing pains. *Perspires much without relief. Worse *at night* and in *damp rainy* weather.

**PULSATILLA.** *Otalgia, with darting, tearing pains, and pulsating at night. *Severe pain in ear, continuing through night, with paroxysms of increasing severity. *Otalgia after measles.*

**LOCAL MEASURES.** A soft sponge wrung out of *hot* water and bound to the ear will often give relief. Two or three drops of *Ether* on a little cotton, inserted in the ear, will in most cases relieve the pain. Take the core of a *roasted onion*, insert the small end in the ear and cover with a compress. Put five drops of *Chloroform* on a little cotton in the bowl of a clay pipe, and blow the vapor through the stem into the aching ear—acts promptly and efficiently. Where an abscess forms, warm poultices, made of *ground flaxseed* or bread and milk, will be found useful.

# OVARITIS.

**THERAPEUTICS.** *Leading indications.*

**ACONITE.** After exposure to *dry, cold winds*, [from *wet weather*, **Dulc. Rhus.**] During the menses, patient is chilled and the flow ceases, or where it results from a fright. *Painful urging to urinate.*

**APIS.** Ovaritis of *right side*, [***Bell.**—*left side*, **Graph.** ***Lach.**] *Stinging pains in ovary, which is swollen and tender to touch. Numbness in right side of abdomen, extending to thigh, [see **Ars.**] *Cough, with soreness in left chest. *No thirst, scanty urine.*

**ARSENICUM.** *Burning, drawing or stitching pains in ovary, with *great restlessness.* The pains extend to thigh, which feels numb; worse from motion.

**BELLADONNA.** *Stitching, throbbing* pains in *right* ovary, which is hard and swollen. Great *heat* and *tenderness* of abdomen; **cannot bear the least jar.* *Constant bearing down as if everything would issue from vagina, [**Plat.**] Glistening eyes, red face and delirium.

**BRYONIA.** *Stitches* in ovaries on taking a deep inspiration, [**Canth.**] *Cannot bear least motion or touch of affected parts.* *Suppressed menses, with bleeding of nose.

**CACTUS GRAND.** *Pulsating pain in ovarian region.* *Pains extend down thighs, return periodically at same time each day. *Painful sensation of *constriction* around pelvis. Organic *diseases of the heart.*

**CANTHARIS.** Stitches or pinching pains arresting breathing, [**Bry.**] *Great burning in ovarian region, [**Plat.**] *Constant desire to urinate*, passing but a few drops, often mixed with blood. *Bearing down* towards genitals, [**Bell.**] *Neck of uterus swollen.*

**CONIUM.** Induration and swelling of ovary, with nausea and vomiting. *Cutting pains in the parts. Dwindling of mammæ. *Vertigo on turning in bed. *Stinging in neck of uterus.*

**HAMAMELIS.** *Ovaritis after a blow*, [***Arn.**] Diffused, agonizing soreness over whole abdomen. Menses irregular; always worse at time of menses. *Phlegmasia alba dolens. *Passive hemorrhages and venous congestions.*

**HEPAR SULPH.** *Where suppuration has occurred or abscess is imminent, [**Lach. Merc.**] *Throbbing* pains, with frequent chills. *Unhealthy skin.*

**LACHESIS.** *Ovaritis of left side*, [*right*, **Apis. Bell.**] Swelling of ovary, with drawing pressing pains. If pus has already formed, [**Hep. Merc.**] Cannot lie on right side, or bear any pressure on uterine region.

**PLATINA.** *Excessive sexual desire*, [**Canth.**] Painful pressing towards the genital organs, [***Bell. Canth.**] Burning in ovarian region, with stitches in the forehead. Profuse or suppressed menses.

**PULSATILLA.** After getting *feet wet, menses are suppressed,* [**Dulc.**] Pains so violent she tosses about in all directions, with cries and tears. Constant *chilliness.* *Craves fresh, cool air; worse in a warm room.

**AUXILIARY MEASURES.** Absolute rest in recumbent position. *Hot fomentations* to ovarian region—in some cases *dry* heat answers best. Copious injections of hot water into the vagina very beneficial. Where suppuration is imminent and abscess points to *outside*, apply warm flaxseed poultices. Usually, however, the pus finds its way through the bladder or rectum.

**DIETETICS.** In *acute stage*, less patient eats the better. Avoid all solid food. Thin gruels, or light puddings of rice, farina, corn-starch, oatmeal, etc. Later, more nourishing diet. Beef-tea, broths, milk, soft-boiled eggs, cream-toast, etc.

---

## PARALYSIS.

**THERAPEUTICS.** *Leading indications.*

**ANACARDIUM.** *After Apoplexy,* [**Bary. c. Caust. Nux.**] *Great weakness or loss of memory. Sensation of weakness in arms, with trembling, numbness of fingers. Knees feel paralyzed, with stiffness and great lassitude. *Sensation as of a hoop or band around the part.

**ARNICA.** Paralysis from concussion, [**Cicu.**] *Hopelessness and indifference. Weary, *bruised* feeling all through the patient. *Everything on which he lies feels too hard, [**Bapt.**] Knee-joints suddenly bend when standing, feet numb and insensible.

**ARSENICUM.** Paralysis, especially of lower limbs, [**Cocc. Gel. Nux. Rhus.**] *Trembling of limbs, particularly of drunkards and after lead-poisoning, [**Nux.**] Sensation as if bruised in the small of back. *Great prostration.*

**BARYTA CARB.** General paralysis in old age, with loss of memory and trembling of limbs. *Paralysis of tongue, with loss of speech, [**Cocc. Dulc. Gel.**] Weariness with constant inclination to lie down.

**CAUSTICUM.** *Hemiplegia of face or tongue, with giddiness, [**Cocc. Nux.**] *Paralysis of single nerves. Tension and shortening of muscles, contracting the joints and bending the limbs. Drawing, lame feeling in affected parts. After exposure to severe cold.

**CHINA.** Paralysis from loss of animal fluids, or after arsenical poisoning, [**Ferr. Nux.**] Numbness of parts on which he lies. Pain in bones and joints as if strained. Worse every other day.

**COLCHICUM.** After sudden suppression of sweat, particularly foot-sweat, by getting wet. *Numbness of hands and feet, with prickling, as if asleep, [**Phos. Sili. Stram.**]

Laming pains in arms, unable to hold anything. Tearing twitches, like electric shocks in one side of body, with sensation of numbness.

**DULCAMARA.** After suppressed eruptions, from cold. *Paralysis of upper and lower limbs and tongue. *The paralyzed arm feels icy cold.*

**GELSEMIUM.** *Paralysis of motion; muscles will not obey the will, and feel bruised. Tingling, pricking, crawling in parts. *Paralysis of lower half of body, [**Caulo. Cocc.**] Trembling of hands when lifting them up. *Adapted to nervous, hysterical females.*

**IGNATIA.** Paralysis after great mental emotions and night-watching. Hysterical paraplegia, [see **Gel.**] Trembling of and languor in the limbs.

**LACHESIS.** Paralysis *left side*, [**Arn. Caust. Rhus.**]. *After apoplexy or cerebral exhaustion, [**Nux.**] Tingling, prickling in limbs, [**Gel.**] *Trembling of hands in drunkards.* *Mind worse after sleep.

**NUX VOMICA.** **Numbness and paralysis* of lower limbs. Parts cold, bluish, emaciated. *Trembling all over, mostly of hands in drunkards*, [**Lach.**] Especially suitable after *apoplexy*, after *sexual excesses*, after abuse of *alcohol*, after *arsenical* poisoning, or after *diphtheria*.

**OLEANDER.** *Spells* of *vertigo* a long time before paralysis is developed. *Numbness of upper lip.* *Painless stiffness and paralysis of limbs. Loss of muscular power, and trembling of knees when standing.

**OPIUM.** *Paralysis of eyelids, tongue, arms and legs. Numbness and insensibility of parts. *Stupefying sleep, eyes half open and snoring. Suitable after apoplexy, to drunkards and old people. Retention of stool and urine.

**PLUMBUM.** *Paralysis of upper or lower limbs, with *wasting of muscular tissues*, loss of motion and sensation. Paralysis preceded by trembling, mental derangement or spasm. *Stools lumpy, like sheep's dung.

**RHUS TOX.** Rheumatic palsies from exposure to wet, strains or excessive exertions, with painful stiffness, tingling and numbness. *Paralysis of one side, (right,) with sensation as if gone to sleep, [see **Colch.**] Paralysis of rectum and bladder, [**Hyos. Opi.**] Restless, must change position often. *Better from warmth and motion.*

**SECALE.** Paralysis after spasms and apoplexy, with rapid emaciation of parts, [see **Plumb.**] Involuntary discharges of fæces and urine, [**Ars. Opi. Rhus.**] Spasmodic twitchings in the paralyzed parts.

**STANNUM.** Paralysis, especially of left side, with a feeling of a heavy load in arm and side of chest. After emotions, spasms or onanism.

For **Paralysis of Eyelids**: Cocc. *Gel. Opi.* Rhus. *Zinc.*

Of **Face**: *Bell.* Caust. Cocc. *Nux v. Opi.*

Of **Tongue**: Ars. *Bell.* Cocc. *Hyos.* Lach. *Opi. Plumb.*

Of **Organs of Deglutition**: *Bell. Canth.* Cup. *Gel.* Lach.

Of **Bladder**: *Bell.* Canth. *Hyos.* Lach. Lyco. *Opi.*

Of **Rectum Sphincter ani**: Caust. *Hyos.* Lyc. *Op.* Ruta. Zinc.

Of **Upper Extremities**: Bell. Caust. Cocc. *Nux. Rhus.* Verat.

Of **Hands**: Ars. Caust. *Cup. Rhus.* Ruta Sili.

Of **Fingers**: Ambra. Calc. *Cup.* Nat. m. *Sec.* Sili.

Of **Lower Extremities**: Alum. Bell. Cocc. *Colch.* Merc. *Nux.* Phos. *Plumb.* Rhus. Sec. Sulph. Verat.

Of **Feet**: Ars. Chin. Oleand. *Plumb.*

**AUXILIARY MEASURES.** First ascertain and remove cause, if possible. Friction and kneading the parts have a beneficial effect. *Electricity,* judiciously applied, is one of best remedies in the treatment of this disease. The alternate use of the faradic and galvanic currents will be found the most successful.

Due attention should be gived the skin. *Tepid sponge baths,* and thorough rubbing of the body with a crash towel very important.

---

## PARTURITION.—LABOR.

When called to a case of labor, go prepared for emergency. Take forceps, blunt hook, fountain syringe, chloroform, ammonia, etc.

**Examination.** Ascertain in first place if woman is in labor. Make out presentation; observe pelvic capacity, the condition of bowels, bladder, rate of progress and probable termination of labor. Deal *frankly* with patient. Make no false promises, but encourage her to bear the pains.

**Rupturing Membranes.** Do not rupture membranes until os is *fully dilated;* if very *tough, notch* finger-nail and scratch through them. Evacuate bladder with *flexible* rubber catheter. Support perineum to *prevent* laceration.

**Protracted Cases.** Tedious cases, attended with much suffering, rigidity of os uteri, etc., may be greatly benefited by one of following remedies.

**ACONITE.** Great *distress, moaning and restlessness.* *Very anxious, is sure she will die. Vulva, vagina, and os dry, tender, and undilatable, [see **Bell.**] *Pains violent.*

**BELLADONNA.** Spasmodic contractions of cervix uteri, which is *hot, dry, tender and rigid,* [**Acon.**] *Pains appear suddenly and disappear as suddenly.

**CHAMOMILLA.** Over-excitement, and excessive sensibility to pain, [also **Coff.**] Anguish and discouragement, with tossing about. *Pains spasmodic and distressing. *Tearing pains in legs.* *She is very impatient, and can hardly answer a civil question.

**CIMICIFUGA.** *Tedious cases caused by rigidity of os, with severe pains, [**Bell. Caul. Gel.**] This remedy, given once daily for ten or twelve days *previous* to the expected confinement, is said to greatly facilitate labor and shorten its duration, [*Caul.]

**COFFEA.** Pains excessively violent, with great mental and nervous excitement, and fear of death. *She weeps and laments fearfully, [Cimi.] *Great sensitiveness of the genital organs, cannot bear them to be touched. *Great wakefulness at night.*

**GELSEMIUM.** *Cutting pains in abdomen from before, backwards and upwards, rendering the *labor-pains useless;* these come on with every pain. *Rigidity of os uteri.*

**IGNATIA.** Hysterical, fitful women, and who are *full of grief.* *Weak, empty feeling in stomach, not relieved by eating. Uterine cramps, with cutting stitches. Convulsive jerking in single parts or limbs. *Patient seems full of grief, with frequent sighing.

**NUX VOMICA.** Pains irregular, and labor does not seem to advance. Drawing in back and thighs with pressure downwards, [Cham.] *Every pain produces a desire to go to stool or to urinate. Habitual constipation, with frequent urging to stool. Irritable.

**OPIUM.** Persons of full habit, and when pains suddenly cease. Determination of blood to head, with bloated, red face, [Bell.] *Drowsiness, and delirious talking. Bed feels so *hot* she cannot lie upon it, [so *hard*, Arn.]

**PULSATILLA.** The pains seem too weak and too far apart, they grow weaker, as if from inactivity of womb. *Pains which excite palpitation of the heart, or suffocating, fainting spells. *Patient craves cool, fresh air; worse in a warm room, [Sec.] Mild, tearful women, with blue eyes and light hair.

**SECALE COR.** *The pain is much prolonged, as if pressing and forcing the uterus. *Constant sensation of bearing down in abdomen; or the pains are too weak or suppressed, [if from *fright*, Opi.] *Thin, scrawny women, subject to passive hemmorhages. *Desire to be uncovered; worse in warm room.*

**ANÆSTHETICS.** *Chloroform* and *Ether* are used by many in protracted cases where there is much suffering and exhaustion. Also where instruments are used, and other cases requiring manual operations. Should be used with *great caution* and only when *absolutely* necessary. We prefer *Ether* on account of it being less dangerous.

**Administration.** Patient in recumbent posture, receives the *Chloroform* from a napkin formed into a cone. Proceed cautiously at first; allow *plenty of air* if *Chloroform* is used. Watch pulse and respiration, if either falter *remove* the napkin. Repeat the dose from time to time as circumstances may require, but do not produce *complete insensibility.* For further details in regard to administration of *Chloroform*, see page 24.

**THE INFANT.** If in a state of *asphyxia*, direct the mother to take *long, deep* inspirations; this failing, wrap infant in warm flannel and dash cold water on face and chest, or close nostrils with thumb and finger, blow in mouth to inflate lungs, then press on chest to expel the air. Have recourse to *artificial respiration*.

Soon as breathing is established, and pulsations in cord *have ceased*, tie and cut the cord.

**WASHING THE INFANT.** Take hog's lard or sweet oil, rub it thoroughly over the entire body, especially in armpits and groins, then with a piece of dry flannel wipe thoroughly clean and dry. After this bathe child daily in tepid water, gradually lowering the temperature from time to time, so that in a few weeks the water may be used cold.

**DELIVERING PLACENTA.** The placenta is usually expelled in 15 or 20 minutes after the fœtus. Should it remain an hour or more, no harm can come of it. Never make *traction* on the cord, unless the placenta is *extruded* from the womb. Make the *womb expel it*. Grasp the fundus of uterus with left hand and press gently downwards and backwards, when in most cases the placenta and membranes will pass out.

**Retention of Placenta.** If retention is due to *uterine inertia*, spasmodic contractions of neck of uterus, or hour-glass contraction, give one of following indicated remedies: **Bell. *Caul. Puls. *Secale.** If it be *adherent*, pass hand into uterus, detach carefully and scoop out all fragments.

In case of *twins* do not attempt removal of placenta of first child until after the birth of second.

**PLACENTA PRÆVIA.** On first appearance of hemorrhage from this complication, place patient on hard mattress with head low, and enjoin perfect quietude. Give the *indicated* remedy. If hemorrhage is profuse, *tampon* at once. Tie two or three handkerchiefs together at corners, insert one end and stuff them in until vagina is full, leaving one end protrude, and remove in 12 hours. When *hemorrhage* can no longer be controlled by these means, proceed to empty uterus.

If *os dilated*, pains vigorous and placenta *central*, pass a female catheter through placenta and membranes during a pain, draw off the water *slowly;* then let finger take the place of catheter and tear the orifice sufficiently large to admit the head, when bleeding will cease. If there is a malpresentation, pass hand through placenta and manage as in other cases.

If *os undilatable*, forcible distension with a dilator will be necessary before the uterus can be emptied.

When placenta is only *partially* over os, it may be pushed aside and the head allowed to descend; but if one-half the os be covered, turn and deliver.

**PROLAPSUS OF CORD.** If pulsations have ceased, no interference necessary. If child be yet alive, take a moist sponge large as hen's egg, make a hole in the centre that will admit the cord, now cut through one edge and place sponge round the cord and sew edges together. This leaves the cord in centre of sponge. Now, oil the surface and push it through the os and well above the superior strait. If labor has advanced so far as to prevent the return of cord, deliver with forceps or blunt hook.

**POST-PARTUM HEMORRHAGE.** Flooding after delivery usually results from a lack of uterine contraction, or may arise from rupture of cervix.

**TREATMENT.** At first alarm of hemorrhage, lower head and elevate the hips. Give one of remedies indicated below and repeat it often. At same time *grasp uterus* with hand, and make firm compression; follow this with copious injections of *hot water*, [110° to 115° F.] into the cavity of uterus. A lump of ice folded in a cloth and laid over the uterus, or a piece of ice passed into the uterus, has been found very efficient.

In urgent cases, apply a ligature about upper part of *left* arm, then one about upper part of *right* thigh; if this does not suffice, bandage *right* arm and *left* thigh in like manner. Soon as bleeding stops, loosen bandages *gradually*.

**REMEDIES.** *Leading indications.*

**IPECAC.** *Constant flow of bright red blood, with cutting about the navel, with nausea. *Patient gasps for breath.* After parturition or miscarriage.

**SECALE.** *Passive hemorrhage, in weak, scrawny subjects. *Want of action in uterus, [Puls.] *Desire to be uncovered.*

**CHINA.** Dangerous cases; discharge of dark clots. *Heaviness of head, ringing in ears, loss of sight, fainting. Wants to be fanned, but not too rapidly.

**SABINA.** Plethoric subjects, [Bell.] *Discharge of bright-red, partly clotted blood, worse from least motion. *Drawing pain from back to pubes* precedes the flow.

**BELLADONNA.** Retained placenta, with profuse flow of hot bright-red blood, speedily coagulating. *Violent bearing down towards the genitals. Plethoric subjects.

**TRILLIUM.** Gushing of bright-red blood from uterus at least motion, [Sabi.] *Pain in back, and cold legs.*

**LOCHIA.** During first day, discharge is bloody and sufficient to soil ten or twelve napkins. After first day or two, it changes in appearance and resembles the menses. About the tenth day red color leaves, and yellowish discharge follows for a few days, which in turn is succeeded by whitish mucus. When patient gets to moving about on her feet, a renewal of discharge is apt to occur for a few days, when it takes final leave.

Deviations from the normal condition call for the following remedies.

**ACONITE**. Discharge continues too long, or is too profuse and red-colored. *Young persons of full habit.* *Fear and anxiety of mind.

**BRYONIA.** *Suppression of discharge, with pain in the head, as if it would split. *Fullness* and heaviness of head; pressure in forehead and temples. *Symptoms all worse by motion.

**CALCARIA CARB.** *Lochia lasts too long, especially in women who menstruate too often and too profusely, [**Bell.**] Persons of a *pallid, flabby state of body.*

**PULSATILLA.** Sudden suppression from any accidental cause, with feverish excitement, but *no thirst.* *Sudden disappearance of the milk. *Mild, tearful persons.* *Worse towards evening.

**RHUS TOX.** Discharge lasts too long and is *black, watery and offensive.* *Sharp pains shoot through the head, which feels too large.

**SECALE COR.** Thin offensive discharge, either painless or accompanied by prolonged bearing-down pains. *Thin, scrawny women.

**LOCAL MEASURES.** In *suppression* of lochia, injections of *warm water* [95° to 100° F.] into the vagina, will often recall the discharge and relieve the difficulty.

---

## PERICARDITIS, ETC.

As Pericarditis, Endocarditis, Myocarditis, and Hypertrophy of the heart involve the same structures, and depend upon the same pathological conditions, we include their treatment under the same general head in order to avoid repetition.

**THERAPEUTICS.** *Leading indications.*

**ACONITE.** *Violent agitation and beating of the heart,* agonized tossing about, violent thirst, red face, and shortness of breath, [**Bell.**] *Great fear and anxiety of mind, *thinks he will die,* [**Ars.**] *Lancinating pain in the chest, hindering respiration. Has to sit straight up, can hardly breathe. After fright, [**Opi.**]

**ARNICA.** *Hypertrophy of heart from over-exertion,* [**Rhus.**] Lancinating pain in region of heart, causing faintness. *Sore feeling all through patient as if from a bruise, [**Bapt.**] *The bed on which he lies feels too hard, causing him to change from place to place.

**ARSENICUM.** *Pericarditis* after suppression of measles, scarlet fever, or drying up of old sores, [**Sulph.**] *Violent palpitation of heart,* particularly at night, and when lying down, [**Aur. *Dig.**] *Great anguish, extreme restlessness, and *fear of death.* Dyspnœa, cannot lie down for fear of suffocation. *Rapid prostration.* *Extreme thirst, drinks little and often.

**ASPARAGUS.** Chronic organic affections of heart. Throbbing of heart, perceptible to the hand and ear, setting in after slight motion, [**Spig.**] *Irregular, quick, double beats of heart, with anxiety.

**AURUM.** Disease consequent upon previously existing rheumatic affections, [**Bry. Spig.**] Distressing, anxious pains, preventing patient from lying down. *Has to sit perfectly quiet, upright. Irregular intermittent pulse, [***Dig. Kali c. Lach.**] *Great melancholy, and loathing of life.

**BELLADONNA.** *Violent palpitation of heart, reverberating in head,* [palpitation, with faintness and dyspnœa, **Verat. v.**—with tingling in fingers, **Acon.**] **Tremor of heart,* with anguish and aching pain, [**Rhus.**] *Throbbing of carotids.*

**BRYONIA.** Where disease is complicated with rheumatism or disorders of pulmonary structure. *Stitching pains in region of heart, aggravated by breathing or motion. *Wants to lie perfectly quiet.* Intermittent pulse, [see **Aur.**] *Hard, dry stools, as if burnt. Exceedingly irritable and snappish.

**CACTUS.** Acute pains in region of heart, with dyspnœa. *Pericarditis and endocarditis,* [**Acon. Bry. Dig.**] *Feeling of constriction at heart, as if an *iron band* prevented its normal action, [as if grasped with an *iron hand,* **Arn.**] Palpitation worse when walking, and at night when lying on left side. Attacks of suffocation, with fainting.

**CANNABIS SAT.** Tensive aching behind sternum. Frequent beatings in both sides of chest, most painful in region of heart. *Sensation as if drops were falling from heart. Violent shocks in region of heart, [**Con. *Nux v.**] as if it would fall out, when stooping or during exertion. Sensation of fullness about heart.

**DIGITALIS.** If caused by protracted grief, care, or anxiety. *Sharp stitches or contractive pains in region of heart, [**Arn. Rhus. Spig.**] *Sensation as if heart would stop beating if one moved. *Palpitation excited by talking, motion, or on lying down. Short, hurried breathing. *Œdema* of feet and legs, [**Ars.**] Bloated, pale face.

**IODIUM.** Scrofulous subjects. *Sensation as if heart were squeezed together.* *Violent palpitation, worse from least exertion. Better when lying perfectly still on back, [worse, **Rhus.**] *Extreme weakness and loss of breath on going up stairs. Fainting spells.

**KALI CARB.** Stitches in region of heart, with frequent and violent palpitation. Crampy pain about heart, as if encircled with bands, [see **Cact.**] *A blowing noise, and a louder second tick of pulmonary artery is heard. *Swelling over upper eyelids, like little bags.

**KALMIA LAT.** **Hypertrophy* and valvular insufficiency, or thickening after rheumatism. Severe pain in cardiac region, with slow pulse. *Palpitation up into throat after going* *to bed.* Trembling all over, worse lying on left side, better on back. *Slow, small pulse. *Neuralgia of heart.*

**LACHESIS.** Constrictive sensation about heart. Palpitation, with much anxiety. Irregular beats of heart, [quick, double beats, **Aspar.**] Sudden oppression of chest, accompanied by cough and palpitation. *Numbness of left arm.* *Cannot lie down, must sit up, bent forwards. *Can bear nothing to touch the throat. Worse after sleep.

**PHOSPHORUS.** *Tightness across chest,* with dyspnœa and great weakness, [***Puls.**] Palpitation, worse after eating, or from mental emotion. Congestion of lungs, tight cough, and spitting of blood. *Hard, *narrow,* difficult stools, or painless diarrhœa.

**PULSATILLA.** Persons of a mild, tearful disposition. Heaviness, pressure, and burning in region of heart. Pain in small of back, and palpitation of heart. *Loose, rattling cough, worse on first lying down at night. Rheumatic pains, which quickly change locality. Nightly diarrhœa. *Scanty or suppressed menses. All worse *towards evening.*

**RHUS TOX.** Sensation of weakness and trembling of heart. *Hypertrophy from violent exercise,* [**Arn.**] Violent palpitation on sitting still, [**Asp. Phos. Spig.**] *Stitches in heart, with painful lameness and numbness of left arm. *Pains worse during rest, has to change position often.

**SPIGELIA.** Organic disease of heart. Rubbing, bellows sound, [**Spong.**] *Palpitation so violent it can be seen and heard at a distance, [**Dig. Verat. a.**] *Can lie only on right side, with trunk well raised. The least motion produces suffocation, anxiety, and palpitation, [see **Iod.**] *Stitching pains in chest from slightest motion. Rheumatic pericarditis.

**SULPHUR.** After suppressed eruptions or piles. Palpitation of heart, especially when going up-stairs. Sensation as if heart was enlarged. Steady pain in left side through to shoulders. *Frequent weak, faint spells. *Constant heat on top of head, [coldness, **Verat.**] *Early morning diarrhœa. Dry, husky, scaly skin.

**TABACUM.** Violent palpitation when lying on left side, [**Baryt. *Cact. g. Nat. m.**] Irregular, generally slow beating of heart. Violent pulsation of heart and carotids. *Muscular relaxation.*

**VERAT. ALB.** Paroxysms of anguish about heart, which beats very strongly. Violent, visible, anxious palpitation. Stitches in sides of chest, worse when coughing, [**Acon. Bry.**] *Cold sweat on forehead. *Exhausting diarrhœa, with great weakness after every stool. Anguish and fear of death.

**CLINICAL MEASURES.** During an acute attack, *absolute rest* in recumbent position. Avoid all mental and emotional excitement, and allow an abundance of *fresh air.* Hot fomentations or warm poultices over region of heart very useful. The diet should be of the simplest kind, and all stimulants discarded.

## PHLEGMASIA DOLENS.—MILK-LEG.

This is most common after parturition, but sometimes occurs in unmarried women and sometimes in males. In the case of lying-in women it usually occurs about a week or ten days after delivery, but may show itself immediately thereafter.

**THERAPEUTICS.** *Leading remedies.*

**ACONITE.** Inflammatory stage. Fever, high temperature, restlessness and thirst. *Fear, anxiety of mind and great nervous excitability.

**ARNICA.** In early stage, after severe and protracted labor, or where *mechanical* means have been employed in delivery. *Sore, bruised feeling all through the body.

**ARSENICUM.** Pale œdematous swelling, with *burning pains* in the parts. Feels cold and chilly, wants to be covered up. *Anxious restlessness and exhaustion.

**BELLADONNA.** Limb very sore, swollen and hot; cannot bear *least jar*, or to be touched. Tearing cutting pains that come suddenly and cease as suddenly. *Back aches as if broken. *Confused, anxious, thinks she will die, [predicts the day, **Acon.**]

**BRYONIA.** Pale-red swelling of leg; pains drawing, lancinating. *Wants to remain perfectly quiet, worse from least motion. *Lochia suppressed, with sensation as if the head would burst, [**Bell.**] Milk suppressed, [see **Cal. c.**]

**CALCARIA CARB.** *Scrofulous subjects*, and in chronic cases, [**Sili. Sulph.**] Whitish swelling of foot and leg, with sensation of coldness. Suppression of milk, with sensation of coldness all through the body.

**HAMAMELIS.** *Milk-leg with swelling of labia, groin and thigh. Painful but *benumbed* sensation in the limb. Swelling commencing at the ankle, with great difficulty in moving the leg. *Veins dilated and very sensitive.

**PULSATILLA.** Leg hot, swollen, with tensive burning pains. Varices on legs, [**Ham.**] Lochia scanty, milk suppressed, [see **Bry.**] *Mild, tearful disposition.

**RHUS TOX.** Loss of power in the limb, cannot draw it up. *Red streaks* run up the veins of the leg. *Short relief from changing position. Wants to be covered up warmly, [**Ars.**] *Rheumatic subjects.*

**LOCAL MEASURES.** Elevate the limb and apply *warm fomentations.* Thick flannel cloths wrung out of a solution of the *indicated* remedy and applied to the parts, then covered with oiled silk, will give good results. Where suppuration is inevitable, poultices made of linseed meal will be found beneficial.

**DIETETICS.** During inflammatory stage diet should be very simple. Later, milk, broths, soft-boiled eggs, fruits, vegetables, etc. Strict attention to cleanliness, and ventilation important.

## PHTHISIS PULMONALIS.

(*Pulmonary Consumption.*)

**HYGIENIC MEASURES.** A person predisposed to phthisis should adopt the most rigid hygienic measures. He should live with great regularity; take *out-doors* exercise in all weather except the very worst; wear flannel next the skin; bathe regularly three or four times a week; make daily use of flesh-brush; sleep in *well ventilated* apartments; take frequent and *full inspirations* to expand the lungs in every part; adopt a regular and systematic course of gymnastics, and cultivate a cheerful, happy disposition.

**CLIMATIC.** Only in the first stage of the disease, as a general rule, can the patient be benefitted by a change of climate. A choice of home for the consumptive is often difficult to make. While some advise a life in the mountains, others send their patients to the lowlands of the south. Our own observations favor an elevated mountainous region, with a *dry cool* atmosphere, plenty of *light* and *sunshine*, and an equitable temperature. Here the patient should eat, sleep and *work* out-doors.

**MEDICAL TREATMENT.**

**ACONITE.** Bright redness of cheeks, particularly of young girls of *full habit*, [Bell. Cal. c.] Short, dry cough, with tickling in larynx. *Hectic fever, with restlessness and anxious expression of face. *Hæmoptisis; pleuritic stitches.*

**BELLADONNA.** *Spasmodic cough, worse at night and after exertion. Congestion to head, with alternate redness and paleness of face. Loss of voice; larynx painful to pressure. *Young girls at age of puberty.*

**BRYONIA.** *Cough at night in bed, compelling one to sit up. Stitches in chest when coughing or breathing deep, [Acon. Bell.] *Dry, hard stools. *Irritable mood.*

**CALCARIA CARB.** *Threatened phthisis, especially in young girls with too frequent and profuse menstruation, [Bell.] *Scrofulous diathesis. Perspires easily and is fatigued from any little exertion. *Losing flesh, yet has a good appetite. Very *sensitive to cold air;* takes cold easily. *Cold, damp feet.

**CALCARIA PHOS.** *Tubercular cough, with soreness and dryness in throat. With the cough, stitches in chest. *Delicate skin with flushed cheeks. Menses *too early*, blood bright-red. Poor digestion.

**CHINA.** Cough worse lying with head low, or on left side. *Loud, coarse rales, great debility, anæmia. Hæmoptisis, with subsequent suppuration of lungs. Œdema of legs, [Iod. Lyc. Kali c.] *Offensive*, chocolate-colored diarrhœa. *Night sweats.*

**FERRUM.** *Anæmic* condition, [Chin.] *Hæmoptisis, with

pain between scapula. Cough dry at night, but with copious expectoration in morning. *The least pain or emotion produces a *flushed* face. Painless, undigested stools, [**Chin. Phos.**] Long-lasting *night sweats.*

**IODINE.** *Scrofulous persons, with swollen glands, general emaciation. Cough from constant tickling in windpipe and under the sternum. Long-lasting hoarseness. *Emaciation with good appetite, [**Cal. c.**] *Morning sweat,* [**Chin.**] Swelling of feet.

**LYCOPODIUM.** After violent or neglected pneumonia. *Hectic fever, with cough and purulent sputa, Fan-like motion of alæ nasi, [**Phos.**] *Night sweats;* gastric irritation.

**PHOSPHORUS.** In threatened and well *advanced* cases. *Dry, tickling cough in evening, with tightness across the chest, [**Puls. Sulph.**] Cough worse from talking, reading, laughing, singing. Pain, soreness, or oppression in chest. Burning between shoulders, [**Bry.**] *Hoarseness with complete *loss of voice.* Night sweats during sleep. Painless diarrhœa, [see **Fer.**] Tall, slender persons with fair skin.

**KALI CARB.** Incipient and advanced cases, [see **Phos.**] Dyspeptic symptoms preceding the development of tuberculosis. Cough, with sputum of pus and blood. Lower part of *right* lung most affected. *Stitches all through the chest and over the body.

**SANGUINARIA.** Cough loose, but expectoration difficult. Sputum *tough,* rust-colored, *offensive,* purulent. Burning in chest, also stitching pains. *Circumscribed redness of cheeks, burning worse P. M. *Hæmoptisis.* Cough worse when lying down.

**STANNUM.** *Cough with copious yellow, green pus, sweetish, putrid, sour or saltish. Cough excited by talking, singing, laughing, or lying on right side, [**Phos.**] Profuse night sweats, [**Chin. Fer. Iod**] *Hectic fever.*

**SULPHUR.** Cough with rattling of mucus in chest, expectoration of greenish lumps of sweetish taste. *Complains constantly of being too hot. *Burning of feet* at night, cannot bear them covered. *Early morning *diarrhœa,* [**Stan.**] *Lean persons who walk stooping.

**AUXILIARY MEASURES.** The troublesome cough may often be palliated by taking a little *rock-candy* in the mouth; sipping gum-arabic water, in which a few drops of lemon juice have been dissolved; or taking teaspoonful doses of *glycerine* and water [drachm to the ounce], as occasion may require.

Inhaling the fumes of *Tar, Benzoine, Resin,* or a few drops *Ether Sulph.,* will often have a good effect. Drinking a cup full of *hot water* will sometimes promptly relieve the cough and oppression.

In the last stage, as a *dernier resort, Morphine* may be given to relieve the terrible oppression and soothe the patient. It may be administered subcutaneously or by the mouth in very *small* doses. Gelatine-coated pills, composed of $\frac{1}{6}$ of a grain *Morphia*, and $\frac{1}{60}$ of a grain *Atropia* are prepared, and furnish a convenient method of administration.

**Night Sweats.** A *hot bath*, 95 to 100° [according to the degree of fever and strength of patient] taken at bedtime will be found very beneficial. Patient should remain in bath from ten to fifteen minutes, then be wrapped in a *clean sheet*, put in bed and allowed to dry *without being rubbed.*

*Sulphate* of *Atropine* or *Picrotoxin* given in doses of $\frac{1}{60}$ of a grain at bed-time, will in most cases check the night-sweats. Taking a glass of milk, or some nourishing food in the night, will often have a good effect.

**DIETETICS.** The consumptive should have the most *nourishing* kind of food, and all he can digest and assimilate. Good fresh *milk, cream*, and *buttermilk* are among the best articles of diet. Rare roast beef, mutton chops, venison, and chicken should enter largely into the bill of fare. Eggs slightly cooked or raw are very nutritious. *Fats* are not only essential as fuel food, but they share largely in the tissue-making process, and should be supplied in the form of cream, butter, fat of meats, etc. Pork, veal, and all *salt* meats should be avoided. Fresh vegetables, as potatoes, carrots, beans, peas, and tomatoes may be eaten liberally. Fresh ripe fruits are not only wholesome, but palatable, refreshing and nutritive. All *alcoholic stimulants* should be discarded.

---

## PLEURITIS.—PLEURISY.

**THERAPEUTICS.** *Leading indications.*

**ACONITE.** Chill and *synochal fever ; full, bounding pulse*, dry, hot skin, agonized tossing about, violent thirst, red face, shortness of breath, and great nervous excitability. *Piercing and stitching pains in chest, hindering respiration, with dry cough. Worse lying on *left* side, [**Phos.**—better on *painful* side, **Bry. Puls.**] General suspension of secretory functions.

**ARNICA.** After mechanical injuries. Sensation as if ribs were bruised. Stitching pains in left chest, with a short, dry cough. *Sore feeling through whole system, as if from a bruise. *Constantly changing about on account of bed feeling so hard.

**BRYONIA.** Cheeks flushed and hot. Position upon affected side, with oppressed breathing. *Stitching pain in affected part, aggravated by inspiration or least motion, [**Acon.**] *Splitting headache. *Cannot sit up on account of nausea and faintness. Thirst for large quantities of water at long intervals. *Hard, dry stools, as if burnt. Exceedingly irritable.

**KALI CARB.** *Darting, stitching, or cutting pains,

especially in right side, [*left* side, **Arn. Phos. Squil.**] Violent palpitation of heart. Dry cough, worse about 3 A. M.

**MERCURIUS.** Soreness and burning in chest. Stitching pain in right chest, through from shoulder-blade, [see **Kali c.**] Cough aggravated at night and when lying on *left* side. Moist tongue, with great thirst. *Much perspiration, which does not relieve. *Symptoms all worse at night.

**PHOSPHORUS.** Short, difficult respiration. Piercing pains, mostly on left side. Sharp pains when pressing upon intercostal space. *Tightness* across chest, with a dry, shaking cough. *Sensation of weakness and emptiness in abdomen. Sharp, cutting pains in bowels, sometimes with vomiting. *Long, narrow, hard stools.

**RHUS TOX.** If the disease has arisen from metastasis of rheumatism, or from exposure to wet, straining, or lifting. Also, where febrile symptoms have subsided, and there yet remain wandering pains in chest, shortness of breath, and general debility. *The pains are worse during rest, [better, **Acon. *Bry.**]

**SQUILLA.** Dyspnœa, with stitching pains in left side when breathing or coughing. Short, rattling cough, disturbing sleep. Inability to lie on left side, [**Acon.**] Twitching of lips, which are covered with thick, yellow crusts, more on the left side.

**SULPHUR.** Where the disease is complicated with pneumonia, or does not yield to well-chosen remedies. Short, dry cough, with stitches in chest, extending through to left shoulder-blade, worse from motion. *Frequent weak, faint spells, and flashes of heat. *Constant heat on vertex.

**TARTAR EM.** Respiration short and difficult. Burning, dry, hot skin, or cold, and covered with perspiration. *Sensation as if the inside of chest were lined with velvet. *Loose cough, as if much phlegm would be expectorated, but nothing comes up. Vertigo, with drowsiness. Threatened paralysis of lungs.

**CLINICAL MEASURES.** Patient should assume the horizontal position and keep still as possible. *Hot fomentations* or poultices to the painful part of great benefit. A gum bag partly filled with *hot water*, or bags of *hot salt*, also very useful. Sponging body with *tepid water*, and drying the skin *without rubbing*, highly important.

**DIETETICS.** During febrile stage, give liberally of cold water to appease thirst. Rice-water, milk, beef-tea, broths, light puddings, etc., soon as depression sets in.

---

## PNEUMONIA.

**THERAPEUTICS.** *Leading indications.*

**ACONITE.** *First stage*, [**Tart. e. Verat. a.**] *High temperature, full, bounding pulse, violent thirst and shortness of breath. *Piercing and stitching pains* in chest, with difficult breathing. *Great fear and anxiety of mind, with nervousness. Worse lying on *left* side, [**Phos.**—better on *painful* side, **Bry. Puls.**] *Fear of death; predicts the day he will die.

**ARSENICUM.** Great anxiety and restlessness, with much tossing about. *Rapid prostration of strength, with clammy perspiration on skin. *Urgent thirst, drinking little and often. Burning pain and heat in chest, [**Sang.**] Coldness of extremities. *Great fear of death.* Worse at night, particularly after midnight. In advanced stages, [**Carb. v. Sang.**]

**BELLADONNA.** *Congestion of brain, with flushed face and throbbing carotids, [**Acon. Gel.**] Violent delirium, with a wild look and desire to escape, strike, bite or quarrel. *Dyspnœa,* with pain in lower and middle portion of chest. Expectoration bloody, scant and difficult. [**Merc. Nitrum. Rhus.**] Dry, cracked tongue and lips, with great thirst. *Starting and jumping during sleep, with moaning. *Sleepiness, but cannot sleep.

**BRYONIA.** Fever moderate. *Cough, with expectoration of tenacious mucus of a *reddish or rusty color,* [***Phos. Sang.**] Great dyspnœa and acute *stitching pains* in side of chest, [**Acon. Bell.**] *The pain is aggravated by *breathing* or least *motion;* better lying on *painful side,* [see **Phos.**] *Wants to lie perfectly quiet. Cannot take a full breath, *lungs feel as if they would not expand.* *Constipation, stools dry and hard. Exceedingly irritable. Delirious talking, with desire to escape.

**CARBO VEG.** Advanced stages, when there is great prostration of vital forces, [***Ars.**] *Sensation of great weakness and fatigue in chest. Cough by spells, with brownish expectoration. Paleness of face and coldness of extremities. Pulse extremely weak. *Craves cold air, and wants to be fanned all the time.

**IPECAC.** *Pneumonia of infants, [**Kali c. Opi.**] Respiration rapid, difficult; surface blue, face pale. *Rattling of mucus in chest. *The chest seems full of phlegm, but does not yield to coughing, [**Tart. e.**] Much nausea and vomiting phlegm, [**Tart. e.**] Suitable to *fat children.*

**KALI CARB.** *Infantile pneumonia during whooping-cough. Great difficulty of breathing, preventing child from sleeping or drinking. *Wheezing, rattling breathing, with choking cough. *Swelling over upper eyelids in morning, like little bags,* [*under* eyes, **Apis.**]

**LYCOPOD.** *Typhoid or neglected pneumonia, [**Phos. Rhus. Sulph.**] Circumscribed redness of cheeks, [**Sang.**] Copious expectoration mixed with pus. *Fan-like motion of nostrils, [**Phos.**] Great fear of being left alone, [**Ars.**] *Red, sand-like sediment in urine.

**MERCURIUS.** *Bilious pneumonia,* [**Tart. e.**] Oppressed

Ether pneu.—give ether 3x

breathing, with stitches in right chest through from scapulæ Cough at first dry, afterwards attended with bloody expectoration. *Great tenderness over region of stomach and liver. *Profuse sweat, affording no relief.

**NITRUM.** Great dyspnœa, must lie with head high. Cough, with cutting, stitching pains in chest, and bloody sputa. Stitches in chest when taking a full breath, [**Bry.**] *Feeling of great heaviness in chest, as if a load were pressing thorax together.

**OPIUM.** *Pneumonia of infants*, where the inflammation is disguised by symptoms of cerebral congestion. *Deep, snoring breathing, with wide-open mouth. Expectoration frothy, containing blood and mucus. *Stupefying sleep.*

**PHOSPHORUS.** In *violent* cases. Stitching pains excited or aggravated by coughing, breathing, or lying on *left side*, [see **Acon.**] *Tightness across chest, dry cough and *rust-colored* sputa, [**Bry.**] *A large portion of lung is involved, and there is great dyspnœa. *Hepatization of right lung.* *Sensation of weakness and emptiness in abdomen. *Long, narrow*, hard stools. Tall, slender persons, with a weak conformation of chest. *Very sleepy.*

**RHUS TOX.** The disease threatens to assume a *typhoid character*. Patient lies in a state of half stupefaction, at times delirious, [**Phos.**] *Terrible cough, as if it would tear something out of chest. Expectoration, color of brick-dust or bloody. *The pains are aggravated by rest, hence patient continually moves about to get relief. Very restless at night, particularly in latter part.

**SANGUINARIA.** Advanced stages, [**Ars. Carb. v.**] Great difficulty of breathing. Position upon back with head well elevated. Stitching, burning pains in chest. *Cough, with tough, rust-colored sputa. Circumscribed redness of cheeks, particularly in afternoon.

**SULPHUR.** Protracted cases, occurring in psoric or scrofulous subjects. The disease threatens to terminate in phthisis. *Much rattling of phlegm in chest. *Frequent weak, faint spells, and flashes of heat. Cough on deep inspiration, with cutting pain in *left* chest, [**Phos.**] Feels suffocated, wants doors and windows open. *Constant heat on vertex.

**TART. EM.** Short, difficult, and oppressed breathing. **Loose cough, as if much would be expectorated, but nothing comes up*, [**Ipe.**] Great dyspnœa and fits of suffocation, [**Sulph.**] *Impending paralysis of lungs, [**Opi. Phos.**] *The inside of chest feels as if lined with velvet. *Bilious pneumonia.* Nausea and straining to vomit.

**VERAT. VIR.** First stage, when congestion and inflammation have fairly set in. High fever, with strong, quick pulse, [**Acon.**] Nausea and vomiting a glairy mucus. *Sinking, faint feeling in pit of stomach. Constant burning distress in cardiac region. Regularly intermitting pulse.

**AUXILIARY MEASURES.** Treat patient in large, airy room. Keep temperature about 70° F. and atmosphere moist. *Hot fomentations* or linseed-meal poultices, applied over the painful part, will frequently relieve the pain. Do not talk to patient, and avoid excitement of every kind.

**DIETETICS.** During the inflammatory stage, only mucilaginous drinks, as gum-arabic or slippery-elm water, and acidulous drinks. As fever abates, give milk, beef-tea, broths and more nourishing diet.

---

## POISONING.

When poison has been taken into the stomach, the main object should be:

1st. To expel it quickly as possible by inducing the patient to vomit or by *pumping* the stomach.

2d. To neutralize its effects by appropriate antidotes.

**EMETICS.** To excite vomiting, administer copious draughts of tepid water, and tickle the fauces. Placing a little salt, snuff or mustard upon the tongue is very efficient. If these fail, give *emetics of pulverized mustard*, [a spoonful in water,] or *sulphate of zinc*, [20 grs. in *warm* water,] and repeat often, until full effect is produced.

The **Stomach-Pump** should be used where promptness is required. In the absence of a pump, pass a *long* rubber tube into the stomach, raise free end, insert a funnel, pour in water until stomach is full, then lower end of tube below the stomach and let contents run out. Repeat the operation until stomach is completely washed out.

**ACIDS.** For poisoning by acids, such as *Acetic, Citric, Muriatic, Nitric, Oxalic, Sulphuric, Tartaric*, etc., give: 1, warm soap-suds; 2, magnesia in water; 3, powdered chalk, mixed in warm water; 4, wood-ashes, soda, potash, gruel, linseed-tea, or rice-water. **Carbolic Acid** is neutralized by *Saccharate of Lime.*

**ACONITUM.** For poisoning by this and other *acro-narcotics*, such as *Arnica, Colchicum, Conium, Digitalis, Ergot, Gelsemium, Helleborus, Hyoscyamus, Veratrum*, etc., use *stomach-pump* or an emetic of mustard. Give strong *coffee* or dilute *vinegar*. Twenty drops *Tr. Belladonna* by mouth or rectum advised. Large injections of soap and water, or of salt and gruel to clear the bowels.

**ALCOHOL.** For poisoning by alcohol, excite vomiting quickly as possible. Give an emetic of *Sulphate of Zinc*, [20 grs.] or use stomach-pump. Milk, mucilaginous drinks. *Black Coffee*, or a few drops of **Ammonia** dissolved in a glass of sugar-water, may be taken in teaspoonful doses every 5 or 10 minutes. The after-effects usually call for **Coff. *Nux v. Opi.**

**ALKALIES.** Poisoning by different preparations of *Am-*

*monia*, *Potassa*, *Soda*, etc., should be treated *without* vomiting. Give: 1, dilute vinegar; 2, lemonade; 3, sour milk; 4, mucilaginous drinks; 5, sweet oil.

**ANTIMONY.** For poisoning by *Tartar Emetic*, *Butter of Antimony*, *Oxide of Antimony*, and other preparations of this metal: Induce vomiting, and give a strong decoction of gall-nuts, oak-bark, strong black tea, strong coffee, and mucilaginous drinks, white of eggs.

**ARSENIC.** Emetics seldom needed; if used, follow by large draughts hot water and salt to wash out stomach. Give *Peroxide of Iron*, a spoonful to an adult, repeated every 5 or 10 minutes; *should be fresh.* (To prepare, add to one ounce of Carbonate of Sodium 2 or 3 ounces Tincture Chloride of Iron.) If this is not at hand, give *iron-rust* stirred in sugar-water; flaxseed tea, flour and water, white of eggs and water, soap-suds or calcined magnesia in water. After alarming symptoms have passed, give **Ipecac.** Apply warm blankets, hot bottles to feet, and friction to extremities. If nausea and vomiting, with heat or chilliness over whole body, and great debility, give **Verat.**

**ATROPIA.** Same as *Belladonna.*

**BELLADONNA.** Stomach-pump, or emetic of mustard-water or *Sulphate Zinc*, [20 grs. in water]. The best antidotes are *strong, black coffee*, or **Opium**; of the latter 30 to 60 drops of the tincture may be given at a dose, and repeated every ten minutes until its influence is apparent. Flagellation with wet towel. Artificial respiration.

**BISMUTH.** For poisoning by *Nitrate* or *Oxide of Bismuth*, *Pearl Powder*, etc., give milk and sweetened mucilaginous drinks.

**CAMPHOR.** Give strong *Black Coffee* until vomiting sets in; after which give **Opi.** in minute doses.

**CANTHARIDES.** Give white of eggs and slimy substances, as gruel, linseed-tea, etc. Afterwards smell **Camph.** or take it internally.

**COPPER.** For poisoning by *Blue Vitriol*, *Verdigris*, *Scheel's Green*, and other preparations of this metal: Excite vomiting. Give white of eggs, sugar-water, milk and mucilaginous drinks.

**CHLORAL HYDRATE.** Strong coffee. Hot bath. Friction. Stimulants. Ammonia. Solution Nitrate of Strychnia [one part in fifty] two drops hypodermically. Hot coffee per rectum.

**CHLOROFORM.** If *inhaled*, see "**Anæsthetics.**" If *swallowed:* Emetics. Stomach-pump. Large draughts water containing carbonate soda. Keep patient *roused.* Employ flagellation.

**CORROSIVE SUBLIMATE.** For poisoning by this substance and other preparations, as *Cyanide* and *Nitrate of Mercury*, *White* or *Red Precipitate*, *Vermilion*, etc.: Excite vomiting *immediately*. Give *white of eggs*, beaten up in water, in large quantities. Next in importance is *sugar-water*, starch boiled in water, flour-paste, and milk in large quantities.

**CROTON OIL.** Stomach-pump. Emetics, [spoonful mustard, or 20 grs. *sulphate zinc.*] Barley-water, white of egg and water, gruel, arrow-root. One-third to one-half grain *morphia*, hypodermically, or 20 drops *laudanum* by mouth.

**DIGITALIS.** Stomach-pump. Emetics. Give 20 grs. tannic acid or gallic acid in *hot water* and repeat frequently. Strong hot tea or coffee. Six drops *Tr. aconite* by mouth or rectum; repeat in half an hour if heart's action is not improved. *Keep in recumbent position.*

**ERGOT.** Evacuate stomach. Active purgative. Tannic or gallic acid in half-drachm doses in water frequently. Inhalations *Nitrite Amyl.* Recumbent position.

**GASES.** If a person has become insensible from inhaling *Carbonic Acid, Carbonic Oxide, Fumes of Burning Charcoal, Chlorine*, or *Sulphuretted Hydrogen*, expose him at once to fresh air, bathe the face and breast with *vinegar*, and give him strong coffee. After he has somewhat recovered, dispense with the vinegar, and give **Opium.** If this does not suffice, give **Bell** or **Nux v.** Dr. Hall's method of inducing artificial respiration, as explained under **Drowning**, should be resorted to if necessary.

**HYDROPHOBIN.** For poisoning from the bite of *Rabid animals:* Excise bitten part at once, if practicable; then immerse in warm water and wash as long as it will bleed; after which cauterize the surface and cover the wound with a poultice. At the same time give a dose of **Bell.** once or twice daily. Try Pasteur's method of *inoculation.*

**IODINE.** For the effects of this poison: Excite vomiting by a weak solution of *Soda.* Give starch stirred in water, starch-paste, flour-paste, linseed-tea.

**LEAD.** For poisoning by *Sugar of Lead, White Lead, Litharge*, and other preparations, *excite vomiting.* Give: 1, Epsom Salts; 2, Glauber Salts; 3, white of eggs; 4, soap-suds; 5, milk.

**NITRATE OF SILVER.** For poisoning by *Lunar Caustic*, give: 1, Common salt dissolved in water, in large quantities; 2, mucilaginous drinks.

**OPIUM.** For poisoning by the different preparations of Opium, excite *vomiting* at once, or use *stomach-pump.* As *Opium* is an antidote to *Belladonna*, so is *Belladonna* an antidote to *Opium.* Give then Tr. *Belladonna*, ten to twenty drops, and repeat every twenty or thirty minutes until desired effect is produced. Strong *Coffee* is also a good antidote; until that can be had, give vinegar and water. Keep patient roused by beating him on back and dragging him about the room. Artificial respiration should be induced, as explained under **Drowning**, if necessary.

**PARIS-GREEN.** See *Arsenic.*

**PHOSPHORUS.** For poisoning by this material, excite

vomiting. Give: 1, Magnesia stirred in water; 2, mucilaginous drinks in large quantities. Chlorine water and magnesia, eight parts of former to one of latter, a spoonful taken every five or ten minutes.

**PRUSSIC ACID.** *Treatment.* Give spirits of Hartshorn to smell, and a weak solution internally. Pour cold water down spine from a height, give strong coffee to drink, and use the same as an injection.

**RHUS RADICANS.** (*Poison-ivy, poison-vine.*) For the external poisoning by this species of *Rhus:* Bathe the parts frequently with *hot water*, and use a little fine soap. Give **Sang. can.** internally. This remedy is regarded as almost specific by some physicians. Other remedies are **Bry. Bell.** ***Ledum.** For poisoning by **RHUS TOX.** (Poison Sumac), give **Cro. tig.**

**SERPENTS.** For bite of venomous serpents, apply a *cupping-glass* over wound, and allow it to bleed all it will. Prof. Bibron's remedy is said to be a *perfect antidote* for bite of *Rattlesnake.* ℞.—Potassi, 4 grs., Hydrar. chlor., 2 grs., Brominii, 4 drachms. Dose, ten drops in a spoonful of brandy or wine, and repeat if necessary. It should be prepared in *glass-stoppered vials.* Others advise large doses of brandy or whiskey as a sure antidote. Dr. E. T. Brown, Mich., advises **Tr. Iodium,** one to four drops every hour, as an effectual antidote for bite of *rattlesnake.*

**STRAMONIUM.** For poisoning by this substance, evacuate the stomach. Give: 1, coffee. 2, vinegar; 3, lemonade in large quantities.

**STRYCHNINE.** For poisoning by strychnine, evacuate stomach as quickly as possible. Administer large doses of *Opium* per *oram* or *anum*, or inject it hypodermically at different points over the body. Other antidotes recommended, are: *Iodine* (30 drops in water), *Camphor*, (5 grains dissolved in mucilage). These, it is said, stop the tetanic spasms, and give time for action of the stomach-pump or emetic.

**TOBACCO.** Emetic of mustard (tablespoonful in water), *Sulphate of Zinc* (20 grains in water), or *Ipecac.* (20 grains in water). Tannic acid, half a drachm in water, repeated frequently. *Cider vinegar* well diluted; give liberally.

---

## PREGNANCY, DISORDERS OF.

Although the state of pregnancy is in accordance with the Divine order of things, it is often attended with many deviations from health which call for special treatment. But before considering these, we wish to call attention to

**DIET IN PREGNANCY.** This is a subject occupying a good deal of attention at the present time. Careful observation has shown that articles of food which contribute largely to the growth of bone and muscle, increase unduly the size of the child in utero, and, to a great extent, the perils and sufferings of the parturient female. Therefore, all articles of food rich in earthy matter, such as beef, pork, mutton, wheat, beans, barley, oatmeal, etc., should be very *sparingly* eaten, and a diet consisting *largely of fruits* and certain vegetables adopted, especially in the latter months of pregnancy.

**MORN.NG SICKNESS,** Treatment of.

**ALETRIS FAR.** Persistent vomiting and obstinate indigestion, with much debility. The least food causes distress in stomach. Nausea and disgust for food. Frequent attacks of fainting, with vertigo. Sleepy all the time.

**ANTIMONIUM.** Eructations tasting of ingesta. Nausea, with vertigo. *Frightful and persistent vomiting, with convulsions. After overloading stomach.

**ARSENICUM.** Excessive vomiting, especially after eating or drinking. *Great desire for water, but can take only a little. *Vomiting fluids as soon as taken. Excessive weakness. *Better from hot drinks.*

**ARS. OF COP.** *Vomiting a glairy froth.* Dull aching over epigastric region. Frequent desire for stool.

**BRYONIA.** Nausea immediately on waking in the morning. Lips dry and parched; dry mouth and tongue, with much thirst. Vomiting food immediately after eating it. *Everything tastes bitter, [Puls.] *She feels better by keeping perfectly quiet. *Dry, hard stools, as if burnt.

**CALC. CARB.** Heart-burn and eructations tasting of food. Soreness of sides or tip of tongue, she can scarcely talk or eat. *Going up stairs puts her out of breath, and causes vertigo. *Cold, damp feet continually. Cannot bear tight clothing around waist. *She cannot sleep after 3 A. M., [***Nux v. Sep.**]

**COCCULUS.** Cardialgia after a meal. In morning, she can scarcely rise up on account of nausea and inclination to vomit; it makes her so faint. *Nausea from riding in a carriage, boat, [see **Nit. ac.**]

**COLCHICUM.** *Loathing and disgust at the thought, sight, or smell of food. The *smell of meats, broth and eggs* is especially repugnant. All attempts to eat cause violent nausea and vomiting.

**CYCLAMEN.** After eating least quantity, disgust and nausea in palate and throat. Much dimness of vision, with fiery specks and sparks before eyes.

**INGLUVIN.** In some cases of *morning* sickness, *Ingluvin,* given in ten-grain doses night and morning, will have a beneficial effect.

**ELECTRICITY.** This agent is highly commended by some practitioners in the vomiting of pregnancy, and succeeds when all others fail. The positive pole is applied at the lower cervicle, and the negative to the epigastrium.

**IPECAC.** Nausea and vomiting, with great uneasiness in the stomach. *Continual nausea all the time, not a moment's relief, [**Tart. e. Verat. a.**] *Vomiting large quantities of mucus. Bilious vomiting, and tendency to relaxation of the bowels.

**LOBELIA.** *Nausea and vomiting, with profuse flow of water from mouth, [**Phos.**] *Feeling of great weakness in stomach.*

**NITRIC AC.** *Much nausea and gastric trouble, relieved by moving about or riding in a carriage, [worse from, **Coco.**] Constant nausea, with heat in stomach extending to throat. *Strong-smelling urine.*

**NUX VOM.** Nausea and vomiting chiefly in morning, while eating, or immediately after eating or drinking. Acrid and bitter eructations and regurgitations. *She feels as if she would be better if she could vomit. *Cannot bear the odor of tobacco. Females of sedentary habits, and who use highly-seasoned food. *Large, difficult stools, with frequent urging.

**PETROLEUM.** Aversion to meat and fat as well as all warm, cooked food. *Nausea and vomiting bitter, green substances; worse from riding in carriage, [**Coco.**] Great weakness of digestion. Diarrhœa only during day.

**PULSATILLA.** Frequent eructations, tasting of ingesta. Vomiting after every meal. *Vomiting mucus. *Bad taste in mouth every morning on waking. No kind of food tastes good. Perceptible pulsations in stomach, [**Sep. Tart. e.**] Diarrhœa, mostly at night. *Mild, tearful disposition.*

**SEPIA.** Nausea in morning as if all the viscera were turning inside out. *Sensation of emptiness in stomach. The thought of food sickens her. *Yellowness of face, particularly across the nose. Painful feeling of hunger.

**TART. EM.** Continuous anxious nausea, [***Ipe. Verat.**] *Vomiting large quantities of mucus. [**Ipe.**]

**VERAT. ALB.** Constant nausea and ptyalism. Excessive vomiting of bile, mucus, and lastly blood. *Cold sweat on forehead. Craves *cold* drinks.

**ZINCUM.** Sweet risings into throat, with sweet taste in mouth, or taste of blood. *Retching, and vomiting bitter mucus. *Soon as first spoonful of food reaches stomach, up it comes. *Fidgety feeling in feet or legs.*

**Nutrient Injections.**

In *severe* cases of vomiting, where the patient is much reduced, starving in fact, *nutrient* injections will often bridge over the danger. Milk, beef-tea, broths, etc., are used for this purpose. Inject about *two ounces* at a time at intervals of two hours. One pint of good broth or milk each day employed in this way, will keep patient alive many weeks. Peptonized foods are valuable for this purpose. SEE PAGE 17.

**Gastric Troubles.**

**NUX VOMICA.** *Heart-burn*, water-brash, worse before

breakfast. Putrid taste in morning, must rinse the mouth, [Puls.] *Craves brandy, beer, fat food or chalk. *Constipation in persons of sedentary habits.

**PULSATILLA**. Aversion to *fat food, pork, meat, milk*, bread. Eructations tasting, smelling of food; bitter, bilious, rancid, sour. *Constant spitting of frothy, cotton-like mucus. *Putrid taste in morning, [**Nux.**] *Obstinate constipation.*

**IPECAC.** *Constant nausea, with copious saliva. Beating in stomach, [**Puls. Sep.**] Full of desires, but knows not for what. *Sweetish taste.*

**SEPIA.** *Yellow streak across the nose. Heart-burn extending from stomach to throat. *Vomiting milky fluid. *Soreness of abdomen. Involuntary weeping and laughter.*

**PHOSPHORUS.** *Regurgitation of food without nausea, [**Nux.**] Aversion to sweets or meat. *Goneness* in region of stomach. *Constipation, stools long, *slender*, tough.

**Pain in Back and Side.**

During pregnancy some women suffer greatly from pain in side and back. They usually occur from the fifth to the eighth month.

**BRYONIA**. Tensive pain in right side below false ribs, worse from deep inspiration. *Better when lying on painful side, or when keeping quiet.

**RHUS TOX**. Pains in small of back, better lying on something hard. *Pelvic articulations stiff when beginning to move. Worse in *stormy weather.*

**KALI CARB**. Back aches as if broken, she must lie down, [see **Bell.**] Stitching pains in region of liver.

**Pruritus Vulvæ.**

Not unfrequently pregnant women are exceedingly annoyed by a troublesome itching of the vulvæ.

**TREATMENT.** **Merc. viv. Lyco. Rhus t. Sep.** and **Sulph.** are the chief remedies in the complaint. Frequent ablutions with *hot water* very beneficial. A solution of *Borax* and water is also very useful in allaying the itching. These failing: Take *Hyposulphite of Soda*, ℥ss, *Camphor water* ℥viij. Mix, and use as a wash three or four times a day—has a salutary effect.

**Itching of the Skin.** During pregnancy some women are greatly annoyed with *itching* of the skin, not confined to any particular parts, but all over the body. This may be relieved promptly by the following lotion:

℞, Acid carbol., ʒij.; *Glycerina*, ℥j.; Aquæ rosæ, ℥viij. Mix and apply with a soft sponge, as occasion may require.

# PREGNANCY, DURATION OF.

Find the date in upper horizontal line when *last* menstruation ceased; the figure *beneath* will give the date of expected confinement—*ten lunar* months or 280 days.

| | | | | | | | | | | | | | | | | | | | | | | | | | | | | | | | | |
|---|---|---|---|---|---|---|---|---|---|---|---|---|---|---|---|---|---|---|---|---|---|---|---|---|---|---|---|---|---|---|---|---|
| Jan. | 1 | 2 | 3 | 4 | 5 | 6 | 7 | 8 | 9 | 10 | 11 | 12 | 13 | 14 | 15 | 16 | 17 | 18 | 19 | 20 | 21 | 22 | 23 | 24 | 25 | 26 | 27 | 28 | 29 | 30 | 31 | |
| *Oct.* | 8 | 9 | 10 | 11 | 12 | 13 | 14 | 15 | 16 | 17 | 18 | 19 | 20 | 21 | 22 | 23 | 24 | 25 | 26 | 27 | 28 | 29 | 30 | 31 | 1 | 2 | 3 | 4 | 5 | 6 | 7 | *Nov.* |
| Feb. | 1 | 2 | 3 | 4 | 5 | 6 | 7 | 8 | 9 | 10 | 11 | 12 | 13 | 14 | 15 | 16 | 17 | 18 | 19 | 20 | 21 | 22 | 23 | 24 | 25 | 26 | 27 | 28 | | | | |
| *Nov.* | 8 | 9 | 10 | 11 | 12 | 13 | 14 | 15 | 16 | 17 | 18 | 19 | 20 | 21 | 22 | 23 | 24 | 25 | 26 | 27 | 28 | 29 | 30 | 1 | 2 | 3 | 4 | 5 | | | | *Dec.* |
| March. | 1 | 2 | 3 | 4 | 5 | 6 | 7 | 8 | 9 | 10 | 11 | 12 | 13 | 14 | 15 | 16 | 17 | 18 | 19 | 20 | 21 | 22 | 23 | 24 | 25 | 26 | 27 | 28 | 29 | 30 | 31 | |
| *Dec.* | 6 | 7 | 8 | 9 | 10 | 11 | 12 | 13 | 14 | 15 | 16 | 17 | 18 | 19 | 20 | 21 | 22 | 23 | 24 | 25 | 26 | 27 | 28 | 29 | 30 | 31 | 1 | 2 | 3 | 4 | 5 | *Jan.* |
| April. | 1 | 2 | 3 | 4 | 5 | 6 | 7 | 8 | 9 | 10 | 11 | 12 | 13 | 14 | 15 | 16 | 17 | 18 | 19 | 20 | 21 | 22 | 23 | 24 | 25 | 26 | 27 | 28 | 29 | 30 | | |
| *Jan.* | 6 | 7 | 8 | 9 | 10 | 11 | 12 | 13 | 14 | 15 | 16 | 17 | 18 | 19 | 20 | 21 | 22 | 23 | 24 | 25 | 26 | 27 | 28 | 29 | 30 | 31 | 1 | 2 | 3 | 4 | | *Feb.* |
| May. | 1 | 2 | 3 | 4 | 5 | 6 | 7 | 8 | 9 | 10 | 11 | 12 | 13 | 14 | 15 | 16 | 17 | 18 | 19 | 20 | 21 | 22 | 23 | 24 | 25 | 26 | 27 | 28 | 29 | 30 | 31 | |
| *Feb.* | 5 | 6 | 7 | 8 | 9 | 10 | 11 | 12 | 13 | 14 | 15 | 16 | 17 | 18 | 19 | 20 | 21 | 22 | 23 | 24 | 25 | 26 | 27 | 28 | 1 | 2 | 3 | 4 | 5 | 6 | 7 | *March.* |
| June. | 1 | 2 | 3 | 4 | 5 | 6 | 7 | 8 | 9 | 10 | 11 | 12 | 13 | 14 | 15 | 16 | 17 | 18 | 19 | 20 | 21 | 22 | 23 | 24 | 25 | 26 | 27 | 28 | 29 | 30 | | |
| *March.* | 8 | 9 | 10 | 11 | 12 | 13 | 14 | 15 | 16 | 17 | 18 | 19 | 20 | 21 | 22 | 23 | 24 | 25 | 26 | 27 | 28 | 29 | 30 | 31 | 1 | 2 | 3 | 4 | 5 | 6 | | *April.* |
| July. | 1 | 2 | 3 | 4 | 5 | 6 | 7 | 8 | 9 | 10 | 11 | 12 | 13 | 14 | 15 | 16 | 17 | 18 | 19 | 20 | 21 | 22 | 23 | 24 | 25 | 26 | 27 | 28 | 29 | 30 | 31 | |
| *April.* | 7 | 8 | 9 | 10 | 11 | 12 | 13 | 14 | 15 | 16 | 17 | 18 | 19 | 20 | 21 | 22 | 23 | 24 | 25 | 26 | 27 | 28 | 29 | 30 | 1 | 2 | 3 | 4 | 5 | 6 | 7 | *May.* |
| Aug. | 1 | 2 | 3 | 4 | 5 | 6 | 7 | 8 | 9 | 10 | 11 | 12 | 13 | 14 | 15 | 16 | 17 | 18 | 19 | 20 | 21 | 22 | 23 | 24 | 25 | 26 | 27 | 28 | 29 | 30 | 31 | |
| *May.* | 8 | 9 | 10 | 11 | 12 | 13 | 14 | 15 | 16 | 17 | 18 | 19 | 20 | 21 | 22 | 23 | 24 | 25 | 26 | 27 | 28 | 29 | 30 | 31 | 1 | 2 | 3 | 4 | 5 | 6 | 7 | *June.* |
| Sept. | 1 | 2 | 3 | 4 | 5 | 6 | 7 | 8 | 9 | 10 | 11 | 12 | 13 | 14 | 15 | 16 | 17 | 18 | 19 | 20 | 21 | 22 | 23 | 24 | 25 | 26 | 27 | 28 | 29 | 30 | | |
| *June.* | 8 | 9 | 10 | 11 | 12 | 13 | 14 | 15 | 16 | 17 | 18 | 19 | 20 | 21 | 22 | 23 | 24 | 25 | 26 | 27 | 28 | 29 | 30 | 1 | 2 | 3 | 4 | 5 | 6 | 7 | | *July.* |
| Oct. | 1 | 2 | 3 | 4 | 5 | 6 | 7 | 8 | 9 | 10 | 11 | 12 | 13 | 14 | 15 | 16 | 17 | 18 | 19 | 20 | 21 | 22 | 23 | 24 | 25 | 26 | 27 | 28 | 29 | 30 | 31 | |
| *July.* | 8 | 9 | 10 | 11 | 12 | 13 | 14 | 15 | 16 | 17 | 18 | 19 | 20 | 21 | 22 | 23 | 24 | 25 | 26 | 27 | 28 | 29 | 30 | 31 | 1 | 2 | 3 | 4 | 5 | 6 | 7 | *Aug.* |
| Nov. | 1 | 2 | 3 | 4 | 5 | 6 | 7 | 8 | 9 | 10 | 11 | 12 | 13 | 14 | 15 | 16 | 17 | 18 | 19 | 20 | 21 | 22 | 23 | 24 | 25 | 26 | 27 | 28 | 29 | 30 | | |
| *Aug.* | 8 | 9 | 10 | 11 | 12 | 13 | 14 | 15 | 16 | 17 | 18 | 19 | 20 | 21 | 22 | 23 | 24 | 25 | 26 | 27 | 28 | 29 | 30 | 31 | 1 | 2 | 3 | 4 | 5 | 6 | | *Sept.* |
| Dec. | 1 | 2 | 3 | 4 | 5 | 6 | 7 | 8 | 9 | 10 | 11 | 12 | 13 | 14 | 15 | 16 | 17 | 18 | 19 | 20 | 21 | 22 | 23 | 24 | 25 | 26 | 27 | 28 | 29 | 30 | 31 | |
| *Sept.* | 7 | 8 | 9 | 10 | 11 | 12 | 13 | 14 | 15 | 16 | 17 | 18 | 19 | 20 | 21 | 22 | 23 | 24 | 25 | 26 | 27 | 28 | 29 | 30 | 1 | 2 | 3 | 4 | 5 | 6 | 7 | *Oct.* |

## PROLAPSUS RECTI.

In ordinary cases, the protruded bowel can be easily replaced; in others, however, the swelling and pain may be so great as to give rise to much difficulty. In this event, a few doses of **Ign.** or **Nux** should be given, and the parts bathed in *Warm Arnicated* water, [ten drops to the ounce] and patient kept at rest for a time. Soon as the swelling and pain have abated, place patient on his knees, hips elevated, lubricate parts with oil, then with finger-tips joined, press firmly on the centre, pushing it up into position. After this, patient should keep horizontal position for a day or two.

In cases where the accident is of frequent occurrence, one of the following remedies should be given.

**BELLADONNA.** The prolapsed rectum is hot, red, swollen and very *tender* to touch. *Spasmodic constriction of sphincter ani.

**HAMAMELIS.** The prolapsus occurs in connection with varices of the rectum, with copious hemorrhage of dark fluid blood.

**IGNATIA.** Prolapsus with every stool, [**Podo.**] *Stitches up the rectum, with itching as from ascarides in anus. Especially suitable to children.

**MERCURIUS COR.** Especially during an attack of dysentery. *Constant tenesmus during and after stool. *Painful bloody, slimy or greenish stools.

**NUX VOMICA.** Persons of sedentary habits. *Habitual constipation in high livers, [see **Sulph.**] Blind or bleeding piles.

**PODOPHYLLUM.** *Prolapsus ani with almost every stool, [**Ign.**] Diarrhœa, stools yellow-colored, with meal-like sediment.

**SULPHUR.** *Blind* or *bleeding* piles, [**Nux.**] *Habitual constipation,* with ineffectual urging, during which the rectum becomes prolapsed.

**DIETETICS.** The diet should be such as to guard against constipation. The use of oatmeal, cracked wheat, bread made of unbolted flour, together with laxative fruits, as apples, peaches, pears, figs, prunes, the most valuable.

---

## PROLAPSUS UTERI, ETC.

**THERAPEUTICS.** *Leading indications.*

**ACONITE.** *Prolapsus occurring suddenly, with inflammation of the parts, and burning pain. Bitter vomiting, cold sweat, or dry, hot skin.

**AMMO. MUR.** Pain in groin, obliging one to walk crooked. Menses appear *too soon,* with pain in belly and small of back, the flow most abundant in night. *Discharge of blood with the stool during catamenia.

**AURUM MET.** Uterus prolapsed and indurated, [see **Con.**] Prolapsus after lifting a heavy load, [**Nux. Rhus.**] Bruised pain, with shooting or drawing. Thick white leucorrhœa; burning, smarting of vulva.

**BELLADONNA.** *Simple prolapsus*, [**Aur. Puls. Pod. Sep.**—*Anteversion*, **Calc. Merc. Nux.** Sep.—*Retroversion*, **Cimi. Helon. Nux. Plat.**] Prolapsus at *climacteric* or after *parturition.* *Pressure towards the genitals, as if everything would protrude, [**Nit. ac. Plat. *Sep.**] *Heat and dryness of vagina*, [**Lyc.**] Feeling in back as if it would break, hindering motion.

**CALC. CARB.** *Palo, flabby state of body. Climacteric period, [**Lach. Sep.**] *Uterus easily displaced by over-exertion.* Stinging in os uteri, [**Con.**] Constant aching in vagina. *Menses too frequent and too profuse, [**Bell.**] *Vertigo on going up-stairs.* *Cold feet, feels as if she had on cold, damp stockings.

**CONIUM.** *Induration and prolapsus at same time, [**Aur. Iod. Plat. Sep.**—Ulceration of cervix, with prolapsus, **Arg. n. Helon. Hydras. Merc.**] Burning, sore aching in region of uterus. *Thick, milky, acrid leucorrhœa, causing burning. *Vertigo, particularly when lying down or turning over in bed. *Scanty* menstruation.

**GRAPHITES.** Anteversion, or standing backwards, can be reached with difficulty. Vagina cold, [heat and dryness of, **Bell. Lyc.**] *Profuse leucorrhœa, occurs in gushes. Dry, unhealthy skin. Itching eruptions.

**HELONIAS.** Prolapsus, with dragging weakness in sacral region. *Prolapsus, with ulceration of cervix, the os protrudes externally, [see **Con.**] Dark, fetid discharge from vagina. "*Consciousness of a womb.*" Greatly depressed in spirits.

**HYDRASTIS.** *Ulceration of cervix and vagina, with prolapsus uteri, [see **Con.**] *Leucorrhœa tenacious, ropy, thick, yellow.* Pruritus vulvæ, with sexual excitement.

**LACHESIS.** *The uterine region feels swollen, will bear no contact, not even the clothing. Uterus feels as if the os was open, [**Kreo.**] Copious leucorrhœa, smarting, and staining linen greenish.

**LILIUM TIG.** Anteversion, severe neuralgic pains in uterus, aggravated by least pressure or jar. *Bearing down in uterine region, as if pelvic contents would issue through vagina, [see **Bell.**] Aching over pubes, with pain in knees. Thin, acrid, excoriating leucorrhœa.

**MERCURIUS.** *Prolapsus uteri et vaginæ*, [**Sep.**] Deep, sore pain in pelvis and dragging in loins. Abdomen weak, as if it must be held up. *Deep ulcers, with ragged edges on os uteri. Leucorrhœa smarting, corroding, causing itching.

**NITRIC ACID.** *Violent pressing down, as if everything

were coming out of vulva, [see **Bell.**] Pain in small of back, through hips and down thighs. Excrescences on cervix uteri, [**Merc.**] Leucorrhœa of ropy or green mucus, [see **Hydras.**] *Hard nodes in mammæ.*

**NUX MOS.** *Prolapsus uteri et vaginæ,* [**Merc. Sep.**] Displacement of uterus, particularly in barren women. *Great dryness in mouth and throat while sleeping. *Enormous distension of abdomen after every meal. Menses irregular in time and quantity.

**NUX VOM.** *Prolapsus uteri from straining or lifting, [**Podo. *Rhus.**] Hardness and swelling of os tincæ. *Bearing down towards the sacrum, with ineffectual urging to stool, [**Puls.**] Burning, heaviness, sticking in uterus. Leucorrhœa fetid, staining yellow.

**PODOPHYLLUM.** *Prolapsus uteri after over-lifting or straining,* or *after parturition.* *Sensation as if genitals would come out during stool. *Prolapsus ani, with every stool. Pain in region of ovaries.

**PULSATILLA.** Chilliness and paleness of face. *Bad taste in morning and dry tongue, without thirst.* *Prolapsus uteri, with pressure in abdomen and small of back as from a stone. Limbs tend to go to sleep. *Menses too late, scanty, flow thick, black, clotted. *Easily moved to tears.*

**RHUS TOX.** *Prolapsus from over-exertion or straining, [***Nux. Podo.**] Bearing down when standing or walking, back aches, better lying on something hard. Amenorrhœa from getting wet, [**Puls.**]

**SEPIA.** Pressing down in uterus oppressing the breathing, seems as if everything would come out of vagina, crosses her limbs to prevent it. *Prolapsus uteri et vaginæ, [**Merc.**] *All-gone feeling in pit of stomach,* relieved by lying down or eating. *Yellow saddle across bridge of nose. *Pot-belliedness.*

**SULPHUR.** *Burning on the vertex, [coldness, **Verat.**] *Bearing down in pelvis, towards genitals.* Weak feeling in genital organs. Burning in vagina, can scarcely keep still. *Frequent weak, faint spells. Flushes of heat, and burning in soles.

**GENERAL MEASURES.** Our chief reliance in the treatment of uterine displacement must rest on suitable hygienic measures and internal medication. The state of general health should be looked after, and the system built up by a nutritious diet, open-air exercise, frequent ablutions, regular habits, etc. Wearing tight clothing, taking long walks, going up and down stairs, lifting heavy weights, and over-exertion of every kind, should be avoided. The use of pessaries should be discarded; as a general thing, they do more harm than good.

# PUERPERAL CONVULSIONS.

**THERAPEUTICS.** *Leading indications.*

**ACONITE.** In the incipiency, when an attack is apprehended. After *fright*, [**Ign.** ***Opi.**] Flushed face; dry, hot skin; thirst and great restlessness. *Great fear and anxiety of mind; thinks she will die, although there is no occasion of alarm. *She dreads too much activity about her. Vertigo on rising up in bed.

**ARGENT. NIT.** The patient has a presentiment of the approaching spasm. Tremor of limbs and faintish, weak feeling. *Sensation as if the body, and especially the face and head, expanded. She feels as if the bones of the skull separated with increase of temperature. *Continually in motion between spasms.

**BELLADONNA.** Red, bloated face, distorted eyes and dilated pupils, [**Opi.**] *She seems to be in a half-conscious state, with disposition to strike and bite. Convulsive jerking of limbs and muscles of face. Foam at mouth, and involuntary escape of fæces and urine, [**Hyos.**] With every pain a spasm comes on, and during interval more or less tossing about. *Sensation as if she were falling down through bed. Grating of teeth, [**Stram.**]

**CICUTA VIROSA.** Violent contortions of upper part of body and limbs. Convulsive tossing of extremities from one side to another. *Bluish face, with interrupted breathing and foam at mouth. *After convulsion she lies motionless, with rigidity of jaws, and as if dead.

**CUPRUM.** The spasm sets in with sudden convulsive jerking of limbs. The arms are drawn in towards body, and fingers tightly clinched. Eyes spasmodically closed, and mouth distorted. *Rigidity of trunk and lower extremities, with closed jaws. *Vomiting and retching, with horrible colic and cramps in legs.

**GELSEMIUM.** *Labor delayed by rigid os, [**Bell.**] Sensation like a wave, from uterus to throat, ending with choking feeling. *Impending spasms, [**Acon.**] Head feels *too large*, speech thick, pulse slow, [see **Opi.**]

**HYOSCYAMUS.** The spasms commence with twitching of muscles of face, and spasmodic motions of eyelids, [see **Stram.**] *Twitching and jerking of all the muscles in body. *Clinching of the thumbs. Complete loss of consciousness, with desire to escape. Oppression of chest, *with stertorous breathing.* Involuntary discharge of fæces and urine, [**Bell.**]

**IGNATIA.** *Sudden starting from sleep, with screams and trembling of body, [**Stram.**] Twitching of muscles of the face and corners of mouth. Convulsive movements of single muscles, or only portions of the body at a time. *Deep sighing and sobbing, with a strange compressed feeling in the brain.

**OPIUM.** Especially after fright, [Acon.] Convulsive trembling of whole body, with distortion of muscles. *The spasm is followed by sopor and stertorous respiration. *Stupefaction of senses, and complete loss of consciousness. Bluish, bloated face, with swollen lips. Pupils dilated and insensible to light. Incoherent and wandering talk. *Slow pulse.*

**STRAMONIUM.** *The patient awakens with a shrinking look, as if afraid of first object seen. The spasm mostly commences with convulsive motions of extremities, especially upper. Grinding of teeth, [Bell.] *Loquacious delirium, with stammering speech. *She makes ridiculous gestures and strange faces; *laughs, sings and sighs.* *The light of brilliant objects, and contact, renew the spasms.

**AUXILIARY MEASURES.** At the first sign of convulsions, the indicated remedy should be given and repeated at short intervals. Soon as os is sufficiently dilated, apply forceps and terminate the labor soon as possible. If os remains unyielding, and convulsions persistent, it is advised by some to *incise* the os, dilate and deliver at once. Others advise *Chloroform* to be given at the very onset of attack to ward off the paroxysm; this sometimes succeeds, but as often fails. Copious injections of *hot water*, [112° to 115°] into the uterus, with *Fountain Syringe*, also recommended as valuable.

*Empty bladder* with catheter, and the rectum with warm water injections, unless they are known to be empty. If patient is in a *comatose condition*, ice-bags to head and spine are advised.

---

## PUERPERAL FEVER.

(*Child-bed Fever, Puerperal Metritis.*)

**THERAPEUTICS.** *Leading indications.*

**ACONITE.** After a violent chill; dry, hot skin, full bounding pulse and intense thirst. Cutting, lancinating, burning and tearing pains in uterus, with anguish and great fear. Suppression of lochia, or too scanty discharge, [Bell.] *Excessive sensibility to touch. *Retention of urine, with stitches in kidneys. *Fear of death, predicts the day she will die.

**ARSENICUM.** Advanced stages. Burning, lancinating pains; the parts *burn like fire.* *Great anguish, extreme restlessness and fear of death, [Acon.] *Rapid prostration,* with sinking of vital forces. *Craves cold drinks, but can take but little at a time. Wants to be covered up warmly, [Rhus.] Aggravation after midnight.

**BELLADONNA.** Great tenderness of abdomen, aggravated by *least motion or jar,* [Bry.] *Violent clutching pains, as if parts were seized with *claws.* *Pains come on suddenly, and cease as suddenly. Great *heat* in abdomen, which imparts a *burning* sensation to the hand. *Almost constant moaning, with starting and jumping while sleeping. Painful bearing down in pelvis. Suppression of lochial or menstrual discharge, or else it is scant and fetid. *Congestion to head, with flushed face and red eyes. Throbbing headache and delirium. *Great intolerance to light or noise, [Acon.]

**BRYONIA.** Stitching, burning pains in abdomen, which is tender to touch. *Lochia *suppressed,* with splitting headache, [Bell.] Lips parched, dry and cracked. Great dryness of mouth, with little thirst, or else drinking large quantities. *Cannot sit up from nausea and faintness. *Wants to remain perfectly quiet; worse from least motion. *Hard, dry stools, as if burnt. Exceedingly irritable.

**CANTHARIS.** Great heat and burning in abdomen, [with lancinating pains, Ars.] Debility, restlessness and trembling of the limbs. *Constant painful urging and tenesmus of the bladder, passing but a few drops at a time, sometimes mixed with blood.

**CHAMOMILLA.** If the disease was induced by a fit of anger. Heat all over, with thirst and red face, or *one cheek red and the other pale,* [Acon.] *Violent labor-like pains in uterus. *Profuse lochia.* Great sensitiveness to pain, becomes furious. *She is very impatient, can hardly answer a civil question. Urine abundant and light-colored. Warm sweat about the head.

**COLOCYNTH.** *Terrible colicky pains, causing her to bend double, with great restlessness. *Feeling in abdomen as if intestines were being squeezed between stones. Vomiting and diarrhœa, worse after eating or drinking, [Ars.] Bitter taste in mouth. Full, frequent pulse and great thirst.

**HYOSCYAMUS.** If the disease assume a typhoid character. *Spasmodic jerking of the limbs, face and eyelids. Furious delirium, with wild, staring look. *Muttering and picking at the bedclothes. *She throws off the bedclothes and wants to remain naked. Complete apathy, or else great excitability.

**IPECAC.** Pain in region of umbilicus, extending towards uterus. Every movement is attended with a cutting pain running from *left to right.* *Continual nausea and vomiting, [Verat.] Discharge from the womb of bright-red blood. *Green, watery, fermented stools.

**KREOSOTE.** Loss of memory, thinks herself well. She has a sick, suffering expression. *Violent burning deep in pelvis, with constant whining and moaning. *Putrid state of the womb, with *offensive, excoriating lochia.* Labor-like pains in abdomen, with drawing in upper abdomen, extending to small of back. Painful sensation of coldness in abdomen.

**LACHESIS.** *Cannot bear any pressure, not even the clothing, over uterine region. *The pain in uterus is relieved for a time by a flow of blood, but soon returns. Repeated chills, livid face, and unconsciousness. Skin alternately hot and cold. Abdomen distended. Lochial discharge thin and ichorous. *Aggravation after sleep, [**Apis. Verat.**]

**MERCURIUS.** Lancinating, boring, or pressing pains in the genital organs. *Very sensitive about the pit of the stomach and abdomen, [**Bell.**] Much saliva in the mouth. *Tongue moist, with great thirst. *Profuse sweat without relief.* Aggravation at night. Green, slimy, or bloody mucous stools, with violent tenesmus.

**NUX VOMICA.** Feeling of heaviness and burning in genital organs and abdomen. Suppression, or else too profuse discharge of lochia, with violent pains in small of back. Pain as if bruised in neck of uterus. *Constipation, with frequent and ineffectual urging to stool. Pain in small of back, worse when attempting to turn in bed. *Ringing in ears and fainting turns.* Aggravation in morning.

**RHUS TOX.** Metritis after confinement. *She cannot lie still, but must change continually to get a little rest. *The lower limbs seem powerless, she can hardly draw them up. *Dry tongue, with red tip.* Typhoid symptoms. Aggravation *during rest*, at night, particularly after midnight, [**Ars.**]

**SECALE.** Tendency to putrescence, [*with dark, offensive discharge*, **Kreo.**] Hot fever, intermingled by shaking chills. Discharge from vagina of thin, black blood, very offensive. Vomiting decomposed matters. Painless diarrhœa, with much debility. She lies either in quiet delirium, or grows wild with great anxiety and desire to escape from bed. *Thin, scrawny women. *Desire to be uncovered.

**VERAT. ALB.** Puerperal metritis, with violent fits *of vomiting and diarrhœa.* *Coldness of extremities, with deadly-pale face, covered with cold perspiration. Suppression of lochial discharge with delirium. *Excessive weakness, [***Ars. Sec.**]

**AUXILIARY MEASURES.** Treat patient on mattress bed with light covering. Apply *hot fomentations* containing indicated remedy, or thin poultices over painful parts. With a fountain syringe wash out *uterus* and vagina thoroughly, two or three times a day, with a solution *Carbolic acid* [gtts. v. aq. ferv. ℥j ] or *Kali. permang.* [grs. jii. aq. ferv. ℥j.] Rectal injections of *hot water*, [110° F.] very useful. Keep patient quiet as possible, and room abundantly supplied with fresh air.

**DIETETICS.** During inflammatory stage, give only the simplest kind of food—thin gruel, rice-water, barley-water, and mucilaginous drinks. Later, beef-tea, animal broths, milk, soft-boiled eggs, cream toast, and ripe fruits.

## REMITTENT FEVER.

(*Bilious Fever; Typho-malarial Fever.*)

**THERAPEUTICS.** *Leading indications.*

**ACONITE.** Chill, *high fever, violent thirst,* red face, shortness of breath, and great nervousness. *Bitter taste of everything except water, [see **Bry.**] *Bitter, bilious vomiting,* [***Cham. Ipe. Nux. Puls.**] Red scanty urine. Stitches in region of liver. *Anxiety and great restlessness.*

**BRYONIA.** Giddiness, nausea, and faintness on sitting up, [**Acon. Puls.**] *Fullness in forehead, as if everything would be pressed out. *Splitting headache,* [***Bell. Puls.**] Lips parched, dry and cracked. Tongue coated white or yellow. *All food and drink taste bitter, [**Colo. Puls.**] *Stitches or burning in region of liver. Constipation; *dry, hard stools. Exceedingly irritable.*

**CHAMOMILLA.** Patient exceedingly *irritable,* can scarcely answer a civil question, [**Bry.**] Thick, white or yellow coating on tongue. *Bitter taste, [***Bry. Nux. Puls.**] *Vomiting food, bile, or slimy substances. *Painful bloatedness of stomach.* Stools green, watery, slimy, or like chopped eggs and spinach. Jaundice-like appearance of face, [see **Merc.**]

**CHINA.** Chills alternating with heat, skin cold and blue, [see **Nux.**] Ringing in ears, with dizziness and a feeling as if the head was enlarged. *Pain in region of liver and spleen, when bending or coughing. Sallow complexion. Miasmatic districts.

**CORNUS.** Dull headache, with aching pains in the eyeballs. Flushes of heat and coldness in alternation, [***Puls.**] Loss of appetite, with aversion to meat and bread. Rumbling of wind in bowels, with emission of fetid flatus. General debility from loss of fluids and night-sweats, [***China.**] Dark, bilious stools.

**GELSEMIUM.** Adapted to nervous, excitable, hysterical females, [**Ign.**] Fullness in head, heat of face, and chilliness. *Heaviness of eyelids, impossible to keep them open. Congestion of liver, with vertigo and blindness. *Aching and soreness in lower legs.*

**IPECAC.** *Headache, as if brain and skull were bruised.* Yellowish or white coating of tongue. Bitter taste in morning, [see **Puls.**] *Continual nausea, with vomiting food, bile, or jelly-like mucus, [**Ant. c.**] Flatulent colic. *Diarrhœa, stools fermented, or like frothy molasses.

**LEPTANDRA.** Constant dull frontal headache. Tongue yellow down the centre, [*white,* **Bell.**] *Vomiting bile, with shooting pains in liver.* *Jaundice, with clay-colored or black stools. Tendency to shiver, with sore, lame feeling in back.

**MERCURIUS.** Pale, yellow, earthy color of face, [**Puls.**] Tongue coated with a dirty yellow fur. *Fetid breath, with ulcers on lips, gums, and cheeks, [Nit. ac. *Nux.] Bitter, sour, putrid, or sweet taste. *Region of stomach sore to touch, [Bry. Nux.] Stinging pains and great soreness in region of liver. *Diarrhœa; stools dark green, frothy,* or yellow like sulphur. Dark-red urine, as if mixed with blood.

**NUX VOMICA.** The patient is very irritable, and wishes to be alone, [see **Cham.**] Head aches, as if skull would split, [**Bry.**] *Bitter or sour taste.* *Bitter, sour eructations, [**Bry. Puls.**] *Vomiting food, or sour-smelling mucus. *Cramp-like* pain in stomach. *Habitual constipation of large, difficult stools. Can't sleep after 3 A. M. Worse in morning.

**PODOPHYLLUM.** *Depression of spirits.* Tongue furred white, moist, shows imprints of teeth, [**Hydras. Merc.**] *Bitter taste and bitter risings from the stomach, [**Bry. Nux.**] Bilious vomiting and purging, with dark urine. *Yellowness of skin, with fullness, soreness and pain in liver.*

**PULSATILLA.** Melancholy, with weeping sadness. *He is disgusted with everything. Vertigo on rising from a sitting posture. **Hemicrania*, as if the brain would burst, worse from stooping, or moving the eyes. Tongue yellow or white, and covered with tough mucus, [**Merc.**] *Putrid taste in mouth, with inclination to vomit, [**Merc. Nux.**] *Every kind of nourishment tastes bitter, [***Bry.**] *Nightly diarrhœa, stools watery, or green like bile.*

**SULPHUR.** Low-spirited, out of humor, inclines to weep, [**Puls.**] Vertigo on sitting up, [see **Bry.**] *Constant *heat* on top of head, [*coldness*, **Verat.**] Putrid taste, with complete loss of appetite. *Sour* eructations, [**Nux.**] *Stitches, or pressing pain in region of liver. *Painless morning diarrhœa*, [**Rumex.**] Lean persons who walk stooping.

**DIETETICS.** In active stage, little food should be taken. Cold water or bits of ice to allay thirst and check vomiting. When improvement sets in, rice, farina, cornstarch, and fresh buttermilk may be taken. Later, broths, beef-tea, fresh vegetables and ripe fruits. A return to the ordinary diet should be very gradual.

Treat patient in a *well ventilated* room, where there is plenty of *sunlight.* Cold or hot compresses may be applied to the painful head, and the body frequently sponged off with tepid water.

---

## ACUTE RHEUMATISM.

**THERAPEUTICS.** *Leading indications.*

**ACONITE.** Synochal fever, with *great agitation of heart.* Red swelling of affected part, *very sensitive to contact and motion.* Stitching pains in chest, hindering respiration, [**Bry.**] *Great fear and anxiety of mind, with nervous excitability. Retention of urine, and stitches in kidneys.

**AMMON. PHOS.** Especially where joints of fingers and hands are involved, [**Caul. Lach.**] Loss of appetite, with emaciation. Sleeplessness and nervous irritability. Mostly the *right side.* Evening fever.

**ARNICA.** Hard, red, shining swelling of the affected parts. *Pains as if sprained or bruised, with a feeling of lameness in limb, [**Rhus.**] *Sensation as if diseased part were resting upon something hard. *Great fear of being struck by persons coming near.

**ARSENICUM.** Burning, stinging, tearing pain, with pale swelling. *Pain relieved by application of warmth, [**Rhus.**] Profuse sweat, which relieves pain, but leaves patient very weak. Frequent chills, alternating with heat. Constantly moving affected limbs. *Extreme thirst, drinking little and often.

**BELLADONNA.** Red, shining swelling of joints, with pressing, cutting, tearing pain, deep in bones. *Frequent darting pains from joint along the limb, [like electric jerks, **Verat. a.**] *Pains which come on suddenly, and leave as suddenly. Fever, with dry, hot skin, thirst, and throbbing headache. Visible pulsations of carotids. Drowsy, sleepy condition, with starting. Aggravation at 3 P.M., and from least motion or touch.

**BRYONIA.** Stiffness, with swelling and a faintish redness of inflamed part, [**Colch.**] *Stitching, tearing pains, worse from least motion. *The patient wants to remain perfectly still. Dry, hot skin, or else perspiration of an acrid character. Bitter taste, dry mouth, and great thirst. *Hard, dry stools, as if burnt. Exceedingly *irritable.* Metastasis to the heart, [***Acon. Colch. Spig. Verat. v.**]

**CACTUS.** The disease is principally confined to the heart and diaphragm. Feeling as if an iron band was around the heart, preventing its normal action. Palpitation of the heart, worse when lying on the left side, [when on the back, ***Ars.**]

**CAULOPHYLLUM.** *Rheumatism of wrists and finger-joints, with much swelling. When disease shifts from extremities to back and nape of neck, with rigidity of muscles. Oppression of chest, high fever, and nervous excitement.

**CAUSTICUM.** Stiffness and swelling of joints, with tearing pains. *Great weakness and lameness of lower limbs, and trembling of hands. Pains worse towards evening, and from exposure to cold; better from application of heat, [**Ars. Rhus t.**] Scrofulous persons, with yellow complexion.

**CHAMOMILLA.** Drawing, tearing pains, with a sensation of numbness or lameness in parts, [**Nux.**] The pains are continuous, and get worse at night, with much tossing about. *Becomes almost furious about pains, can hardly endure them. *Great irritability of temper, is very cross and snappish. Hot perspiration, especially about head, *Redness of one cheek and paleness of other, [**Acon. Nux v.**]

**CHELIDONIUM.** *Rheumatic swelling, with a *stone-like hardness* of the affected parts. Constant pain under the lower, inner angle of the right shoulder-blade. *Stools like sheep's dung, [**Plum. Ruta.**]

**CHINA.** Violent tearing, sticking, drawing pains, increased by pressure or motion. Bruised pains in the small of the back, with painful jerks in the region of the os sacrum. *Debilitating morning and night sweats.* *Weakly persons, who have lost much blood.

**CIMICIFUGA.** Articular rheumatism of lower extremities, with much swelling and heat of parts. Pain worse from motion, extorting screams. Delicate hysterical females who suffer from uterine diseases.

**COLCHICUM.** Moderate swelling with pale redness of affected parts, [**Bry.**] Pains burning, tearing, or jerking, frequently shifting about, [**Bell. Puls.**] *Chilliness even near hot stove, intermingled with flashes of heat, [**Puls.**] Metastasis to heart, with stitches and tearing in chest and region of heart. Strong and fluttering beating of heart. Profuse *sour-smelling sweats.* *Urine dark and scanty, depositing a whitish sediment.

**DULCAMARA.** *After exposure to wet,* [**Merc.**] The parts feel as if bruised, [**Arn.**] The pains are mostly in back, joints of arms, and legs. When the disease sets in after acute cutaneous eruptions. *Aggravation after every cold change in weather.

**FERRUM.** Little or no swelling, but a constant drawing, tearing pain, especially in deltoid muscle. Pain worse in bed; has to get up and walk slowly about. *Least emotion or exertion produces a red, flushed face. Palpitation of heart, and dyspnœa.

**HAMAMELIS.** Pains unbearable, with great sensitiveness to touch, and fear of exciting new pain on moving. *Great soreness of affected parts. Articular rheumatism, with swollen, painful joints, [**Cimi.**]

**KREOSOTE.** Pain in joints, especially in hip and knee-joints, [**Ledum**], with a feeling of numbness or loss of sensation, as though the whole limb were going to sleep. *Wretched livid complexion.

**LACHESIS.** Swelling of index-finger and wrist-joint. Stinging, tearing in knees, with a sense of swelling. Left side generally affected. No relief from profuse sweating, [**Merc.**] *Patient worse after sleeping.

**LEDUM.** Rheumatic pains in the lower extremities, especially in the hip and knee-joints, and when it commences from below and goes upwards. *Great want of vital heat, [**Sep.**] Pains grow worse in the evening in bed, and last till midnight.

**LYCOPODIUM.** Drawing and tearing pains, worse at night and during rest, [**Rhus.**] Painful rigidity of muscles and joints, with sensation of numbness in part. The disease is mostly on right side, with or without swelling. Chronic forms, especially of old people. *Urine dark and turbid, or with *sediment of red sand.* *Constant sensation of satiety, feels so full can eat nothing. Constipation, much sour belching.

**MERCURIUS.** Shooting, tearing or burning pains, worse at night, from warmth of bed or exposure to damp or cold air, [**Dulc.**] Puffy swelling of the affected parts, of a pale or slight pinkish color. Green, slimy diarrhœa, with griping and tenesmus. *Much perspiration, affording no relief, [**Lach.**]

**NUX VOMICA.** Especially in back, loins, chest or joints, with pale, tensive swelling, [**Bry.**] Tensive jerking or pulling pains, aggravated by contact or motion. Numbness or lameness of affected parts, with twitching in muscles. Aversion to open air, and great sensitiveness to cold. Heat mixed with chilliness, especially when moving. *Perspiration relieves the pain, [see ***Merc.**] Dyspeptic symptoms. *Habitual constipation. Persons of intemperate habits. Irritable mood.

**PHOSPHORUS.** Tearing, drawing and tensive pains setting in when taking cold. Lameness and weakness in lower limbs, [**Nux Puls.**] *Sensation of weakness and emptiness in abdomen. Belching large quantities of wind after eating, [**Bry. Nux Puls.**] *Long, narrow, hard stools, very difficult to expel.

**PHYTOLACCA.** Pains shoot from one part to another, [**Puls.**] *Joints swollen and red.* *Pains in middle of long bones or attachments of muscles. Worse in damp weather and at night.

**PULSATILLA.** Not much swelling or redness of the affected parts. *Pains which shift rapidly from one part to another, [**Bell. Rhod.**] Sensation of weight in the disordered structure. *Chilliness, even in a warm room. *Craves cold, fresh air; feels worse in a warm temperature. *Persons of a mild, tearful disposition. *Bad taste in the mouth in the morning.

**RHODODENDRON.** Drawing, tearing pains in joints and limbs. Pains worse during rest, and in rough, stormy weather, [**Rhus.**] Swelling and redness of single joints. *Rheumatism of knee*, [**Verat. v.**]

**RHUS TOX.** Swelling and redness of affected parts. Pains drawing, tearing, burning, or as if sprained, with sensation of lameness and creeping in the parts. *Pains worse during rest and when first commencing to move, [**Ars. Sulph.**] *Better from continued motion and external warm applications, [**Ars.**]

**SPIGELIA.** Rheumatic pericarditis, [see **Bry.**] Dull stitches in region of heart. Violent palpitation of heart, with great anxiety. Dyspnœa, he can lie only on right side, with trunk raised. *The least motion produces great suffocation.

**SULPHUR.** Chronic form, and for secondary effects of acute rheumatism. Tearing, stitching, or dull aching pains. *Constant heat in top of the head, [coldness, **Verat.**] *Frequent weak, faint spells.

**THUYA.** Tearing and beating pains, as if from subcutaneous ulceration. Feeling of coldness and numbness in parts, [**Nux v. Puls.**] Rheumatism in syphilitic subjects, [**Phyto. Merc.**] Symptoms worse in a warm room.

**VERAT. ALB.** Pains as if bruised, worse from the heat of the bed; better from rising and walking about. *Electric jerks in the affected limbs. Painful heaviness in the knees and lower legs.

**VERAT. VIR.** Rhematism, especially of left shoulder, hip, and knee, [**Rhod.**] *Aching in all the bones.* Advised in endocarditis and pericarditis.

**AUXILIARY MEASURES.** Persons subject to rheumatism should wear *flannel* next the skin as a preventive. They should avoid *over-exertion*, and especially should they guard against the sudden checking of perspiration.

During an attack patient should rest on a soft bed and between *blankets*. *Hot fomentations* applied to painful parts will often afford great relief. Enveloping the parts in *raw cotton* is also very useful. The room should be light and well *ventilated*, and the temperature about 70° F.

**DIETETICS.** Only plain, simple food. Light puddings, made of rice, tapioca, sago or corn-starch; plain toast and good ripe fruits. The drink should be pure fresh water, lemonade, or water with a little jelly added. All alcoholic beverages should be strictly avoided.

---

## SCABIES.—ITCH.

Scabies, or *common itch*, is a disease characterized by a *vesicular* eruption which is produced by an *animal parasite*. It is a *contagious* disease, easily communicated, may last for years, and seldom gets well without treatment.

### INDICATED REMEDIES.

**SULPHUR.** This is the principal remedy for *acarous itch*, or true scabies. *Voluptuous tingling, itching, with burning or soreness after scratching. Excoriation of skin; glandular swellings.

**MERCURIUS.** Itch-like eruption in bends of the elbows. *Scabies, where some of the vesicles become pustular. Itching all over, worse at night when warm in bed.

**CAUSTICUM.** After abuse of Sulphur or Mercury, [**Sep.**] *Involuntary urination when coughing, sneezing or walking. Sensitive to cold air.

**ARSENICUM.** *Inveterate cases.* *Itch-like eruptions in bends of knees, [see **Merc.**] Pustular eruptions, burning and itching, better from external warmth,

**LOCAL MEASURES.** Give two or three doses of *Sulphur* daily for a week before using external applications. Rub patient thoroughly with *Soft-soap* for half an hour, then give a *warm bath*, and when *dry* rub all over with a solution of two parts *Liquid Storax* and one part *Glycerine*. Two or three operations of this kind will suffice for a cure in nearly all cases.

Take *Balsam of Peru* ℨj, *Glycerine* and water āā ℥ji. Mix and rub well on all parts that are the seat of the eruption. Before applying this patient should take a warm bath, using plenty soap and friction; should be repeated three times a day for two days. This is an efficient remedy.

---

## SCARLATINA.

**THERAPUETICS.** *Leading indications.*

**ACONITE.** In commencement, before the eruption makes its appearance. **Dry, hot skin*, full, frequent pulse, *great restlessness*, violent thirst and hurried breathing. *Great fear and anxiety of mind, with nervous excitability. Pain in stomach, with nausea and vomiting.

**AILANTHUS.** Small, rapid pulse, [full, frequent, **Acon. Bell.**] Severe headache, with hot, red face. Very drowsy and restless, with muttering delirium. *Skin covered with a miliary rash, with efflorescence between the points of a dark, livid color, [*smooth, bright-red*, ***Bell.**] The livid color, when pressed out with the finger, returns very slowly, [*very quickly*, **Bell.**] Violent vomiting, with inability to sit up.

**AMM. CARB.** Hard swelling of parotid and lymphatic glands of neck, [**Bary. c.**] The rash continues out longer than usual period. Tendency to gangrenous ulceration.

**APIS MEL.** Fever of a typhoid character. *Rash hard, sharp, pointed, [*smooth*, **Bell.**] Tongue of a *deep-red color* and covered with blisters. *Nose discharges a thick, white fetid or bloody mucus, [a thin, purulent matter, **Nit. ac.**] *Ulcerated throat.* Abdomen sore to touch. Dropsical symptoms during desquamation. Child lies in a stupor.

**ARSENICUM.** The eruption delays or grows suddenly pale, *with rapid prostration. Putrid sore throat*, [**Arum. t. Apis.**] *Great anguish, extreme *restlessness*, and fear of death. *Intense thirst, drinking little and often. *Wheezing respiration. Fetid diarrhœa.

**ARUM. TRI.** Corners of mouth and lips sore and cracked. Redness of tongue, with elevated papillæ. Putrid sore throat, [**Ars. Nit. ac.**] *Submaxillary glands swollen.* *Nose stopped, or discharging a burning, ichorous fluid, *excoriating* nostrils and upper lip, [**Mur. ac.**] Eruption all over body, with much itching and restlessness. *Scarlatina maligna.

**BAPTISIA.** *Typhoid character,* [**Ars. Lach. Rhus.**] *Fauces dark red, tonsils swollen and covered with dark putrid ulcers. *Eruption resembles measles,* [*bluish-black eruption, **Argen. n.**] *Great fetor of breath,* [**Ars. Nit. ac.**] *Tongue cracked, sore, ulcerated. Slight delirium, and burning heat of face. *Sordes on teeth and lips.*

**BARYTA CARB.** Parotid and submaxillary glands swollen, with much saliva, or else dryness of throat. Tonsils swollen, and of a pale red color, with a pressing, stinging pain on swallowing. Breath putrid. *Scrofulous children that grow but little.

**BELLADONNA.** *The eruption is *perfectly smooth* and *scarlet red,* [purple colored, **Ailan. Mur. ac. Rhus.**] Skin so hot it imparts a burning sensation to the hand. Tongue white, with red edges and prominent papillæ. Fauces and tonsils inflamed of a *dark red color,* with *burning, stinging pain,* [**Acon. Apis. Cap.**] *Congestion to brain, with delirium and throbbing carotids. *Starting and jumping while sleeping. Springs suddenly up in bed, and attempts to escape. *Use as a prophylactic.*

**BRYONIA.** The eruption does not come out fully, or suddenly disappears, [**Cup. act. Ipe.**] Congestion to chest, with difficult, anxious breathing. Sensation of weight upon chest, with troublesome cough. Splitting headache, worse by motion. Lips parched, dry and cracked. *Patient wants to lie perfectly still.

**CALCARIA CARB.** Protracted cases, where glands of neck are swollen and hard, [**Bary. c.**] Throat greatly inflamed, with aphthæ on tonsils and roof of mouth. Does not convalesce after regular recession of eruption. Face pale and bloated, showing no signs of rash. *Scrofulous children with large heads and open fontanelles. *Otorrhœa and parotitis* following scarlatina, [**Bary. c. Bell.**]

**CAMPHOR.** In desperate cases. Extremities cold and purple. Rattling in throat, and hot breath. Hot perspiration on forehead; the child refuses to be covered. Sudden retrocession of eruption.

**CARBO. VEG.** Usually in last stage. *Putrid sore throat, with sloughing of fauces. Rattling in throat. Great prostration of strength and coldness of extremities, [see **Ars.**] *Craves cold air.*

**CUPRUM ACET.** *When *metastasis to brain is apprehended,* or eruption suddenly disappears, followed by convulsions, vomiting, [see **Opi.**] Rolling of eyes, distortions of face and all the flexor muscles. Great restlessness and tossing about. Sopor and delirium.

**IPECAC.** Slight fever through the day, increased in the evening. *Constant nausea and vomiting of green, bilious, or slimy matter. Great uneasiness in the stomach and epigastrium. Violent itching of the skin. Sleeplessness, with sadness and despondency.

**LACHESIS.** Scarlatina maligna, with external swelling of neck and glands. Diphtheritic inflammation of throat, with great difficulty in swallowing. *External throat very painful to touch. Ulcers on tongue, [**Bapt.**] *Aggravation after sleeping, [**Apis.**]

**LYCOPODIUM.** Inflammation of throat of a brownish red color, with stitches on swallowing. *Ulceration of tonsils, beginning on right and spreading to left, [beginning on left side, **Lach.**] Obstruction of nose. Rattling in throat, and hawking up bloody mucus. Dryness of mouth and tongue, without thirst. *Red sediment like sand in urine.

**MERCURIUS.** Ulcers in mouth, throat and upon tonsils, covered with ash-colored sloughs. Deglutition very difficult, attended with stinging pain. Fluids escape through mouth and nose when attempting to swallow, [**Bell. Lach.**] Very fetid breath. *Profuse secretion of saliva, often offensive. Acrid discharge from nose.

**MURIATIC ACID.** Malignant cases; tonsils and throat swollen, inflamed, and covered with dark-colored ulcers, [**Phyto.**] Great tendency for sloughs to extend and run together. Dark-redness of face, and purplish color of skin. Discharge of thin, acrid pus from nose, excoriating the parts, [**Arum.**] *Sliding down in bed.

**NITRIC ACID.** Putrid sore throat extending up into nose. Profuse discharge of thin, purulent matter from nostrils. *Putrid-smelling breath; mouth full of fetid ulcers.* Swelling of the parotid and submaxillary glands, [**Bary. c. Merc.**] Ulceration of the corners of the mouth and lips. After abuse of mercury.

**OPIUM.** *Extreme drowsiness, stertorous breathing, and vomiting. Delirious talking, with eyes wide open, face red and puffed up, [see **Zinc.**] *Impending paralysis of brain. *Spasms, with loud screams.*

**RHUS TOX.** The rash is *dark-colored* and *itches violently*, [*scarlet-red*, **Acon. Am. c. Bell.**] *Drowsy state, with delirium. Tongue red and smooth, with *triangular, red tip.* Much fever and *restlessness, particularly after midnight.* *Pain in limbs and joints. Ichorous or yellow, thick discharge from nose. *Constantly changing position.

**SULPHUR.** *Bright-redness of whole body.* *Violent itching, tingling of skin, with burning after scratching. *Child jumps, starts, and screams fearfully. Where other well-chosen remedies have failed to have the desired effect.

**ZINCUM.** *Threatening paralysis of brain. The child lies in a state of unconsciousness. Jerking of whole body, or twitching of single limbs. Grating of teeth, and shrill, frightful screams during sleep. Small, frequent pulse, and fixed, stupid expression of the eyes. Icy coldness of skin from sunken vitality.

**PREVENTIVE MEASURES.** During the prevalence of scarlet fever use **Belladonna** as a prophylactic. Look well after drainage and sewer-pipes, and use disinfectants. In case of *death* disinfect body and place in coffin soon as possible. *Private funeral.*

**AUXILIARY MEASURES.** Isolate patient, if possible, in a *light, airy, upper* room. Send other children from house, and have few *nurses* as possible. Divest room of all needless furniture—curtains, carpet, rugs, etc. Secure free *ventilation.* Disinfect all excretions. See article **Sick-Room.** Keep patient scrupulously *clean.* Change body-linen and bed-clothing often. Sponge body off two or three times a day with water at 90° F., wrap in dry sheet, and let the skin dry *without* being rubbed. Keep sharp lookout for kidney complications.

For the troublesome itching of skin, anoint the surface with *cocoa-butter,* or reasty bacon. The tenacious phlegm that accumulates in throat may be loosened and removed by taking teaspoonful doses of equal parts *Glycerine* and water. *Hot fomentations* or poultices to the swollen throat often very valuable.

**DIETETICS.** During violence of attack, fresh milk, ice-cream, thin gruels, orange juice, etc,, will suffice. Pure *fresh* water may be drank liberally. After the crisis, beef-tea, mutton or chicken broth, cream toast, light puddings and ripe fruits may be taken. All alcoholic stimulants should be discarded.

---

## SCIATICA.—COXALGIA.

**THERAPEUTICS.** *Leading indications.*

**ARGENT. NIT.** Periodical drawing cramp-like pains, from hips down to knee. *During paroxysm, sensation of expansion of limb. Paralytic weakness of limbs, with emaciation. Worse in morning, and *after dinner.*

**ARNICA.** *If caused by over-exertion, lifting, straining,* [**Ars. Rhus.**] *Tearing, drawing pains, insufferable, drive him crazy. Constantly changing position of limbs. Everything on which he lies feels too hard, [**Bapt.**]

**ARSENICUM.** Violent shooting, tearing pain in hip, thigh, groin and left foot. *Severe pain extending from hip down posterior part of thigh to knee. Pain least felt when moving affected part. *After great exertion, etc.*

**BELLADONNA.** Pain in hip-joint, especially at night, has to change position often. *Worse from least jar, even to stepping of other persons in room. Cannot bear least draught of air. Better from warmth, and letting limb hang down. *Wants to sleep, but cannot.

**BRYONIA.** Stabbing pain in hips, pain comes from head of femur, extends along anterior surface of thigh to knee.

*Lies best on painful side, [Calc. Ign.] Worse from least motion; often relieved by cold water.

**CHAMOMILLA.** *Violent drawing, tearing pains*, from left ischium to heel and sole of foot, with cramp-like tension of muscles. Numb feeling in affected parts after motion. *Becomes almost furious about the pains. *Worse at night in bed*, and from motion.

**COCCULUS.** *Pain as if hip was screwed together, [see Colo.] *Shooting pain like lightning down whole limb*, [Colo.] Pains worse from motion, and attended with cold extremities. After the pain, parts feel numb.

**COLOCYNTH.** Crampy pain in hip as if screwed in a vice, lies upon affected side, with knee drawn up. *Shooting pain, like lightning, down whole limb. Pain sets in suddenly, is constant in character, becoming intolerable in paroxysms. Worse from touch, cold, and motion. Better from perfect rest or warm applications.

**EUPATO. PUR.** *Severe shooting pains in course of left sciatic nerve, producing a palsied sensation, especially after motion. Gnawing in hip-bone; legs feel tired, particularly left. *Neuralgia of right shoulder*, pains come instantly, and go as quickly, [Bell.]

**HEPAR SULPH.** Pain in left hip as if sprained, worse from motion, touch, and exposure to air. *Better from being wrapped up and keeping quiet.

**IGNATIA.** *Throbbing pain in hip as if joint would burst, accompanied by chilliness. In chronic cases, and where the disease is intermitting, occurring every day or every other day. *Better* in summer, *worse* in winter.

**IRIS VERS.** *Sudden shooting along the sciatic nerve, causing lameness, worse from least motion. Shooting, burning pain in right shoulder. **Gastric sick-headache*, with vomiting sweetish water or bilious matter.

**LACHESIS.** *Sciatica of left side, pain as from a hot iron, worse after sleep. Pain constantly changing locality, now in head, now in teeth, now in sciatic nerve, [see Puls.] Nervousness and palpitation of heart.

**LEDUM.** Pinching, drawing pain in hip-joint, descending along posterior surface of thigh. The pain frequently *runs from below upwards*, [Nux.] Affected limb cooler than rest of body.

**LYCOPODIUM.** *Coxalgia, with violent jerks of the limbs. Stiffness, weakness and formication in affected limb. *Constant sense of fermentation in abdomen. *High-colored urine, with red, sandy, sediment. *Constipation*, almost impossible to void the stools.

**MENYANTHES.** Stitching, contractive pain in region of hip-joint. *When sitting, thighs and legs are spasmodically jerked upwards. Pain relieved by motion and pressure. *After abuse of quinine.*

**NUX VOMICA.** *Darting pains from below upwards, [see

Ledum.] Stiffness and contraction of the limb. Can lie best on *painless* side, [see **Bry.**] *Pain relieved by hot water.*

**PHYTOLACCA.** *Neuralgic pain on outer side of thigh, shooting, drawing and aching. Worse from motion and pressure, and at night. *Rheumatic diathesis.*

**PLUMBUM.** Drawing, pressive pains in sciatic nerve, in posterior part of thigh, down to knee. Great exhaustion after walking. Tubercular diathesis, hacking cough.

**RHUS TOX.** If caused by exposure to wet or straining in lifting, [see **Arn.**] Sciatica of right side, dull, aching pain, worse at night, in cold or damp weather. Numbness and formication of parts, [**Lyc.**] *Pains relieved by rubbing, heat, and when warmed by exercise.*

**TELLURIUM.** *Pain in sacrum, passing into right thigh down sciatic nerve. *Worse when lying on painful side,* [better, **Bry. Ign.**] Chilly, with the pains, [**Ars. Bell.**]

**VALERIANA.** *Pain in hip and thigh, intolerable whilst standing, with a feeling as if the thigh would break off.

**AUXILIARY MEASURES.** Electricity often gives good results. Place positive pole over point where nerve emerges from sciatic foramen, and the negative where most pain is felt along the nerve. Bags of *hot* salt often relieve. Covering the part with flannel, and running a hot iron over, very beneficial. In some cases *cold* applications give most relief. The operation of *nerve-stretching* has proved successful.

---

## SMALL-POX.—VARIOLA.

### PREVENTIVE TREATMENT.

**VACCINATION.** A person should be *vaccinated* at least twice—in *infancy* and at *puberty*, and on other occasions when exposed to the *contagion*. Only the purest *vaccine* or *bovine virus* should be used. We prefer a *scab* from off the arm of a *healthy* child who has been vaccinated with *bovine* virus.

**Operation.** Take a small piece of the crust and moisten with water till of the consistence of cream. Now with the point of a lancet make several slight horizontal and transverse cuts in the skin, and rub the virus in, or, if points used, moisten and rub on in same manner.

**COURSE OF VACCINE DISEASE** is as follows:—

On 3d day.—A small, red, elevated spot appears.

On 6th day.—A pearl-colored vesicle, centre depressed.

On 8th day.—Vesicle distended with lymph, surrounded with red areola.

On 10th day.—Areola begins to fade.

On 14th day.—A dark-brown scab will have formed.

On 21st day.—The scab usually drops off.

On the evening of the 8th day it is best to give a dose of *Sulphur* or * *Thuya*, to abort any tendency to eruptive disease.

## MEDICAL TREATMENT.

**ACONITE.** At the commencement, during the febrile stage, especially if there be congestion to the head or lungs. Headache, bleeding at the nose, and injected eyes. Fullness in the chest, with increased action of the heart. Pain in the back, and aching in the limbs.

**AMM. CARB.** *Hemorrhagic diathesis*, [**Ham. Phos.**] Bleeding from nose, gums and bowels. *Putrid sore throat*, and tendency to gangrenous ulcerations.

**APIS MEL.** Erysipelatous redness and swelling, with stinging, burning pains. *Stinging and burning pains in throat, [**Acon.**] *Sensation in abdomen as if something tight would break.

**TARTAR EM.** This remedy has been found to greatly ameliorate the disease. It reduces the fever, and the pustules run their course, leaving scarcely a mark behind. Especially suited where there is much irritation of the respiratory organs.

**ARSENICUM.** The eruption is dark, and skin turns blue or livid. Great sinking of strength; small, frequent pulse and restlessness, [**Camph.**] *Extreme thirst, drinking little and often. *Great anguish and fear of death. Hæmorrhagic variola, [***Ham.**]

**BELLADONNA.** Congestion to head, with throbbing or stitching pain in forehead. High fever and sore throat. *Starting, jumping during sleep. Restless tossing about, cannot get to sleep. *Pain in back as if it would break. *Ophthalmia.*

**CAMPHOR.** Sudden desiccation of pustules and disappearance of swelling. *Extreme prostration and sinking of vital forces, [***Ars.**] *Great coldness of skin, but cannot bear to be covered.

**CIMICIFUGA.** *General bruised, sore feeling. Exhaustion, with nausea. Reduces the danger of pitting.

**HAMAMELIS.** *Hæmorrhagic variola. Blood, *dark, venous* and oozing from nose, gums, etc., [see **Amm. c.**] *Hæmatemesis*, bloody stools, uterine hemorrhage. Typhoid condition.

**HYDRASTIS.** Great redness, swelling and itching of skin, with very sore throat. *Intense aching in small of back, legs feel very weak and ache. It is said to prevent pitting to a great extent, [**Cimi.**]

**MERCURIUS.** During suppurative stage. *Moist, swollen tongue. *Ulcerated throat, with profuse flow of saliva.* Diarrhœa with green or bloody mucous stools, with tenesmus. *Perspiration without relief.

**OPIUM.** If brain becomes oppressed, and there is great *drowsiness, with stertorous breathing.* *Complete loss of consciousness. Dilated pupils.

**RHUS TOX.** The disease has assumed a typhoid character. Tongue dry and cracked, with red tip; corners of the mouth sore and ulcerated. Sordes on the lips and teeth, mind wandering. Great debility and restlessness. *Worse after midnight.

**SARRACENA.** It is claimed by some that this remedy exerts a salutary effect over all forms of the disease. But as we have no proving of it, there is no reliable data for its application.

**SULPHUR.** In early stage, and about the perid of desiccation; also as an intercurrent remedy when others seem to fail. *Metastasis to brain.*

**VACCININ and VARIOLIN** have been highly extolled as remedies in this disease. It is said, by those who have used them extensively, that all stages of the malady are shortened, and the disease rendered mild and harmless. *They promote suppuration and exsiccation, and prevent all scars.

**AUXILIARY MEASURES.** Complete isolation in upper airy room. The freest possible *ventilation.* Temperature of room at 60° F. *Cleanliness* of great importance. *Burn* all soiled rags, and disinfect all discharges and soiled linen. Sponge body frequently with *warm* water, and *dry* in a sheet *without rubbing.* Keep room dark, and protect pustules from injury. Cover the face with cloths saturated with *milk*, or a thick mucilage made of *starch* to prevent pitting. For ulcers in the mouth and throat, use gargle of *kali chlo.*, [8 grs. to ounce of water.]

**DIETETICS.** During inflammatory stage, milk, ripe fruits and mucilaginous drinks should constitute the chief articles of food. Later, a more nutritious diet must be allowed, animal broths, beef-tea, eggs, oysters, rice-puddings, toast, etc.

**FUMIGATION.** The room should be thoroughly *fumigated* after patient has left it, and the clothing destroyed or *buried* for a time in the earth.

---

## SORE NIPPLES.

**TREATMENT.** During the last few weeks of pregnancy the nipples should be manipulated with the thumb and finger wet with cold water, to accustom it to the friction of nursing. A weak solution of *Alum* or *Borax* is very good to harden the skin and prevent tenderness.

Where the skin has become excoriated and the nipples sore, as if bruised, bathing the parts with a solution of *Arnica* [20 drops to the ounce] will be found very useful. If ulcers form and incline to suppurate and bleed, use a lotion of *Calendula,* [30 drops to the ounce.] Anointing the parts with *Tr. Benzoin* and *Glycerine*, equal parts, valuable in the cure of fissures.

Where any of the above remedies have been applied, the nipples should be well washed off with *warm* water before allowing the child to nurse, and a rubber shield should be used to protect the parts until entirely healed.

Where the morbid condition depends upon a scrofulous taint, or some latent eruption, like tetter, erysipelas, etc., one of the following remedies should be exhibited.

**CALCARIA CARB.** Unhealthy skin, very little injury inclines to suppurate, [**Graph. Sulph.**] Sore, chapped nipples, with deep cracks. *Cold, damp feet.

**GRAPHITES.** The chapped nipples burn and ache, and are tender to touch. *Eruptions on skin oozing a sticky fluid. Skin dry, inclines to crack.

**HEPAR SULPH.** Deep cracks in the parts, which incline to suppurate. *Burning, stinging in the ulcers, which bleed easily. *Unhealthy skin.*

**SULPHUR.** Sore, chapped nipples, with deep fissures around the base, which bleed and burn. *Dry, scaly skin. *Scrofulous habit.*

---

## SORE THROAT.—ANGINA FAUCIUM.

**THERAPEUTICS.** *Leading indications.*

**ACONITE.** *Febrile excitement*, with anxiety and restlessness. *Dark redness of soft palate and uvula, with pricking, burning in throat. *Feeling of dryness, as if something had stuck in throat, and hoarseness.*

**ÆSCULUS HIP.** Tonsils dark, congested and swollen. *Dryness, burning and constriction in fauces. Pricking pain in fauces. *Hawks up ropy mucus* of a *sweetish taste*, [see **Kali b.**] *Hemorrhoids, with dull backache.

**AILANTHUS.** *Throat livid, swollen, tonsils studded with deep, angry-looking ulcers, with scanty, fetid discharge. *Neck tender and very much swollen.

**AMM. CARB.** Putrid sore throat, with burning pain, [**Apis. Arum. Bapt.**] Gangrenous ulcerations of tonsils.

**APIS MEL.** *Tonsils bright red, stinging when swallowing, [**Acon.**] Deep ulcers on tonsils or palate. *Great dryness of throat, [**Bell. Phos.**] *Erysipelatous and œdematous* appearance of throat. Hoarseness and difficulty in swallowing.

**ARGENT. NIT.** *Uvula and fauces dark red, [**Bell. Bapt. Cap.**—*bright red*, **Acon. Apis.**] *Thick, tenacious mucus in throat, obliging him to hawk, [**Cimi. Phos. ac. Kali. c.**] Sensation as if a *splinter had lodged in throat* when swallowing, [**Hepar. Nit. ac.**] *Head feels too large.

**ARUM TRI.** *Throat and tongue very sore, burning pains, putrid ulcers in fauces. Buccal cavity raw, sore, bleeding. *Refuses all food and drink on account of soreness.* *Lips as if scalded. *Acrid discharge from nose, excoriating nostrils and upper lip.

**BAPTISIA** *Fauces dark red, studded with dark putrid ulcers, [see **Ailanth.**] *Liability to quinsy from every slight cold*, [**Baryta.**] *Tongue cracked, sore, ulcerated.* *Throat feels as if constricted, [as if *expanded*, **Hyper.**] Tickling in throat provoking cough; uvula elongated, [**Cap.**]

**BARYTA CARB.** **Chronic induration of tonsils*, [**Lyc.**] Sensation as of a plug in throat, [**Bell. Lach. Merc. Nux.**] Smarting in throat when swallowing. *Scrofulous subjects.*

**BELLADONNA.** *Inflammatory redness of soft palate, uvula and tonsils. *Great dryness of throat*, [**Apis. Bry. Phos.**] Burning, shooting pains in throat when swallowing. *When drinking, fluids return through nose, [**Lach. Merc.**] *Constant inclination to swallow or hawk up something.* *Spasmodic constriction of fauces.

**CACTUS GRAND.** **Constriction of throat*, exciting a constant desire to swallow, [**Bell.**] Must take large draughts of water to force the fluid into stomach.

**CALC. CARB.** Inflammatory swelling of palate and uvula or tonsils, with constrictive sensation in throat when swallowing. Pain in throat, extending to ears. *Scrofulous diathesis.*

**CANTHARIS.** Burning in mouth, extending down pharynx, œsophagus and stomach, [**Gel.**] *Throat feels as if on fire, is inflamed and covered with plastic lymph.

**CAPSICUM.** *Inflammation, with dark redness and *burning in throat*, [**Acon. Bell.**] *Soreness, smarting, burning and biting in throat.* *Uvula elongated, feels as if pressing on something hard. *Chilliness in the back.*

**CHAMOMILLA.** *Soft palate and tonsils dark red*, [see **Arg. n.**] Sore throat, with swelling of parotid or submaxillary glands. **Catarrhal hoarseness of trachea*, with dryness of eyelids. *Redness of cheeks, or one red and the other pale, [**Acon.**]

**CIMICIFUGA.** *Dry spot in throat, causing cough. Dryness of pharynx, with constant desire to swallow. Sensation of *fullness* in throat, [**Gel. Glon. Sili.**] Uvula and palate swollen. Hawks up a viscid, coppery-tasting fluid, [soft *fetid tubercles*, color of peas, ***Mag.** c.—*hard, greenish lumps*, **Merc. iod. rub.**]

**GELSEMIUM.** *Fauces dry, burning, irritated, sore.* Tonsils inflamed, swollen, mostly in or beginning on *right* side, [**Bell. Lyc.**—*left side*, **Lach.**] *Throat feels as if filled up, [see **Cimi.**] Burning in œsophagus from mouth to stomach, [see **Canth.**] Hawking up bloody water, [*bloody mucus*, **Mag. m.**]

**HEPAR SULPH.** *Scraping in throat*, impeding speech. *Sensation in throat as if caused by a splinter or a fish-bone, [**Arg. n. Nit. ac.**] *Stitches in throat*, extending to ear when swallowing, or when turning the head, [see **Nux.**] *Hawking up mucus*, [see **Gel.**] *Unhealthy skin.*

**IGNATIA.** *Stitches in throat *when not swallowing*, [when swallowing, **Bry. Lach.**] Choking sensation from stomach up into throat. *Sensation of a lump in throat, [**Bell. Hep. Lach. Merc. Nux.**] *Better when swallowing food.*

**IODIUM.** *Swelling and elongation of uvula,* [**Bapt. Cap. Merc.**] Inflammation of throat with burning pain. Sensation of fullness in larynx, impeding deglutition, [see **Cimi.**] Ulcers in throat, with swelling of glands of neck.

**KALI BICHRO.** Fauces and palate erythematous, bright, or dark-red, or coppery. *Œdematous uvula. *Ulcers in fauces, discharging *cheesy lumps* of offensive smell, [hawks up soft, fetid tubercles, color of peas, ***Mag. c.**]

**LACHESIS.** Uvula elongated, fauces purplish, swollen or ulcerated. *Pain and soreness begin on *left* side, [*right* side, **Bell. Lach.**] When swallowing, pain shoots into ear, [**Apis.**] *Can bear nothing to touch the neck, [see **Phyto.**]

**LYCOPODIUM.** *Chronic enlargement of tonsils,* [**Bary. c.**] *Swelling and suppuration of tonsils, going from right to left, [see **Lach.**] Hawking bloody mucus, or hard, greenish-yellow phlegm, [**Mag. m.**—hawking yellow, tough mucus from posterior nares, **Hydras.**]

**MANCINELLA.** Angina following scarlatina. Great elongation of uvula, [**Bapt. Cap. Lach.**] Yellowish-white ulcers on tonsils, with violent burning pain. Choking sensation rises in throat when speaking.

**MERCURIUS.** *Uvula swollen, elongated.* *Rawness, roughness, and burning in throat. *Swelling and inflammatory redness of the affected parts.* *Difficult deglutition, especially of liquids, which frequently return through nose, [**Bell. Lach.**] *Tonsils dark-red, studded with ulcers. Painful dryness of throat, with *mouth full of saliva.* *Profuse sweating without relief. Worse at *night* and in evening.

**MERCURIUS COR.** *Uvula swollen, elongated, dark-red.* Throat intensely inflamed, preventing swallowing and causing suffocation. *Tonsils swollen and covered with ulcers.* *Pricking in throat as from needles. *Retching and vomiting on attempting to swallow.

**NUX VOMICA.** *Throat raw, sore, rough, as if scraped. Pain as if pharynx was constricted, or as if a plug was sticking in throat, during empty deglutition. *Stitches into the ear when swallowing,* [see **Lach.**] Irritable mood, sedentary habits.

**PHOSPHORUS.** *Rawness and scraping in pharynx,* worse towards evening, [in morning, **Nux.**] *Hoarseness with *loss of voice.* Dryness of throat day and night, it fairly glistens. Sensation as of cotton in throat.

**PHYTOLACCA.** Sore throat, worse on right side. Fauces dark, bluish-red, [purplish, **Lach.**] *Feels as if a red-hot ball was lodged in fauces. Cannot bear touch of clothing about neck, [**Lach.**] Uvula large, transparent *Cannot drink hot fluids.*

**PULSATILLA.** *Throat sore, and feels raw. *Veins prominent,* throat inflamed, bluish-red, [see **Phyto.**] Cutting, burning when swallowing. *Mild, tearful disposition.*

**RHUS TOX.** *After straining* the throat, it feels sore and stiff. *Erysipelatous inflammation of throat. [**Bell. Merc.**] Sticking or stinging pain, worse when beginning to swallow. *Throat feels swollen.* Rheumatic subjects.

**SILICEA.** Sore throat, with tough slime in the fauces. Tonsils swollen, each effort to swallow distorts face. *Throat feels as if filled up, [see **Gel.**] Pricking in throat as from a pin, causing cough. Frequent cough, bringing up white, frothy, saltish mucus.

**CLINICAL REMARKS.** In some cases of sore throat, especially where there is laryngeal complications, the use of the voice should be interdicted. When local suffering is severe, demulcent drinks as *hot gum arabic* or *ulmus fulva*-water will palliate. Drinking *hot water* or frequently gargling throat with the same will be found beneficial.

Persons subject to sore throat should wear good heavy shoes to protect the feet, flannel next the skin, and be careful to avoid draughts. [Comp. **Chronic Catarrh, page 62.**]

---

## SPOTTED FEVER.

(*Meningitis Cerebro-spinalis.*)

**THERAPEUTICS.** *Leading indications.*

**ACONITE.** Chill, fever, restlessness, and great thirst. Crawling or numbness in spine. Despairing mood and fear of death. *Painful stiff neck.

**ARNICA.** *Soreness in all the limbs as if bruised. Ecchymosed spots on skin, [**Crotal.**] Stupid, apathetic condition. *Great weakness of cervical muscles.*

**BELLADONNA.** *Violent throbbing headache, [**Chin. s.**] Great soreness and stiffness of neck, [**Bry.**] *Dilated pupils*, with double vision, [**Gel. Hyos.**] Delirium, with frightful figures before the eyes.

**BRYONIA.** *Splitting headache*, worse from motion, [**Bell.**] Stiffness of neck, [**Acon.**] Pain in joints and limbs, [**Crotal.**] Soreness of stomach.

**CHIN. SUPLH.** Involuntary closing of eyelids from prostration, [see **Gel.**] Violent throbbing headache, [**Bell.**] Redness of face, and vertigo. Great *prostration.* *Pain in dorsal vertebra on pressure.

**CIMICIFUGA.** Intense pain in head, as though a bolt were driven from neck to vertex with every throb of the heart. *Sensation as if top of head would fly off, and as if the cerebellum was too large for skull. Stiffness of the back, [**Bell. Bry.**] *Tonic and clonic spasms*, [**Hyos.**] Intense pain in eyeballs. Tongue swollen.

**CROTALUS.** *Horrid headache*, with feeling of *tightness* in brain, [**Opi.**] Red face and delirium, with open eyes, [**Opi.**]

Red spots on all parts of body. Pain in all the limbs, [**Bry.**] *Heart-beat feeble.*

**GELSEMIUM.** Dull pain in back part of head. *Feels as if intoxicated.* *Paralysis of eyelids. Double vision and dilated pupils, [**Bell. Hyos.**] *Complete loss of muscular power.* Pulse very feele, [*very slow*, **Opi.**] Labored breathing. Nausea and vomiting.

**LYCOPODIUM.** Stupor and delirium, [**Opi.**] *Stupefying headache extending down the neck.* *Fan-like motion of nostrils. Sinking of lower jaw, [**Opi.**] Jerkings of limbs and body.

**OPIUM.** *Stupor, and deep, slow breathing. *Congestion to head, occiput feels heavy as lead.* *Very quick or very *slow pulse.* Drawing the body backwards and rolling it from side to side. Spasms, with tossing of limbs. *Worse while sweating,* [better, **Gel.**]

**AUXILIARY MEASURES.** Free *perspiration* is advised in the *early* stage. Put two teaspoonfuls of *Alcohol* in a gill of water, and give teaspoonful doses every half hour until desired effect is produced. Others advise *hot baths*, and wrapping in warm blankets to induce perspiration; while others again use hypodermic injections of *Pilocarpin* [1/6 of a grain] or Fl. Extr. *Jaborandi* [10 to 30 drops] every half hour until free sweating occurs.

**DIETETICS.** Plain, simple food should be given during the stage of excitement, as in other febrile diseases. During the stage of depression, beef essence, broths, milk, eggs, oysters, etc., should be served liberally.

---

## SPRAINS.

**THERAPEUTICS.** If case is seen early, and before inflammation has set in, apply compresses wet in *cold Arnicated* water. These must be changed frequently and the limb kept elevated and at perfect rest. Should the parts become *inflamed* and swollen, substitute *hot Arnicated fomentations* for the cold compresses, and give *Arnica* internally.

Other remedies as **Rhus. Ruta** and **Hyper.** are valuable in some cases, and may be used externally and internally when properly indicated.

**LEADING INDICATIONS.**

**ARNICA.** Chief remedy in injuries of this kind. *Much swelling, with bluish redness and intense soreness. Pains almost insufferable.

**RHUS TOX.** Especially for sprains from over-liftng, particularly where tendons are involved. *Pain as if the flesh was torn from the bones. Worse *after* midnight and in *dump weather.*

**HYPERICUM.** Sprains or lacerations where *nerves* are

severely involved. The parts feel as if dislocated; pains excruciating. Threatened lockjaw.

**RUTA GRAV.** Sprains and other mechanical injuries where *periosteum* is especially involved. Bruised feeling all over, [**Arn. Hyp.**] Worse in *wet, cold weather.*

**ACONITE.** High fever; restlessness, and nervous excitability. Pains insupportable, especially at night.

---

## STOMATITIS.

**THERAPEUTICS.** *Leading indications.*

**ARSENICUM.** *Aphthæ in mouth, they become livid or bluish. Painful blisters in mouth and on tongue burning like fire. Edge of tongue red, takes imprint of teeth, [***Merc.**] *Swollen, bleeding gums,* [**Bapt.**]

**BAPTISIA.** Putrid ulceration of buccal cavity with salivation, [**Merc. Phyt.**] Gums loose, flabby, dark-red, purple, fetid. *Fauces dark-red, studded with dark, putrid ulcers. *Stomatitis materna,* [**Bapt. Carb. v. Hydras.**]

**CANTHARIS.** *Mucous membrane, red, and covered with small blisters. Burning pain in mouth, throat, and stomach. *Copious, disgusting, sweet saliva.* *Urging to urinate, with painful emissions by drops.

**CAPSICUM.** Small, flat, *burning ulcers* in mouth and fauces. *Fetid breath, smelling like carrion. *Throat inflamed, dark-red, burning, biting. Viscid, offensive saliva.

**CARBO VEG.** Mouth hot, tongue almost immovable, saliva bloody. *Gums loose, receding, ulcerated, and bleeding. *Greatly troubled with flatulence.*

**DULCAMARA.** Stomatitis after abuse of *mercury,* [**Carb. v. Iod. Iris. Nit. ac.**] Gums spongy, saliva tenacious, and cervical glands swollen. Rheumatic diathesis.

**HELLABORUS.** Mouth, gums, and tongue full of flat, yellow ulcers, with elevated gray edges. Carrion-like odor from mouth, [**Cap.**] *Tongue trembling, numb.*

**HYDRASTIS.** *Stomatitis after mercury,* or *chlorate of potash,* [see **Dulc.**] *Ulcers in mouth of nursing women, or weakly children. *Peppery taste;* tongue as if burned, or raw, with dark-red appearance and raised papillæ. *Rawness of fauces, and ulcers in throat.

**IODIUM.** Gums red and swollen, receding from teeth, bleeding slightly. *Painful ash-colored ulcers in mouth. *Profuse fetid ptyalism.* Ulcers in throat, with swelling of glands of the neck.

**IRIS VERS.** Burning in mouth and fauces, as if on fire. Ulcers on mucous lining of checks. Saliva tastes greasy. *Tongue feels as if scalded, [**Hydras.**]

**KALI IOD.** *Irregular ulcers, looking as if coated with milk. Bloody saliva, with sweetish taste in mouth. Burning of the tip of the tongue.

**MERCURIUS.** Mouth inflamed, with burning, aphthous ulcers. *Copious, fetid, ropy salivation. *Red, spongy, receding, ulcerated gums, with burning pains at night. *Teeth loose and gums painful to touch.* *Tongue swollen, flabby, taking imprint of teeth, [**Ars.**] *Glands swollen.*

**MERC. CORRO.** Mouth feels as if scalded, [*tongue*, **Iris. Hydras.**] *Corroding, eating ulcers* in mouth, throat, and on gums, with fetid breath. *Ptyalism*, with salty taste; saliva bloody, yellowish, tough, acrid. Painful burning in mouth, extending to stomach.

**NITRIC ACID.** Mucous membrane swollen, ulcerated, with burning pains, especially after abuse of mercury. *Gums white, swollen, bleeding. Teeth loose, [***Merc.**] *Cadaverous smell from mouth*, [**Merc.**] Corners of mouth ulcerated. Parotid glands swollen.

**NUX VOMICA.** Roof of mouth, throat and gums inflamed, swollen. *Small aphthous ulcers in mouth, with putrid smell. Gums white, putrid, bleeding. *High livers and persons of sedentary habits.*

**PHYTOLACCA.** Inflammation and ulceration of buccal cavity. *Small ulcers on inside of cheek, very painful. Tonsils enlarged, bluish, ulcerated. Yellow saliva, of a metallic taste. Teeth feel sore.

**SILICEA.** Stomatitis, mouth gangrenous, with perforating ulcer on palate. *Gums inflamed, and very sore. *Constipation, stool recedes after being partially expelled. *Throat feels as if filled up.*

**AUXILIARY MEASURES.** As local applications in the severer cases, some advise a weak solution *Sulphite of Soda*, [a drachm to ounce water,] rinse mouth three or four times a day. *Carbolic Acid* one drachm, *Glycerine* two ounces, water six ounces. Mix and wash the mouth out several times a day. A solution of *Kali Chlo.* [8 grains to the ounce] is also recommended.

**DIETETICS.** Strict attention should be given to diet. Well boiled rice, oatmeal gruel, farina, fresh milk, mutton broth, cracker gruel, barley water, and in some cases beef tea. Acids of all kinds, sweets, and condiments must be avoided.

---

## STYE.—HORDEOLUM.

A small inflammatory tumor located on the free edge of eyelids, usually near the inner angle of the eye. It is often very painful, and attended with headache.

**TREATMNET.** *Special indications.*

**PULSATILLA** This remedy given in the early stage will usually disperse it. *Especially adapted to styes on *upper* lid, [**Phos. ac. Lyc.**—on *lower* lids, **Rhus.**] Lids swollen, itch, burn.

**STAPHYSAGRIA.** Frequently appearing styes. Margins of lids dry, with *hardened* styes, or tarsal tumors, sometimes ulcerating.

**HEPAR SULPH.** Where there is a tendency to a *recurrence* of the complaint; suppuration inevitable. *Unhealthy skin, every little injury inclines to suppurate.

**MERCURIUS.** Tumor *hard*, inflamed and painful. The abscess *matures very slowly*, [Hepar.] *Profuse sweating without relief.

**LOCAL MEASURES.** Some cases require mild flaxseed meal poultices or *hot* fomentations to relieve the pain. Soon as abscess points open with *sharp* lancet.

---

## SUNSTROKE.—COUP DE SOLEIL.

**THERAPEUTICS.** *Leading indications.*

**ACONITE.** *If the head has been exposed to direct rays of sun, or body to excessive heat.* Arteries of head throb violently. Violent thirst, red face, shortness of breath, and great nervous excitability.

**AMYL NITRITE.** *Congestive stage of sunstroke.* Great anxiety, and longing for fresh air. Head confused and giddy, as if intoxicated. *Head feels full to bursting, with sensation of blood rushing upwards. **Red face, with flashes of heat, particularly up sides of head.* Dyspnœa and constriction in chest and heart, [Cact.]

**BELLADONNA.** *Severe headache and fullness as if head would split; worse when stooping. Feeling in forehead as if brain would be pressed out. *Vertigo when stooping or rising from a sitting posture.

**BRYONIA.** *Splitting headache*, aggravated by the least motion, [Bell.] Very peevish in morning, is more passionate and cross than plaintive. *Cannot sit up from nausea and faintness. *Dry, hard stools, as if burnt. Head feels *too full*, [*too large*, *Glon.]

**CAMPHOR.** Sunstroke or inflammation of brain arising from exposure to sun. *Throbbing*, like beats with a hammer, in cerebellum, [see Glon.] Eyes fixed, staring, turned upwards or outwards. *Skin icy cold, covered with cold sweat. *Sinking of vital forces.*

**GLONOINE.** Intense congestion to head. *Feeling as if temples and top of head would burst open. *Violent *throbbing headache*, with increased action of heart. Fullness and pressure in forepart and top of head, with confusion of senses. *Sensation of balancing, requiring a constant effort to keep head erect Undulating sensation, increased by every turn of head. Sick, faint, death-like sinking at epigastrium, with nausea.

**GELSEMIUM.** Severe pain in forehead and vertex, dim

sight, roaring in ears. *Head feels enlarged, [Glon.] Great fullness in head, heat in face with chilliness. Pulsations of the carotids; thick speech. Brain feels as if bruised.

**AUXILIARY MEASURES.** Place patient at once in the shade or in a cool room. Have but few persons about. Loosen the body clothing and envelope the whole head in clothes wrung out of *hot water* and change them often. Sponging the body off quickly with *warm* water, then wrapping it in a *dry sheet without* rubbing will be found of great value. If the feet are cold immerse them in *hot water*, or apply warm bricks to them.

If patient is in a syncopal state, the inhalation of a few drops of *Amyl Nitrite*, or the holding of spirits of *Ammonia* under the nostrils will give good results.

Soon as patient can swallow, give a little beef-tea, milk, or warm coffee to drink.

---

## TETANUS AND LOCKJAW.

**THERAPEUTICS.** *Leading indications.*

**ACONITE.** Frequent alternation of redness and paleness of face, and distortion of eyes, [Glon.] Tetanus in which the body is bent backwards, [Cicu. Ign. *Nux. Opi.—bent *forward*, Cup. Hydro. ac.—*backwards and forwards*, Bell.] Face covered with cold sweat. *Rigidity of muscles of jaws and neck.*

**BELLADONNA.** Great restlessness, with convulsive twitching of muscles of face, jaw, and limbs. *Sudden jerks and shrieks during sleep. *Inability to swallow. Clinched teeth*, with painful stiffness of muscles of mastication. *Lock-jaw, [Cicu. *Hydro. ac. *Opi. Verat. a.] Spasmodic motions of body, generally backwards. *Throws body forwards and backwards. Involuntary discharges of fæces and urine, [Hyos. Verat. a.]

**CAMPHOR.** Tetanic spasms, with loss of consciousness. *Limbs extended and fixed, head bent sideways, lower jaw rigid and wide open. Oppressed, anxious, panting breathing. *Great coldness of external surface.

**CICUTA VIROSA.** *Lockjaw and tetanic rigidity from injuries inflicted upon head and spinal column.* *Convulsions, with loss of consciousness, frightful distortions of limbs and whole body. Deadly paleness of face. *Body bent backwards, [see Acon.] Inability to swallow.

**CUPRUM.** *Jaws closed, with loss of consciousness, and foam at mouth. Twitching, jerkings, or startings during sleep, [Bell.] *Body bent forward, [bent *backwards*, Cicu. *Nux. Opi.] Stiffness of whole body, [Bell.]

**HYDROC. AC.** *Tetanic spasms, with *lockjaw*. Bloating of face and neck. Protruded glistening eyes, with dilated pupils, [Bell. Hyos.] Blackish-red color of face. Trunk bent forward or backward, [Bell.] *Irregular pulse.*

**HYOSCYAM.** *Dark-red, bloated face, with protruding eyes. *Clinching of teeth and foam at mouth.* Alternate convulsions of upper and lower extremities. Drawing of neck to one side. Rigidity of hands, contortions, and spasmodic curvings of body. *Involuntary discharges of fæces and urine.

**NUX VOMICA.** *Intermittent fits of spasms, with bending of body backwards,* and disturbed respiration. *Extreme *stiffness of limbs,* with great hardness of muscles. Spasmodic attacks from the merest touch. *Full consciousness during the spasms, [loss of, Camp. Cicu. Cup.]

**OPIUM.** *Staring, glistening eyes, pupils dilated and insensible to light, [Hydro. ac.] Red, bloated, swollen face, [see Hyos.] *Lockjaw. *Tetanic spasms, with rigidity of neck, or whole body,* the trunk curved in form of an arch. *Urine suppressed,* bowels constipated.

**PHYTOLACCA.** Reddish-blue swelling of eyelids, *pupils contracted.* *Chin drawn closely to sternum by convulsive action of muscles of face and neck. *Lips everted and firm.* Extremities stiff, hands firmly shut, feet extended, and toes flexed. General muscular rigidity. Respiration difficult.

**STRAMONIUM.** Eyes wide open, rolling, squinting. Lockjaw, mouth spasmodically closed. Bending of neck backwards, [see Cup.] Hands clinched. Violent motion of limbs, with stretching and trembling of hands.

**VERAT. VIR.** Twitching, contortion of eyes, rolling of balls. Cold, bluish face, covered with cold sweat. *Muscles of back contracted, drawing head backward. Shocks in limbs, [Nux.] Head jerking or continually nodding.

**AUXILIARY TREATMENT.** *Chloral Hydrate* is highly commended in the treatment of this distressing malady, especially in the subacute form. It may be administered hypodermically, and also by the mouth and rectum. Hypodermic dose 5 grs. dissolved in glycerine. By the mouth, average dose 10 to 30 grs. [in syrup with a little peppermint water] repeated every hour or two. As an enema, 15 to 60 grs. in a little water, rubbed up with the yolk of egg, and mixed with milk.

Atropia, administered hypodermically in $\frac{1}{10}$ grain doses, has cured many cases. The *hot* bath, or *hot-water* bags to the spine, and prolonged *sweating* has given good results.

Keep temperature of room at about 70° F. and patient very quiet; allow free *ventilation* but avoid drafts and cold air.

**DIETETICS.** Nourish well with beef-tea, animal soups, milk, soft eggs, oysters, etc. In some cases it may be necessary to give nutrient enemata, [see page 17.]

# TINEA CAPITIS.—SCALD HEAD.

**THERAPEUTICS.** *Leading indications.*

**ARCTIUM LAPPA.** Head covered with a *grayish-white crust*, and most of hair gone. Moist, bad-smelling eruptions on heads of children, [**Brom. Lyc.**] Crusta lactea, with swelling and suppuration of axillary glands.

**ARSENICUM.** *Dry, scald head,* [**Calc. Merc. Sep. Sili. Sulph.**—*moist eruptions,* **Clem. Graph. Hepar. Lyc. Rhus. Staph.**] Scalp covered with *dry scales and scabs,* sometimes extending to forehead and face. *Burning, itching eruption, *better from warmth.*

**BROMIUM.** Malignant scald head, with dirty-looking and *offensive-smelling* discharge, [**Psor.**] In places where eruption is dry, skin throws off flakes. Scalp tender to touch. *Swelling and induration of glands.

**CALC. CARB.** *Thick scabs, with yellow pus, spreading to face. Whitish-yellow scales of dandruff, hair dry and falls out on sides of head, [**Graph.**] **Scrofulous children,* with large heads and open fontanelles, [**Sulph.**]

**CLEMATIS.** Tinea on back part of head and neck. Eruptions moist and sore, often drying up in scales. Parts itch violently, worse on getting warm in bed, [**Merc.**] Temporary relief from scratching, [**Sulph.**]

**DULCAMARA.** Ringworm on scalp, glands of throat swollen. *Thick crusts on scalp, causing hair to fall out. Tinea oozing a *watery* fluid, [a *sticky* fluid, **Graph.**—a *corroding* fluid, **Nat. m.**] *Worse in damp, cold weather.*

**GRAPHITES.** Vesicular eruption of entire scalp, forming dirty crusts, matting hair together. *The eruption exudes a *sticky glutinous* fluid. *Rawness in bend of limbs, groins, neck, behind ears. *Unhealthy skin.*

**HEPAR SULPH.** *Humid eruptions* on scalp, feeling sore, of fetid odor, [**Lyc.**] Falling out of the hair, with very sore, painful pimples, and large bald spots on scalp.

**LYCOPODIUM.** *Eruption, beginning on back of head; crusts thick, easily bleeding, oozing a fetid moisture, [see **Rhus.**] Worse after scratching and from warmth.

**MERCURIUS.** *Pustular, fetid eruption on scalp, with yellow crusts. Parts bleed when scratched, [**Lyc. Sulph.**] Hair falls out on temples and sides, [**Graph.**] Itching worse at night, when warm in bed.

**MEZEREUM.** Head covered with a thick, leathery crust, under which pus collects and mats the hair, [see **Viola.**] *Elevated, white chalk-like scabs, with ichor beneath, breeding vermin. *Burning, biting, itching* on scalp, scratching changes locality.

**RHUS TOX.** *Eruption suppurating, moist, forming thick crusts, offensive, itching. Hair is eaten off and drops out. Intolerable itching of parts, worse at night.

**SILICEA.** *Eruption on back of head, moist or dry,

offensive, scabby, burning, itching, discharging pus. Eruption in patches on scalp, exfoliating thin, dry, bran-like scales. Glands of neck swollen. *Constipation, stools recede after being partially expelled.

**STAPHISAGRIA.** *Humid, itching, fetid eruption on occiput, sides of head, and behind ears. Scratching increases the oozing. *Teeth turn black.*

**SULPHUR.** *Humid, offensive eruption, with thick pus, yellow crusts, itching, bleeding, and burning. Scalp sore to touch, itching violently in evening, when getting warm in bed. After other well-chosen remedies have failed to produce desired effect.

**VIOLA TRICO.** *Thick incrustations, pouring out a large quantity of thick yellow fluid, which agglutinates the hair. Tinea capitis, with frequent involuntary urination. *Urine smelling like cat's urine.

**AUXILIARY MEASURES.** The hair should be kept closely trimmed, the head frequently washed with warm water, and the whole person kept scrupulously clean. A little *Olive oil* or *Vaseline* may be applied to the parts to soften the dry scabs and facilitate their removal. In some cases it may be necessary to apply flaxseed meal poultices to remove the crusts, after which dress with a little *Vaseline.*

---

## TONSILLITIS.—QUINSY.

**THERAPEUTICS.** *Leading indications.*

**ACONITE.** Tonsils swollen, inflamed, and of a dark red color, with fever, [Bell.] Pain and great difficulty in swallowing or in speaking. Burning, pricking or contracting sensation in the throat. *Great restlessness and nervous excitability.

**AMM. MUR.** Swelling and inflammation of both tonsils. The patient can neither swallow, talk, nor open his mouth. *After taking cold,* [Merc.] *Tendency to gangrenous ulceration. Hawking up *tough* phlegm.

**APIS MEL.** *Red and highly inflamed tonsils,* with dryness in mouth and throat. *Burning, stinging pain in throat when swallowing, [Acon.] Can bear nothing to touch his neck, [Lach.] *Throat swollen outside.* Aggravation from heat, better from cold.

**BARYTA C.** Raw, scraping or shooting pain when swallowing. Sensation of a plug in throat. *The tonsils incline to suppurate, [Hepar.] *Chronic induration of tonsils, [Lyc.] *Scrofulous diathesis,* [Hep. Sil. Sul.]

**BELLADONNA.** Tonsils *swollen, inflamed, and of a dark red color;* ulcers soon forming, [Merc.] Burning and shooting pains in throat when swallowing. *The throat feels as if a plug were in it. *Drinking produces spasms in throat, fluids return through nose, [Lach. Merc.] Constant inclination to swallow or hawk up something. Especially *right* side, [*left*, **Lach.**]

**HEPAR SULPH.** Where there is a frequent recurrence of the disease. Sticking pain as from a fish-bone in throat when swallowing. Sensation of a *lump in throat*, [**Bell. Merc. Nux.**] ***Inclination to suppurate.** Persons of a scrofulous habit. After abuse of mercury.

**LACHESIS.** Tonsillitis, especially on left side. When swallowing, pain extends to ear. Fluids escape through nose when being swallowed, [**Apis.**] Sensation of a plug in throat, [see **Hepar.**] ***Cannot bear anything to touch the neck, not even bedclothes.** ***Worse in afternoon, and after sleep.**

**MERCURIUS.** Tonsils swollen, inflamed, and dark red, or become ulcerated. Offensive odor from mouth. Aphthæ, or thick yellow coating on tongue. Violent pricking pains when swallowing, extending to ears or glands of throat. Gums and back part of tongue swollen. ***Profuse discharge of saliva.** ***Much perspiration, which does not relieve.** *Worse at night.*

**MERC. IOD. RUB.** Slimy or metallic taste. Tongue furred, wrinkled, feels scalded. ***Left tonsil swollen, fauces red, and submaxillary glands painfully enlarged.** Hawks and spits a tough white phlegm. ***Difficult deglution, with ulcers in the throat.** Will often *prevent* suppuration.

**NUX VOMICA.** If derangement of stomach be predisposing cause. Sensation as if a lump were in throat when swallowing. The throat feels raw, or as if scraped, [**Hepar.**] ***Patient very irritable, and wishes to be alone.** Dyspeptics and persons who have been drugged with mixtures. Symptoms worse in morning.

**SILICEA.** When the appearance of throat indicates the *formation of an abscess*, attended with stitches and throbbing pain, [***Hepar.**] ***Throat feels filled up.** Mostly on left side. Scrofulous persons.

**SULPHUR.** Where there is a frequent recurrence of the disease. ***After suppuration parts remain sore, and heal slowly,** [***Hepar.**] Scrofulous persons troubled with boils; every little scratch of skin suppurates. ***Lean persons who walk stooping.** ***Frequent weak, faint spells.** *Chronic enlargement of tonsils* require: ***Baryta c. Cal. c.** ***Calc. iod.** ***Cal. phos. Hepar. Ign. Lyc.** ***Merc. Iod. Sulph.**

**AUXILIARY MEASURES.** Inhaling the vapor of *hot water* in which the *indicated* remedy has been dissolved will greatly relieve the suffering. Holding *hot milk* or *hot gruel* in the mouth will also be found valuable. When suppuration becomes inevitable (indicated by throbbing pain, swelling and tenderness externally), *warm* flaxseed meal poultices will relieve the pain and hasten suppuration. Gargling the throat with *hot milk* or *hot water* after the abscess has burst, will be beneficial. In *follicular tonsillitis*, or where the discharge is *offensive*, gargling throat with a solution of *Permanganate of potash* (4 grs. to the pint) will be found very useful.

**DIETETICS.** Hot milk, beef tea, mutton broth, and oatmeal porridge, blanc-mange, or any nourishing food that can be swallowed.

---

## TOOTHACHE.

**THERAPEUTICS.** *Leading indications.*

**ACONITE.** The patient is almost frantic with pain, which is indescribable. Stitching or throbbing pain, with congestion to head, and great restlessness. *Constant fear and anxiety of mind, with great nervousness.

**ANTIMONIUM.** Pains in carious teeth, followed by jerking and gnawing, extending up to head, especially in evening, in bed. Pains worse after eating, or from cold water, [**Bry. Cham. Nux v. Merc.**] The gums bleed readily, and recede from the teeth.

**ARSENICUM.** Elongation and painful looseness of teeth. Drawing, jerking pains in teeth and gums, extending to ears, cheeks and temples. Pains intolerable, driving patient to despair, [**Acon. Cham.**] *Prostration, restlessness, drinking often, and but little.*

**BELLADONNA.** Drawing, tearing pains in teeth, face and ears, with swelling of cheek. Ptyalism or dryness of throat and mouth, with great thirst. *Pains which come on suddenly, and leave just as suddenly. Face flushed, and eyes red. Pains worse after lying down at night, or in cold air.

**BRYONIA.** Pains in carious, and still more in sound teeth. *Sensation of elongation* in teeth, with jerking drawing pains. Worse at night, or from taking anything warm in mouth, [**Cham. Nux v. Puls.**] Mouth unusually dry, with thirst. *Constipation, stools dry and hard, as if burnt. Exceedingly irritable. Wants to be perfectly still.

**CALC. CARB.** Beating, stitching, boring pains, or soreness of teeth. *The pains are aggravated by a draught of air, by drinking anything *warm* or *cold*, or by the slightest change, [**Nux m. Puls.**]

**CHAMOMILLA.** After taking cold when in a perspiration. The pains are drawing, jerking, or *beating* and *stitching*. Intolerable pains, especially at night, driving one to despair, [see **Acon.**] Hot swelling of cheeks, and red, swollen gums. Worse in open air and at night, [**Bell. Merc. Phos. Rhus.**] *Very impatient, can scarcely give a civil answer.

**COFFEA.** Insupportable pains, which drive patient almost frantic, [**Acon. Cham.**] *The pain is relieved by ice-cold water, [**Bry. Cham.**] *Head feels contracted or too small. *Excessive wakefulness.

**DULCAMARA.** Toothache from taking cold in damp or wet weather, and if accompanied by diarrhœa. Confusion of head, and profuse salivation. The teeth feel blunt, [**Acon. Chin. *Nux m. *Puls.**] *Symptoms always worse by a cold change in the weather.

**MERCURIUS.** Tearing pains in several teeth at the same time, [**Cham. Rhus.**] Drawing and stinging pains, which extend to ear, especially in *carious* teeth, worse at night. *The pains are excited by cool, damp air, or by eating anything hot or cold, [***Bry. Nux. Puls.**] *The teeth feel sore, loose and too long. *Perspiration does not relieve. *Much saliva in mouth.*

**MEZEREUM.** Mostly in *carious* teeth, [**Merc.**] *Pains boring, stinging, extending to malar bones and temples. Teeth feel dull and elongated, [**Bry. Cham. Rhus.**] Worse by contact, motion, or in the evening, with chilliness.

**NUX MOS.** Suitable to children, and women during *pregnancy*, [**Cham. *Sep. Puls.**] After taking cold in damp, wet weather, [**Rhus.**] Better from warm water or warm applications, [**Rhus. Staph.**] *Great dryness of the mouth, and disposition to faint.

**NUX VOMICA.** Sore pains or jerking, drawing, with stitches in teeth and jaw. Pains extending to head, ears, and malar bones, with painful swelling of submaxillary glands, [**Merc.**] Worse at night, or in *morning*, from mental labor, cold or cold things; better from warm drinks. *He feels cross and irritable. *Persons of sedentary habits, and who live on stimulating food.

**PULSATILLA.** Suited to persons of a mild, tearful disposition. *Toothache, with otalgia and hemicrania. Pains tearing, drawing, stitching, or jerking, as if the nerves were put upon the stretch, and then suddenly let go again. *Better from cold things, and worse from warm, [**Bry. Cham. Coff.**] *Chilliness even in a warm room. *Scanty or suppressed menses.*

**SEPIA.** Toothache *during pregnancy*, [of *nursing* females, **Chin.**] The pains are beating, stitching, and extend to ears, and along arm to fingers, where they terminate in a creeping sensation. *Swelling of cheeks* and submaxillary glands, [**Merc. Nux.**] *Sallow complexion, with spots on face. *Profuse leucorrhœa* having a fetid smell.

**SPIGELIA.** *Throbbing pains in decayed teeth; dark redness of the affected side. Flow of water from the eyes and nose, [**Merc. Puls.**] Pains worse from cold water or going into open air. *Palpitation of heart, chilliness, restlessness.

**STAPHISAGRIA.** *Black, crumbling, carious teeth, [**Kreo.**] *Pale, white, ulcerated, swollen, and painful gums.* *Gnawing, tearing in decayed teeth; shooting into ear; throbbing in temples. Worse early in morning, and after drinking anything cold. Cold sweat in face, and cold hands.

**SULPHUR.** Jumping pain in hollow teeth, extending to upper jaw, or to ears. Looseness, elongation, or dullness of teeth, [see **Mez.**] Aggravation or renewal of pains in open air, at night in bed, or from *cold water.* *Burning heat in top of head, and cold extremities. *Scanty, black menstrual discharges.

**AUXILIARY MEASURES.** Where the pain is caused by exposure of the nerve, saturate a pledget of lint in a mixture of equal parts *Carbolic ac.* and *Iodine*; introduce this into the tooth, then close the cavity with a little beeswax, and allow it to remain a few hours. A little *Chloroform* applied in the same way will also have a happy effect. Warm fomentations or hot salt bags applied to the painful jaw will often relieve.

---

## TYPHOID FEVER.

(*Enteric Fever ; Abdominal Typhus.*)

**PROGNOSIS.** Coma; convulsions; marked picking of bedclothes; subsultus tendinum; persistent delirium; pulse frequent and feeble, first sound of heart notably weak; great prostration; intestinal hemorrhage, are omens of *great danger.* In case of pregnancy, abortion generally takes place, and death follows. Temperature 105°, grave; 106° or 107°, mostly fatal. On the other hand, a *decrease* of temperature much below normal, is extremely ominous.

*Prognosis favorable* so long as pulse not above 110 or 115, and resistive; temperature not over 104°; no serious complications; abdominal symptoms mild; carphologia, subsultus, etc., not marked.

**THERAPEUTICS.** *Special indications.*

**ACONITE.** Chill and synochal fever, with full, bounding pulse, great heat, dry, burning skin, and violent thirst. *Great fear and anxiety of mind, with much nervous excitability. *Headache as if everything would press out of the forehead, with vertigo on rising up. Mostly in the first stage.

**BAPTISIA.** *Incipient stage,* [see **Gel. Merc.**] Face dark red, with a besotted expression. Dull, stupefying headache, with confusion of ideas. *Head feels as if scattered around, patient tosses about to get pieces together. Tongue coated *brown, dry,* particularly in centre, [*clean, parched, dry,* **Hyos. Rhus.**] Sordes on teeth; very offensive breath. Offensive and exhausting diarrhœa. *Sweat, urine and stools all extremely fetid.

**BRYONIA.** Face red, burning and swollen. *Lips dry, brownish and cracked. Tongue coated with a thick, white or yellowish fur; *later brown and dry,* [dry, red and cracked, **Rhus.**] *Oppressive, stupefying headache,* or pain as if head would split, *worse from least motion.* *Delirium day and night, with strange fancies, and desire to escape and go home, [Bell.] Constant desire to sleep, with *sudden starting and strange dreams*, or sleeplessness, with restless tossing about. *Dryness of mouth without thirst, or with thirst, drinking large quantities at a time. *Cannot sit up from nausea and faintness. Great soreness in stomach. *Constipation, stools dry and hard.

**BELLADONNA.** Face flushed and bloated, with red, sparkling eyes and dilated pupils. *Throbbing headache, with violent pulsation of carotids.* *Intolerance of noise or light, [**Acon.**] Delirium, with a wild look; *he wishes to strike, bite, or quarrel.* Starting, jumping during sleep, with desire to escape. *Sleepiness, but cannot sleep, [***Lach. Opi.**] Tongue dry, red and cracked, or red on edges and white in centre. Tenderness of abdomen, the least jar of bed painful.

**RHUS TOX.** *Prostrate and stupid.* Face red and swollen, with blue circles around eyes. Lips dry, brownish, or black. *Tongue dry, red and smooth, or *red at tip in shape of triangle.* Muttering delirium, or talking to himself. Stoppage of the ears and dullness of hearing. Dry, troublesome cough, with *oppression of chest.* *Severe pains in limbs, worse during rest. Diarrhœa, with profuse, watery, sanguineous, or jelly-like evacuations. *Involuntary stools, with great exhaustion, [see **Hyos.**] *Worse at night, particularly after midnight.

**ARSENICUM.** *Face pale, shrunken, hippocratic.* Cold sweat on forehead, [**Verat. a.**] Constant licking of lips, which are dark, dry and cracked. *Sordes on teeth,* [**Bapt. Hyos. Stram.**] Tongue dry, shriveled, bluish or black, with inability to protrude it. *Intense thirst, drinking little and often, [**Apis. Chin.**] Coma or low muttering delirium, and trembling of limbs. *Extreme prostration. *Great anguish, extreme restlessness and fear of death. Ileo-typhus, [**Carb. v. Phos. ac. Rhus.**]

**APIS MEL.** The patient remains in a stupid, unconscious state, with muttering delirium. Inability to talk or put out tongue, which is cracked, ulcerated, or covered with vesicles, [**Nux. Puls.**] Dryness of mouth and throat, with difficulty of swallowing. *Great soreness in pit of stomach and abdomen. Constipation, or frequent, foul, bloody mucus and involuntary stools. White miliary eruptions on chest and abdomen. *Great weakness and sliding down in bed. [***Mur. ac. Zinc.**]

**ARNICA.** Stupid, apathetic condition, with greatest indifference, [**Phos. ac.**] Tongue dry, with a *brown* streak in middle, [*red* streak, **Verat. v.**—red edges, *white* centre, **Bell. Gel.**] Confusion of thought, when speaking forgets the word, [falls asleep in midst of a sentence, ***Bapt.**] *Sore, bruised feeling all through patient, which compels him to constantly change position. *If conscious, he complains of bed being too hard, [**Bapt.**] Involuntary discharges of fæces and urine.

**LYCOPODIUM.** Earthy, yellow complexion. Tongue dry, black, cracked, or covered with tough mucus. Sopor, delirium, slow breathing, with open mouth, [**Opi.**] Prostration, and depression of lower jaw. *Circumscribed redness of cheeks. He uses wrong words when expressing an idea. Fan-like motion of alæ nasi. *Bowels much distended, with rumbling, particularly in left hypochondria. *Constant sensation of fullness in stomach, extending up to throat. *Great fear of being left alone. *Red, sand-like sediment in urine. Indisposed to lie on left side. He awakes from sleep very cross and irritable. *Worse from* 4 to 8 P. M.

**MERCURIUS.** In early stage. The patient does not complain of anything in particular, yet feels so weak and ill all over is obliged to go to bed. Tongue dirty-yellow, or clean, with bitter, foul taste. Gums swollen and ulcerated, with offensive breath. Headache, especially in forehead and on the vertex. *Region of stomach and liver very sensitive and painful, [**Bell. Bry.**] Dry, hot skin, or *copious perspiration.* *Green-yellow stools, with tenesmus. Dark urine. *Symptoms all worse at night and in rainy weather.

**PHOS. ACID.** *Complete indifference. Does not wish to talk, and answers very slowly, [*wants to talk,* **Stram.**] Tongue dry and cracked, teeth covered with sordes, [see **Ars.**] Fixed look, with hollow, glassy eyes. Continual delirium or dull mutterings. Subsultus tendinum. *Great rumbling in bowels, and painless watery diarrhœa, [**Hyos.** ***Mur. ac. Opi. Stram.**] Cold perspiration on face, hands, and pit of stomach. Pulse frequent, feeble, and intermittent.

**CALC. CARB.** Persons of a *scrofulous habit.* Palpitation of heart, with tremulous pulse, anxiety and restlessness. [**Ars.**] Despairing mood, with fear of death, tormenting all around him. *As often as he falls asleep, the same disagreeable feelings rouse him. Constant tickling under sternum, causing a dry, hacking cough, [**Rhus.**] *Persistent diarrhœa,* [**Ars. Sulph.**] After great anxiety and worriment of mind.

**CARBO. VEG.** Mostly in last stages of abdominal and putrid typhus. Face pale, sunken, hippocratic, cold, [**Ars. Colch.**] Eyes sunken, dull, without lustre, and insensible to light. Tongue dry, dark and tremulous, or sometimes moist and sticky. *Complete torpor of the vital functions. Colliquative diarrhœa, brownish, grayish or bloody, of a cadaverous smell and involuntary, [**Ars.**] *Great prostration, wants more air and to be fanned all the time. *Extremities cold and covered with cold perspiration.*

**OPIUM.** Face swollen and of a purplish color. *Extreme drowsiness and coma, with stertorous breathing. Delirious talking, with eyes wide open, [with *eyes closed,* **Hyos.**] Pulse full and labored, *or slow and feeble.* Impending paralysis of brain. Involuntary stools and retention of urine, [**Bell. Hyos.**]

**PHOSPHORUS.** *Typhoid pneumonia.* *Soporous condition, dry, black lips and tongue, open mouth. Great depression of mental faculties, mild delirium and grasping at flocks. *Thirst for very cold drinks.* *Vomiting what has been drunk soon as it becomes warm in stomach. Painless diarrhœa, discharges watery, greenish, or black, decomposed blood, [**Chin.**] *Great sense of weakness and emptiness in abdomen.

**COCCULUS.** Loss of nervous strength, feeling weak and badly all over, but no place in particular, [see **Merc.**] Slow to comprehend; he cannot find right word to express himself, [forgets the word, **Arn.**] He talks in a muttering tone, requiring much effort to speak plainly. *Vertigo, especially when rising up in bed, with nausea, compelling him to lie down again. *Head and face hot, while extremities are cold.

**COLCHICUM.** Face sunken and hippocratic. Lips, teeth and tongue covered with a thick brown coating. Intellect beclouded, though he gives correct answers to questions. Region of stomach extremely sensitive to pressure. Diarrhœa; stools whitish, watery, offensive, involuntary, [**Calc. c.**] *Cold surface, tongue and breath; mottled skin and bluish nails.

**GELSEMIUM.** *In early stage.* *Typhoid fever, when so-called nervous symptoms predominate. Great fullness in head, with heat of face and chilliness. *Head feels too big,* [**Cimi.** ***Nux.**] Tongue yellowish white or thick brown. *Nervous chills, with chattering of teeth, and fever without thirst, [see **Puls.**]

**HAMAMELIS.** *Typhoid fever, with bloody crisis. *Profuse hemorrhage from bowels, blood black, partly coagulated and offensive, with a *bruised, sore feeling* in abdomen and hips, [see **Nit. ac.**] *Epistaxis, flow passive.*

**HYOSCYAMUS.** Brown-red, swollen face. Tongue, red, brown, dry and cracked. Lips look like scorched leather. *Furious delirium, which continues while awake.* *Loss of *speech* and consciousness, [**Bell. Stram.**] *Muttering, with picking at bedclothes, [**Mur. ac. Opi.**] Great restlessness, jumping out of bed, and endeavoring to escape, [**Bell. Bry.**] Eyes red and sparkling, staring, rolling about in their orbits. *Twitching and jerking of limbs; *subsultus tendinum.* *Paralysis of sphincter ani and vesicæ.

**LACHESIS.** Dry, red or black tongue, cracked at tip, and bleeding; it trembles when being protruded. Lips dry, cracked and bleeding. *Stupor, and muttering delirium.* Depression of lower jaw, [**Lyc. Mur. ac. Opi. Stram.**] *Cannot bear anything to touch the throat, it is so sensitive. *Symptoms all worse after sleeping, [**Apis. Opi.**] Thinks he is dead, and that preparations are being made for the funeral.

**STRAMONIUM.** Loss of consciousness, with involuntary motions of limbs. Earnest and ceaseless *talking,* [not disposed to talk, **Bell. Nit. ac. Phos. ac.**] Constant and repeated *jerking of head up from pillow.* *Loquacious delirium, with a desire to escape from bed. Tongue yellowish-brown, and dry on centre, [see **Bapt.**]. *Lips sore and cracked, and sordes on teeth.* *No desire for water, although mouth is very dry. *Blackish diarrhœa, smelling like carrion, [**Ars. Carb. v. Chin.**] Loss of sight, hearing, and speech. Copious involuntary discharge of urine.

**PULSATILLA.** In early stage, and where there is much gastric disturbance. Febrile heat, mingled with chilliness. *Thickly-coated tongue, with bad taste in morning, [*bitter* taste, **Bry. Merc. Nux.**] *Taste as of putrid meat in mouth, with inclination to vomit.* Symptoms very changeable, feeling well one hour, and very miserable next. *Craves fresh. cool air. is worse in a warm room. *Mild, tearful persons.* Symptoms all worse towards evening.

**MURIATIC ACID.** Advanced typhus; patient stupid, unconscious, and *extremely prostrate.* *Constant sliding down in bed, [**Apis. Zinc.**] *Low, muttering delirium, groaning in sleep, and picking at bedclothes. Inability to protrude tongue, which is very dry. Depression of lower jaw, boring head into pillow, turning up whites of eyes, slavering. *Involuntary stools and urine,* [**Ars. Hyos. Rhus.**] *Bleeding from anus.*

**NITRIC AC.** Mostly in advanced stages of disease. Inclination to looseness of bowels, with green, slimy, acrid stools, accompanied by severe pain. **Hemorrhage from bowels, and great sensitiveness of abdomen.* [Rapou gave **Nit. ac.** and also **Phos. ac.** as injections to arrest intestinal hemorrhage; four drops in two or three ounces of water.] *Extremely offensive urine. Irregular pulse, failing strength.

**TARTAR EM.** Typhoid pneumonia, with great rattling in chest, and dyspnœa. *Loose cough, without expectoration, [**Ipc.**] *There is apparent danger of suffocation. Acute œdema of the lungs.

**ZINCUM.** Entire loss of consciousness; does not recognize his relations. Delirium, with staring eyes and efforts to get out of bed, [**Mur. ac.**] Position on back, and sliding down in bed. Subsultus tendinum, grasping at flocks, and feeling around as if in search of something. *Constant trembling of the hands, and coldness of the extremities. Small, intermittent pulse. *Impending paralysis of brain.

**CLINICAL OBSERVATIONS.** Quarantine patient in an upper airy room. Provide for *free ventilation.* Look after sewer-pipes. Disinfect all discharges and soiled clothing immediately, [see article "Sick-Room."] Use hair mattress; have two if possible, that patient may be frequently changed, Guard against bed-sores. Observe the strictest regard to cleanliness, and exclude all persons from room not absolutely needed.

**AUXILIARY MEASURES.** If fever runs high, put patient

in a bath or sponge him off in *warm* water, [90° to 100°, the higher the fever the hotter should be the water.] After the bath, wrap in a *clean dry* sheet, place him in bed and allow him to dry *without being rubbed;* repeat two or three times a day. If the head is *hot* and painful, or patient *delirious*, envelop the whole head in cloths wrung out of *hot water*, and change them often. Where there is great pain and tenderness of the abdomen, *hot fomentations* or thin poultices should be applied to the parts and frequently changed.

In *obstinate constipation*, enemas of *warm* water will afford the best means of relief, and where *diarrhœa* occurs, lavements of *starch water* [about two ounces] administered after every stool will have a salutary effect.

**DIETETICS.** Diet of the greatest importance. It should consist mainly of *fresh sweet milk*, given in moderation and at regular intervals. Good *fresh buttermilk* is also excellent, and may be taken ad libitum. Thin gruel made of farina, corn-starch, or oatmeal may be allowed for a change. *Beef-tea, mutton- or chicken-broth* should be given later for the prostration, and to build up the vitality of patient. No *solid food* should be taken so long as any *tenderness* of abdomen or *looseness of bowels* are present.

Water may be drank at pleasure, and the mouth washed frequently to prevent the accumulation of *sordes*. *Sweet* cider, fresh from the press, is an excellent beverage in fevers, and may be taken in moderate quantities.

---

## ULCERS.

**THERAPEUTICS.** *Special indications.*

**ARSENICUM.** Irritable ulcer in exhausted, impoverished constitutions, [see **Lach.**] *Ulcers with high edges, pains *burning* or tearing, discharge greenish, thin, acrid or bloody. The surface round sore bluish, inflamed and œdematous.

**ASAFŒTIDA.** Nervous individuals. *Ulcers with high hard edges, sensitive to touch, easily bleeding, [**Ars.**] Pus profuse, greenish, thin, offensive, even ichorous, [**Ars.**]

**CARBO VEG.** Sensation of tension around the sore. *Ulcers varicose, scorbutic, livid, easily bleeding, fetid. Ulcers on leg, burn, especially at night, [**Ars.**] Bottom of sore has a bluish tinge.

**HEPAR SULPH.** *The ulcer discharges bloody pus, smelling like old cheese. The edges are very sensitive, and have a pulsating sensation; discharge corroding. *Unhealthy skin, every little injury inclines to suppurate.

**LACHESIS.** Gangrenous ulcers on legs and toes. *Phagedenic and sloughing ulcers. Large ulcers tending to spread rapidly. Specially adapted to old persons.

**MERCURIUS.** Ulcers *superficial*, *flat*, readily bleeding, tendency to spread. Worse from heat of bed or from hot or cold applications. Sensation as if the parts were corroded by insects. *Dripping night-sweats.

**NITRIC ACID.** Ulcers with irregular edges and luxuriant granulations. *Stinging* or *pricking pains, intolerable.* Foul-smelling foot-sweats, [**Sili.**] After the use of *mercury*, or in *secondary syphilis.*

**SULPHUR.** Ulcers with raised swollen edges, surrounded by pimples. Stinging, lacerating pains. *Proud flesh in the ulcers, readily bleeding.

**AUXILIARY MEASURES.** Remove the cause of irritation. Observe *perfect cleanliness.* Keep limb in horizontal position.

**Healthy** ulcers should be dressed with compresses wet in solution of **Calendula,** [ ʒji. to ℥vi. *warm water*] keep sore clean and renew dressings often.

**Indolent** or unhealthy ulcer may often be cured by attention to *diet, cleanliness* and internal medication. In other cases it may be necessary to freshen the sore with *Carbolic ac.* [10 drops to the ounce] by applying it on lint to the ulcer, then poultice, after which draw the parts together with adhesive plasters and apply a roller from the foot to the knee.

**Irritable** ulcers mostly require *poulticing,* followed by *hot water* dressings, frequently changed, and the limb kept at rest.

**DIETETICS.** Hygienic precautions. Nutritious, easily digested food, such as rare beef, mutton-chop, soft eggs, fresh vegetables, ripe fruits, milk, Graham bread, rice, etc. All alcoholic beverages must be strictly avoided.

---

## URINARY DIFFICULTIES.

**THERAPEUTICS.** *Leading indications.*

**ACONITE.** *Fever, anxiety, restlessness and fear of the future.* *Scanty, red, hot urine, without sediment. Retention of urine, with stitches in kidneys. *Consequent upon taking cold,* or *from exposure to dry, cold winds.*

**APIS MEL.** Renal pains, soreness on pressure or when stooping. Frequent sudden attack of pain along ureters. *Frequent desire, with passage of only a few drops of dark-colored urine. *Eyelids œdematous.

**ARNICA.** Urinary difficulties after mechanical injuries, [after getting *wet,* **Rhus.**] Tenesmus of the neck of bladder, with ineffectual efforts to urinate. Urine brown, with brick-red sediment.

**ASPARAGUS.** Slight, febrile excitement. Rapid and irregular pulsations of the heart, especially on exercising. Pains in kidneys just under short ribs. Frequent and painful micturition. Urine scanty, brown and without sediment, [see **Acon.**] After urinating, burning in urethra.

**BELLADONNA.** *Back feels as if it would break, hindering motion. *Sensation as of a worm in bladder,* [of a *ball,* Lach.] *Retention of urine, passing off drop by drop, [Canth. Nux.] *Inability to retain the urine.* Wets the bed, restless, starts in sleep.

**BENZOIC AC.** Soreness, or hot, burning pain in left kidney. Frequent desire to urinate. *Urine contains mucus and pus, (with enlargement of prostate gland.) Urine dark-colored, has an exceedingly strong smell, [like that of *horses,* Nit. ac.] *Rheumatic, gouty subjects.*

**BERBERIS.** Violent sticking pains in bladder, extending from kidneys into urethra, with urging to urinate. *Stitches in urethra, extending to bladder.* *Muco-purulent discharge from bladder, with enlarged prostate, [Benz. ac.] Blood-red urine, which soon becomes turbid and deposits a thick mucus or bright-red, bran-like sediment.

**CALC. CARB.** Frequent micturition, also at night. *Urine dark, brown, with white sediment, [Brom.] The urine has a *putrid* smell, [see Nit. ac.] During micturition, burning in urethra. *Cold, damp feet continually.

**CANNABIS IND.** Aching in kidneys, keeping him awake at night. *Burning in kidneys,* [Canth.] The urine passes freely at times, then again in small quantities. *Urine dribbles out after the stream ceases.

**CANTHARIDES.** Cutting and burning pains in both kidneys, the parts being snsitive to touch. *The urine scalds, and is passed drop by drop, with extreme pain. *Constant desire to urinate, passing a few drops at a time, sometimes mixed with blood. *Vomiting, with violent retching.*

**CHAMOMILLA.** Dragging down the ureters, like labor-pains, with frequent urging to urinate. Burning in neck of bladder during micturition. *Urine yellow, with flaky sediment.* *The urine becomes turbid, clay-colored soon after passing. *Patient very irritable and snappish.*

**CONIUM.** Suited to old people troubled with frequent urination at night. Urine thick, white and turbid, with gray or white sediment. *During micturition flow intermits. *Vertigo, especially when lying down or turning over in bed.

**DIGITALIS.** *Inflammation of the neck of bladder,* [Acon. Cann. in. *Canth.] Throbbing pain at neck of bladder when straining to pass water. Urine dark-brown, hot and burning. Can retain urine best in recumbent posture.

**DULCAMARA.** *Catarrh of the bladder,* [Acon. Merc. Puls.] Urine scanty, fetid, turbid; on *standing gets oily, containing a tough, jelly-like, white or red mucus mixed with blood.* *Gets worse from every cold change in weather.

**EQUISETUM.** *Difficulty in passing urine during pregnancy and after confinement. Urging and severe pain immediately after the urine is voided. *Incontinence of urine at night, [Bell. Nit. ac. *Puls. *Sep.]

**GELSEMIUM.** Incontinence of urine from *paralysis of sphincter*, [**Hyos.**] Alternate dysuria and enuresis. Spasms of bladder. Suitable to nervous children.

**HELIONIUS.** *Mind dull and inactive.* Constant aching and extreme tenderness of kidneys, especially the right. *Burning in kidneys*, [**Cann. in. Canth.**] *Weariness, languor, weight in renal region. Burning scalding when urinating. Urine clear, profuse, light-colored.

**HYDRASTIS.** Dull aching in region of kidneys. *Catarrh of bladder, with thick ropy mucus sediment in urine. *The urine has a decomposed smell.*

**LACHESIS.** Stitches from kidneys through the ureters. Copious emissions of *foaming* urine, [**Lyc. Seneg. Spong.**] Urine dark, almost black. *Sensation of a *ball* in bladder when turning over, [see **Bell.**] Catarrh of bladder.

**LYCOPODIUM.** Severe backache, relieved by passing urine. Urging to urinate, must wait long before it will pass. Urine turbid, milky, with an offensive, purulent sediment. *Red sandy sediment in urine, [**Phos. Sep. Sili.**] *Urine copious at night, scanty through the day.* *Child cries before passing urine.

**MERCURIUS.** Region of bladder sore to touch. *Urine passes in a thin stream or in drops, containing blood and pus. *Scanty, fiery-red urine. *Turbid and fetid urine.*

**NATRUM MUR.** *Involuntary discharge of urine when walking, coughing or laughing, [**Puls. Verat.**] During urination, stitches in bladder, smarting, burning in urethra. Urine dark, like coffee, [see **Tereb.**]

**NITRIC AC.** While urinating, smarting, burning in urethra. Urine turbid, looks like remains in a cider barrel. *Scanty, dark brown, smelling strong, like *horse's* urine, [**Chin. s.**—smells like *cat's urine.*—**Viola.**—like *violets*, **Nux m. Tereb.**—like *ammonia*, **Asaph. Iod.**] Enuresis.

**NUX VOMICA.** Painful ineffectual urging to urinate. *Urine passes in drops, with burning, tearing in neck of bladder, [see **Canth.**] Reddish urine with brick-dust sediment. When caused by *abuse of spirits*, [**Lach. Merc. Puls.**]

**PAREIRA BRAVA.** Great difficulty and pain in passing the urine; he cries out, and can only emit urine when on his knees, pressing his head against floor. Urine smells strongly of ammonia, and contains a quantity of viscid, thick, white mucus. Pain in thighs.

**PHOS. ACID.** *Frequent micturition. Urine milky, with bloody, jelly-like lumps, or as if stirred with flour. *Great indifference to the affairs of life.

**PHYTOLACCA.** *Weakness, dull pain and soreness in region of kidneys. Uneasiness down the ureters. Pain in bladder before and during micturition. *Dark red urine, which leaves a stain on vessel color of mahogany, [see **Sep.**] Urine deposits a *chalk-like sediment.*

**PULSATILLA.** *Nocturnal enuresis*, particularly of little girls. Cannot retain urine, it is involuntary when coughing, walking or during sleep. *Colorless watery urine *Scanty, brown-red urine*, with brick-dust-like sediment, [**Dig. Lyc. Nux. Phos. Sep.**]

**SARSAPARILLA.** Tenderness and distension over region of bladder. Tenesmus of bladder, with discharge of *white acrid pus and mucus.* Urine bright and clear, but irritating. *Severe pain at *conclusion of urination.* Child *screams before and while passing urine*, [see **Lyc.**] Pale sand in the urine.

**SEPIA.** Involuntary urination at night, especially in first sleep. Urine turbid, with sediment of red sand, [see **Lyc.**] Blood-red urine, with white sediment and a cuticle on surface. *Fetid urine depositing a clay-colored sediment, which adheres to vessel with great tenacity, [see **Phyto.**]

**TEREBINTH.** Burning and drawing from right kidney to hip. Frequent urination at night, with intense burning. *Urine black, with coffee-grounds sediment, [**Hell.**] Blood thoroughly mixed with the urine. *Urine smells like violets*, [**Nux m.**] Great emaciation and weakness.

**AUXILIARY MEASURES.** In some cases warm *sitz* baths, or *hot* fomentations to the region of bladder has a happy effect. *Hot salt* pads or rubber bags partially filled with *hot* water and applied to the region of the kidneys very beneficial. Adopt measures to keep skin active and promote perspiration. Frequent bathing and open-air exercise important.

**DIETETICS.** Regulate diet carefully. Eat sparingly of meat. Adopt a mixed vegetable diet, with fresh ripe fruits. Avoid all highly-seasoned food, and all *alcoholic stimulants* of every kind. Let fresh *soft* water be the principal drink.

---

## URTICARIA.—NETTLE-RASH.

**THERAPEUTICS.** *Special indications.*

**APIS MEL.** Stinging, burning, prickling, smarting, or itching of the skin. *Body covered with large white wheals, deep scarlet interspaces. *Uterine catarrh.*

**CALCARIA CARB.** *Nettle-rash which always disappears in cold air, [see **Caust.**] White nettle-rash of children which itches intolerably. Unhealthy, ulcerative skin. *Cold, damp feet. *Scrofulous diathesis.*

**CAUSTICUM.** Chronic nettle-rash, coming out more fully in fresh air, with decided aggravation and itching from heat of bed.

**CHLORAL.** Nettle-rash in large raised wheals, with intense irritating, itching œdematous swelling of face, cheeks, eyelids and ears. Coming on from a chill.

**COPAIVA.** Violent chills, headache and general malaise. Red, hot skin, nettle-rash all over body, delirium, drowsiness, scanty urine, which is dark, with brick-dust sediment.

**RHUS TOX.** *Nettle-rash from getting wet, during rheumatism, with chills and fever, worse in cold air, [*better*, Cal. c.] Itching all over, worse on hairy parts, burning after scratching,

**URTICA URENS.** A valuable remedy. Itching and burning of skin as if scorched. *Raised red blotches, with fine stinging points. Pale rash requiring constant rubbing.

**LOCAL MEASURES.** To allay the intense itching and burning, apply *hot* water to the affected parts, sopping it on freely, or give patient a *warm* bath, and dry *without* rubbing. As the disease usually arises from some derangement of the digestive organs, measures should be taken to correct this by suitable diet, and the observance of regular habits.

---

## VERTIGO.—DIZZINESS.

**THERAPEUTICS.** *Leading indications.*

**ACONITE.** *Vertigo from heat of sun, [Bell. Glon.] Vertigo from a fall or contusion, [Arn.] *Vertigo on raising the head, with nausea and vanishing of sight.

**AMM. CARB.** *Giddiness, especially in morning*, when sitting and reading, better when walking.

**APIS MEL.** Vertigo when sitting, standing, lying, when closing the eyes, with nausea and headache. Brain feels tired, as if "gone to sleep."

**ARGENT. NIT.** *Vertigo with headache. *Head feels much too large. [Cimi. Gel. Glon. *Nux.] *Buzzing in ears.*

**BELLADONNA.** *Vertigo, as if everything turned in a circle.* *Vertigo, as if he would fall to one side or backwards, with flickering before the eyes, especially when stooping, or rising from a stooping posture, [see Puls.]

**BRYONIA.** *Giddiness*, with sensation of looseness in brain when stooping, or raising the head. *Hard, dry stools.

**CALCARIA CARB.** *Vertigo when ascending a height*, [see Ferr.] walking in open air, turning head quickly, or looking upwards. Head feels too full, [Acon. Bell.] *Cold, damp feet continually.

**CICUTA.** *Giddiness, with falling forwards*, [Phos. ac. Graph. —falling *backwards*, Bry. Nux. Rhus.—falling *sideways*, Ipe. Sili. Sulph.] *Vertigo, reeling as if everything turned around him.

**CONIUM.** *Vertigo, particularly when lying down and when turning over in bed, [Sang.] *Vertigo on looking round, as if he would fall to one side.* Suitable to old people.

**FERRUM.** Vertigo when *descending* a height, [see Calc. c.] Vertigo on seeing flowing water, with sickness at stomach when walking. Sensation as if the head would constantly incline to one side.

**GELSEMIUM.** *Giddiness, with confusion of head, dim

ness of vision, chilliness, and accelerated pulse. Intoxicated feeling, and tendency to stagger, [**Amm. c. Bry. Kreo. Nux.**] *Head feels light and large.

**GLONOIN.** *Vertigo, with confusion of head, faintness, black spots before eyes. *Worse from stooping or moving head,* [better from *stooping,* **Indigo.**] Head feels too large, constant effort to keep it erect.

**GRAPHITES.** Dizziness during and after stooping, with inclination to fall forward. *Vertigo on looking upwards, and in morning on awaking. Feels as if drunken when rising from bed in morning.

**INDIGO.** *Excessive giddiness, with headache, better from stooping or leaning forwards. *Cannot look up, and staggers when rising from a sitting posture.*

**LEDUM.** *Vertigo, as from intoxication,* especially when walking in open air, [**Calc. c. Nux v.**] Feels dull after eating; head inclines to fall backwards.

**MERCURIUS.** Dull and stupid feeling, with dizziness. *Vertigo, as if in a swing, everything turns black before the eyes. Vertigo after stooping, when lying on the back, with nausea and headache.

**NUX MOS.** *Vertigo, as if drunk, staggering;* reeling when walking in open air. Weak, limbs numb, feels as if floating in air. Head feels full, and as if expanding. *Sleepiness and inclination to faint. *Hysterical subjects.*

**NUX VOMICA.** Stupefaction, confusion, as from nightly reveling. *Reeling vertigo, in morning and after dinner, with vanishing of sight and loss of hearing. *Worse when stooping,* in morning and from use of wine.

**OPIUM.** *Vertigo when rising from bed, compelling one to lie down. *Vertigo after fright,* [**Acon.**] Dizziness, with sensation as if he were flying or hovering in the air, [see **Nux m.**] *Dull, stupid, as if drunk.

**PHOSPHORUS.** *Vertigo from abuse of narcotics, coffee, [**Cham. Nux.**] *Vertigo on rising from bed, or a seat,* with faintness, worse mornings and after meals. *Constipation, stools long, narrow, and hard, like a dog's.

**PULSATILLA.** *Vertigo, as if intoxicated, when rising from a seat,* [**Podo.**] *Vertigo when stooping, lifting up the eyes, or after eating. *Giddiness, particularly in evening.* *Menses scanty or suppressed. *Derangement of stomach.*

**RHUS TOX.** *Giddy, as if intoxicated, when rising from bed, [**Acon. Opi.**] Vertigo in the aged, worse when rising from lying, and from turning or stooping, [see **Con.**] Chilliness and pressure behind eyes. *Brain feels loose when stepping or shaking head, [see **Bry.**]

**SANGUINARIA.** *Vertigo, with long-continuing nausea, debility and headache.* Dizziness when quickly turning head and looking upwards. *Vertigo on lying down at night, or on rising from stooping, [**Con. Rhus.**] *Vertigo in cold weather. Circumscribed redness* of the cheeks.

**SILICEA.** *Vertigo, as if one would fall forwards, [see **Cicu.**] *Worse from motion or looking upwards.* *Constipation, stools recede after being partially expelled.

**SPIGELIA.** Vertigo when looking *downwards*, [**Kalm Olean.**—when looking *upwards*, **Calc. c. Graph.** ***Indigo.** ***Puls. Sang.**] Vertigo in open air when turning head while walking, [comp. **Sang.**]

**THUYA.** *Vertigo, with eyes shut, ceases on opening them. Vertigo when rising from sitting, on stooping, looking upwards or sideways, [**Puls.**]

**CLINICAL OBSERVATIONS.** If the vertigo is associated with disease of the ears, that affection should first receive attention. If the stomach is at fault, correct the abnormal condition of that organ by appropriate remedial agents. If the dizziness is caused by uterine derangement, this should receive due consideration.

Persons subject to vertigo should eat and drink moderately, take suitable out-door exercise, use the flesh-brush frequently, and adopt such measures as will promote the general health.

---

## VOMITING.

**THERAPEUTICS.** *Leading indications.*

**ANTIMONIUM.** Nausea and vomiting from *overloading stomach*, or after drinking sour wine, [**Ipe. Nux. Puls.**] *Terrible vomiting which nothing can stop, [**Tart. e.**] *Thick milky coating on tongue.

**ARSENICUM.** *Vomiting immediately after eating or drinking, [**Bry. Nux. Puls.** ***Verat.**] *Vomiting black bile and blood,* [**Ipe. Sec.** ***Verat.**] *Great restlessness, thirst and prostration.* *Pressure in stomach as of a stone.

**BRYONIA.** Vomiting immediately after eating or drinking, [**Ars.**] *Bitter bilious vomiting. Stitches in left side when vomiting. *Constipation, stools hard and dry.

**CHAMOMILLA.** Vomiting food, tastes bitter or sour. *Bitter bilious vomiting. *Pain in belly just above the navel, running from side to side. Suitable to children.

**COCCULUS.** *Nausea and vomiting from *riding in a carriage, on a boat*, or from swinging, [**Nux m. Pet.**] *Sea-sickness.* Nausea and inclination to vomit on taking cold.

**CONIUM.** *Violent vomiting of black masses, like coffee-grounds, in clear, sour water, [see **Ars. Phos. Verat.**] Frequent vomiting with *heart-burn.* *Spasmodic pains in stomach. *Tremulous weakness after every stool.*

**IPECAC.** Nausea, as if proceeding from stomach. **Constant and continual nausea*, [**Lobe.** ***Tart. e. Verat.**] *Vomiting large quantities of mucus, [**Tart. e.**] *Vomiting food, bile, sour fluid or blood.* Vomiting a dark, pitch-like substance,

[**Ars. Sec. Verat.**] *Stomach feels relaxed, as if hanging down, [**Staph.**] *Beating* in stomach, [**Puls. Rhus.**]

**LOBELIA.** *Nausea and copious vomiting, with profuse perspiration. Incessant violent nausea, [see **Ipe.**] Vomiting, with cold perspiration on face, [**Verat.**] Feeling of great weakness of stomach, extending through chest.

**NITRUM.** *Nausea, with cold sensation from throat to stomach. Choking faintness, bruised headache and burning in eyes. Vomits mucus with blood.

**NUX VOM.** *Nausea after eating.* *Empty retching of drunkards. *Vomiting sour-smelling and sour-tasting mucus, [see **Phos.**] *Region of stomach sensitive to pressure.* Victims of intemperance or drug medication.

**OPIUM.** *Vomiting fæces, or a fecal-smelling substance, [**Acon. Bell. Nux v. *Plumb. Thuy.**] Hiccough, great thirst, cold limbs, distorted face, [ileus or incarcerated hernia.]

**PHOSPHORUS.** Vomiting sour, offensive fluid in large quantities, looking like water, ink and coffee-grounds. * *Vomiting bile,* [see **Acon.**] Very drowsy *after meals,* particularly after dinner. *Constipation, *long, narrow,* hard stools.

**PHYTOLACCA.** *Violent vomiting of clotted blood and slime, with retching, intense pain and desire for death to relieve.

**PULSATILLA.** *Vomiting after taking cold, or from suppression of menses. Vomiting, caused by disordered stomach, [**Ant. Ars. Ipe. Nux.**] Vomiting mucus, bile, or bitter-sour fluids, especially in evening or at night.

**TARTAR EM.** *Violent straining to vomit, with sweat on forehead,* [**Lob. *Verat.**] *Continuous nausea, vomiting and diarrhœa, [**Verat.**] Vomiting green, tough, watery mucus, followed by great drowsiness and *prostration,* [**Ars. Verat.**]

**VERAT. ALB.** Violent vomiting, with continuous nausea. *Vomiting food, acrid, bitter, foamy, white, or yellow-green mucus. Vomiting *black bile and blood,* [**Ars. Ipe.**] *Vomiting whenever he moves or drinks.* Great prostration.

**AUXILIARY MEASURES.** If the vomiting is due to the presence of *poison* or irritating substances, evacuate the stomach at once. Give freely of *tepid water* containing powdered *mustard,* and tickle the fauces with a feather or something similar to excite vomiting.

In vomiting caused by reflex action or gastric irritation, great benefit will be derived from taking frequent draughts of *hot water.* In some cases, swallowing *bits of ice* will give prompt relief. In *excessive, obstinate* vomiting, equal parts of *Ether* and *Spt. Lavender,* given in teaspoonful doses, well diluted with *cold* water, is an efficient remedy.

**Sea-Sickness.** This is often very intractable. Patient should assume *horizontal* position, with *head lower* than the body, and on frequent occasions take *exercise* by *walking,*

Drinking *largely* and *repeatedly* of *tepid* water is said to be beneficial. Partaking freely of nutritious food, even if the stomach rejects it, is highly commended. *Cocculus* is one of the principal remedies, and should be administered in repeated doses.

---

## WORM AFFECTIONS.

**THERAPEUTICS.** *Leading indications.*

**ACONITE.** Febrile disturbance. The region around umbilicus is hard, and the whole abdomen distended. Frequent ineffectual straining at stool, or nothing but slime is passed. Itching of anus, worse at night, with restlessness, [Merc.] *Much fear and anxiety, child is even afraid to go to bed.

**BELLADONNA.** Flushed face and red eyes. *Violent starting and jumping during sleep. Involuntary discharge of fæces and urine. Grating of teeth, moaning and uneasy sleep. *Picking at bedclothes.*

**CALC. CARB.** Headache, dark rings around the eyes. Pale, bloated face and distension of abdomen. Pain around the navel, [Cina.] Itching of anus, particularly in the evening. Scrofulous persons.

**CHINA.** If the patient has had much diarrhœa or taken aperient medicine. The child frequently passes worms, picks its nose much, and the belly is distended, [*Cina.] Painless diarrhœa of undigested stools. Pain in abdomen, worse at night, aud after eating.

**CINA.** *Constant boring at nose. Frequent swallowing, [Spig.] Restless sleep, with rolling of eyes. *Dark circles around eyes.* Short, hacking cough, particularly at night. Abdomen hard and distended, with frequent pain in umbilical region. *The urine turns milky after standing a short time.

**LYCOPODIUM.** Earthy, yellow complexion, with blue circles around eyes. Much flatulent distension in stomach and bowels. Sensation as of something crawling and moving in abdomen. *Ascarides*, with much itching about anus, [Merc.] *Red, sandy sediment in urine. Constipation of hard stools.

**MERCURIUS.** *Ascarides*, with troublesome itching of the anus; the worms crawl out, and can be seen on the perineum, [Stan.] Continual greediness for eating, yet grows weaker withal. Offensive breath.

**SANTONINE.** Many prefer this preparation to Cina. The symptoms indicating its use are the same as enumerated under Cina. A dose of the $1^x$ trit. given thrice daily for two or three days, will usually suffice.

**SPIGELIA.** Sensation of a worm rising in throat, [of a worm in bladder, Bell.] Nausea every morning before breakfast, better after eating. Vomiting, with sour eructations. Very pale face, and a yellow margin around the eyes, [see Cin. Lyc.] *Violent palpitation of heart.

**STANNUM.** Discharge of mucus from bowels, mingled with ascarides, [*Lyc. Merc.] Soreness and smarting at anus. *Frequent spells of pain in abdomen, during which child wishes to lean against something hard for relief.

**SULPHUR.** Frequent passage of lumbricoides, ascarides and tænia. Creeping and biting in rectum. *Gets very hungry about 11 A. M. *Frequent weak, faint spells through the day. Rawness and excoriation of anus much of the time. Pustular eruptions on the skin.

**HYGIENIC MEASURES.** The best preventives of worms are *cleanliness*, regular habits, open air exercise, suitable diet, and such other measures as will improve the general health.

**DIETETICS.** Persons subject to worms should have a good, wholesome, nutritious diet. Well-cooked beef, mutton, fowl, eggs, bread and butter, ripe fruits, fresh vegetables, etc. All *pastry*, *sweet cakes*, *pies*, *sweetmeats*, uncooked vegetables and the like should be avoided.

**TAPEWORM.** The first step in treatment is to get rid of the "critter." The following remedies will be found efficient.

**FILIX MAS.** This is an old and popular remedy. A drachm of the *ethereal extract* should be given in capsules at bedtime, twelve hours after fasting, followed by an ounce of castor-oil in the morning.

**KOUSSO.** This is safe and efficient in tænia. To two drachms of powdered flowers, add four ounces *boiling* water, and when cold administer without being strained. Patient should fast the day before using the medicine. The worm is generally discharged in 24 hours.

**PEPO SEMEN.** Is one of the best remedies for *tapeworm.* Take from one to two ounces fresh, dry pumpkin-seeds, freed of their shells, *powder* finely and mix in a little milk. Give this in the morning after fasting 24 hours. Three hours later take an ounce of Castor-oil. If the first dose is not sufficient it may be repeated the following morning.

**PUNICA GRANATUM.** *Pomegranate bark.* This has long been celebrated as a *tænicide.* Use fresh bark of the *root.* Take two ounces of bark hashed, soak over night in a pint and a half of water, then boil down to one pint. Strain and administer lukewarm in three doses, at intervals of an hour, after having fasted.

**ROTTLERA.** *Kamala.* This is highly commended in *tænia.* The *dose* of powdered kamala is about two drachms, prepared in gum-arabic emulsion, and repeated every three hours if necessary. If two or three doses prove inefficient, add a drachm of the oil of *male fern*, and repeat.

# WOUNDS.

*General Considerations.*

**ARTICLES OF DRESSING.** A great variety of dressings are employed in the treatment of wounds, as Lint, Bran, Compresses, Bandages, Adhesive Strips, etc.

**Lint.** One form of lint is made by scraping old linen cloth, and using the soft substance thus obtained. Another variety, called *patent lint*, comes in packages prepared for use.

**Bran.** This article being cleanly and easily obtained, makes a good dressing in compound fractures and in all cases where there is much oozing or suppuration. It also makes an excellent packing in fracture-boxes.

**Compresses.** These are made of cotton or linen cloth, folded to any desired shape or thickness. Used to make and equalize pressure, and as a means for applying medicated lotions.

**Bandages.** These are made of cotton or linen cloth, cut three inches wide, and about three or four yards long, rolled tightly. In applying the bandage, every succeeding turn should overlap the one immediately below it, and where there is any inequality of surface, the *reverse* turns must be made.

The *many-tailed*, or Scultetus bandage, is made of roller strips three inches wide and long enough to encircle the limb once and a half. These are placed on a table side by side, overlapping each other about an inch. Then a strip of roller is laid in the centre at right angles, and stitched to the pieces to hold them in place.

To apply the bandage, place it under the limb with the central piece extending along the posterior surface of the leg. Now beginning at the lowest end, bring the tails one over the other until the last strip is reached, and secured with a pin.

**Adhesive Plaster.** Cut in strips from a quarter to half an inch or more wide, and in direction of long fibres of cloth. To apply, hold the unspread surface of plaster against a tin vessel filled with *hot* water, and when sufficiently warm apply quickly. In wounds of scalp or other hairy parts, skin must be shaved before applying the plaster.

## GENERAL RULES OF TREATMENT.

**INCISED WOUNDS.** The first step in the treatment, is to arrest the hemorrhage; this in slight cases may be done by *compression* or *torsion*. If large vessels are severed, tie both extremities with silk or cat-gut ligature. 2d. Remove all foreign bodies with finger, forceps or sponge and water. 3d. Bring edges of wound together and secure with cross-strips of adhesive plaster, or sutures of *silk* or *cat-gut*. If wound is deep and extensive, provide drainage by twisted horse-hair, cat-gut, or perforated rubber tube. If much oozing of blood, apply solution of *Tannin* or *Per Sulphate of Iron.*

**Dressings.** The wound should be dressed with compresses saturated with *Aqua Calendula*, [half ounce to pint], kept constantly wet, and the wound kept scrupulously clean. If patient has fever, is restless, and wound painful, give **Aconite.** **Staphisagria** is a valuable remedy in injuries from *sharp-cutting* instruments. The *Calendula* dressings have given us the most satisfactory results, while others speak in highest praise of the

**Antiseptic Dressings.** A favorite method of applying these is as follows: The operator's hands, instruments, sponges, etc., are all soaked in a solution of *Carbolic Acid*, [1–40] before commencing. The wound is frequently irrigated with a solution of *Corrosive Sublimate*, [4 grs. to the pint.] For ligatures, *carbolized cat-gut* or fine *carbolized silk* is used. For drains, *carbolized* horse-hair, [twisted together] cat-gut or perforated rubber tubes; these are placed in bottom of wound, and the ends cut off flush with the skin. After the final washing, wound is sprinkled with *Iodoform* and protected by a strip of prepared oiled silk, placed over the sutured margins. Over this is placed *eight* layers of antiseptic gauze, larger than the oiled silk, wet with 1–40 Carbolic solution, and on this a layer of MacIntosh cloth, [glazed side down], and on this a layer of dry gauze. The whole is then secured by a neatly-fitting bandage.

In most cases the first dressing may remain on four or five days, the indication for their earlier removal being a higher temperature. When oozing of blood and serum has ceased, drainage tubes may be removed and dressings replaced.

**PUNCTURED WOUNDS.** These when slight are not dangerous, but when extensive are always serious. Great care should be taken to remove all foreign matter or portion of broken instrument that inflicted the injury. It may be necessary to enlarge the wound for this purpose, after which dress as advised for **Incised Wounds.** *Ledum* is an excellent remedy in wounds of this character, also *Hypericum.*

**LACERATED WOUNDS.** These present a torn and ragged appearance. The wound should be *carefully cleansed* of all foreign matter. Then draw parts together and secure by adhesive plaster, leaving sufficient space between for exit of matter. The *Calendula* dressings should be applied, and *Calendula* given internally. *Hypericum* is a valuable remedy, especially when *nerves* are *lacerated* and pains are excruciating. If there be great weakness, offensive discharge, extreme thirst, *restlessness*, threatened gangrene, give *Arsenicum.* Watch patient closely, as hæmorrhage or tetanus may ensue.

**CONTUSED WOUNDS.** The principal remedy in this form of injury is **Arnica.** It should be used both *externally* and *internally*. If case is seen early and before *inflammation* supervenes, apply compresses saturated with *cold Arnicated*

water. If the parts are *inflamed*, swollen and painful, apply compresses saturated in *hot Arnicated* water, and change them often. Should fever, restlessness, and nervous excitability occur, give **Aconite.** Where the *joints* or *tendons* are injured, pains worse at night, particularly after midnight, give **Rhus t.** If *periosteum* or *tarsal* and *carpal* joints are contused, give **Ruta g.**

**GUN-SHOT WOUNDS. Prognosis.** Wounds of *heart, lungs*, and *brain* generally fatal if injury reach centre of organ.

Wounds of *spinal marrow* mostly cause death.

Penetrating *wounds of abdomen* most always fatal.

Wounds of *liver dangerous*, but not always fatal.

*Laceration of bladder* generally causes death.

*Diagnosis* often difficult. The *orifice* of wound is no *guide* to *course* of ball. A bullet may strike middle of forehead, and instead of going through the brain, pass round the skull under the integuments and emerge at the occiput. Again, a ball may strike near the breast-bone and pass round the ribs and come out near the spine.

The *orifice of entrance* of ball is always *smaller* than that of *emergence*. The *latter* has *ragged, everted* edges. In searching for ball, place patient near as possible in position he was when wound was inflicted. The *finger* is the best probe, but if object cannot be reached with this, use long *silver* probe. For extracting balls many ingenious instruments have been devised, but want of space forbids their mention here. The surgeon will realize the importance of *removing* the *ball, shot, fragments of clothing*, splinters of bone, etc.

The remaining treatment should be the same as prescribed for *incised* and *lacerated* wounds; *Aqua Calendula* being the principal remedy with which to dress the injured parts. Many eminent surgeons, however, prefer the antiseptic treatment, believing it preferable.

---

## YELLOW FEVER.

**PROGNOSIS.** Great yellowness of the skin, *black vomit, suppression* of urine, abundant hemorrhage, jactitations, hiccough, coma and convulsions are bad omens.

A *favorable* prognosis cannot confidently be entertained. An *active* state of the kidneys, with *free flow* of urine, is a favorable sign.

**THERAPEUTICS.** *Leading indications.*

**ACONITE.** Mostly in first stage, when there is burning heat and dry skin; full, hard and rapid pulse. Agonized tossing about, violent thirst, red face, shortness of breath and great nervous excitability. *Headache as if everything would press out of forehead, with vertigo on rising. Eyes injected and sensitive to light. Vomiting mucus and bile.

**BELLADONNA.** In early stage. Glowing redness of face, with red, sparkling eyes, or fixed look. *Throbbing headache, with visible pulsations of the carotids. *Furious delirium, wishes to strike, bite, or quarrel. Tongue coated white, yellowish, or brown. Painful heaviness and cramp-like pains in back, loins, and legs. Cramp-like, contractive pains in stomach. Vertigo, with vanishing of sight, stupefaction, debility.

**BRYONIA.** Mostly in second stage. Splitting headache, aggravated by motion, opening eyes, or stooping, [**Bell.**] Eyes red, or dull and glassy, or sparkling and filled with tears. Tongue coated white or yellow, with *dry, parched, and cracked lips.* *Sitting up in bed causes nausea and faintness. Food is thrown up immediately after eating. *Patient wants to keep perfectly quiet. *Great irritability.* Everything tastes bitter.

**CAMPHOR.** Severe and long-lasting chill at commencement. *Great coldness of skin, yet cannot bear to be covered, [**Verat.**] *Retention of urine. *Prostration.*

**CANTHARIS.** Complete insensibility, cramps in abdominal muscles and legs; *suppression of urine.* Hemmorrhage from stomach and intestines, [from all the organs, **Crotal.**] Cold sweat on hands and feet. *Constant desire to urinate.

**ARGENT NIT.** Suitable in second stage, when there is vomiting of a *brownish mass mixed* with *coffee-ground-like flakes.* Dizziness and much confusion in head. Time seems to pass *very slowly.* *Green, fetid stools, passing off with much flatulence.

**ARSENICUM.** Face yellowish or livid, with distorted features and death-like countenance. *Nose pointed, eyes sunken and surrounded by dark margins.* Burning or sharp and darting pain in epigastrium or in region of liver. Limbs feel stiff and useless. Frequent stools, with tenesmus, or painless and involuntary. *Violent vomiting immediately after eating or drinking. *Vomiting a brown and *black substance,* [**Arg. n. *Verat.**] *Burning in stomach, with great thirst, drinking little and often. *Rapid prostration.* *Extreme restlessness and fear of death.

**CARBO VEG.** Last stage; hemorrhages, with great paleness of face, violent headache, great heaviness in limbs and trembling of body. *Patient wants more air, and to be fanned. *Great foulness of all the secretions.

**CROTALUS.** *Hemorrhages from the eyes, nose, mouth, stomach, and intestines, [***Ham.**] Tongue scarlet-red, or brown and swollen. Fetid diarrhœa.

**IPECAC.** First stage, when there is vertigo, chilliness, pain in back and limbs; uncomfortable feeling in epigastrium. *Continual nausea, with vomiting glairy mucus, [see **Tart. e.**] Diarrhœa, *stools fermented.*

**MERCURIUS.** Skin yellow, red, injected; eyes sensitive to light. Paralysis of one or more limbs. Drowsy, or sleepless from nervous irritation. Dizziness, or violent pain in head. Violent vomiting of mucus and bilious matters, [Ipe. Nux.] Burning pain and tenderness of stomach. Diarrhœa, with discharges of mucus, bile, or blood, with tenesmus. *Much perspiration without relief. Great weakness of memory. Aggravation at night and in damp weather.

**NUX VOMICA.** Yellow skin, pale or yellowish face, especially around nose and mouth. Eyes injected, yellow, and watery, encircled by dark rings. Tongue slimy, or dry, cracked, and red on edges. Burning pains in stomach; pressure or cramp-like pains in epigastrium. *Vomiting acid, bilious matters. Burning pains at neck of bladder, with difficulty in urinating, [Canth.] Coldness, paralysis, and cramps in legs. *Very irritable, and wishes to be alone. Persons of *intemperate habits.* Aggravation in morning.

**QUININE.** In latter stages, when there are regular intermissions and remissions of fever from the admixture of *malarial* influences, this is a valuable remedy. If not tolerated by the stomach, give it by injection.

**TART. EM.** Nausea or vomiting, with a sense of sinking at the stomach, as if he could not survive a moment. General prostration of the whole system. Profuse cold sweat, rapid and weak pulse, [Verat.] Drowsiness and disposition to go to stool.

**VERAT. ALB.** Yellowish or bluish face, cold, and covered with *cold perspiration.* Lips and tongue dry, brown, and cracked. Trembling and cramps of feet, hands and legs. *Violent vomiting of green or black bile, with great weakness after. Diarrhœa, stools thin, blackish, or yellow. *Intense thirst for cold drinks. Excessive weakness.* Pulse almost imperceptible. *Cramps of the limbs, with cold sweat.

**AUXILIARY MEASURES.** *Isolate patient.* Provide for free *ventilation.* Disinfect all discharges. Keep patient in *horizontal* position. Permit but two or three persons in room, and *forbid* talking. Change sheets and clothing daily. If fever runs high, sponge body frequently with *warm* water and let dry *without* being *rubbed.* If convulsions threaten, give *hot* foot bath, or wrap limbs to the knees in blankets wrung out of *hot* water. For obstinate constipation, give enemas of warm soap-suds.

**DIETETICS.** Highly important. In early stage, give food sparingly. As a drink, fresh soft water, weak black tea, orange-juice, rice-water. If patient can take nourishment, fresh milk, thin gruels, buttermilk, toast-water. Later, milk, beef-tea and chicken-broth, [all fat skimmed off,] oyster soup, well-boiled rice, ice-cream. Give food in small quantities and at short intervals. Return to ordinary diet cautiously.

# PART III.

# POST-MORTEM EXAMINATIONS.

## GENERAL DIRECTIONS.

**CONSENT OF FRIENDS.** Sometimes there will be great difficulty in obtaining consent of friends for a post-mortem examination. In such cases it will be better to speak to those interested separately or together, and not allow one member of the family to decide the matter. Point out the peculiarity of the disease, the satisfaction it may afford the friends, and the benefit that others may derive from such a procedure.

**PRELIMINARY PREPARATIONS.** Make preparation at place of operation for hot and cold water, slop-buckets, sponges, towels, soap, bran or saw-dust, old newspapers and some stout twine.

**INSTRUMENTS.** An ordinary *Dissecting Case* will contain all the instruments necessary, except a small saw, which can usually be obtained at a carpenter's shop. Instruments employed in post-mortem examinations should be repolished or disinfected before being used on the living.

Notes should be taken on the spot, in ink, by an assistant, especially in *medico-legal* cases; heading these by name, age, and brief sketch of disease.

**PRECAUTIONARY MEASURES.** Guard against absorption of *virus* in all malignant cases. If any abrasions on hands, touch with *Nitrate of Silver*, and cover with collodion. Smear hands with lard or olive oil before commencing. Should skin be then cut, wash, squeeze and suck immediately, then apply *Carbolic Acid* or cauterize with *Nitrate of Silver.*

## OPERATION ON THE HEAD.

The body lying on a board, place a thick block under the occiput. The hair being turned aside, make an incision through scalp, over top of head, from ear to ear. Turn flaps aside, anterior over face, posterior on back of neck. Now, with saw, make a circular incision through skull bones, [being careful not to injure *dura mater*,] using a chisel to pry off *calvarium.* This being done, open *longitudinal sinus*, and with scissors cut through *dura mater* on a line with division of bone; it may now be lifted up, when adhesions will be found beneath its under surface and pia-mater along either side of *falx cerebri.* These being divided, the whole may be turned back, exposing the brain.

To remove the brain, raise anterior lobes, divide the several pairs of nerves, the tentorium on either side, passing knife down into foramen magnum, divide medulla oblongata and vertebral arteries, when the organ may be lifted out.

Having examined external surface, the hemispheres may be sliced off down to *corpus callosum;* this being removed, *lateral ventricles* will be exposed. Removing other portions in this way, the *fornix, velum interpositum, third* and *fourth ventricles*, and all parts of organ will be exposed.

*Base of skull* should next be inspected; open lateral and other sinuses, tear away dura mater, and examine for fractures, etc. Examination completed, replace brain, put on calvarium, bring scalp over same, and unite with stitches.

---

## REMOVAL OF SPINAL CORD.

Place body in prone position, make incision whole length of back over spinous processes; then turn aside the integument and muscles, exposing laminæ of vertebra. Now, divide the latter on each side with saw and chisel, when laminæ and spinous processes can be removed. By dividing roots of nerves on either side, cord enclosed in its sheath may be taken out.

The *dura mater* may now be opened and cord examined. If a portion of cord is desired for microscopic examination, put it in a solution of *Kali bichro.* [20 grs. to ounce water] and after *three* days, transfer to solution *Chromic acid,* [2 grs. to ounce water] and let remain till hard enough to cut in thin slices.

---

## EXAMINATION OF THE NECK.

Make an incision in *median line* of neck from chin to sternum. Turn aside integuments, separate muscles of tongue from jaw, and divide mucous membrane on each side of tongue. The latter being well drawn down beneath the jaw with tenaculum, carry knife back on either side, dividing muscles, mucous membrane, palatine arches and tonsils, including posterior walls of pharynx. The slight adhesion to spinal column being divided, the tongue, larynx, trachea and œsophagus may be removed together.

The œsophagus and trachea being divided at point of entrance to chest, may be opened and examined.

## EXAMINATION OF THE CHEST.

Make an incision in *median line* through the skin and superficial tissues, from upper end of the sternum to umbilicus. If abdomen is to be examined at same time, extend incision to the pubes; otherwise, make a transverse cut from navel to border of chest on either side. These being made through muscles and peritoneum, the flaps may be turned up on the chest and peritoneum divided along the cartilages of the ribs. The skin and muscular tissues of chest should now be dissected up together and turned aside. Then, with a strong knife, divide the cartilages at their union with ends of the ribs, also the ligaments which connect sternum with clavicle. Now raise sternum from below, divide the mediastinum, and remove it, exposing internal organs.

**THE HEART,** which will first engage attention, is about 5 inches long, 3½ broad, and weighs about 10 ounces. The *pericardium* which envelops the heart contains about a drachm of *liquor pericardii.* It may be drawn out with a *syringe* and measured.

The heart may be removed by dividing the larger vessels at its base. To examine it internally, open the *right* auricle first by an incision along its base, another meeting this at *right angles* will expose its interior. Next open ventricle by an incision running parallel with the groove, dividing right from left ventricle; now make another incision along *posterior* groove meeting former at apex, thus making a triangular flap, which if turned aside will expose its interior.

The *left side* of the heart may be opened in same way. *Semilunar valves* may be exposed by opening pulmonary artery and turning aside its walls.

**THE LUNGS.** Generally the lungs will be found in a *collapsed* state unless extensive *adhesion* prevents this. They may be examined *in situ,* unless a careful inspection is desired, in which case divide trachea and œsophagus, which draw down, and divide posterior mediastinum, also aorta and œsophagus as they pass the diaphragm, and remove the whole *en masse,* when they may be opened and examined in detail.

All blood should be absorbed, organs replaced, and incisions sewed up.

---

## OPERATION ON THE ABDOMEN.

Make an incision through the skin and superficial structure from sternum to pubes. Carefully divide peritoneum at a given point, so as to admit two fingers to serve as a guide in completing the incision. Next make a cross incision at umbilicus, then turn the angular flaps aside exposing the abdominal viscera. In many cases it will not be necessary to remove any of the organs, while in others the whole viscera must be examined.

**SMALL INTESTINES.** These are about 20 feet long; they may be removed *en masse* or in sections. Apply double ligature at lower end of ilium and just below duodenum, divide bowel between these, and clip off the mesentery along intestinal border, when they may be removed and opened for inspection.

**LARGE INTESTINE.** The *colon* is about 5 feet long; any portion of it may be removed by observing same care in the application of ligatures as above suggested.

**THE STOMACH.** This organ varies greatly in size; when moderately distended, the *transverse* diameter is about 12 inches, and the vertical about 4 inches. If it is to be examined *internally*, it should be removed from the body. Detach both omenta with fingers or scissors, place a ligature round œsophagus at cardiac end of stomach, and double one just below *pyloric* orifice; now divide œsophagus and bowel between ligatures, and stomach may be removed. If the *contents* are to be analyzed, place the organ at once in a clean jar, seal, label, and hand over to the chemist. If only the inner surface of organ is to be examined, open along one of curves, remove contents and cleanse thoroughly.

**THE KIDNEYS.** These may be removed by tearing open peritoneum with fingers and dividing vessels with knife. To examine the gland, make longitudinal incision along *convex* border and expose its interior.

Each kidney is about 4 in. long, 2 in. broad, 1 in. thick; weighs from 4 to 6 ounces.

**THE SPLEEN.** This is a ductless gland, situated in *left* hypochondriac region, embracing cardiac end of the stomach. It is of *bluish-red* color, about 5 in. long, 3 in. broad, 1 in. thick, and weighs about 7 ounces.

**THE PANCREAS.** This is situated transversely across the posterior wall of abdomen, in front of aorta. To remove it, raise the liver, draw down the stomach, and tear through gastro-hepatic omentum. The gland is 6 to 8 in. long, 1½ in. broad, from half an inch to an inch thick; weighs about 3 ounces.

**THE LIVER.** In most cases this organ may be examined *in situ.* Where removal is necessary, first draw down the organ and divide suspensory ligament, then with fingers carefully separate the gland from diaphragm, using knife to divide *vena cava,* which it will be necessary to sever at upper and lower border of the gland, together with portal vessels, hepatic artery and duct. This done, it may be lifted out.

The liver is the largest gland in the body, weighs from 3 to 4 lbs. The **gall-bladder**, lodged in a fossa on the under surface of *right* lobe, is about 4 in. long, and holds from 8 to 10 drachms.

**THE PELVIC VISCERA.** These with external genitals may

be removed together. Apply *double* ligature to the upper portion of rectum, and cut between. Next divide peritoneum around border of pelvis, round and broad ligaments of uterus in female; then strip the bladder down from inner side of pubes, and tear rectum loose from sacrum. Now flex the thighs upon abdomen, make incision through skin of mons veneris just over *anterior* commissure of vulva or penis of male, then carry knife on either side of genital organs *meeting behind* the anus. Carry incision back until parts are all detached, when the whole may be removed.

---

## MEDICO-LEGAL AUTOPSY.

(*Method of Conducting the Examination.*)

It may be necessary to examine the *spot* and *locality* where the body was found, position it occupied, and make *careful inspection* of clothing and surroundings.

Where death is thought to result from *poisoning*, all the *viscera* must be examined. The stomach and intestines, with their contents, must be removed, put in clean and separate vessels, and after being *carefully* examined, placed in clean *glass jars*, securely corked, *labeled* and given to the chemist for analysis. Portions of the *liver*, *spleen*, *kidneys*, and brain, should be preserved for *future* analysis.

**RECORD.** An *assistant* should make a careful record of *post-mortem* appearance at the time—in ink—which must be *read* and *endorsed* by the physician.

**EXTERNAL INSPECTION.** Divest the body of all clothing, and note especially:

1. **The Sex.** If external genitals are destroyed, sex can still be ascertained by size, shape of pelvis, etc. A circumscribed arc of hair on *mons veneris* is distinctive of *female*. While its projection *upwards in angular* form marks the male.

2. **The Age.** This can only be conjectured, and it is best to allow a wide margin.

3. **The Size.** Measure length accurately from crown of head to sole of heel.

4. **General Condition of Body.** Lean or fat, etc.

5. **Color and Condition of the Hair.**

6. **Color of Eyes.** Open or shut, etc.

7. **Teeth.** Number and condition. Accurate description advisable for identification.

8. **Special Marks or Deformities.** All *scars*, *tattoo-marks*, ulcers, etc., should be noted.

9. **Injuries or Wounds.** Describe their position, dirction, length, breadth, etc.

10. **Natural Openings.** Examine ears, nose, mouth, anus and female genital organs.

**INTERNAL EXAMINATION.** Open the head, chest and abdomen; that part most likely to reveal the cause of death, open first. In case of new-born infants, however, open *abdomen first*, in order to determine the *natural position* of diaphragm. Note position of organs, appearance of each, amount of fluid effused, blood, etc. Examine wounds far as possible *before* disturbing any organs.

In presenting a report to court, describe only post-mortem appearances, *give no opinion* unless required by the court.

---

## DEATH OF NEW-BORN INFANTS.

(*Medico-Legal Questions.*)

The physician may be called upon to answer the following questions after the body of a dead infant has been found.

**WAS CHILD MATURED?** The most positive proof, is *ossification of central* epiphysis in *lower end* of the femur. Open knee-joint by cross section, and expose end of the bone, then remove cartilage by *thin* slices till greatest diameter of bony nucleus is reached, which if visible will appear as a *bright* red spot. If this centre of ossification is absent, fœtus is not more than 36 or 37 weeks old, but if it shows a diameter of 2 or 3 lines, fœtus has arrived at *full term*, and if more than 3 lines, child has lived after birth.

**WAS CHILD BORN ALIVE?** Signs from position of diaphragm. Open abdominal cavity well up into chest, so as to measure *highest* point of *concavity* of diaphragm; this is found between 4th and 5th ribs in children *born dead*, and between 5th and 6th in those *born alive*.

**Hydrostatic Test.** Use large deep vessel, filled with pure, cold water. If respiration *has* taken place, lungs will *float*—buoyancy depending on completeness with which air has penetrated the tissues. Only one lung or lobe, or part of such may float.

Bluish-red insular patches in the lungs are *proof* of child *having breathed*.

Lungs of a *live-born* child are *crepitant* and *spongy*, those of a still-born *resistant, liver-like.*

Buoyancy of lungs arising from *gases* caused by putrefaction, must not be mistaken for that due to respiration.

**HOW LONG DID CHILD LIVE AFTER ITS BIRTH?** If no blood or unctuous matter on body, time and opportunity must have been afforded to remove these.

Contraction of umbilical arteries in *living child* does not take place for 8 or 10 hours.

If umbilicus has cicatrized, child must be at least 5 days old.

At birth stomach contains a little white, transparent, tough mucus, or a small quantity *liquor amnii*. If milk be found, child probably lived 3 days.

*Meconium* is found in *large intestines* 2 to 4 days after birth.

**WHAT WAS THE CAUSE OF DEATH?** Death may occur

during labor from cerebral hyperæmia, or injuries to cranium, due to imperfect ossification of bones; in which case there will be no marks of violence on the body.

Death may result from *coiling of cord* around the neck, producing *strangulation.* In this case, the mark on neck will be *broad, soft,* circularly depressed, grooved, *never* excoriated. Whereas, if child was *purposely* strangulated, mark will be *deep, hard,* interrupted, and *excoriated.*

Prolapsus and pressure of the cord may cause death with all appearances of suffocation. The absence of any marks of violence must decide the question here.

Death may occur at time of birth, by child falling on floor, striking the head. Probable result of such a fall, would be *rupture of cord,* fracture of skull, and concussion of brain. Fracture of *several* bones of head, and signs of violence on other parts, speak *against* accidental death from such a fall.

The child may be suffocated by the mother in attempting self-delivery. In this case, only *scratches* or *marks* on face or neck would be visible. *Severe injuries* are never produced in this way.

---

## THE PERIOD WHEN DEATH OCCURRED.

We can only approximate the period of death by noting the phenomena which occurs previous to putrefaction.

1. The complete cessation of respiration and circulation.
2. General relaxation of muscles immediately after death.
3. No vital reaction to stimulants.
4. Body grows ashy-white, [A *very florid* complexion may retain its color some *days* after death.]
5. The red or *livid edges* of ulcers, and tattoo-marks do not disappear after death.
6. An icterus hue, or ecchymosis existing at death, remains the same.
7. Body becomes *cold* in 8 or 12 hours. Fat persons and those killed by lightning, or suffocated, retain heat longer than others.

A body presenting only the above signs, has not been dead more than 8 or 12 hours.

8. In from 12 to 18 hours, the eye-balls become soft, inelastic, and feel flaccid.
9. In from 8 to 12 hours after death, *hypostasis,* or the settling of blood in capillaries, begin to form in all depending parts. External hypostasis must not be mistaken for ecchymosis. If an incision be made in the former, no effused fluid or blood will escape, while in the latter it will be otherwise.

**RIGOR MORTIS,** or stiffening of dead body, begins on back of the neck, passes over facial muscles, neck, chest, upper extremities, and last of all, lower extremities. It begins after 8, 10 or 20 hours, and may last 9 days. A *low* temperature, and the effects of *alcohol* retard stiffening.

**PUTREFACTION.** The progress of this is modified by age, condition and circumstances.

Bodies of *new-born* infants putrefy *rapidly*, while those of quite *old people* very slowly.

Fat, flabby, lymphatic bodies putrefy quicker than lean ones. It is rapid after death from injuries with much mutilation, from suffocation, and narcotic poisons.

It is slower after death in healthy persons, and from poisoning by *Phosphorus*, *Sulph. acid*, and *Alcohol*.

When a body is excluded from air by earth, water, clothing, etc., decomposition is retarded.

Bodies exposed to the air begin to putrefy externally, with greenish coloration of abdominal coverings, in from 24 to 72 hours after death.

Bodies lying in water, putrefaction begins in face, head, ears, neck, with a livid bluish tinge, soon turning red.

After from 3 to 5 days discoloration has spread over whole abdomen and external genitals.

After from 8 to 10 days it has spread over whole body; abdomen distended with gas, the peculiar odor developed, and *cornea* sunken, *concave*.

In 14 to 20 days the whole body is bright green, mixed with red and brown; epidermis raised and blistered here and there, nails loose, and maggots cover the body.

---

## PROBABLE CAUSE OF DEATH.

*Wounds* inflicted during life always show signs of *vital reaction*, as swelling, inflammation, bleeding, etc., while such signs are absent in wounds made *after* death.

A *contused* wound seldom represents exact *size of weapon* used. Examine *depth*, *breadth*, *direction* and *number* of wounds; they often furnish a clew to *position* and object of perpetrator.

*Gun-shot* wounds made after death are never so deep as similar ones made in live body, and their *track* can be distinctly traced.

*Burns* on dead body never produce vesication, except by *intense* heat, then *bulla* never contains *serum* or has boundary line of redness.

*Apoplexy* may be distinguished from *cerebral hemorrhage*—the result of injuries—by small amount of blood effused in former case, while in the latter it will be much more extensive.

**Body found in water.** Was it dead or alive when it entered therein? If some of the fluid in which the body was lying be found in the stomach, and is such as never voluntarily drank, it is the surest sign that body was alive. Examination will reveal the cause of death.

# DEATH FROM POISONING.

*Post-Mortem Appearances.*

**ALCOHOL.** The morbid appearances are: *hyperæmia* of brain, sometimes cerebral hemorrhage. Also hyperæmia of large abdominal veins, heart and lungs. *Fluidity* and *dark color* of blood; odor of brandy; body *slow* to putrefy. From 2 to 6 ounces have proved *fatal.*

**ARSENIC.** *Inflammation* of alimentary canal; inner surface of stomach *red* or *blackish* from extravasation of blood, sometimes thickened, with *rugæ raised,* corrugated. Sanguinolent fluid or actual blood is often found in the stomach. Blood in a state of great *fluidity.* There are some cases in which no morbid appearances are to be seen. Arsenic, like alcohol, *retards* putrefaction. From 2 to 3 grains have proved fatal. Death may ensue in half an hour, or be delayed for 2 or 3 weeks.

**CARBONIC OXIDE.** After death from this gas, a bright *cherry-red* color of the heart is characteristic. Also hyperæmia of lungs and right side of the heart.

**CORROSIVE SUBLIMATE.** Appearance very similar to that of *Arsenic,* but *mouth, throat* and *gullet* more affected, being white or bluish-gray color. Coats of stomach and intestines, particularly the colon and rectum, congested and inflamed. Bladder *contracted;* kidneys congested and inflamed. *Three* grains have proved fatal.

**HYDROCYANIC ACID.** The lesions produced are uncertain. The spine and neck are stiff, abdomen contracted, skin livid. On opening the body, *odor* of the *acid* is observed. Turgescence of veins and *emptiness* of arteries. Stomach and intestines congested and red. Liver and lungs gorged with blood. This *acid* in $\frac{9}{10}$ of a grain has proved fatal.

**NITRIC ACID.** Appearances similar to those described under *Sulphuric Acid.* Only marked difference is, *Nitric ac.* produces *yellow* color of the skin, lips, mouth, etc., which it touches, while *Sulphuric ac.* colors the parts *brownish. Two drachms* have caused death.

**OPIUM.** The skin is usually *livid.* Vessels of brain turgid, and watery effusions in *ventricles.* Lungs gorged with blood, stomach sometimes *red.* Blood always *fluid,* and putrefaction *rapid. Four* grains have proved fatal.

**OXALIC ACID.** The mucous membrane of the mouth, throat, and gullet looks as if scalded. Stomach contains thick fluid, dark like coffee-grounds; inner coat pulpy, some points black, others red. *Sixty* grains have proved fatal.

**PHOSPHORUS.** After death from *Phos.,* stomach is found contracted, mucous membrane inflamed, partly ash-colored, partly dark purplish red, and exhibits gangrenous ulcers. On opening stomach, strong smell of *garlic.* Fatty degeneration of liver, heart and kidneys. *Two* grains of *Phos.* have caused death.

**STRYCHNIA.** The *rigidity* of body which existed before, often remains for hours *after* death. Hands are *clenched*, feet *arched*, or turned inwards. Congestion of membranes of brain and spinal cord. Very slight irritation is found in the stomach or intestines. *Half* a grain has proved fatal.

**SULPHURIC ACID.** On the lips, fingers and other parts of the skin where the *acid* has touched, spots and streaks of a brownish or yellowish-brown color are to be seen. The lining membrane of mouth and fauces whitish, while that of the throat and gullet is brown or ashy-gray and corroded. The stomach, if not perforated, is collapsed and contracted, and contains yellowish-brown or black matter. If the stomach be perforated, holes are *roundish*, with vascular margins. Inner coat of duodenum often resembles that of stomach. Bladder usually empty. Blood thicker and of *acid* reaction. Bodies *slow* to putrefy. *One drachm* of acid has proved fatal.

---

## DEATH FROM SUFFOCATION.

Death from impeded respiration, or inhaling noxious gases, presents the following appearances: Face bluish-red, swollen, with protruding eyes. Froth often issues from mouth. Mucous membrane of larynx and trachea injected and of *blood-red color*. Trachea contains frothy mucus, or bloody foam; more gradual suffocation has been, greater quantity of this fluid. Unusual *fluidity* and *dark color* of blood. Hyperæmia of lungs and congestion of pulmonary artery. *Right* side of heart gorged with blood, *left* empty.

---

## DEATH FROM HANGING, THROTTLING, ETC.

In these cases death may result from dislocation of neck, *cerebral* congestion, *thoracic* congestion, and from neuro-paralysis. The internal appearances will vary accordingly.

The face may be livid, with protruding eyes and tongue, or be like any other corpse.

The mark of cord on neck may be a dirty, yellowish-brown color, *cutting hard* and leathery, or of a blue or dirty-reddish color soft to cut. If cord has been *hard* or *rough* excoriation will be visible. Similar marks of cord may be made after death.

In case of *throttling*, finger-marks will be visible of a dirty, *brownish-yellow* color, hard to cut, not ecchymosed.

---

## DEATH FROM DROWNING.

In death from *drowning* the appearances upon dissection are almost *identical* with death from asphyxia or strangulation. The cutaneous surface resembles "goose-skin." Face pale, *not* swollen, eyes *closed*. If body has been in water several days, face will be reddish, or blue-red; putrefaction begins in head, and extends downwards. [See Putrefaction].

Feet and hands have a livid, grayish-blue color, and skin corrugated in longitudinal folds, if body has not been taken out of water within 8 hours after death.

Penis and scrotum *contracted*, if body entered the water alive.

Dissection reveals *cerebral* congestion, the rarest form; thoracic congestion, or *neuro-paralysis*, the last two are of equal frequency in drowning.

Lungs increased in volume, all cavity of chest, are not crepitating, feel like sponges.

Trachea and bronchial tubes mostly filled with frothy mucus. Very little water enters the lungs or stomach.

---

## PRESERVING SPECIMENS OF MORBID ANATOMY.

That the fullest benefit may be realized from a post-mortem examination, any rare specimens found should be carefully preserved.

**SOFT TISSUES.**—All specimens of *soft* tissues to be preserved should be thoroughly washed and soaked in water, which is freqently changed until all blood is removed. In *warm* weather it will be necessary to add a little alcohol, carbolic acid or common salt to the water to prevent putridity.

All blood having been removed, place the specimen in alcohol, slightly diluted, and let it remain until thoroughly "cured." Small specimens will not require the alcohol so strong to cure them as larger ones. After being *well "cured,"* equal parts of alcohol and water will be sufficient to preservo all specimens except large ones, which will require two-thirds alcohol to one of water.

**GLASS JARS.**—The best form of vessel for preserving specimens in is a glass jar with a ground stopper; the latter should have a hook in the centre from which to suspend the specimen.

Where the common jar is used, great care will be required to make it tight so as to prevent evaporation. Take a piece of *thick* sheet lead, cut round to fit on top of the jar; make two small holes near the centre through which to pass a string to suspend the specimen. The holes and string on top of lead should be well covered with sealing-wax to prevent the alcohol from escaping. Then take a piece of moistened bladder, place it over the lead, and with strong twine tie it down tightly around the neck of the jar. When dry cover with a coat of black varnish, then another layer of bladder and another coat of varnish.

Preparations of this kind should be kept in a well lighted room and not in a dark closet.

**SPECIMENS FOR MICROSCOPICAL EXAMINATION.**—To preserve sections of tumors, glands, membranes, spinal cord, brain, etc., for microscopic examination, take Bichromate of Potassa, 75 grains; Sulphate of Soda, 35 grains; dissolve in six ounces of water. Suspend the specimen in this solution until it is sufficiently hardened to be cut into thin sections.

---

## PREPARATION OF BONES.

In preparing pathological specimens of bones, two methods are employed. The boiling process may be used where the texture of the specimen is firm and solid. Maceration is the better method, especially in all cases where the bone is softened by caries or necrosis. Strip off the soft tissues and place the bone in a vessel of water; change the latter daily, so long as it becomes colored by the blood. Then let it remain in the water until the putrefactive process softens the tissues so they may be easily removed, after which thoroughly wash in *soda water*. If the weather is cold the macerating must be conducted in a *warm* room.

To remove the grease and improve the color of bones, they may be bleached by covering them for a few days with Sulphuric Ether. Such specimens should be mounted to expose their interesting points.

# CHARACTERISTIC SYMPTOMS

OF THE MOST IMPORTANT

# HOMŒOPATHIC REMEDIES

---

## ACONITUM NAPELLUS.

**MIND.** Fear and anxiety of mind, with great nervous excitability, [see **Bell.**] ***Fear** of death; predicts the day he will die; [desires death, **Aur. Bell. Phos.**] **Anxiety, restless, agonized tossing about.* Over-sensitive, cannot bear light or noise. Fitful mood, changing from one thing to another; sings, whistles and weeps, [**Bell.**] *Delirium, especially at night,* [**Bapt.**]

**HEAD.** Vertigo on rising from a seat, stooping, or looking up, [**Bry. Podo.** ***Puls.**]. *Congestion of head, with great heat and redness of face, [***Bell.** ***Bry.**] *Fulness and heaviness* in forehead, as if the brain would start out of the eyes, [***Bell.** ***Bry. Merc.**—Sensation of *emptiness* in head, **Carol. r. Cocc. Ign. Opi.**] *Piercing, throbbing pain in forehead; worse from motion. Burning headache, as if brain were moved by boiling water, [**Indigo.**] *Hair feels as if standing on end, [**Bary. c. Dulc.**—As if a cluster were *pulled out* of vertex, **Mag. c. Indigo.**]

**EYES.** *Acute ophthalmia,* with burning, shooting pains. Aversion to sunlight, [***Bell. Con. Euph.**—Candlelight, **Gel.** —Desires light, **Stram.**] Hard, red swelling of lids, [with scurfs and ulcers on edges, **Merc.**]

**EARS.** *Roaring in ears, [see **Chin.**] *Acuteness* of hearing; noise is intolerable, [**Mag. c. Phos. ac.** ***Sil.**—Dulness of hearing, **Ars. Bell.** ***Calc. Phos. Stram.**] *Inflammation of external ear.*

**NOSE.** *Bleeding of nose, especially of plethoric persons, [**Bry.** ***Bell.**] *Acuteness of smell.*

**FACE.** *Swollen, red and hot,* [dark-red, bloated, ***Bell. Hyos. Opi.**—See **Merc.**] On rising, the red face becomes pale, [the least emotion produces a red-flushed face, ***Ferr.**—Pale, death-colored face, with distorted features, ***Ars. Canth. Phos.**] *Neuralgia,* left side.

**MOUTH and THROAT.** *Lips dry and black,* [***Ars. Bry.** ***Merc.** — *Continually licking his dry, parched lips, **Ars.**] Great dryness of mouth and tongue,[***Ars. Bry. Cham.**— *Without thirst,* **Bell. Lyc.** ***Nux m.**] Tongue coated white. *Inflammation of throat, (palate, tonsils, fauces), with high fever, dark redness of parts, burning, stinging pain, [***Apis. Bell.**

**Merc.**] Stinging in throat when swallowing, [**Apis.**—*Burning, shooting*, **Bell.**]

**STOMACH and ABDOMEN.** *Bitter taste of everything except water, [all food and drink taste *bitter*, ***Bry. Colo. Chin. Puls.**] *Unquenchable thirst*, but drinks *little and often*, [***Ars. Apis. Chin. Hyos.**—Takes large draughts at long intervals, **Bry.**] Bitter, bilious vomiting, with cold perspiration, [with cold sweat on forehead, ***Verat.**—See **Ipec.**] *Inflammation of stomach, [***Ars. Canth.** ***Phos. Nux.**] Violent pains in stomach after eating or drinking, [***Ars. Ferr.** ***Nux. Puls.**] *Acute hepatitis.* *Pressure in *region of liver. Inflammation of bowels, with sharp, shooting pains in whole abdomen, which is very tender to touch.* *Inflammation of hernial stricture, with bilious vomiting, [see **Nux.**]

**STOOL.** *Frequent, scanty stools, with tenesmus*, [**Ars. Bell. Colch. Merc.** [*Green, watery stools, like chopped herbs, [like scum on frog-pond, ***Mag. c.**] *White stools*, [**Calc. Chin. Hep.**—*Black*, **Camph. Chin.** ***Lept.** ***Verat.**] *Seat-worms, with nightly itching at the anus.*

**URINE.** *Retention of urine, with stitches in kidneys, [see **Canth.**] Difficult and scanty emissions of bright red urine, [brown, blackish, **Colch. Nat. m. Tereb.**] *Burning and tenesmus at neck of bladder.*

**SEXUAL O'S.** . Piercing, pinching in glans penis when urinating. *Bruised pain in testicles.*

*Ovaritis* after sudden checking of menstrual flow. **Menses* too profuse and protracted, especially in young and plethoric women, [***Bell. Calc.**—See **Puls.**] *Suppression of menses from fright, [**Lyc.**—From cold, ***Dulc. Podo.** ***Puls. Sulph.**] Too scant, or suppressed lochia, [with splitting headache, ***Bry.**] Rigidity of os uteri, [**Bell.** ***Caul. Gel.**]

**RESPIRATORY O'S.** Inflammation of larynx and bronchia, [**Bell. Dros. Phos.**] *First stage of croup, with dry cough and loud breathing during *expiration* [see **Spong.**] *Every expiration ends with hoarse, hacking cough. *The child grasps at the throat* with every coughing fit. Shortness of breath when sleeping or rising up. Paroxysms of suffocation, with anxiety, [**Ars. Hep. Lach.**] **Pleurisy and Pneumonia*, with great heat, much thirst, dry cough and nervous excitement, [***Bry. Kali c. Phos.**] *Hot feeling in lungs. Stitches* in chest, with dry, hacking cough. **Palpitation of the heart, with great anguish.*

**SLEEP.** *Sleeplessness, with restless tossing about*, [**Ars. Bell. Cham.**—*Sleepy*, but cannot sleep, ***Bell. Ferr.** ***Opi.**] Dreams with a sort of clairvoyance, [**Phos.**] *Nightly delirium.

**FEVER.** *Pulse hard, full, frequent*, [**Bell. Bry. Hyos. Stram.**—*Slow*, full, **Dig. Merc.** ***Opi.**—*Small, contracted, weak*, **Ars. Carb. v. Phos. ac.** ***Verat.**] *Chill and synochal fever, with dry, hot skin, violent thirst, red face, shortness of breath and great nervous excitability, [see **Bell. Bry.**] *Sensation of coldness in the blood-vessels*, [**Verat.**—As if hot water were coursing through them, ***Ars.** ***Rhus.**] Perspiration over whole body, [only on upper part, **Sep.**] *Bad effects from suppressed sweat.*

**SKIN.** Red, hot, swollen, shining skin, [**Bell.**] *Morbilli.* Purpura millaris. **Rubeola, Variola.*

**CHARACT. PECULIARITIES.** Adapted to sanguine, plethoric persons, [**Arn.** ***Bell. Hepar. Merc.**—Leucophlegmatic persons, **Ars. Calc. c. Nit. ac. Sulph.**] Congestions of head, heart, chest, [***Bell. Bry.**] Complaints arising from exposure to cold, dry winds, [**Hepar.**] Excessive sensibility to least touch, [**Agar. Bell. Bry. Nux m.**] Attacks of pain, with thirst and redness of face, [with *chilliness*, **Ars.** ***Bell. Sep.** ***Puls.** —Chilliness after pains, [**Kali c.**] Stinging pains in affected parts, [***Apis.**] *Pains insupportable, especially at night, [***Ars.** ***Cham. Coff. Lach.**] *Stitches* here and there, [**Bry.**]

*Aggravation* in evening (chest symptoms) when lying on left side; [**Cact. Phos.**] *in a warm room*, [**Croc.** ***Puls. Sec. Verat.**]

*Amelioration* in open air, [**Puls.**] nervous symptoms; when sitting still, [**Bry.**] rheumatism.

## ANTIMONIUM CRUDUM.

**MIND.** *Loathing of life. *Sentimental mood. Conduct like that of an insane person, [gesticulates, dances, sings and laughs, **Bell.** ***Stram.**] *Child cannot bear to be touched or looked at, [cries if spoken to, **Sil.**—Cries if *touched*, **Cina. Tart. e.**]

**HEAD.** Vertigo, with nausea, or bleeding of nose, [with nausea and headache, **Apis.**] Congestion of blood to head, followed by bleeding of nose, [headache, with nosebleed, **Alum. Carb. a. Coff. Dulc.**] Stupefying headache, with nausea; worse in evening; after eating or drinking, [see **Puls.**] *Headache from bathing, [**Calc. c. Puls.**—From use of tobacco, **Acon. Ant. Ign.**] *Headache from deranged stomach.*

**NOSE.** *Coldness in nose when inspiring. *Sore, cracked and crusty nostrils, and corners of mouth, [cracks in point of nose, **Carbo a.**] Epistaxis after headache, [with headache, **Alum. Carbo a. Dulc.**]

**MOUTH.** *Thick, *milky-white* coating on tongue, [**Arn.** ***Bry, Nux v. Sep.**—*Coated as if with fur,* ***Merc. Puls.**] *Saltish tasting saliva.* Decayed teeth ache worse at night, and from contact and cold water, [better from cold water, ***Coff. Puls.**] *Profuse bleeding of gums,* [**Ars.** ***Merc. Nit. ac. Phos.**]

**STOMACH.** *Derangement from overloading stomach,* [**Ipec. Nux. Puls.**—From eating fat food, pork, etc., **Carb. v. Ipec.** ***Puls.**] *Stomach very weak, easily deranged.* *Fluid eructations *tasting of ingesta,* [**Calc. c. Chin. Con.**] *Violent nausea.* *Terrible vomiting which nothing can stop, [**Lob. in. Tart. em.**] Vomiting slime and bile, [**Ipec.**] Violent vomiting and diarrhœa, [***Ars. Jatropha. Tart. e.** ***Verat.**] *Cramp-like pain in stomach* from indigestion, [**Chin. Nux.** ***Puls.**]

**STOOL.** *Sensation as if a copious stool would take place, when only flatus is passed; finally, a hard stool is voided. *Alternate diarrhœa and constipation, especially of aged persons, [**Bry. Lach. *Phos. Rhus.**] *Watery diarrhœa*, with cutting pain in bowels, [without pain, **Ars. Ferr. *Podo.**]

**FEVER.** *Pulse very irregular*, [**Ars. Dig. Lauro. Merc.**] Chilliness preponderates, even in a warm room, [**Anac, Mez. *Puls.**] **Intermittent fever*, with great sadness and a woeful mood; desire to sleep, and no thirst. *Heat*, especially during night, with cold feet. *Perspiration* when awaking in morning.

**CHARACT. PECULIARITIES.** Disposition to grow fat, [**Bary. c. *Calc. c. Sulph.**—To grow *lean*, **Ars. Chin. *Iod. Phos.**] When the symptoms reappear they change their locality, or go from one side of body to the other.

## APIS MELLIFICA.

**MIND.** *Absent-mindedness. Inability to fix the thoughts on any subject, [confusion of mind, cannot connect his thoughts, ***Gels.**—Anxiety, with fear of losing one's mind, **Merc. v.**] *Delirium*, after suppressed scarlet eruptions, [**Bell. Bry. Opi.**]

**HEAD.** *Vertigo, with nausea and headache*, [with nausea and nosebleed, **Ant. c.**] Pressing pain in forehead and temples; worse when rising, and in a warm bed, relieved by pressure, [**Puls.**] *Pain in occiput, with sudden screams.* *Hydrocephalus in children. *Sudden shrill screams.*

**EYES.** Inflammation of eyes, with intolerance of light, and increased secretions, [**Ars. Bell. *Euph. Merc.**] *Œdematous* swelling of eyelids, [**Ars. Cro. t. Kali hy.**—Swelling over upper lid, like a little bag, in morning, **Kali c.**]

**MOUTH and THROAT.** Swelling of lips, especially of upper. *Dry, swollen, inflamed tongue, with inability to swallow, [**Bell. Merc.**] *Stinging, burning in throat*, [**Acon.**] *Red and highly-inflamed tonsils, [**Acon. *Bell. Cap.**] *Diphtheria; the pseudo-membrane assumes at once a dirty grayish color*, [see **Kali b.**] Ulcerated sore throat, in scarlet fever, where eruption does not come out, [**Bell. Merc. Mur. ac.**] *Can bear nothing to touch the neck, [***Lach.**]

**STOMACH and ABDOMEN.** Vomiting, with inflammation of stomach. *Burning heat in stomach. Violent pain and *sensitiveness of the stomach.* *Sensation in abdomen as if something tight would break if much effort were made to void a stool. *Great soreness of abdomen, [**Acon. *Bell. Merc. Nux.**]

**STOOL.** *Greenish, yellowish, slimy mucus; or yellow, watery, *painless* diarrhœa; worse in morning. Involuntary, as though anus stood open, [***Phos.**] *Hemorrhoids, with stinging pains, [**Ars. Nit. ac. Sulph.**] *Prolapsus ani*, [**Calc. *Ferr. Mur. ac. *Pod.**]

**URINE.** *Strangury.* *Urine dark-colored and scanty,

[Bell. Lyc. Nit. ac.—Black like coffee, Colch. Nat. m. Tereb.] Incontinence of urine, worse at night, and when coughing. Involuntary emissions of urine when coughing, sneezing, etc., [*Caust. Puls. Verat.]

**SEXUAL O'S.** *Swelling of testicles*, [Acon. *Merc.] *Inflammation, induration, swelling and dropsy of the *right ovary*, with sharp, cutting, stinging pain, [*Bell.—*Left ovary* swollen, with pressing, stitching pains, Graph. *Lach.] *Miscarriage.*

**CHEST.** Hoarseness, especially in morning, [*Caust. *Iod. Phos. Sulph.—In evening, Calc. c. Brom. Kali b.] Soreness in chest, as from a bruise, [*Arn. Kreo. Lyc. Phos.] Rapid, painful, spasmodic respiration, worse when lying down. Hydrothorax, with a sensation as if he would not be able to breathe again. *Cough after sleeping*, [*Lach.]

**EXTREMITIES.** Hands bluish and inclined to be cold. **Panaritium.* Legs cold, [Amb. Nux. Sil.—Burning, Agar. Borax. Lyc.] *Swelling of feet, ankles and legs, [Bry. Calc. c. Merc. Puls.]

**FEVER.** Pulse full and rapid—small and trembling—intermitting, [see Dig.] Chilliness from least motion, [Merc. c. *Nux v. Rhus. Podo.—From warmth of stove, Cina. Dulc. Merc. Ruta.] **Intermittents;* chill about 4 P. M.; worse in a warm room or near stove, [chill relieved by heat, Ars. Coral. r. *Ign.—Increased by, Apis. Ipec.] After fever paroxysm, deep sleep. *Perspiration*, alternating with dryness of skin, [Nat. c.]

**SKIN.** *Red spots on skin, with stinging, burning pains, [Dulc. Rhus. *Urt. u.] Scarlet eruptions, [Bell. Sulph.] *Skin white, and almost transparent, with ovarian dropsy. *Dropsy* without thirst.

**CHARACT. PECULIARITIES.** *Stinging pains in affected parts, similar to bee-stings, [burning, stinging pains, Merc. Puls.] Great sensitiveness to touch, [*Acon. Agar. *Bell. Bry.—Strong pressure relieves, Nat. c. *Nux.] *Burning, stinging pains.

*Aggravation*, in morning, (diarrhœa) from heat, especially in warm room, [better from heat, Ars. Hepar. Kali b. Rhus.] Wants to be in the cold air.

*Amelioration;* cold water relieves pain, swelling, burning. Pressure relieves the headache, [Arg. n. Puls.]

## ARGENTUM NITRICUM.

**MIND.** *Falters in speech, cannot find right word. No inclination to work, is melancholy, and thinks about killing himself. *Time seems to pass very slowly*, [Cham.—Very *quickly*, Cocc. Ther.] Faint feeling.

**HEAD.** *Vertigo, with *buzzing in ears.* Staggers when walking in the dark. *Congestion of head, with throbbing of carotid arteries*, [Acon. *Bell. *Glon. Opi.] *Screwing, *throbbing* pain in frontal protuberance, temple, or bones of face. Headache, with chilliness, or trembling of the body. The headache is relieved by tying head up tightly, [**Apis. *Puls.**] *Head feels much enlarged, [***Cimi. Gel. *Glon. *Nux.**—Too *small*, **Coff.**—As if *elongated*. **Hyp. per.**] *Sensation as if bones of skull separated. Crawling in scalp, as from vermin.*

**EYES.** *Itching and smarting of canthi.* Conjunctiva of ball and lids intensely congested. *Bright-red granulations in lids. Lids crusty, swollen, thick.

**EARS.** Dull hearing. *Ringing in ears*, [see **Chin.**] Whizzing and feeling of obstruction in ears.

**FACE.** Face sunken, pale, bluish; leaden colored. *The face has an old look, [***Opi.**] Circumscribed red cheeks.

**MOUTH.** Fetor from mouth in morning. *Tip of tongue red, painful, papillæ prominent. Red streak down middle of tongue, [**Verat. v.**—Dry, *brown streak*, **Bapt.**]

**THROAT.** *Uvula and fauces dark red, [**Acon. Bapt. Bell.**] *Sensation as if a splinter had lodged in throat*, [**Hepar. Nit. ac.**] *Hawks up thick, tough mucus, [**Kali c. Kobal. Lobe. Phos. ac.**—Tasting *coppery*, **Cimi.**—Tasting *greasy*, **Asaf.**—*Hawking up *lumps* of phlegm, **Chel.**—Hard, *greenish lumps*, **Merc. iod.**—Soft, *fetid tubercles*, color of peas, ***Mag. c.**—Bloody mucus, **Lyc. Mag. m.**]

**STOMACH.** *Sweetish taste*, [**Cup. Merc. Sulph.**] *Metallic* taste, [**Cocc. Merc. Plumb.**] *Irresistible desire for sugar, [for *acids*, **Bry. Chin. Nux.**] *Belching after every meal, stomach as if it would burst with wind, [see **Chin.**] Regularly towards midnight, attacks of pain preceded by vomiting slimy and bilious fluids. *After ice-cream, gastralgia, pain radiating in all directions, worse after food. Rumbling, gurgling in abdomen. Flatulent dyspepsia.

**STOOL.** *Diarrhœa soon as he drinks, [**Ars. Cro. t.**] Stools *green, fetid mucus*, with noisy flatus at night. *Green*, brown, bloody, fetid mucus, worse after midnight. *Emissions of much noisy flatus.*

**URINE.** Urine dark-red, deposits red crystals of uric acid. *Urine passes unconsciously and uninterruptedly. *Incontinence of urine at night.*

**SEXUAL O'S.** *Impotence in men.* Organs shrivelled. *Women.* *Coition painful, followed by bleeding from vagina. *Prolapsus, with ulceration of os or cervix uteri*, [**Arum. *Hydras, Kreo. Merc. Sep.**] *Menses irregular*, too soon or too late, too copious or too scanty, but always with thick, coagulated blood. *Metrorrhagia at change of life. Leucorrhœa, copious, yellow, corroding.

**RESPIRATORY O'S.** *Chronic laryngitis of singers, raising the voice causes cough. *Rawness, soreness* in larynx, [**Gel. Phyto.**] Short breathed, with deep sighs. Spasmodic asthma, forcing him to rise and walk about. *Palpitation of heart, with nausea. Pain about heart, can hardly breathe.

**CHARACT. PECULIARITIES.** *Convulsions preceded by great restlessness. *Periodical trembling* of body. *Paralysis of lower half of body, from debilitating causes. *Septic forms* *of scarlet fever, eruption bluish-black.* Sensation of *expansion* of head, face, etc.

## ARNICA MONTANA.

**MIND.** Depression of spirits and absence of mind. *Hypochondriacal anxiety,* peevishness, [**Aur. Nux. *Puls.**—Gaiety, cheerfulness, **Croc. Lach. Oxal. ac.**] Declines answering questions; [indisposed to talk, ***Phos. ac. Stan.**—Talks continually, **Stram.**]

**HEAD.** Vertigo, with nausea; better when lying down, [worse lying down or turning over in bed, ***Con.**] *Heat in head, while body is cool,* [**Bry. Hyos.**—*Cold limbs,* with hot head, **Bell.**] *Stitches in head, especially forehead and temples. *Headache as from a nail thrust in temple, with sweat and faintness. *Bad effects from concussion of brain, [***Cicu.**]

**EYES.** Contraction of pupils, [**Cicu. Phos.**—Pupils dilated, ***Bell. Hyos. Opi. *Stram.**] Eyes half closed.

**NOSE.** *Frequent bleeding of nose, [**Acon. *Bell. Bry.** —See ***Phos.**] *Swelling of the nose, end cold.*

**STOMACH.** *Putrid, slimy taste, [***Merc. Nux v. Puls.**] Aversion to meat or broth, [see **Hepar.**] **Eructations tasting like rotten eggs,* [**Mur ac. Sep. Sulph.**] *Feeling of nauseous repletion after eating, [immediately after eating, abdomen is bloated full, [***Chin. *Lyc. Nux v. Phos.**] *Vomiting coagulated blood, renewed by eating or drinking. Vomiting after drinking, [**Ars. Verat.**]

**STOOL.** Diarrhœa, stools *slimy, mucous; brown, fermented,* [*like yeast.*] *Stools of mucus, blood and pus, with tenesmus, [**Acon. Cap. *Merc. Nux.**]

**URINE.** Involuntary discharges of urine at night, when asleep or when coughing, [see **Caust.**] *Brown urine, brick-red sediment,* [white sediment, **Calc. c. Sep.**] Bloody urine, [**Ipec. Millef. Nit. ac. *Uva ursi.**]

**SEXUAL O'S.** *Cannot walk erect on account of a *sore, bruised* feeling in uterine region. Too long and violent after-pains, [**Bell. Puls. *Sec.**] *Great soreness of parts after labor. *Prolapsus uteri from concussion.*

**RESPIRATORY O'S.** Cough in children, excited by crying, [by laughing, talking, singing, etc., **Chin. Dros. Phos.**] **Whooping-cough;* every coughing-spell is preceded by crying, [**Tart. e.**—Cries after coughing, **Bell.**] *Asthma, with inclination to move about. Stitches in the left chest, with a short cough; worse from motion, [see **Bry.**] *Soreness in the intercostal muscles after severe exertion, ribs feel as if bruised.

**EXTREMITIES.** Sensation as if joints of arms and wrists *were sprained,* [**Rhod. Ruta.**—As if dislocated, **Bry. Merc. Ruta.**] *Limbs ache as if beaten.* *Gout, with great fear of being touched.

**FEVER.** *Chilliness* internally, with external *heat,* [**Ars.**

**Calc. c. Thuya.**—External heat, with internal coldness, **Cham. Ign. Nit. ac. Sulph.**] *Intermittent fever;* chill in morning; drawing-pains in bones before fever, [during chill, pain in back and limbs, as if *bones were broken*, ***Eup. per.**] Dry heat over whole body, or only in face and back. **Typhoid fever*, with the greatest indifference; putrid breath, and red, black or yellow spots on body; *while speaking forgets the word, [falls asleep in midst of a sentence, ***Bapt.**—After a correct answer relapses into delirium and unconsciousness, ***Hyos.**—Thinks another person is in same bed, ***Hydras.**—See ***Stram.**] Continually changing position, the bed feels too hard, [**Bapt.**—See **Rhus.**]

**CHARACT. PECULIARITIES.** Adapted to sanguine, plethoric persons, [**Acon. Bell. Hepar.**] *Sore, aching pains, as if from a bruise, [**Cicu. Rhus t.** ***Ruta.**] *Bad effects from *mechanical injuries*, [**Symph. of.**—Punctured wounds, when nerves are injured and lockjaw is threatened, **Hyper. p.**] *Everything on which he lies feels too hard, [**Bapt.**] Heat in upper parts of body, while lower parts are cold.

*Amelioration*, in the evening or at night; from contact and motion; even from noise.

## ARSENICUM ALBUM.

**MIND.** *Great anguish, extreme restlessness, and fear of death, [***Acon. Bry. Rhus t.**—Desires death, ***Aur.** ***Bell. Creo. Sil.**] Fear of being alone, [**Lyc.**—Wants to be alone, ***Nux v.**] Delirium; springs up from bed and hides; [springs out of bed and tries to escape, ***Bell. Bry.**] *Cannot find rest anywhere, wants to go from bed to bed.

**HEAD.** *Periodical headache*, better from application of cold water, [periodical nervous headache, worse from heat of bed and when lying down, **Bell. Spig.**] *Throbbing* in head, with inclination to vomit, [**Bell. Sep.**] *Great weight, particularly in forehead, [on vertex, **Cact. Cann. s Kali b.**]

**EYES.** Inflammation of eyes, with severe burning pains, [stinging pains, **Apis. Calc. c.**] **Scrofulous ophthalmia*, [**Arum. Hepar.** ***Merc. sub. Sulph.**—*Syphilitic ophthalmia*, **Arg. nit.** ***Nit. ac. Phyto.**] *Specks or ulcers on cornea*, [**Calc. c.** ***Merc.** ***Sil. Sulph.**]

**NOSE.** Cancer of nose, with severe burning. *Profuse fluent coryza, with discharge of burning, excoriating water, [***Arum t.**—*Dry coryza*, **Dulc. Nit. ac.** ***Nux v. Sep.**] *Cannot bear smell of food.*

**FACE.** Puffiness of face, especially around the eyes. *Pale, death-like color of face, with distorted features, [**Canth. Chin.**—*Cold, collapsed face;* pinched-up, bluish nose, ***Verat.**—Distorted, bluish face, with mouth wide open, **Hyos.**] *Lips dark, dry and parched, which he constantly licks.*

**MOUTH and THROAT.** *Swollen, bleeding gums. Mouth reddish-blue, inflamed, burning. Tough, fetid, bloody saliva,

[**Hyos. Nit. ac. Nux. Rhus.**] *Tongue bluish* or white; *brown or blackish*, [see **Lyo.**] *Burning* in throat, [***Acon. *Bell. Lach. Nit. ac.**—*Coldness* in throat, **Carb. v. Laur. *Verat.**] **Angina gangrenosa*, [**Amm. Lach. Merc.**]

**STOMACH and ABDOMEN.** Food has no taste, [tastes like straw, ***Stram.**—All food and drink taste bitter, ***Bry. Colo. Puls.**] * *Violent thirst, drinking often, but little at a time*, [**Apis. Chin. Hyos.**—Often, and much at a time, **Acon. Bell. Nat. m.**] *Vomiting, especially *after eating or drinking*, **Bry. Nux v. Puls. *Verat.**—Vomiting renewed by least motion, ***Verat. Zinc.**] Vomiting *black bile and blood*, [**Hyd. ac. Ipec. Sec. *Verat.**] *Vomiting, with diarrhœa and great prostration*, **Jatro. Tart. e. *Verat.**] *Morning vomiting of drunkards. *Violent burning in stomach, [**Canth. Nux v. *Phos. Sec.**—Great burning distress in epigastric region, ***Iris v. *Verat. v.**—Coldness in stomach, **Colch. Laur. Phos.**] *Pressure in stomach as from a stone, especially after eating, [***Bry. Merc. *Nux v. Sep.**] *Stomach very painful to touch*, [**Bry. Lyc. *Merc. *Nux v.**] *Disordered stomach from eating fruit, ice-cream, drinking ice-water, [**Chin. *Puls. Nux.**] Spasmodic colic, with a sensation as if intestines became twisted, [as if tied in knots, **Verat.**—As if squeezed between stones, ***Colo.**] *Burning in abdomen, [**Lach. Phos. Sec. Sep.**—*Coldness*, **Calc. c. Colch. Plumb. Podo.**]

**STOOL.** *Dark-green, mucous stools*, [***Arg. n. Cro. t. *Merc.**—*White, jelly-like mucus*, ***Colch. *Hell.**] *Dark or black watery stools, very offensive*, [**Kali b. Lep. *Verat.**] *Corrosive*, watery stools, [***Cham. Merc. Sulph.**] *Cutting pain in bowels, with tenesmus.* Painless watery stools. **Sudden and rapid prostration*, [**Acon. *Camph. *Verat.**] *Burning in anus and rectum during and after stool. *Worse after eating or drinking*, [***Cro. t. Ferr. Podo. *Verat.**]

**RESPIRATORY O'S.** Cough, as if caused by *smoke of sulphur*, with a sense of suffocation, [**Chin. Ign.**—As if from *dust in throat*, **Bell.**—As if caused from a feather in throat, **Am. c. Cal. c. Dros. Ign.**—From tickling under sternum, **Rhus r. Rumex.**—From *tickling in chest*, **Phos. *Rhus r. Stan. *Verat.**] *Dry, hacking cough, with *soreness of chest.* Difficult, scanty expectoration, sometimes *streaked with blood.* *Anxious and oppressive shortness of breath, particularly when *ascending an eminence*, and at *night* when *lying down.* *Cannot lie down for fear of suffocation, [**Acon. Eup. per. Samb. Tart.**] Constriction of chest, with anguish, [**Cact. g. Nux. Phos. *Sulph.**—Sensation of expansion, **Olean.**—Of extension, **Cap.**] Sensation of *coldness* of chest, [**Carb. a. Lach. Ruta. Sulph.**—*Burning* in the, **Am. c. Calc. c. Merc. Spong. Sulph.**] **Palpitation of heart, especially at night*, and when lying on back.

**EXTREMITIES.**—*Arms* swollen, with *black blisters*, having a fetid smell. Burning ulcers on the tips of fingers, [burning, itching and redness, *as if frozen*, ***Agar. m. Carb. an.**]

*Legs* feel so heavy, can hardly raise them, [**Bell. Calc. c. Nit. ac. Rhus.**] ******Ulcers on legs*, with burning, lancinating pains, [***Lach. *Lyc. Merc.**] *Varices, burn like fire.*

**SLEEP.** *Sleeplessness, with constant tossing about, [***Acon. Bell. Cham.**] Starting of the limbs when falling asleep, [**Lyc. Opi. Puls. Sep.**], *grasping at flock*, [**Zinc.**]

**FEVER.** *Pulse* small, frequent, intermittent. *General coldness, with parchment-like dryness of skin, or with profuse, cold, clammy perspiration. **Chilliness*, particularly after drinking, [**Cap. Chin. *Nux. Verat.**] Chilliness relieved by external heat, [***Ign. Kali c.**] Chills *intermingled* with heat, or *internal coldness* and external heat, [**Arn. Calc. c. Thuj.**—*External coldness* and internal heat, **Cham. Ign. Nit. ac. Sulph.**—Chills and heat alternating, **Lach. Nux v. Phos. Verat.**] *Burning heat, as from hot water coursing through veins*, [**Bry. Rhus.**] *Intermittent fever*, chill every 3 P.M., [**Apis. Chin. Nux v. Puls. *Saba.**] *Blue nails and lips during chill. *Thirst only during hot stage, drinks often, but little at a time, [**Apis. Chin.**] During fever, great restlessness, pain in bones, small of back and forehead. *Perspiration* at beginning of sleep, cold, clammy, smelling sour. *Great weakness following paroxysm.

**SKIN.** Dry, parchment-like skin. *Black blisters*, burning and painful. *Red pustules, changing to ichorous, crusty, burning and spreading ulcers. **Putrid ulcers, with fetid ichor and proud flesh*, [**Carb. v. *Creo. *Sil. Sulph.**] *Ulcers feel as if burnt, [***Sec.**] *Ulcers discharging a *thin, bloody pus*, [**Asaf. Bell. Con. Hep.**—Corroding, acrid, **Caust. *Merc. Rhus. *Sil.**] **Carbuncles, which burn like fire*, [**Caust. Merc. Rhus. Sil.**] *Herpes*, red and burning.

**CHARACT. PECULIARITIES.** **Rapid prostration of strength*, [**Acon. *Camph. *Verat.**] *Extreme restlessness, and fear of death, [**Acon. Bry. Rhus t.**] *Extreme thirst, drinking little and often*, [**Apis. Chin.**] **Burning* pains, [**Carb. a. Carb. v. Phos. *Sec.**—*Stinging* pains, ***Apis. Merc. Sulph.**] Wants to be in a warm room, [**Hep. Kali b. Rhus.**—In a cold room, **Croc. *Puls. *Sec. Verat.**]

*Aggravation*, at night, particularly after midnight, [**Bell. Rhus.**] From cold in general; eating cold food.

*Amelioration*, from *heat* in general; lying with head high; *warm applications relieve.*

## BAPTISIA TINCTORIA.

**MIND.** *Confusion of ideas*, [**Bell. *Gel. Rhus.**] Excitement of brain, especially at night. Stupor and delirium, especially at night, with frightful dreams. Want of power to think.

**HEAD.** *Dull, stupefying headache*, [**Con. Dulc. Gel. Hydras.**—Beating, pulsating headache, ***Bell. Kalm. Nat. m. *Puls.**] *Head feels too heavy*, [**Calc. c. Phos. ac. Rhus. Sulph.**—Too *light*, *Stram. Hipp.] *Head feels as if *scattered about;* she tries to get the pieces together, [see **Stram.**]

**FACE.** Burning heat of face, cheeks burn. *Face dark-red, with a besotted expression; flushed.

**MOUTH and THROAT.** Tongue feels as if it had been scraped, [as if scalded, **Colo. Merc. Verat. v.**] Tongue coated *brown* and *dry*, particularly in the centre, [**Ars.**] *Putrid ulceration of buccal mucous membrane, with salivation, [**Merc. Nit. ac. Nux v.**] *Diphtheria*, the disease assumes a putrid character, the ulcers dark and breath fetid, [see **Kali b.**] Oesophagus as if *constricted.*

**STOOL.** Very fetid, exhausting diarrhœa, excoriating. Stools *dark, thin, fecal.* **Dysentery;* stools of pure blood or bloody mucus. Before stool, severe colic; during and after stool, *tenesmus*, [see **Merc.**]

**CHEST.** Congestion of lungs, with oppressed breathing; rising up in bed does not relieve; must go to window for fresh air, [**Sulph.**—Wants to be fanned all the time, ***Carb. v.**] Can't get a full breath; want of power in respiratory organs. Constriction and oppression of chest. Pain in right lung. Heart seems to *fill the chest.*

**EXTREMITIES.** Stiffness of the joints, as if sprained, [***Arn. Rhod. Ruta.**—As if dislocated, **Bry. Merc. *Ruta.**] *The hands feel too large*, [**Diad. Nitr.**—Too heavy, **Bry. Nitr. Puls.**] Severe drawing-pains in the calves. Limbs tremble and are very weak.

**FEVER.** Typhoid fever, wild delirious stupor. *While answering a question falls into a deep sleep, [after a correct answer relapses into delirium and unconsciousness, ***Hyos.** —See **Arn.**] *Head feels as if *scattered about*, tries to get the pieces together. *Face dark-red, with a besotted expression. *Soreness of flesh; the bed on which he lies feels too hard, [***Arn. Rhus.**] *Scarlet fever*, of a typhoid character, ulcerated sore throat, fetid breath, dry, sore tongue and vomiting.

**CHARACT. PECULIARITIES.** Pains of a *pressing, drawing* character, [**Bell. Mez. *Nux. Rhus.**] *All discharges from mucous surfaces have a fetid odor, [**Carb. v.**] *Right* side most affected, [**Bell. Iris. *Lyc.**—*Left* side, ***Lach.**] Pains *worse* from motion, relieved by rest, [**Acon. *Bry. Merc.**—Better from motion, worse during rest, **Con. Lyc. *Rhus. Sep. Sulph.**]

## BELLADONNA.

**MIND.** *Delirium*, with wild manner; he tears his clothes, and tries to injure himself, [wants to cut up everything, **Verat.**] **He tries to strike, bite and injure those around him,* [fury, with impulse to strike and kill, ***Hyos. *Stram.**] *Delirium, with frightful figures and images before eyes, [**Opi. *Stram.**] **Loquacious delirium, with desire to escape,* [**Bry. Hyos. *Stram.**—Tries to hide, ***Ars. Cup. Puls.**] *Al-*

*ternate laughing and crying*, [**Aur. Hyos. Ign. Stram.**] *He sings and tries to compose songs. Great irritability of all the senses, [**Nux. Stram.**] *Picking at bedclothes.*

**HEAD.** *Vertigo, with vanishing of sight and stupefaction. Vertigo when stooping or rising from a stooping posture, [**Bry. *Puls.**] **Throbbing headache*, with congestion of blood to head; throbbing of carotids, and great intolerance of light and noise, [**Acon. *Glon. Opi.**—See **Kali c.**] Pressing headache, as if a heavy weight were pressing upon forehead, [***Bis. Puls. Sulph.**—On vertex, ***Acon. Cann. Phos. *Sep.**] *Periodical, nervous headache;* worse about 3 P.M., from heat and when lying down. *Boring pain in right side of head, (neuralgia) increased by motion. *Sick headache; head feels as if it would burst; worse* from motion, a bright light, noise, or in a draught of air. *Hysteric headache*, [gastric sick headache, **Ipec. *Iris. Nux. *Puls.**] *Sense of great *fulness* in head, [***Acon. Bry. *Glon. Rhus.**—Of *emptiness*, **Cocc. Ign. Oxal. ac. Sep.**—Of a *lump* in brain, **Con.**—As if everything were alive, **Pet. Sil.**] *External heat* and soreness of head, [burning on the vertex, **Graph. Nat. m. *Sulph.**—*Coldness*, **Calc. c. Sep. *Verat.**] Sensation of swashing in head, [**Hepar. *Hyos. Nux v.**] **Boring* head into pillow, [**Apis. *Hell.**—Rolling head, **Podo.**—Frequent jerking head up, ***Stram.**] Shaking the head, [**Hyos.**]

**EYES.** *Eyes red, glistening, sparking; wild and unsteady, [**Hyos. Stram.**] Congestion to the eyes, with bright redness of vessels; "one gore of blood," [**Kali c. Thuya.**] *Great intolerance of light, [**Acon. Euph. Graph. Sulph.**—Desires light, ***Stram.**] *Objects appear *inverted*, [appear *double*, **Hyos. Stram. Thuya.**] *Pupils dilated*, [**Acon. Hyos. *Opi. *Stram.**—*Contracted*, **Ars. Cicu. *Laur. Phos.**]

**EARS.** *Inflammation* of external and internal ear. *Stitches* in ear, with hardness of hearing, [**Cham. Merc. Nat. m.**] *Humming and roaring in ears, [see **Chin.**] *Tingling in the ears.*

**NOSE.** **Bleeding* of nose, with red face. [***Acon.**—Bleeding of nose, when menses should appear, ***Bry. Ham. *Puls.**—See **Phos.**] *Ulcerated nostrils.*

**FACE.** **Glowing redness* of face, or else great paleness, [**Acon. Bry.**—Dark-red, swollen face, **Bry. *Hyos. Opi.**] **Erysipelas, with smooth, shining skin;* the redness runs in streaks from a centre, [*vesicular erysipelas*, **Rhus.**] *Swelling of upper lip.* Inflammatory swelling of submaxilliary glands.

**MOUTH.** *Dryness* of mouth, without thirst, [***Apis. Lyc. *Nux m.**—*Particularly after sleeping*, ***Nux m.**] **Tongue red, hot and dry*, with red edges and white in middle; papilla bright-red, prominent, [yellow, with *red streak* down middle, **Verat. v.**—Dry, black, cracked, **Ars. Merc. Verat.**—*Clean*, smooth, parched, dry, **Kali b. Hyos. *Rhus.**] **Tremor of tongue, stammering speech*, [**Ars. Lach.**] *Profuse ptyalism*, [see **Merc.**] *Grinding of teeth, with moaning, [see **Stram.**] *Soreness* of inner cheeks.

**THROAT.** *Violent burning in throat,* [**Acon. Ars. Canth. Lach. Merc. Nit. ac.**—*Coldness,* **Carb. v. Laur. *Verat.**] **Inflammation of tonsils, with dark redness of the parts,* [a similar inflammation, with *burning stinging pain,* **Acon. *Apis, Cap.**] *Suppuration of tonsils;* the parts are covered with a tenacious skinny substance, [see **Kali b.**] *Difficult deglutition; liquids swallowed return by nose, [**Lach. Merc.**] Constriction of throat; it feels too narrow, [**Ars. *Hyos. *Nux. Stram.**]

**STOMACH and ABDOMEN.** Putrid taste in mouth, [***Arn. Merc. Nux. *Puls.**] *Bread tastes and smells sour,* [everything tastes *bitter,* ***Bry. Colo. Puls.**] *Vomiting* undigested food, or *mucus and bile,* [see **Ipec.**] *Cramp-like* pain in stomach, [**Chin. *Cocc. *Nux.**] **Constriction* of abdomen around umbilicus, as if a ball would form. **Clutching in abdomen, as if a spot were seized with talons,* [as if grasped with a hand, ***Ipec.**] *Colic, with padshaped protrusion of transverse colon. *Great tenderness and heat* in abdomen; cannot bear least jar.

**STOOL.** *Thin, green mucous stools,* with griping colic, [***Colo. Laur. *Mag. c. Nux v.**—*Thick, green* mucus, ***Ars. Ipec. Merc.**] *Dysentery, with bloody, mucous* stools; griping colic, and *tenesmus* during and after stool, [**Bapt. Cap. *Merc. *Nux. Sulph.**] *Griping pains in hypogastric region, better from *holding breath and bearing down.* *Paralysis of sphincter ani, [**Acon. Colo. *Hyos. Laur. *Phos.**—Anus remains *open,* **Apis. *Phos.**]

**URINE.** *Frequent desire to urinate. The urine becomes turbid like yeast, *with reddish sediment,* [**Con. Sep.**—Dark urine, with white sediment, **Calc. c. Sep.**] *Inability to retain urine. *Sensation of a worm in bladder, [of a ball, ***Lach.**]

**SEXUAL O'S.** *Orchitis,* with great hardness of drawn-up testicles, [**Aur. Clem. Merc. *Nux.**] *Ovaritis* of right side, with great tenderness, [***Apis.**—*Left side,* **Graph. *Lach.**] **Menses* too *early* and too profuse, [**Am. c. *Calc. c. Cimi. Nux m. *Plat.**—*Too late* and too scanty, **Con. *Dulc. *Phos. Sulph.**—See **Puls.**] **Great pressing towards genitals,* as if everything would protrude, [**Nat. m. *Nit. ac. Plat. *Sep.**] *Heat and dryness* of vagina, [**Lyc.**] Rigidity of os uteri, [***Acon. Caul. Cimi. Gel.**]

**RESPIRATORY O'S.** Laryngitis and tracheitis, parts very painful to touch, [***Acon. Hepar. Lach. *Spong.**] *Barking cough, pain in larynx, headache, fever, [**Dros. *Nit. ac. Rumex. *Spong. *Verbas.**] *Dry, spasmodic cough; worse at night and from motion, **Dros. *Hyos. *Ign.**] *Distressing dry cough, excited by a tickling in larynx,* [**Acon. Ipec. Phyto. Phos.**—Excited by *creeping* sensation from chest to throat, **Nux m.**—By a tickling under *upper half* of sternum, ***Cham. Plat. Rhus. *Rumex.**] *Pertussis, cough preceded by crying,* [***Arn.**] Breathing labored, unequal, quick, with moaning.

*Stitches in chest when coughing, or taking a deep breath, [*Acon. *Bry. Phos.] *Palpitation of heart,* reverberating in neck and head.

**BACK.** Painful stiffness between the scapulæ and in the nape of the neck, [**Kali c. Phos. Sep.**] **Back aches* as if it would break, [as if broken, **Mag. c. Graph. Phos.**] *Glandular swelling* on the neck.

**EXTREMITIES.** *Feeling of weight* in both arms, [***Mur. ac. Nat. m. Puls. *Stram.**] *Lameness, with tearing pain in arms, [**Bry. Rhus.**] Coxalgia, with stinging pain or burning in hip-joint; worse at night and from least motion, [**Bry. Calc. c. Puls.**—Pulsating pain, with formation of pus, ***Hep. Mur. ac. *Sil. Staph.**] **Phlegmasia alba dolens.*

**SLEEP.** *Sleepy, but cannot sleep, [**Apis. *Lach. Opi.**—Drowsiness in daytime, sleepless at night, **Lyc. Merc. *Sulph.**] *Drowsiness, with almost constant moaning.* *Starting as in fright on falling asleep, [**Ars. Bry. *Nux v.**—Starts with screaming in sleep, ***Bell. *Cham. Stram. *Zinc.**—Starting of *limbs* when falling asleep, **Ars. Caust. *Lyc. Puls.**—Awakens with a start, **Cham. Sam. Sil. *Sulph. *Stram.**—With a *shrill shriek,* **Apis.**]

**FEVER.** *Pulse* frequent and full, or slow and full, [see **Acon.**] Chilliness in evening, especially of extremities, with heat in head, [heat in head, while rest of body is cold, **Arn. Bry. Hyos.**] Chilliness not relieved by heat of stove, [**Phos. Nux v.**—*Reverse,* **Ars. *Ign. Kali c.**] *Chilliness as soon as he moves under covers, [**Nux v. Puls.**] *Internal and external burning heat, with restlessness. Dry, burning heat, with perspiration only on head. **Typhoid fever,* with prominent cerebral symptoms. **Scarlet fever, with smooth, shining redness of skin.*

**SKIN.** **Smooth, shining redness* of skin, with *bloatedness,* [miliary rash, with efflorescence between the points of rash of a dark, almost livid color, ***Ailanthus. Rhus t.**] *Erysipelas, with *smooth, shining* skin, not much swelling, [see **Rhus.**] *Skin so hot, it imparts a burning sensation to hand.*

**CHARACT. PECULIARITIES.** *Right side* most affected, [**Bapt. Canth. Iris.**—*Left side,* **Lach.**] *The pains appear suddenly, and disappear as suddenly as they come, [*reverse,* **Plat. *Stan.**] Pains in joints, flying from one place to another, [**Kali b. *Puls. Sulph.**] *Spasms renewed by contact, or bright light, [**Stram.**] *Stiffness of whole body. Pains worse* at night, or in afternoon; sometimes from contact or *least jar;* from *noise or bright light. Better* wrapped up warmly in room, [see **Ars.**]

## BRYONIA ALBA.

**MIND.** **Exceedingly irritable,* everything makes him angry, [***Cham. Hep. Kali c. Lyc.**—Happy, cheerful, **Croc. Lach. Sabi.**] Delirium at night; talking of business. *Desire to *escape* from bed, and go home, [see **Bell.**] *Desire for things*, which are refused when offered, [see **Cham.**]

**HEAD.** *Vertigo, nausea, and faintness on rising up*, [**Acon. Puls.**] *Fulness in forehead, as if everything would be pressed out, [***Acon. *Bell. Merc. Rhus t.**—Sensation of *emptiness* in head, ***Carol. r. *Cocc. Ign. Opi.**—Of a great *lump* in brain, **Con.**—As if everything in brain *were alive*, **Pet. Sil.**] **Splitting* headache, [***Am. c. *Bell. Cap. Merc. Puls.**] Headache *worse from motion*, stooping, or opening eyes; relieved by pressure, [**Bell. Nux v. Puls.**] *Heat in head*, with dark-red face, with coldness of rest of body. *Headache on waking in morning.

**NOSE.** *Frequent bleeding of nose when menses should appear, [**Bell. Ham. Puls.**] *Dry coryza*, [fluent during day; dry at night, ***Nux v.**]

**FACE.** Pale, hot, bloated, or red face, [**Bell.**—*Dark-red*, swollen face, ***Hyos. Opi.**]

**MOUTH.** *Lips parched, dry, and cracked, [dry, parched, and black, **Acon. *Ars. *Hyos. Merc.**] Great dryness of mouth, tongue and throat, [**Acon. *Ars. *Bell.**] *Tongue coated white or yellow.* *Tongue rough, cracked, and often *dark-brown. Toothache, worse* from taking *warm* things in mouth, [**Calc. c. Merc. Puls.**—Better from *cold water*, ***Bry. Coff. Puls.**] Teeth feel *elongated.*

**THROAT.** Sore throat, with difficult deglutition and hoarseness. *Sticking sensation* when swallowing, [as of splinters, **Arg. n. *Hepar. Nit. ac.**—Feeling as if a ball of red-hot iron had lodged in fauces, **Phyto.**] Sensation of constriction in throat, [**Ars. *Bell. *Hyos. *Nux.**] *Scraping in throat*, [raw, sore, rough, as if scraped, **Nux.**]

**STOMACH.** Abnormal hunger, must eat often. *Loss of taste*, [**Anac. Hep. Lyc. Nat. m.**] *All food and drink taste *bitter*, [**Colo. Puls.**—Taste *sour*, ***Chin. Lyc. Nux.**—Taste *sweet*, **Mur. ac. Squill.**] Putrid taste, [**Arn. Merc. Nux.**] *Thirst; takes large draughts at long intervals, [drinks often, but little at a time, ***Ars. Apis. Chin. Hyos.**] *Vomiting immediately after eating, [***Ars. Nux. Puls.**] *Vomiting bile and water*, [see **Ipec.**] Great pressure in stomach after eating, [**Ars. Merc. Nux. Sep.**] *Stomach sensitive to touch or pressure, [**Ars. Lyc. *Merc. *Nux.**]

**LIVER.** *Tensive, burning pains in hepatic region, which is swollen, sore. *Stitches in liver, worse from pressure, coughing, breathing, [***Merc. *Nux.**]

**STOOL.** *Constipation; stools *dry, hard, as if burnt.* Stools too large in size, [**Calc. c. Kali c. *Nux. v.**—Composed of *small, hard, black balls*, **Chel. *Opi. Plumb.**] *Diarrhœa in hot weather, or from taking cold drinks when system is heated, [see **Dulc.**] Stools brown, thin, fecal, or thin, bloody; worse in morning and from motion; cutting colic before stool.

**URINE.** Hot urine, *red, brown and scanty*, deposits white sediment. Burning in urethra, [see **Canth.**] Cutting in urethra during micturition.

**SEXUAL O'S.** Menses too early, too profuse, dark-red; worse from motion, [**Croc.** ***Saba.**] *During menses, tearing pains in legs, [**Cham.**] Stitching pains in ovaries on taking a deep inspiration; parts very sensitive to touch, [see **Apis.**] *Suppressed lochia, with splitting headache, [with fulness and burning in uterus, **Puls.**] **Stone-like hardness* of breasts, which are hot, painful, but not very red, [***Phyto.**] Abscess of mammæ.

**RESPIRATORY O'S.** Hoarseness, particularly in open air. *Cough, worse after eating or drinking, with vomiting food, [cough relieved by eating or drinking, **Spong.**—By a sup of cold water, ***Caust. Cup**]. Cough, with vomiting food, [***Dig.** ***Ferr. Dros.** ***Rhus.**] *Cough, at night in bed, *compelling one to assume an erect posture at once,* [and to hold head with both hands, ***Niccol.**—To hold chest, **Nat. sul.**] *Cough, with stitches in chest and expectoration of tenacious, *rust-colored sputa,* [***Phos. Rhus. Sang.**—With bloody expectoration, **Bell. Merc. Nitrum.**] *Quick, anxious, difficult breathing, caused by stitches in chest; aggravated by every movement,* [**Acon. Bell.**—*Pneumonia* (right side), with stitches in lung —**Bell. Merc.**—*Left* side, ***Phos. Rhus.**] *Typhoid pneumonia.*

**BACK.** *Painful stiffness* in nape of neck [see **Bell.**] Burning between the scapulæ, [**Lyc.**—*Coldness*, **Amm. m.**] Stitches in lumbar region. Pain in *small of back.*

**EXTREMITIES.** Shining, red, rheumatic swelling of joints, with stitches and lacerating in upper arms; worse from least motion, [**Acon. Bell.**—Better from motion, **Con. Lyc.** ***Rhus. Sep.**] *Hot, inflammatory swelling of feet, [**Arn. Cocc.** ***Puls.**] *Painful stiffness of knees.*

**SLEEP.** Great drowsiness in daytime, [**Merc. Nux.** ***Phos. Sep.**] **Starting* when falling asleep, [see **Bell.**] **Delirium* as soon as he awakens.

**FEVER.** *Pulse* full, hard, tense and quick. Chilliness, with a muddled condition of head, red cheeks and thirst. *Intermittent fever;* chill predominant, thirst during cold and hot stages; dry cough, with stitches in chest, [a dry, teasing cough just before and during chill, **Rhus t.**] *Chills beginning on lips, fingers and toes. Dry, burning heat, mostly internal, as if blood were burning in veins, [see **Ars.**] Typhoid fever, with great irritation of nervous and vascular system.

**SKIN.** Yellowness of skin, (jaundice.) *Rash of lying-in women and infants, [**Acon.** ***Cham.**] *Erysipelas,* particularly of joints, [**Puls.**] *Arthritic nodosities.*

**CHARACT. PECULIARITIES.** Adapted to rheumatic and gouty subjects. **Stitching, tearing pains;* worse from least motion, [worse during rest and on first moving after rest, **Con. Lyc.** ***Rhus t. Sep. Sulph.**] *Nausea and faintness from sitting up. *Pale-redness* of inflamed parts, [bright redness, **Acon. Bell.**]

*Aggravation,* in morning; (diarrhœa) during hot weather, from motion. *Gets *faint and sick on sitting up.*

*Amelioration*, by keeping *perfectly still;* while lying on painful side, [**Calc. c. Ign. Puls.**—*Worse* on painful side, **Ars. Hepar. Iod. Nux m. Sil.**] Better from eating cold things.

## CACTUS GRANDIFLORUS.

**MIND.** Sadness, bad humor, melancholy, [**Lyc. *Plat. Puls.**—Gay, cheerful, **Croc. *Lach. Oxal. ac.**] *Cries and knows not why, [rage, with weeping sadness, **Puls.**]

**HEAD.** Pulsating pain, with a sense of weight in right side of head. Heavy pain, like a weight on the vertex, [**Aloe. Cann. s. Kali b.**—See **Bell.**]

**NOSE.** Profuse bleeding from nose, [**Bell. Ham.**—In plethoric persons, **Acon. *Bell.**] Fluent coryza, corroding nose, [**Arum t. Lyc. Kali b.**]

**THROAT.** Constriction of œsophagus, which prevents swallowing, [**Alum. Bell. Hyos. Stram.**] Frequent swallowing of saliva, [**Bell.**]

**STOMACH.** Constriction, pulsation or heaviness in stomach, [see **Puls.**] **Sensation as if a rope were being drawn tighter and tighter around her*, [see **Nux v. Plat.**] Vomiting blood, [**Ars. Ham. Hyos.**]

**STOOL.** Hard, black stools, [in balls, ***Opi.**] Diarrhœa in morning; stools watery, mucous, bilious. Copious hemorrhage from the anus, [see **Calc. c. Cascarilla. Ham.**] Sensation of great weight in anus, [***Sepia.**] Swollen, painful varices of the anus.

**URINARY O'S.** Constriction of neck of bladder, [**Clem. Pet.**] Constant irritation in the urethra, as if he would pass water. Urine passes by drops, with much burning, [see **Con.**] Straw-colored urine, depositing a *red sand*, [***Lyc. Sil.**—*Brown* sand, **Lach.**] Bloody urine, [**Ipec. Millef. Nit. ac. Sec.**]

**SEXUAL O'S.** Pulsating pain in uterus and ovaries, [stitching pains, **Bell. Bry.**] Sensation of constriction in uterine region, [of heaviness, **Gel.**] *Very painful menstruation, [***Cham. Cupr. *Nux v.**]

**CHEST.** Feeling of constriction in chest, as if bound; hindering respiration, [see **Ars. Phos.**] Difficulty of breathing; attacks of suffocation, cold perspiration on face, and loss of pulse, [**Verat. al.**] Acute pains and stitches in heart, [**Spig.**—See **Dig.**] *Constrictive sensation in heart, *as though it were grasped by a hand of iron;* [as if squeezed together, **Iod. Arn. Kali c.**] Palpitation of heart; worse when walking, and at night when lying on left side, [worse when bending chest forward, **Spig.**] *Pain in heart, shooting down left arm to fingers. Spitting of blood, with convulsive cough, [**Ipec.**] Spasmodic cough, with copious expectoration. Pricking pains in chest, with oppression.

**EXTREMITIES.** Œdema of the hands; worse in left. Œdema of feet, extending to knees, [**Apis.**]

**SLEEP.** Can't sleep on account of pulsation in different parts of body. Delirium at night, on waking up, [see **Bry.**] Sleepless, without cause.

**FEVER.** Slight chilliness about 10 A. M.; chattering of teeth. Burning heat, with shortness of breath; headache, followed by perspiration. *Intermittent fever; chill every day at same hour, [**Saba.**] 1 P. M., followed by burning heat, dpspnœa, pulsating pain in uterine region, no perspiration, and much thirst.

**CHARACT. PECULIARITIES.** *Sensation of constriction in different parts of the system. Aggravation,* in forenoon; [diarrhœa] at night; [palpitation, headache.] Lying on left side, [palpitation.] After eating, [weight in stomach.]

## CALCAREA CARBONICA.

**MIND.** Low-spirited, inclines to weep, [**Puls. Staph. Sulph.**] *Forgetfulness.* *Apprehensive of some misfortune. Afraid he will lose his senses. Disinclined to every kind of work, [**Con. Nit. ac. Phos.**—Indisposed to talk, **Dig.** ***Phos. ac. Stan.**]

**HEAD.** *Vertigo on ascending a height, [on descending, **Ferr.**—On stooping, or rising from a seat, **Bry. Podo.** ***Puls.**] *Throbbing headache in middle of brain, every morning, worse from mental exertion. Headache, with nausea, vertigo; worse from mental exertion, stooping or walking in the open air, [see **Nux.**] Heat in vertex, [**Graph. Nat. m.** ***Sulph.**—*Coldness,* **Sep.** ***Verat.**] Sensation as of a *piece of ice* lying on right side of head, [*on the vertex,* ***Verat.**] *Enlargement of head, with open fontanels, [***Sil. Sulph.**] **Perspiration* in drops on head, when child sleeps, [see **Merc. Sil.**]

**EYES.** Ophthalmia of infants or scrofulous subjects. Redness and swelling of lids, sticking together at night. *Ulcers and specks on cornea,* [**Ars.** ***Merc.** ***Sil. Sulph.**] Sees things as through a gauze, [**Caust. Kreo. Phos.**] *Fistula lachrymalis,* [**Nitr. ac.** ***Petro.**] Fiery sparks before the eyes.

**EARS.** Stitches or pulsations in ears, [**Kali c. Nit. ac.**—*Darting, tearing* pains, **Puls.**] Discharge of pus from ears, [**Lyc.** ***Merc. Sulph.**] Hardness of hearing after abuse of quinine, [after mercury, ***Hep. Nit. ac.**] *Polypus of the ear.

**NOSE.** Great dryness of nose. Sore, ulcerated nostrils, [with yellow, fetid discharge, **Alum. Nat. c. Nit. ac.**] Stoppage of nose, also with yellow, fetid pus, [green, fetid discharge, **Merc. Puls. Sulph.**] Fetid odor in nose, [like old cheese or brimstone, **Nux v.**] Fluent coryza, with headache. *Nasal polypi.*

**FACE.** Yellowness of face, [across nose, *resembling a saddle,* ***Sep.**—*Pale, death-like,* **Ars. Verat. al.**] Circumscribed redness of cheeks, [**Lyc. Phos.**] *Crusta lactea,* with violent itching; burning after washing; [thick crusts, and fetid, bloody ichor, **Rhus t.**] Painful, hard swelling of submaxillary glands.

**MOUTH.** Dryness of tongue at night and after awaking, [ ***Nux m.**] Difficult dentition, [in scrofulous children.] Toothache, drawing, stinging pains; aggravated by noise, cold drinks, after the catamenia, [better from cold water, **Coff. Bry. Puls.**] Toothache of *pregnant* females. Bleeding of the gums, [**Ars.**]

**THROAT.** Stitches in throat when swallowing, [as if constricted, **Bell. Nux.**] Swelling of tonsils. Swelling and inflammation of palate; uvula dark-red and covered with blisters, [with dirty-yellow coating, **Merc. iod.**] Stinging pain in throat when swallowing, [burning, **Merc. v.**]

**STOMACH and ABDOMEN.** No appetite. *Aversion to anything boiled, [**Puls.**] Aversion to meat, [**Merc. v. Puls.**] Craves salt food and eggs, [everything tastes too salty, **Sep.**] Milk disagrees with him, [ ***Puls. Sulph.**] Frequent eructations, tasting of ingesta; also sour eructations, [bitter eructations, **Bell. Chin. Hyos. Nux v.**—Tasting like garlic, **Mosch.**—Without taste or smell. ***Hepar. Kali c. Merc.**] After eating, heartburn and loud belching of wind. Sour vomiting, especially in children, [**Hepar.**] *Swelling over pit of stomach, like a saucer turned bottom up, [pad-shaped protrusion of transverse colon, **Bell.**] *Stinging pain in liver when stooping. *Cannot bear tight clothing around waist, [ ***Lyc. Nux v.**] Sensation of coldness in abdomen, [**Ars. Phos.**—Burning in, **Lach. Phos. Sec. c. Sil.**] Enlargement of abdomen and mesentery glands. Incarcerated flatulence, [**Chin. Carb. v.**] *Inguinal glands swollen, painful.

**STOOL.** Constipation of *hard, undigested stools, clay-colored,* [**Hepar.**—Black-colored, **Opi. Phos. Verat. a.**] *Diarrhœa;* stools whitish, watery, smelling sour, [during dentition.] Involuntary, frothy stools. *Pricking* in rectum, ascarides. Violent itching of anus, [**Caust. Nit. ac. Sil. Sulph.**] Varices swollen, protruding, burning, [**Caust. Nit. ac.**]

**URINARY O'S.** Urine *dark-brown* and fetid, with white sediment, [**Colch. Nit. ac.**] *Bloody urine.* *Involuntary emissions of urine when *walking,* [**Nat. m.**—When *coughing,* ***Caust. Puls. Verat.**]

**SEXUAL O'S.** *Catamenia too early and too profuse, [ ***Bell. Croc. Phos.**] *The least excitement causes menses to return. During menses vertigo, rush of blood to head, toothache, and *cold, damp feet.* *Leucorrhœa, *like milk,* with burning, itching in parts, [**Graph. Puls.**] Stitch-like pains in os uteri. Itching or pressing in vagina, [burning, **Sulph.**] *Constant aching in vagina. Prolapsus uteri, [see **Merc.**]

**RESPIRATORY O'S.** *Painless hoarseness,* [painful, **Bell. Phos.**] Tickling cough, caused by a sensation of dust in larynx, [**Bell.**—As from vapor of sulphur, **Ars. Chin.**] Cough at night, while sleeping, with expectoration only during day, [expectoration only at night, **Staph. Tart. e.**] Tightness in chest, as if full of blood, and not room to breathe, [sensation of emptiness, **Cocc. Stan.**] Burning in chest, [*coldness,* **Ars.**

**Sulph.**] Soreness in chest when drawing a deep breath. Shortness of breath when going up-stairs, [**Merc.**] *Stitches in chest when moving or taking a deep breath, [**Bry. Lyc. Puls.**] *Palpitation of heart at night or after eating, with anguish, [after drinking, **Con.**] Secretion of milk too abundant, [**Acon. Phyto. *Uran.**—Deficiency of milk, **Caust. Puls.**]

**BACK.** Pain in small of back, as from a bruise. [**Merc. Nux v.**] Pressing pain between scapulæ, impeding respiration, [pain under lower, inner angle of right shoulder-blade, ***Chel. m.**] Curvature of dorsal vertebra, [**Puls. Sil. Sulph.**] Painful swelling of cervical glands, [**Bell. Merc. Sil.**]

**EXTREMITIES.** Cramp in hands at night, [**Nat. m.**] Arthritic nodosities on hand and finger-joint, [**Graph. Ledum.**] Sensation of deadness in fingers, [**Sep.**] Hip-disease, with stitches and cutting in joints, [with stinging, pulsating, **Merc. v.**] *Children late learning to walk*, [early learning, **Sil.** —Early learning *to talk*, **Nat. m.**] *Phlegmasia alba dolens, [***Bell.**] Burning of soles of feet, [**Cham. *Sulph.**] *Cold feet, feel as if they had on damp stockings.

**SLEEP.** Tired and sleepy all day; [sleepless at night, **Coff. Hyos. Sulph.**] *Cannot sleep, ideas crowd his mind so*, [**Chin. *Nux.**] Horrid visions when *opening* eyes from sleep, [when *closing* eyes, **Bry.**]

**FEVER.** Pulse full, frequent or tremulous. Chilliness, mostly in evening; *chills* and *heat* simultaneous, [**Arn. Ars. *Thuya.**] Frequent flashes of heat, with anxiety and palpitation, [flashes of heat, beginning in hands, **Phos.**] Heat, with thirst, followed by chilliness. Sweats from least exertion, even in cold air. Perspiration in first sleep. Night-sweat, especially on *head, neck* and *chest*, [see **Merc.**]

**SKIN.** Unwholesome, readily ulcerating skin; even small wounds suppurate and do not heal, [**Graph. Hepar. Sil.**] *Hard, white, elevated eruptions. Burning, itching herpes; chapped. Deep fistulous ulcers, with red, hard, swollen edges, [see **Lach.**]

**CHARACT. PECULIARITIES.** Persons of *scrofulous* habits, [**Bary. c. Ferr. Merc. Sulph.**] *Very sensitive to least cold air; great liability to take cold, [**Graph. Sil. Sulph.**] *Children and young persons incline to grow *fat* [too *fast*, **Phos. ac.**] *Great *emaciation, with swollen abdomen and good appetite*, [**Iod.**] *Pulsating pains, [*stinging*, ***Apis. Merc.**] Internal chilliness, [internal *heat*, **Ars. Cicu.**] Arthritic nodosities, [**Graph. Ledum.**]

*Aggravation*, in morning, evening, after midnight. In cold air, in wet weather and from washing, [**Sil. Spig.**]

*Amelioration*, after breakfast, on rising, in dry weather. When lying on painful side, [**Bry. Puls.**]

## CANNABIS SATIVA.

**HEAD.** Sensation as if intoxicated, [**Bell. Gel. *Nux.**

**Rhus.**] Sense of weight on vertex, and as if cold water were falling on it, [as if ice were lying on it, **Verat. a.**] Crawling sensation in scalp.

**CHEST.** Asthma, can only breathe when standing up, [better lying down, **Psor.**] Difficult respiration when lying down. Cough dry, or with green, viscid expectoration, [**Carb. v. Dros. Lyc.**] *Frequent, tearing, hard, dry cough. Violent palpitation of heart, [**Cact. Dig. Spig. Verat. a.**] Shocks and beats in region of heart, [**Caust. Nux v.**—Stitches, **Cap. Caust. Kreo.**] Sensation as if water were dropping from heart, [burning at heart, **Opi. Puls. Verat. v.**]

**URINARY O'S.** Soreness in region of kidneys, [burning, stinging, ***Canth.**—Pulsative pains; *urine bloody and contains large quantities of albumen*, ***Berb. Ocim. can.**—*Sugar in the urine*, ***Uranium.**] *Strangury, with painful urging to urinate, passing only a few drops of bloody, burning urine, [***Canth. Nux v.**] *Burning while urinating, but especially after, [**Canth. Cap. Nit. ac.**] *Gonorrhœa*, with discharge of watery mucus, [white discharge, *like cream*, **Cap.**—Yellow purulent, **Agnus.**—*Yellowish-green*, **Merc.**—*Thin, greenish*, **Thuya.**] The urethra feels sore, [with bloody discharge, **Canth.**] *Dark-redness of glans and prepuce.

**GENITALS.** Great swelling of prepuce, approaching phymosis, [**Thuya.**] *Penis *feels sore*, as if burnt; *hurts him to walk*. ·Painful erections, [**Canth. Nit. ac. Thuya.**] Sexual desire increased. Swelling of prostate gland, [**Puls.**]

**CHARACT. PECULIARITIES.** Acts especially on the urinary and genital organs, [see **Canth.**] on the lungs, heart and cerebro-spinal system. Great debility after a meal, or from exertion; from talking or writing. *Feels as if hot water were poured over him.*

## CANTHARIDES.

**MIND.** Great restlessness. *Furious delirium.* *Paroxysms of rage, with crying, barking, etc., renewed by touching larynx or drinking water, [see **Bell.**] Amorous frenzy, [see **Hyos.**]

**HEAD.** *Stitches* in back part of head, [in forepart, **Dig. Sil. Sulph.**—In top of head, **Ipec.**—In temples, **Kali c. Lyc. Sil.**] Soreness and burning in brain. Burning in sides of head, ascending from the neck, [coldness on right side, **Calc. c.**] *Throbbing* in temples, [**Acon.** ***Bell.**—See **Kali c.**]

**EYES.** Spasmodic movements of eyes, with fiery, sparkling, staring look, [see **Bell.**] Burning and soreness in eyes. *Objects look yellow.*

**FACE.** Pale, wretched, death-like appearance, [see **Ars.**] Bloated, red face. Itching vesicles on face; burning when touched (erysipelas). Lockjaw, with grinding of teeth, [see **Hyos.**]

**MOUTH and THROAT.** Burning in mouth, pharynx,

œsophagus and stomach, [**Ars. Iris. Nux v.**—Coldness, **Hydro. ac. Verat. a.**] Inflammation of mouth and pharynx, [see **Ars. Bell.**] Inflammation of tonsils, with great difficulty of swallowing liquids, [***Bell. Hyos.**] Expectoration of frothy saliva, streaked with blood, [see **Hyos.**] *Vesicles* in the mouth.

**STOMACH.** Aversion to food. Burning thirst, with aversion to all fluids, [see **Ars.**] **Gastritis*, with violent burning pains in stomach, [**Ars. Nux. Phos.**] Great *sensitiveness* of stomach, [**Bry. Nux. Merc.**] *Vomiting, with violent retching.* Vomiting mucus and blood. *Hepatitis.

**STOOL.** **Dysentery*, with white or pale-reddish mucous stool, like scrapings of intestines, [**Colch. *Colo.**] *Green or bloody mucous stools;* before stool, violent colic; during stool, *burning at anus;* after stool, *tenesmus, burning, biting, stinging at anus.*

**URINARY O'S.** *Nephritis*, with burning, stinging and tearing in kidneys, [**Tereb.**—Dragging or shooting pains along ureters to groin, **Cann.**—Cutting or tearing pulsative pains in *region of kidneys;* worse when stooping, ***Berb. v.**] *Pressing pain* in kidneys, along ureters to bladder. **Constant desire* to urinate, passing but a few drops at a time; sometimes mixed with blood, [***Cann. Cap. Tereb.**—*Urine bloody and intensely albuminous*, ***Berb.**] After micturition, burning, cutting in urethra, [**Cap. Nit. ac.**] *Gonorrhœa, with soreness of urethra and bloody discharge, [discharge like cream, **Cap.**—Yellowish-green or purulent, **Merc. Thuya.**]

**SEXUAL O'S.** Painful erections, (in gonorrhœa). Strong sexual desire, [see **Phos.**] *Menses* too early and too profuse; black discharge, [see **Puls.**]

**CHARACT. PECULIARITIES.** Acts especially on *urinary* and sexual organs. *Burning pains, with soreness in the cavities of the body. *Right* side most affected, [**Bapt. *Bell. Iris.**—Left side, **Lach.**] *Worse* from drinking coffee; better from lying down.

## CAPSICUM ANNUUM.

**MIND.** Sense of intoxication, [**Cann. Gel.**] Increased acuteness of the senses, [dulness of, **Hell.**] Peevish, easily offended. Homesickness.

**HEAD.** Beating, throbbing headache, especially in the temples, [**Bell.**] Headache, as if the skull would burst, when moving the head or walking, [**Bry.**—Better from motion, **Rhus t.**] Darting pain through the head; worse from rest and better from motion.

**EYES.** Burning of the eyes, with redness and lachrymation, [**Ars. Phos.**] Objects appear black before the eyes, [appear *red*, **Bell.**—Yellow, **Canth.**]

**MOUTH and THROAT.** Burning blisters in the mouth. Stomacace, with fetid odor from the mouth. Spasmodic contraction of the throat, [**Bell. Ipec.**] Throat inflamed, *dark-red*, with burning, [see **Bell.**] *False membrane on tonsils in diphtheria. Soreness, *smarting, biting* and *burning* in throat.

**STOOL.** *Dysentery, with bloody mucous stools;* also mucus, *streaked with black blood.* Before stool, cutting colic. After stool, tenesmus; thirst, drinking causing shuddering. Hemorrhoidal tumors, with burning pain in anus. *Bleeding piles,* with sore feeling in anus.

**URINARY O'S.** Strangury, with tenesmus of the bladder. Spasmodic contraction of neck of the bladder, [**Cact.**] Burning while urinating, [**Caust.**] Discharge of blood from the urethra, very painful, [**Canth.**]

**SEXUAL O'S.** Coldness of scrotum, with impotence. Atrophy of testes, [swelling of, **Merc.**] *Intense burning in urethral canal, [stitches in, **Chin.**] Purulent discharge from urethra, [**Agnus.**—Yellowish-green discharge, **Merc. Thuya.**]

**CHEST.** Deep breathing, almost like a sigh, [almost imperceptible, **Lauro.**] Pain, as if the chest were constricted, oppressing the breathing. Throbbing pain in the chest, [cramp-like pain, **Nit. ac.**] Dry, hard cough in the evening and at night, with pain in distant parts, [bladder, knees, legs, ears, throat.]

**FEVER.** Pulse irregular and often intermittent. Shuddering and chilliness in back. *Intermittents; chill commences in back, and from thence spreads over entire body, [**Eupa. pur.**] During chill, thirst followed by fever, with or without thirst. Chill worse after drinking, [**Ars. Chin. Nux. Verat.**] Sensation over body as if the parts would go to sleep.

**CHARACT. PECULIARITIES.** Affects particularly the throat, alimentary canal and urino-genital organs. Stiffness and pain in joints. *Worse* from eating and drinking; during first motion after rest, [see **Rhus.**] *Better* from continued exercise.

## CARBO VEGETABILIS.

**MOUTH and THROAT.** Looseness of the teeth; gums recede from the teeth and bleed easily, [**Merc.**] Dryness of mouth, without thirst, [**Bell. Nux m.**—With thirst, **Nit. ac. Rhus t.**] *Profuse salivation of stringy saliva. Tongue coated white or yellow-brown. The throat feels constricted, [**Bell.** ***Hyos.**] Feeling of coldness in throat, [**Laur.**—Burning, **Ars. Canth.**] Scraping and rawness in the throat.

**STOMACH.** Great hunger or thirst. Craves coffee, [aversion to, **Nux v.**] Aversion to meat and fat things, [desire for, **Nit. ac. Nux v.**] Bitter or salty taste. Food tastes too salty, [**Sep.**—Craves salt food, **Calc. c.**—Craves chalk, lime, earth, etc., **Nit. ac.**—Brandy, **Nux v.**] *Weak digestion, the simplest food disagrees. *Eructations of sour, rancid food. *Great fulness* after eating or drinking, [**Chin. Lyc.**—Emptiness after, **Sang. Sarsa.**—Hunger after, **Phos. Staph.**] Burning, pressing pain in stomach, and is sore to pressure. Stitches

> from eructa.

under the ribs, in region of liver. Pain in liver, as if bruised, [as if grasped with a hand, **Lyc.**] Can bear nothing tight around waist or abdomen, [***Lyc. Nux v.**] *Cardialgia in nursing women. *Incarcerated flatulence.*

**STOOL.** Constipation; stools hard, tough, scanty, [see **Caust.**] Diarrhœa, of thin, pale mucus. *Involuntary, cadaverous-smelling stools, [last stage of acute disease.] Stools of *foul blood and mucus.* Large, blue, burning varices, [**Mur. ac.**]

**SEXUAL O'S.** Involuntary seminal emissions, without sensation; [without erections, **Canth. Gel.**—Especially after onanism, **Chin. Gel. *Phos. ac.**] *Menses* too early, too profuse; blood thick, corrosive and of an acrid smell, [**Am. c. Nat. s.**—Too late, too scant, acrid, corroding the thighs, **Kali c. Sars. *Sulph.**] *Morning leucorrhœa,* very acrid, excoriating the parts, [**Ars. Con. Kreo.**] *Aphthæ of the vulva.

**RESPIRATORY O'S.** *Long-lasting hoarseness; worse from talking and in evening; [worse in morning, **Caust. Phos.** Loss of voice, [see **Phos.**] Short, spasmodic cough, with retching, [with vomiting food, ***Dig. Ferr. Rhus.**] *Greenish, fetid expectoration, [**Sil. *Stann.**] Cough, with spitting blood and burning in chest, [with bursting headache and soreness in chest, **Phos.**] Cough, with expectoration only in morning, [expectoration only at night, **Caust. Staph. Tart.**] *Cough, worse* after eating, drinking or talking, [*better* after a swallow of cold water, ***Caust. Cup.**— *Worse* after, **Dig. Sul. ac. *Verat.**] Wheezing and rattling of mucus in chest, in the bronchia, [***Ipec. Tart.**] *Rawness* and *soreness* in chest, [**Æscul. Iris.**] *Sensation of weakness in chest.* Violent burning in chest, **Am. c. Lach. Merc.**—*Coldness,* ***Ars. Ruta. Sulph.**]

**EXTREMITIES.** Pain in elbow-joint, as if contused, [as if dislocated, **Bry. Ruta.**] Drawing, tearing pain in forearm and wrists, [see **Bry.**] Icy cold hands, [with blueness, **Verat.**] Lameness and heaviness of lower extremities, [**Ars.**] Cramps in legs and *soles* of feet, [in toes, **Lyco.**]

**FEVER.** *Pulse* frequent, very *feeble; collapsed,* [in cholera.] Chilliness, mostly in evening; sometimes only on one side, [left side, **Caust.**] Intermittent fever, with thirst only during chill, followed by burning heat, then sweat, [thirst before chill and during sweat, **China.**] *Night-sweats.*

**SKIN.** Readily bleeding ulcers, with burning pain; *putrid ulcers,* [black-looking ulcers, with bloody pus, ***Ars.**] Lymphatic swellings, with suppuration and burning pain. *Dry, rash-like itch.*

**CHARACT. PECULIARITIES.** *Burning pains, [the parts burn like fire, **Acon. *Ars.**] Great debility and weakness from least exertion. *Wants more air and to be fanned all the time. *Great foulness of all the secretions, [**Bapt.**] Bad effects from loss of animal fluids, [**Chin. Phos. ac.**]

## CAUSTICUM.

**HEAD.** Vertigo, with sensation of weakness in the head, [with vanishing of sight and loss of hearing, **Nux v.**] Stitches in temples, [**Kali c. Lyc.**—In forehead, **Arn. Dig. Sil.** —In back of head, **Canth.**—In vertex, **Ipec.**] *Throbbing in vertex. Sensation of tightness in head and of scalp, [**Carb. an. Merc.**—Sensation of looseness in the head, **Nat. sul. Nux m.**]

**EYES.** Eyes feel as if sand were in them, [**Euph.**—Burning, smarting, as from salt, **Nux v.**] Ophthalmia, with burning, itching of eyes and lids, [**Ars.**—Ulceration of margins of lids, **Sulph.**] *Cannot keep upper eyelids up; they fall down over eyes, [***Gel.**] Sudden loss of sight, as if a film were before the eyes. Movements before eyes, as of a swarm of insects, [of black motes, **Acon. Merc. Phos.**]

**EARS.** Buzzing and roaring in ears and head, [roaring and humming, **Coni. Croc.**] Stitches in ears, [**Chin. Nit. ac.** —*Pulsations*, **Rhus.**]

**FACE.** Yellow complexion, [pale, bloated face, **Ars. Calc. c.**] Neuralgia, mostly on right side, cheek-bone to temple, [cramp pain, with numbness on left side, **Plat.**] Tightness of jaws, with difficulty in opening mouth. Burning, itching eruption in face, with acrid discharge, forming crusts.

**MOUTH and THROAT.** Bites inside of cheek when chewing, [the tongue, **Ign.**] Paralysis of tongue, with indistinct speech, [**Hyos.**—Heaviness and numbness of tongue, **Kali c.**] When swallowing, pain as if a tumor were in throat, [as if a splinter, **Arg. n.**] Cracking in throat when swallowing, [**Ign.**] Sensation of something cold rising in throat, [of hot vapor, **Merc.**—As of a ball, **Kal. lat.**]

**STOMACH and ABDOMEN.** Aversion to sweet things, [desire for, **Lyc.**] Greasy taste. *Sensation as if lime were being burned in stomach. Colic, with heat in head; chilliness over body; better when lying down; [colic, compelling one to walk about, **Rhus t.**—To bend double, **Chin. *Colo.**]

**STOOL.** Constipation, hard, tough stools, covered with mucus, and shine like grease, [*lumpy, covered with mucus*, **Hydras.**] The stool is, too, *small-shaped*, [see ***Phos.**] Bloody stools, with soreness and burning of rectum. Large, painful varices; burning when touched; increased by walking. *Fistula in ano.*

**URINARY O'S.** Difficult, frequent and painful urination. Involuntary emissions of urine night and day; when coughing, sneezing, [**Puls. Verat.**—Involuntary stools when coughing, **Phos.**] .

**SEXUAL O'S.** Menses too late, but profuse, [too early and profuse, **Bell. Calc. c.**] Discharge clotted and passed only during day, with pain in small of back, as if bruised; [discharge principally at night, **Am. m.**] Difficult first menstruations, [see **Puls.**] *Leucorrhœa at night, [**Amb.**] Sore, cracked nipples, surrounded by herpes, [itching and burning, **Sulph.**] Deficiency of milk, [abundance, **Calc. c.**]

**RESPIRATORY O'S.** Hoarseness and roughness of the throat, in morning, [in evening, **Calc. c.**] Loss of voice, [**Bell. Merc. Phos.**] Soreness in larynx. *Catarrh, with cough and rawness in throat. Asthma, especially when sitting or lying down, [better when lying down, **Psorin.**—Can only breathe when standing up, **Cann. s.**] Dry, hollow cough, with soreness in chest, caused by tickling and mucus in throat; expectoration only at night. Cough, with pain in hip, [**Bell.**] *Cough, worse in evening till midnight; *relieved by drinking cold water.* Stitches deep in chest during inspiration. Palpitation of heart; stitches about the heart, [shocks and beats in heart, **Cann. s.** ***Nux v.**]

**BACK.** Painful stiffness between scapulæ, [soreness between, **Sil.**] Pain as from a bruise in nape of neck, [as from a sprain, **Coni.**] Swelling, like goitre on throat, [with sense of constriction, **Iodi.**]

**EXTREMITIES.** Dull tearing in hands and arms, [jerking in, **Cup.**] Great heaviness and weakness in arms. Tearing in right wrist-joint, [pain as if sprained, **Arn. Calc. c.**—As if dislocated, **Bry. Ruta.**] Hip-joint feels as if dislocated when walking, [as if sprained, **Mez.**] Swelling of feet.

**FEVER.** *Pulse* only accelerated towards evening, [fast in morning; slow in evening, **Ars.**] Coldness frequently on left side. Internal chilliness, followed by perspiration without heat. Flushes of heat, followed by chilliness.

**CHARACT. PECULIARITIES.** Adapted to weak, scrofulous persons, with yellow complexion, [see **Calc. c.**] Glandular indurations, **Baryt.**] *Great sympathy for others. Epileptic spasms at night during sleep, [**Calc. c. Cup.**]

## CHAMOMILLA.

**MIND.** Great restlessness, and tossing about, [**Ars.**] Exceedingly irritable, everything makes him angry, [**Bry. Hep. Kali c. Lyc.**] *Very impatient, can hardly answer one civilly. *Child *very fretful*, must be carried all the time to be quieted. **Child wants different things, which it repels when offered*, [***Bry. Staph.**—Cries if spoken to, **Sil.**—Cries if touched, **Cin. Tart. e.**—Can't bear to be looked at, **Ant.**]

**HEAD.** Vertigo after lying down, [when lying down or turning over in bed, **Coni.**] Throbbing headache, mostly on one side, [see **Puls.**] Headche felt even during sleep. Headache from drinking coffee, [**Nux v.**] *Warm sweat about head.

**EYES.** Burning heat in eyes, [smarting as from *sand*, **Euph. Caust.**—As from *salt*, **Nux v.**] Inflammation, especially of edges of lower lids, [ulceration of, **Euph. Merc.**] Yellowness of the whites, [blood-red, **Thuya.**] Twitching of eyelids. Bleeding from eyes, [**Carb. v.**]

**EARS.** **Otalgia*, with stitches and tearing pains, [**Merc. Nat. m.**—Shooting pains, ***Puls.**—*Cracking* in ears, **Kali c.**—When moving jaws, **Graph. Nat. m.**] *Swelling* of parotid gland.

**MOUTH and THROAT.** Putrid smell from the mouth. *Toothache, with, hot, red, swollen cheeks; *pain worse* from drinking anything warm, especially coffee, [temporary relief from cold water, ***Bry. Calc. c. Merc. Puls.**] Dry mouth and tongue, with thirst, [**Nit. ac. Rhus.**—Without thirst, **Bell. *Nux m.**] Tongue red, cracked, [**Bell. Rhus.**—See **Lyc.**] Inflammation of *soft palate and tonsils*, with dark-redness, [***Acon. *Bell.**] Sensation as of a plug in throat, [***Hepar. Ign. *Nux.**—As of a ball of red-hot iron, **Phyto.**—As of a splinter, **Arg. n. Hepar. Nit. ac.**]

**STOMACH and ABDOMEN.** Aversion to food, [see **Rhus.**] Great thirst for cold water. Bitter taste in mouth in morning, [**Puls.**] *Bitter, bilious vomiting, [*green, jelly-like mucus*, **Ipec.**—Vomiting black bile and blood, **Verat. a.**—See **Ipec.**] Colic after anger, [**Colo.**] Oppression in stomach as from a stone, [**Ars.**—Especially after eating, **Nux v.**] Burning in stomach, [**Ars. Nux v.**—*Coldness* in, **Colch. Sulph.**] Pressing towards the abdominal ring, as if hernia would protrude, [see **Nux.**]

**STOOL.** *Hot, diarrhœic stools, smelling like bad eggs*, [**Psor.**—Yellow mucus, smelling like carrion, ***Podo.**] *Stools green, watery, and slimy, or like chopped eggs and spinach, [*green, slimy, like scum of a frog-pond*, ***Mag. c.**] Green, watery, *corroding stools*, with colic, [**Ars. *Merc. Sulph.**] Diarrhœa *during dentition*, [**Calc. Colo. Dulc. Merc. Podo. Sulph.**]

**SEXUAL O'S.** *Burning in vagina, as if excoriated, with yellow, smarting leucorrhœa, [**Sulph.**] *Dysmenorrhœa, with *labor-like pains;* discharge *dark and clotted*, with tearing pains in legs, [**Aloe. Cimi.**] *Metrorrhagia*, blood passed in clots and smells putrid, [bright-red blood flowing in a gush, ***Ipec.**] Violent after-pains; she can hardly endure them. Suppression of milk, [**Puls.**—Too abundant, **Calc. c.**] Induration of mammæ, [falling away of, ***Iodi.**]

**RESPIRATORY O'S.** *Catarrhal hoarseness.* Hoarseness and cough, from rattling mucus in trachea, [see **Ipec.**] *Dry, tickling cough at night, (even during sleep) in children, [cough with stitches in the chest, back, hip, uterus, **Bell.**] Burning in chest, [**Lach.**—Coldness, **Ars. Sulph.**] Stitches in sides of chest, [about the heart, **Caust.**] Rattling mucus in chest, [in bronchia, **Ipec.**—The chest seems full of phlegm, ***Ipec. *Tart.**]

**EXTREMITIES.** Convulsions of arms, with clasping in of the thumbs, [hands closed to a fist, **Stram.**] Cracking of knee-joint during motion, [**Con, Ign.**—Of all the joints, **Kali c.**] *Cramp in the calves*, [**Cup. *Hyos. Nit. ac. Nux.**]

**SLEEP.** Starts in his sleep, uttering sudden cries, [see **Bell.**] Sleepy, but cannot sleep, [**Bell.**]

**FEVER.** Pulse small, tense, and frequent. *Chilliness* and coldness of some parts, while others are hot. Chilliness of whole body, with burning hot face and breath. *Heat* with chills; one hot red cheek, the other pale, [**Acon. Nux.**] Hot perspiration about the head and face.

**SKIN.** Rash of infants and nursing females, [**Acon.**] *Jaundice. Unhealthy skin, every injury ulcerates.

**CHARACT. PECULIARITIES.** *Especially suitable to children, [**Rheum. Pallad.**] *Excessive sensibility to pain, [**Coff.**—*Indifference* to pain, **Jatro. Laur. Merc.**] Great debility as soon as pain begins. Pains are worse at night, are accompanied by thirst and heat. **One cheek* red and hot, the other cold and pale, [**Acon. Mosch. Nux v.**—*One hand* hot, the other cold, **Dig.**—*One foot* hot, the other cold, **Lyc.**]

## CHINA.

**MIND.** *Discouragement,* [**Iris v.**—Great cheerfulness, **Croc. Lach.**] Indifference and apathy, [**Merc.** ***Phos. ac.**—High spirits, **Kobal.**] *Indisposed to perform any kind of labor, or to talk.

**HEAD.** Vertigo on raising the head, [*when rising from a seat, with chilliness, ***Puls.**] *Heaviness* of head, with reeling sensation, [lightness of head, ***Stram.**] *Pressure in head, from within outwards, as if it would burst, [**Acon. Bell. Bry.**] Soreness of brain as if bruised, aggravated by *contact* or mental exertion. *Throbbing headache after excessive depletion, [after a blow or concussion, **Arn. Cicu.**] The headache is worse in a draught of air, by the slightest contact, and is *relieved by hard pressure.*

**EYES.** Redness of eyes with heat and burning. Pressure in eyes as from sand, [**Caust. Euph.**—Burning, smarting, as from salt, **Nux v.**] Yellowness of the whites, [blood-red, **Thuya.**] When reading, letters run together, [seem to move about, **Cicu.**]

**EARS.** Ringing in ears, [**Calc. c. Graph. Nux v.**—Roaring humming, **Bell. Lyc. Nit. ac.**—*Singing,* snapping, **Calc. c.**—Cracking in ears, **Bary. c. Kali c. Nit. ac.**—Stoppage of ears, which open at times with a loud report, **Sili.**] Stitches in ears, [**Kali c. Nit. ac.**—Pulsations in ears, **Calc. c. Phos. Rhus.**—Whizzing in ears, **Phos. Rhus. Sulph.**] *Hardness of hearing.*

**NOSE.** Frequent bleeding of nose, [when menses should appear, **Bry. Ham.**] Fluent coryza, [with watery discharge, excoriating nostrils, **Ars.** ***Arum t.**]

**FACE.** Pale face, pointed nose, sunken eyes with blue margins, [**Ars. Verat.**] *Neuralgia, mostly of infraorbital and maxillary nerves, worse from *least touch,* or when lying down at night.

**MOUTH.** Lips dry, parched and chapped, [***Bry.**] *Blackish lips. Throbbing toothache,* worse from *contact* and better from hard pressure. *Ptyalism,* also from abuse of mercury. Thick, dirty coating of tongue.

**STOMACH and ABDOMEN.** *Weak digestion.* Milk deranges stomach easily, [**Sulph.**—Fat food, pork, ice cream, ***Puls.**] Eructations, tasting of ingesta, [**Calc. c. Chin. Con.** ***Puls.**] Bitter eructations after a meal, [sour, **Kali c. Nux v.**] Vomiting sour mucus, water, food, bile, blood, [see **Ipec.**] *After eating, abdomen feels full and tight, as if stuffed, [feels *empty* after eating, **Sang. Sars.**] *Incarcerated flatulence,* [**Carb. v.**] Pinching colic, obliging him to bend double, [see **Colo.**] Liver swollen and painful to touch.

**STOOL.** Difficult passage of fæces, even when soft, [**Phos. ac.**] *Painless, very debilitating diarrhœa, stools undigested, [***Ars. Ferr. Podo.**] Diarrhœa, stools watery, white, blackish, or yellow; worse after a meal, at night. Diarrhœa after eating fruit, [**Puls.**]

**URINARY O'S.** Urine dark, turbid, scanty, [brown, black urine, **Colch. Nat. m. Tereb.**—Like milk, **Phos. ac.**—*Urine turns milky after standing a short time, **Cina.**] Stitches in the urethra, [burning, **Cap.**]

**SEXUAL O'S.** *Nocturnal emissions, after onanism, very debilitating, [**Gel. Phos.** ***Phos. ac.**—Involuntary, without erections, **Canth. Gel.**] Sense of heaviness in genital organs when walking, [when standing, **Sulph.**] *Menses profuse, black and clotted, [with labor-like pains, **Cimi.** ***Cham.**] Hemorrhage unto fainting, after miscarriage. *Leucorrhœa before menses, with pressure towards groin; bloody leucorrhœa.

**RESPIRATORY O'S.** Cough, excited by laughing, talking, or drinking, [**Dros.** ***Phos.**] Cough, with expectoration of *clear, transparent mucus,* or blood-streaked mucus. Hemorrhage from lungs, [after loss of much blood.] Oppression of chest at night, while lying down, [better lying down, **Psor.**] Inclination to take a deep breath, [like a sigh, **Cap.**] Stitches in chest, above the heart; *under sternum.*

**BACK.** Pressure as from stone between scapulæ. Pain in small of back at night. Stitches in the back.

**EXTREMITIES.** Coldness of one hand, while other is warm, [**Dig. Puls.**] Hot swelling of right knee, with tearing pains, [painful swelling above knee, **Rhus.**] Arthritic swelling of feet.

**FEVER.** Pulse small and rapid, less frequent after eating. **Chilliness* over whole body, worse from drinking; *thirst before* and *after* chill, [thirst only during chill, **Cap.**] During the *chilly stage,* headache, nausea, absence of thirst. During *hot stage,* dryness of mouth and lips, with burning; red face and headache. After *heat, thirst* and profuse sweat. **Acute fevers, with profuse sweat. Typhoid fever,* after loss of much blood. *Exhausting night-sweats,* [**Phos. Phos. ac.** ***Sil.**]

**CHARACT. PECULIARITIES.** *Patient worse every other day, [**Amb.**] *Neuralgia of a periodical character, aggravated by slightest contact, [**Colo.**] *Bad effects from loss of animal fluids, [**Calc. c. Phos. ac.**] Least draught of air causes suffering. Pains *darting, tearing;* worse at night, after a meal, or from contact, [vide **Bell.**]

## CIMICIFUGA RACEMOSA.

**MIND.** Desire for solitude, [**Chin. Mag. m. *Nux.**] Declares she will go crazy. Fear of death, thinks she will die, [see **Acon.**] Mental depression, with suicidal tendency. *Very irritable, least thing makes her angry, [see **Cham.**]

**HEAD.** *Vertigo, head feels *large* and heavy, [**Gel.**] Dull frontal headache relieved by pressure. Severe pain in head and eyeballs, increased by slightest motion, [see **Bry.**] *Top of head feels as if it would fly off. *Head feels too large and throbs, [**Gel. *Gloin.**]

**EYES.** Dark spots before eyes, dilated pupils. *Intense pains in eyeballs, worse moving head or eyes.

**EARS.** Sensitive to least noise, [**Acon. Bell. Bry.**] Singing in left, later in both ears, [see **Chin.**]

**FACE.** Wild, fearful expression. Forehead feels cold. *Neuralgia affecting malar bone, pain goes off at night, reappears next day. Wants to be in open air.

**MOUTH and THROAT.** Breath offensive. Tongue light-brown, more in middle. Mouth and tongue feel hot and dry. *Feeling of fulness in pharynx,* [see **Gel.**] Dry spot in throat, causing cough. *Hawks up a viscid, coppery-tasting mucus, [see **Arg. nit.**]

**STOMACH.** Vomiting a green substance; groans, raves, presses both hands to head for relief. Acute, darting pains in stomach, [cramping pains, **Bell. Nux.**] Sinking or "goneness" in epigastrium, [**Hydras.**]

**SEXUAL O'S.** *Great tenderness over uterine region, [**Apis. Bell. Lach.**] Menses *too early, profuse, dark, coagulated.* Sharp pains across abdomen, has to double up. Labor-like pains, [**Cham. Nux m.**] *Rheumatic dysmenorrhœa, causing patient to *cry out and weep. Membranous dysmenorrhœa.* Leucorrhœa, with sensation of weight in uterus. False labor-like pains during pregnancy. After-pains, worse in groins, with over-sensitiveness, nausea and vomiting. Lochia suppressed by cold or emotions.

**CHEST.** Pain in right side of chest, must lie quietly on back and press with hand. Pains from region of heart, all over chest and down left arm. Palpitation of heart, face livid, cold sweat on hands, left arm numb and as if bound to the side.

**BACK.** Stiff neck, with pain on moving even the hands. *Sensitiveness of spine, especially in cervical and upper dorsal regions. Head and neck retracted, (in spotted fever.) Severe pain in back, down thighs, and through hips.

**CHARACT. PECULIARITIES.** Adapted to persons at "change of life," [**Lach. *Puls.**] Nervousness from anxiety or over-exertion. *Whole body, especially arms, feel numb.

General bruised feeling, as if sore, [**Arn. Bapt.**] Pains come on suddenly, [see **Bell.**] Closely allied to **Caulo.**, in uterine and rheumatic affections.

## CINA.

**MIND.** *Pitiful weeping.* *Child extremely cross, must be carried and nursed all the time, [***Cham.**] Rejects everything offered it, [see **Cham.**] *The child will not be touched, [**Tart. e.**—see **Cham.**]

**EYES.** *Dilatation of pupils, [contraction of, **Cicu.**] Squinting, [**Bell.**] When looking steadily at an object, sees it as through a gauze, relieved by wiping eyes, [**Phos. Puls.**]

**NOSE.** *Constantly picking and rubbing the nose [**Phos. ac. Selen.**] Bleeding of nose, [**Acon.** ***Bell.**]

**FACE.** *Bloated, pale face, with blueness around mouth. Pale, cold face, with cold perspiration.

**MOUTH.** *Grinding of teeth, especially during sleep, [**Ars. Cicu. Podo.**—With foam at the mouth, **Bell.**] Dryness of mouth. *Tongue slightly coated white, with *papillæ raised, and red on the edges.*

**STOMACH.** Loathing of food, or canine hunger. Hunger soon after a full meal, [**Merc. Staph.**] Child refuses the mother's milk. *Vomiting* and diarrhœa after drinking, [after eating, **Ars.**] *Vomiting worms*, food, mucus, and bile. Pinching pain in region of navel, from worms, [**Spig.**] Abdomen *bloated and hard* in children. *Gnawing in stomach*, [when it is *empty*, **Puls.**]

**STOOL.** Diarrhœa, stools *watery, white*, [**Chin. Phos. ac. Rhus.**] Stools mixed with lumbrici. *Itching of anus.*

**URINARY O'S.** Involuntary emissions of urine (at night). *The urine turns milky after standing a little while, [like curdled milk, **Phos.**]

**RESPIRATORY O'S.** Short, hacking cough. Dry, spasmodic cough, preceded by rigidity of body and unconsciousness. Whooping-cough, violent attacks in morning, without expectoration; in the evening difficult expectoration of white, sometimes blood-streaked mucus. Worse morning and evening; better during night. Cough excited by drinking, walking in open air, pressing on larynx, [see **Lach.**]

**FEVER.** Chill, with a cold, pale face, and hot hands. *Chill*, mostly in evening, not relieved by external heat, [relieved by external heat, **Ign.**—*Increased*, **Ipec.**] *Heat*, mostly in face and head. *Sweat*, generally cold, on forehead, around nose, and on hands. Vomiting and great hunger during paroxysm. *Thirst*, only during chill or heat. *Trembling* motion of heart.

**CHARACT. PECULIARITIES.** **Especially adapted to children troubled with worms*, [**Spig.**] Epileptic attacks, mostly at night, with screams and violent jerks of the hands and feet. *Restless tossing about *during sleep.*

# COCCULUS.

**HEAD.** *Vertigo on sitting up in bed, or riding in a carriage, [*when lying down or turning in bed, **Coni.**] *Stupid feeling* in head, as from *intoxication*, [**Gel. Nux v.**] Sensation of emptiness in head, [**Ign.** ***Oxal. ac. Sep. Puls.**—*Fulness* and heaviness, **Bry. Rhus.**] *Sick headache from riding in a carriage, on a boat, etc., [**Bell.**] Headache, worse from lying on back part of head; must lie on side.

**STOMACH and ABDOMEN.** Repugnance to food, at same time hunger, [aversion to meat and boiled food, **Calc. c.**] Intense thirst while eating. Nausea, with tendency to faint, [great drowsiness and tendency to faint, ***Nux m.**] *Nausea and vomiting when riding in a carriage, [**Ars. Petro.**—Better riding in a carriage, **Nit. ac.**] *Seasickness.* *Cramp in stomach during and after a meal, with oppressed breathing, [see **Nux v.**] Sensation of emptiness in stomach, [***Ign. Pet. Sep.**—Fulness, **Chin.** ***Lyc.** ***Nux m.**] Abdomen distended, and feeling as if full of sharp stones when moving, [intestines feel as if *squeezed* between stones, ***Colo.**]

**SEXUAL O'S.** *Menstrual colic; pains spasmodic, irregular. Dysmenorrhœa, always followed by hemorrhoids. *Leucorrhœa in place of menses; so weak, can scarcely speak, [leucorrhœa worse during menses, **Iod.**] Discharge of bloody mucus from the vagina during pregnancy.

**CHEST.** Cough, as if the throat were irritated by smoke, with oppressed breathing, [as from smoke of sulphur, **Ars. Chin.**] Tightness and constriction in right side of chest, [in region of heart, **Lach.**] Burning in chest, extending to throat, [coldness, **Ars.**] Sensation of emptiness in chest, [**Cro. tig. Zinc.**—Of fulness, **Calc. c. Ferr. Nux m.**] *Palpitation of heart.*

**BACK and EXTREMITIES.** Painful cracking of cervical vertebra, [on bending backwards, **Sulph.**] Pain in shoulder and arms, as if bruised, [in wrist, as if dislocated, **Bry.**] The hands are alternately hot and cold, [heat of one and coldness of the other, **Dig. Chin. Puls.**—Heat of one *foot* and coldness of the other, **Lyc.**] Cracking of knee during motion.

**FEVER.** Chilliness alternating with heat. Chill in afternoon and evening, principally on legs and in back, not relieved by heat, [relieved by heat, ***Ign.**] Flushes of heat, with hot cheeks and cold feet. *Typhoid fever, where there is great slowness of comprehension; he don't find right words to express himself; cannot remember what has passed, and talks muttering, mumbling, [see **Arn.**]

**CHARACT. PECULIARITIES.** Disposition to tremble, [**Ign.**] *Hysterical spasms, [**Ign.**] *Worse* after eating, drinking and talking; from riding in a carriage, [better from riding in a carriage, **Nit. ac.**]

## COLCHICUM.

**MIND.** Dissatisfied with everything, [disgusted with everything, **Puls.**] His sufferings seem intolerable, [**Cham. Coff.**] *Forgetfulness*, [**Arg. n. Calc. Canth.**]

**HEAD.** Vertigo when sitting down, after walking, [vertigo on rising, **Bry. Puls.**] Sensation of constriction over eyes. Pulsations in the head, [**Puls.**]

**SOMACH.** Bitter taste, [everything tastes bitter, **Bry. Chin. Puls.**] *The smell of fish, eggs, fat meats, etc., causes nausea even to faintness. Profuse secretion of saliva. Vomiting mucus, bile, or food, with trembling, [vomiting green, jelly-like mucus, or blackish substance, **Ars. Ipec.**] Every motion excites or renews the vomiting, [riding in a carriage or becoming cold, ***Cocc.**] *Great coldness in the stomach, [**Laur. Phos.**—Violent *burning*, ***Ars. Canth. Nux. Sec.**] *Stitches* in the stomach.

**STOOL.** Extremely painful, scanty stools. Diarrhœa, with *transparent, jelly-like, mucous stools*, [**Aloe. *Hell. Kali b.**] *Fall dysentery; white mucous stools with violent tenesmus. *Bloody stools, mingled with a *skinny substance*, [stools like scrapings of the intestines, **Brom. *Canth. *Colo.**] During stool, sensation as if anus were being torn. Prolapsus ani, [with every stool, **Podo.**]

**URINE.** Frequent micturition. *Brown, black urine, with whitish sediment, [**Calc. c. Sep.**—Urine like milk, with bloody, jelly-like lumps, ***Phos. ac.**] Burning in urinary organs, with scanty secretion.

**CHARACT. PECULIARITIES.** Great weakness, with sensation of lameness in limbs. Rheumatism in warm weather, [in cold or wet weather, **Dulc.**] Tingling in different parts, as if frost-bitten, [itching, burning, and redness of parts as if frozen, ***Agar. m.**] Pains increase towards evening, [**Puls.**—Diminish, **Lyc.**]

## COLOCYNTHIS.

**MIND.** *Don't wish to talk or answer questions, [don't wish to be spoken to, **Gel. Sil.**] Inclines to be angry and indignant. Delirium, with open eyes and desire to escape, [see **Opi.**] Very impatient, [**Cham.**]

**HEAD.** One-sided headache, with nausea and vomiting, [**Con. Puls.**] Pressing headache in forehead, worse when stooping or lying on back, [pressing headache on vertex, worse stooping or lying down, **Lyc.**]

**FACE.** Dark-redness of the face. *Neuralgia*, with tearing, burning, and stinging pain on left side, *extending to ear and head*, [drawing pains on *right* side from cheek-bone to temple, **Caust.**] Cramp-like pain in left cheek-bone, extending into eye. The pains are worse from motion or contact, [see **Chin.**]

**STOMACH and ABDOMEN.** *Tongue feels as if scalded*, [**Verat. v.**] *Bitter taste* of all food and drink, [***Bry. Puls.**] *Bitter taste* after eating, [**Nit. ac.**—*Sour*, **Nux v.**] Vomiting, without nausea, [nausea, without vomiting, **Ign.**] *Colic and diarrhœa after taking least nourishment. *Bruised feeling in bowels.* *Feeling in whole abdomen as if the *intestines were being squeezed between stones*, [abdomen feels as *if full of sharp stones*, **Cocc.**] Terrible colicky pains, *causing him to bend double*, with great restlessness and lamentation, [**violent colic*, the abodomen drawn in to spine, **Plumb.**] The colic is relieved by *bending double, external pressure*, and coffee, [*pinching* in abdomen, relieved by bending double, **Chin.**—*Clutching*, griping in bowels, worse from pressure, ***Bell.**] *Cutting, as from knives, [**Con.** ***Verat.**]

**STOOL.** *Diarrhœa* after vexation, grief; stools green, [diarrhœa from fright, ***Gel. Opi.**—From drinking impure water, **Zing.**—Limestone water, **Camph.**] *Dysentery-like diarrhœa, renewed each time after taking the least food or drink, [***Ars.** ***Crot. t. Ferr.**] **Dysentery;* stools bloody, slimy, *like scrapings*, with tenesmus; relief after stool, [***Canth.**] Bloody diarrhœa, with *violent pain in bowels*, extending down the thighs, [see **Merc.**] Paralysis of the sphincter ani, [see **Phos.**]

**URINARY O'S.** Scant emissions of urine, fetid, thick, viscid, jelly-like, [dark urine, with white sediment and putrid smell, **Calc. c.**—*Urine bloody, and containing albumen.* ***Berb.**] Urine of a faint flesh color, with a whitish-brown sediment.

**CHARACT. PECULIARITIES.** *Complaints arising from indignation or grief, [from *bad news*, ***Gel.**—From *fright*, **Opi.**] Stiffness of joints, [stitches in the joints, **Bry.**] Pulsations through the body, [**Puls.** ***Zinc.**—In the head, **Colch. Puls.**] The extremities are contracted, [the whole body is *relaxed and limber*, **Nat. c.**] Pains worse during rest.

## CONIUM MACULATUM.

**MIND.** Depression of spirits [**Lyc. Plat. Puls.**—Gay and cheerful, ***Croc. Lach.**] Great difficulty of recollecting things. *Indisposed to work, [**Nit. ac. Phos.**—To *speak*, **Dig. Phos. ac.**] *Inclination to start.*

**HEAD.** *Vertigo, particularly when lying down or turning over in bed, [on sitting up in bed or riding in a carriage, **Cocc.**—On *going up-stairs*, **Calc. c.**] One-sided headache, with sick stomach, [see **Kali c.**] Tearing pain in occiput and nape of neck. Headache, as if the head were too full and would burst, [**Bell. Bry. Merc.**] Sharp, darting pain in forehead. Falling off of the hair.

**EYES.** Sensation of *coldness in the eyes*, [*burning*, itching, **Ars. Caust.**] Yellowness of the whites, [**Cham. Chin.**] Things look red, [**Bell.**—*Yellow*, **Canth.**—*Black*, **Cap.**] *Obstruction of sight.*

**EARS.** Stitches in both ears, [**Kali c. Nit. ac.**—*Pulsations* in ears, **Hepar. Phos. Rhus t.**—Vide **Merc.**] Roaring and humming in ears, [see **Chin.**] Painful sensitiveness of hearing, [**Acon. Bell. Phos. ac.**—Hardness of hearing, **Ars.** ***Calc. c. Hep.** ***Phos.**]

**FACE.** Neuralgia at night, tearing pains in right side of face, [on left side, extending to ear and head, **Colo.**] Cancer of the lips, [with burning pain, ***Ars.**] Drawing pain in lower teeth, extending to cheek-bone. Constriction of the throat, [of the chest, ***Cact.**]

**STOMACH and ABDOMEN.** Sour eructations, with burning in stomach. *Eructations tasting of the ingesta, [**Ant. c. Calc. c.** ***Chin.** ***Puls.**] *Desire* for coffee, acids, salt food, [see **Hepar.**] *Vomiting a substance like coffee-grounds, [see ***Ipec.**] *Spasmodic or pinching* pain in stomach, [**Colo. Nux.**] Cutting pain in abdomen as from knives, [***Colo. Verat.**] *Stitches extending from abdomen to right side of chest. *Rumbling* in the abdomen.

**STOOL.** *Constipation*, with frequent urging without stool, [**Anac. Lyc.** ***Nux.**] **Diarrhœa*, stools liquid, fæcal; mingled with hard lumps, [**Lyc. Nux v.**] Watery, undigested stools, [**Chin.** ***Ferr. Iris.** ***Podo.**] During stool, heat and burning in the rectum; after stool, weakness and trembling, [see **Verat. a.**]

**URINE.** Urine thick, white and turbid, [see **Phos. ac.**] *Much difficulty in voiding urine, the flow intermits, [passed in drops, sometimes mixed with blood, [***Canth. Nux.**] Cutting pain in urethra when urinating, [burning, cutting after urinating, **Cap. Nit. ac.**] *Old men and others suffering from sexual excesses.

**SEXUAL O'S.** Menstruation too early and too scanty, [too early and too profuse, ***Bell.** ***Calc. c.**—See **Puls.**] Catamenia, *brownish* blood. *During menses, stinging pain in uterus and vertigo while lying down. *Leucorrhœa of white, acrid mucus, burning and smarting*, [**Kreo. Puls.**] *Prolapsus uteri, with induration, ulceration and leucorrhœa, [prolapsus from *overlifting*, ***Rhus Nux.**—From *concussion*, **Arn.**—From *fright*, **Gel. Opi.**] *Burning, sore, aching pain in region of uterus. Induration and swelling of ovary, [see **Apis.**] **Indurations of mammæ*, very painful just before menstruation, [dwindling away of the mammæ, ***Iodi.**]

**RESPIRATORY O'S.** *Dry, hacking cough at night;* worse while lying down, [***Hyos.** ***Puls.**] Cough during pregnancy, [cough excited by a crawling, tickling in the larynx, especially during pregnancy, ***Nux m. Sabi.**—Threatened miscarriage from cough, or *after a fright*, **Acon.**] Shortness of breath when walking, [when going up-stairs, **Ars.** ***Calc. c.**]

**EXTREMITIES.** Cracking in wrist-joint, [in elbow-joint, **Kalm.**—Wrist feels as if dislocated when moving it, ***Bry. Ruta.**] Cracking of knee-joint when moving, [**Cocc.**—Cracking in left hip-joint, **Cocc.**] Coldness of the feet.

**FEVER.** Pulse irregular; generally slow and full. Coldness in morning and forenoon, [in afternoon and evening, **Lyc.** ***Puls.**] Chilliness, with desire to be in sunshine. Heat, with great nervousness. Perspiration, particularly when sleeping.

**SKIN.** Swelling and induration of glands, painful in evening. *Blackish ulcers*, with bloody, fetid, ichorous discharge, [see **Ars.**—*Sticky, glutinous discharge*, ***Graph.**] Cancerous ulcers, [*mortifying ulcers*, **Ars.**] *Humid* tetters, [**Calc. Dulc. Graph.**]

**CHARACT. PECULIARITIES.** Especially adapted to the diseases of debility of old people. *Bad effects from sexual excesses, [**Phos. ac.**] *Induration of the mammæ; hard as a stone, [**Bry. Phyto.**] *Great soreness of breasts, preceding the menses.

## DIGITALIS.

**MIND.** Desponding and fearful. Anxious about the future, [great fear of death and of being alone. ***Ars. Lyc.**] Indisposed to speak, [**Phos. ac. Stan.**—Wants to talk continually, ***Stram.**]

**HEAD.** Vertigo with trembling, [*with chilliness, **Puls.**] Stitches in forehead and temples, [in back part of head, **Canth.**—In vertex, **Ipec.**—See **Canth.**] When stooping, sensation as if brain fell forward, [to left side, **Nat. s.**] Sudden cracking in head, with starting as in a fright.

**EYES.** Throbbing in the orbits. Inflammation of the meibomian glands, [***Puls. Rhus.**] Agglutination of lids in the morning, [**Caust.** Dimness of vision. *Things appear green or yellow, [appear *red*, **Bell.**—*Black*, **Cap.**] *Various colors* before the eyes.

**STOMACH.** Sweet taste, with constant ptyalism, [vide **Merc.**] Gulping up a sour or tasteless fluid, [a bitter fluid, **Ign. Pet.**] Excessive nausea, as if he would die, [**Ipec. Lobe.**] Not relieved by vomiting. *Morning vomiting*, [**Kreo. Nux v. Puls.**] Vomiting of the ingesta, [*vomiting large quantities of mucus, **Ipec. Tart.**—Of bitter, sour fluids, **Puls.**] *Great sense of weakness in stomach* Frequent pressure in stomach, [as from a stone, **Cham. Nux v.**] Burning in stomach extending to œsophagus, [in pit of the stomach, **Ars. Nux v.**] Cramp in stomach, [**Ars. Nux.**]

**STOOL.** Watery diarrhœa. * White or ash-colored stools, [**Cist. Kali c.**]—White, chalk-like stools, [***Calc. c.** ***Podo.**] Chilliness *before* stool, [*during* stool, **Ars.** ***Merc.** ***Verat.**—*After* stool, **Canth.**] *Diarrhœa during jaundice*, [**Nux v.**]

**URINE.** Continual desire to urinate, only a few drops being emitted each time. Urine dark, brown, hot and burning, with *sharp cutting pains* at neck of bladder. *Inflammation of neck of bladder, [**Canth.**]

**RESPIRATORY O'S.** Cough, with expectoration looking like boiled starch; raw, sore feeling in chest. Dyspnœa when walking and in a recumbent position, [better when lying down, **Iodi. Psor.**] The least movement produces *violent palpitation* of heart, [**Iodi.**—Violent palpitation, particularly at night and when lying down, ***Ars.**—Better when lying quiet on back, **Iodi.**—Worse when lying on left side, **Cact. Lyc.**] Sensation as if heart would stop beating if one moved, [*feeling as though an iron band was around the heart, preventing its action, **Cact. g.**—As if squeezed together, **Arn. Iodi.**] Frequent stitches in heart [**Caust. Ign.** ***Spig.**—Frequent shocks in heart, **Coni.** ***Nux v.**—Painful jerking in heart, **Fluor. ac.** *Burning* in region of heart, **Kali c.**—*Coldness* in, **Nat. m.**—See **Spig.**]

**EXTREMITIES.** Heat of one hand and coldness of the other, [**Chin. Ipec. Puls.**—One hand burning hot and pale, other cold and red, **Mosch.**—One *foot* cold, other hot, **Lyc.**] Heaviness or paralytic weakness of left arm, [of *right*, **Caust.**—Of both arms, **Dulc. Nat. m.**] Great weakness of lower extremities. *Dropsy of knee-joint. Swelling of feet during the day, diminished at night.

**FEVER.** *Slow* and irregular pulse, [full, frequent, ***Acon.** ***Bell.**] The slow pulse is accelerated by slightest motion. Internal chilliness, with external heat, [**Calc. c.**—External coldness, with internal heat, and *vice versa*, **Ign.**—See. **Ars.**] *Sudden flushes of heat, followed by great debility.

**CHARACT. PECULIARITIES.** *All diseases where the *heart* is more or less involved, and there is irregular or intermittent pulse. Great nervous weakness. Dropsy of external and internal parts. Symptoms *worse* in a warm room, [***Puls. Sec. Verat.**—*Better* in a warm room, ***Ars. Hep. Rhus.**]

## DULCAMARA.

**HEAD.** *Vertigo on awaking in morning and when rising from bed, [when rising from a sitting posture, ***Puls.**] Boring headache in forehead and temples, [on right side, **Bell.**] worse before midnight and when lying quiet; better when talking. Digging pain in forehead, with a sensation as if the brain were too large, [as if the head were too large, **Arg. n. Glon. Lactu. Nux.**] Stupefying pain in back part of head, ascending from nape of the neck. *Chilliness* in back part of head. *Heaviness* of the head, [lightness, **Hipp.** ***Stram.**—Hollowness, **Coral. r. Ign. Opi.**] *Ringworm* of the scalp.

**MOUTH and THROAT.** Bitter taste. *Dry, rough* tongue. Paralysis of the tongue, [**Bary. c.** ***Hyos.**—Paralysis of the œsophagus, **Hyd. ac.**] *Sore throat after taking cold*, [**Cham.** ***Merc.**] Rough *scraping* in throat.

**STOMACH and ABDOMEN.** Vomiting white, tenacious mucus, [sweetish water or bilious matter, **Iris v.**—See **Ipec.**] *Sensation of fulness in stomach and emptiness in abdomen.

Colic from cold, as if diarrhœa would set in. Dropsy of abdomen. Swelling of the inguinal glands, [*Merc.]

**STOOL.** Diarrhœa from *taking cold;* stools *mucous, green, watery,* and *whitish,* [from *fright,* ***Gel. Opi.**—From impure water, **Zing.**—Calcareous water, ***Camph.**] Diarrhœa, with colic; stools watery, especially in summer and when the *weather suddenly becomes cool,* [diarrhœa from *cold drinks in hot weather,* ***Bry.**] *Diarrhœa from repelled eruptions, chills, or dentition.

**URINARY O'S.** Urine turbid and white, [*turns milky soon after being passed, **Cina.**] Sediment at times red, at times white; urine fetid, [see **Nit. ac.**] Strangury, painful micturition.

**SEXUAL O'S.** Retarded flow, blood watery, thin, [see **Puls.**] Suppression of menses from cold, [**Merc.** ***Podo. Sulph.**—See **Puls.**] *Always as a forerunner of the catamenia, a rash appears on skin, [previous to the menses, violent itching of old tettery eruptions, **Carb. v.**—*Before* and *during* the menses has a fatiguing cough, **Graph.**] *Lochia suppressed by cold or dampness, [from *fright,* **Opi.**] Suppression of milk from cold, [**Puls.**]

**CHARACT. PECULIARITIES.** *Especially adapted to catarrhal and rheumatic diseases in damp, cold weather, [diseases induced by dry, cold, west winds, **Acon. Hepar.**] Symptoms aggravated at every cold change in weather. Increased secretion of the mucous membranes and glands; those of skin being suppressed. Symptoms better from moving about, [***Rhus t.**—Worse by movement, ***Bry.**]

## FERRUM.

**HEAD.** *Vertigo* when descending a height, or seeing flowing water, [from ascending a height, **Calc. c.**—When rising from a seat, stooping, or looking up, **Bry. Puls.**—When turning round, **Coni.**] Congestion to the head, with *throbbing headache and flushed face,* [**Acon. Bell.**] Pain in back part of head when coughing.

**FACE.** Ashy-pale or greenish color of face, [pale, sickly appearance, as after excesses, **Chin.**] Pale, bloated face, especially around eyes. *Pale face and lips, with great debility. *Least emotion or exertion produces a red, flushed face. Yellow spots in face, [across nose, like a saddle, ***Sep. Sulph.**]

**STOMACH.** Aversion to, and bad effects of, meat, beer, acids, [craves acids, **Chin. Verat.**—*Brandy, chalk,* **Nit. ac. Nux v.**—Salt food, **Calc. c.**] Can neither eat nor drink anything hot, [worse from anything *cold,* **Ars.**] All food tastes *bitter,* [***Bry. Chin. Puls.**] Bitter eructations after fat food, Vomiting food soon as it is eaten, [**Ars. Bry.**] Everything vomited tastes sour. Pressure in stomach after taking least food or drink, [feels full up to throat, ***Lyc.**—Abdomen feels as if *stuffed,* ***Chin.**]

**STOOL.** *Watery* diarrhœa, burning, corroding anus, [**Iris v.**] **Painless diarrhœa;* stools of undigested food, [**Chin. Phos. Phos. ac. *Podo.**] Frequent diarrhœic stools of slimy mucus mingled with ascarides, [***Cina. Spig. *Sulph.**] Stools with blood and mucus.

**SEXUAL O'S.** Impotence in men, [after onanism, **Phos.**—After gonorrhœa, **Thuya.**] Nocturnal emissions, [very debilitating, **Chin. *Phos. ac.**] Menses too frequent, too profuse, and lasting too long, [***Bell. Calc. c. Ign.**] *Previous to the menses, has stinging headache, ringing in ears, and discharges long pieces of mucus from uterus. Uterine hemorrhage in weakly persons, with labor-like pains, blood partly fluid and partly clotted, [***Sabi.**] Leucorrhœa like watery milk, smarting, corroding the parts, [**Coni.**]

**RESPIRATORY O'S.** *Spasmodic cough, with expectoration of tough, transparent mucus, [**Chin. Sil.**] Cough in morning, relieved by eating, [relieved by drinking, **Caust. Spong.**—Excited by eating or drinking anything cold, **Hepar.**] When coughing, stitches and soreness in chest. Cough after eating, with vomiting the ingesta, [**Dig. Rhus t.**] *Hæmoptysis, with pain between scapulæ; better from walking slowly about, [worse from least exertion, **Ipec.**] Fulness and tightness of the chest, [**Calc. c. *Phos. Puls. *Staph.**—*Emptiness,* ***Cocc. Graph.**]

**EXTREMITIES.** Paralytic pain in left shoulder-joint, preventing motion of arm, [right shoulder, **Sang.**] *Sticking and tearing in shoulder-joint.* Nightly tearing and stinging from hip-joint to thigh, better from slow motion, [**Rhus t.**] Painful cramps in the calves, while at rest. Œdematous swelling of the feet.

**FEVER.** Pulse full and hard. Frequent short shudderings. Chilliness and want of animal heat, [**Lead.**] *Intermittent fever* (after abuse of quinine) with congestion of head, distention of the veins, vomiting the ingesta and swelling of the spleen. Profuse and long-continued perspiration.

**CHARACT. PECULIARITIES.** Weakly persons, with *fiery-red face.* *The least pain or emotion produces a flushed face. Leucophlegmatic constitution, [**Calc. c.**] General hemorrhagic tendency. *Always better from walking slowly about, although he is very weak, [better from being perfectly still, ***Bry.**]

## GELSEMIUM.

**MIND.** Confusion of mind; cannot collect his thoughts, [**Bapt.**] Great irritability, does not wish to be spoken to, [don't wish to speak, **Dig.**—Talks continually, **Cicu. *Stram.**] Liveliness, followed by depression of spirits, [**Lach.**]

**HEAD.** Staggering, as if intoxicated. *Vertigo, as if intoxicated, [**Cann. s. Croc. *Nux.**] Fulness in head, with heat in face and chilliness, [sensation of emptiness or hollowness in the head, **Coral. Ign. Oxal. ac.**] Pain as from a tape around the head, [**Merc. Sulph.**—Headache relieved by compression, [**Cinna. *Puls.**] Dull pain in occiput after breakfast, worse when moving and stooping. Headache, with giddiness, faintness, pain in neck. Sensation as if the brain were bruised, [**Chin. Hell.**]

**EYES.** * *Great heaviness of eyelids*, cannot keep them open, [**Rhus. Sep.**—Eyes *open and staring*, **Laur. Stram.**] Dimness of vision [during pregnancy.] Eyes feel bruised, [feel too large, **Mez. Phos. ac.**] Pupils dilated, [**Bell. Croc.**—Contracted, **Cicu. Phos.**] Great aversion to light, [see **Bell.**]

**MOUTH and THROAT.** Lips dry, hot, and coated. Tongue coated yellowish-white, with fetid breath, [**Merc. pro.**—Dry, hard, coated black, **Merc. v.**] Burning in mouth, extending to throat and stomach, [**Canth.**—*Burning* in stomach, ascending to throat, **Merc.**—Coldness in throat, **Carb. v. Laur.**] Sensation as if a foreign body were lodged in throat, [see **Hepar.**] *Throat feels as if filled up*, [**Eupa. pur. Glon. Sil.**]

**STOMACH.** Sour eructations, [**Nit. ac. Nux v.**—*Bitter*, **Bell. Chin.**—*Without taste or smell*, **Hepar.**] Nausea, (with giddiness and headache.) Sensation of emptiness in stomach, [**Ign. Sep.**—*After eating*, **Sang. Sars.**—Great *fulness after eating*, **Chin. *Lyc. Nux v.**]

**STOOL.** The soft stool is passed with difficulty, as if owing to contraction of sphincter ani, [from inactivity of rectum, **Alum.**] * *Diarrhœa from sudden depressing emotions, fright, grief, bad news*, [**Opi.**—From anger, **Cham.**—Indignation, **Colo.**] Stools *yellow, fecal; cream-colored; bilious. Paralysis* of sphincter ani, [**Bell. Hyos.**]

**SEXUAL O'S.** Involuntary emissions, with or without erections, followed by great debility and lowness of spirits, [after onanism, ***Chin. *Phos. ac.**] Sensation of heaviness in uterus, [**Nux v.**—Of fulness, **Chin.**] Suppressed menstruation, with convulsions, [**Cocc. Nux m.**—With *semi-lateral headache*, ***Puls.**] * *Rigidity of os uteri*, [***Acon. *Caul. Cimi.**] During pregnancy, violent pains in uterus, headache, etc.

**RESPIRATORY O'S.** Spasm of glottis, threatening suffocation, [with crowing inspiration and expiration, ***Chlorine.**—With blueness of face and lips, convulsions, **Cup.**] Roughness of throat, as if ulcerated. *Sensation of constriction* in lower part of chest, [***Cact. Puls. Verat.**] Stitches in region of heart, [***Dig. Caust. Ign.**] *Sensation as if heart would stop beating if she would cease walking*, [see **Dig.**]

**FEVER.** Pulse slow, accelerated by motion, [accelerated only towards evening, **Caust.**—Fast in morning, slow in evening, **Ars.**] *Chills begin in hands. Chilliness every day at same hour, especially in morning, [at 10 A.M., **Nat. m.**, at 4 P.M., **Lyc.**—Every evening, same hour, ***Saba.**] Chill followed by heat, and later by perspiration. Feet cold, as if in ice-water, [as if they had on *cold, damp stockings*, **Calc. c.**] *Nervous chills*, "chatters." *Fever without thirst, [**Puls.**]

**CHARACT. PECULIARITIES.** *Prostration of whole muscular system*, [**Cimi.**—Of the nervous system, **Phos. Verat. a.**] Feeling of lightness in body from spinal exhaustion, in onanists. *Great depression of spirits in onanists, with excessive languor. Headache, worse from smoking tobacco, [relieved by smoking, **Diad. ar.**] *Bad effects from sudden emotions, joy, grief, fright, [**Ign. Opi.**]

## GRAPHITES.

**MIND.** *Great tendency to start.* Want of disposition to work. Easily vexed; *out of humor*, [exceedingly irritable, ***Bry. Nux.**] *Ailments from grief.

**HEAD.** *Feeling of intoxication in head, [**Bell. Nux. Puls.**] Headache in morning on waking, mostly on one side, with inclination to vomit, [pressing pain in temples after rising, **Lach.**] Rheumatic pains on one side of head, extending to teeth and neck. *Burning on vertex*, [**Nat. m.** ***Sulph.**—*Coldness*, **Sep.** ***Verat.**] Humid, itching eruption on hairy scalp, emitting a fetid odor, [**Lyc.** ***Rhus. Sulph.**]

**EYES.** Ophthalmia, with intolerance of light; eyelids red and swollen. *Dryness of the eyelids*, [increased secretion in the eyes, **Euph.**]

**EARS.** Dryness of inner ear, [**Carb. v. Lach.**—Accumulation of wax, **Coni. Sil.**] *Moisture and eruptions behind the ears, [**Bary. c. Calc. c. Hepar.**] Hardness of hearing, [with sensation as if stopped up, **Calc. c.** ***Puls. Sulph.**] *Cracking* in ears when chewing, [when *not* chewing, **Kali c.**] *Hissing in the ears. Detonation* in ears like report of a gun, [see **Sil.**]

**STOMACH and ABDOMEN.** Nausea and vomiting after each meal, [after eating or drinking, **Ars. Bry. Verat. a.**] *Morning sickness during *menstruation*. *Pressure in stomach*, [as of a stone, after eating, ***Ars. Bry. Merc.**] Burning in stomach, causing hunger, [sensation of emptiness in stomach, with *hunger*, ***Sep.**] Nauseous feeling in *abdomen*. *Fulness and hardness* in abdomen, as from incarcerated flatulence. Croaking as of frogs in abdomen, [gurgling and rumbling, **Lyc.**—Sensation of something *alive* in abdomen, ***Croc.**]

**STOOL.** *Constipation;* large, difficult, knotty stools, united by mucous threads, [stools of *hard, black balls*, ***Opi.**—In lumps, like sheep's dung, **Chel. m.** ***Plumb. Ruta.**—*Long, narrow*, like a dog's, ***Phos.**] *Diarrhœa;* stools of brown fluid, mixed with undigested substances, *very fetid. Varices of the rectum*, [see ***Carb. v.**]

**SEXUAL O'S.** Soreness of vagina. Painful swelling of left ovary, [**Lach.**—Of right, ***Apis.** ***Bell.**] *Menses *too late*, pale and scanty, [***Puls. Sulph.**] *During menses, severe tearing pain in epigastrium*, [in liver, **Phos. ac.**] Suppression of menses, with heaviness in arms and lower limbs, [with chilliness and pale face, ***Puls.**] *Profuse leucorrhœa; discharge white, thin, excoriating, with great weakness in back.

**RESPIRATORY O'S.** *Scraping* in trachea and *roughness* of throat. Oppression of the chest—Asthma. *Violent throbbing about the heart*, [see **Dig.**] Swelling and induration of mammary glands, [**Bell. Carbo a. Coni.**—*Dwindling* of, **Iod. Nit. ac.**] Soreness of nipples, having deep cracks and blisters, [*cracked, stinging and burning*, ***Sulph.**]

**EXTREMITIES.** Pains as if sprained in joints of fingers, [as if dislocated, **Bry. Ruta g.**] Gouty nodosities on finger-joints, [**Calc. c. Dig. Led. Staph.**] Numbness and stiffness of thighs and toes, [**Nux v.**] Stiffness of knees when bending them, [cracking, **Cocc.**] *Herpes in bend of the knees and groins.* *Ulcers on legs, discharging a *glutinous* fluid, [old *ulcers*, with *burning*, cutting pains, **Ars. Lyc.**]

**SKIN.** Swelling and induration of glands, [**Bary. c. Calc. c.**] *Rawness in bends of limbs, groins, neck, behind the ears, especially in children. Ulcers, with fetid pus, [**Ars. Carb. v. Sulph.**] **Eruptions, oozing out a sticky fluid*, [*watery* fluid, **Dulc.**] Humid tetters and eruptions, [**Calc. c. Merc.**—Herpes dry, scabby and scurfy, **Clem. Phos. *Sulph.**] *Unhealthy skin; every little injury suppurates, [**Calc. c. Hepar. Sil.**]

**CHARACT. PECULIARITIES.** Adapted to females inclined to obesity, [see **Calc. c.**] Liability to take cold; very sensitive to a draught of air, [**Calc. Caust. Sil.**] *Disposition to delaying menstruation, [**Puls. Sulph.**] *Aggravation* at night, during and after menstruation.

## HEPAR SULPHUR.

**MIND.** Great anguish in the evening, [gaiety, mirth, joking, **Croc.**] The slightest cause irritates him, [he seeks a cause for quarrel, ***Cham.**] Dejected, sad, inclined to shed tears, [**Dig. Graph.**]

**HEAD.** *Vertigo when riding in a carriage or shaking head, [**Cocc.**] Headache when shaking the head, with vertigo. Boring pain in the right temple, [**Bell.**—In forehead and temples, **Dulc. Merc. Puls.**—In *vertex*, **Mag. m.**] Boring pain in root of nose every morning. Sensation of swashing in head, [**Hyos. Nux v.**—Of looseness of brain, when walking, **Cicu. Graph. Nux m. Rhus.**—As if falling to left side, **Nat. s.**] Humid scald head, itching and burning, [dry, scabby, easily bleeding, offensive, **Sulph.**]

**EYES.** Pain in the eyes as if pulled back into the head. *Boring pain* in upper bones of the orbits. Erysipelatous inflammation of the eyes; they ache from a bright light Objects appear red, [**Bell.**—*Blue*, **Stram.**—*Black*, **Cap.**—*Yellow*, **Canth.**] *Things look too large, [***Hyos.** – *Too small*, **Plat Stram.**]

**EARS.** Scurfs on and behind the ears, [see **Graph.**] Discharge of fetid pus from ears, [**Carb. v. Merc. Sulph.**—After scarlet fever, ***Bell.**—Bloody pus, **Rhus.**] Whizzing and throbbing in ears, with hardness of hearing, [see **Merc.**]

**FACE.** Vesicular erysipelas, with prickling in parts, [burning, tingling, stinging; the vesicles containing yellow water, ***Rhus.**] *Pains in bones of face, especially when being touched, [**Chin. Colo.**] Ulcers in corners of mouth, [**Calc. c. Graph. Sil.**—Cracks in lips and corners of mouth, **Merc. Nit. ac.**]

**MOUTH and THROAT.** Gums and mouth painful to touch and bleed readily, [gums swollen, white, bleeding, **Nit. ac. Nux v.**] Toothache worse in a warm room, and when pressing teeth together, [see **Puls.**] When swallowing, sensation as if a plug were in throat, [**Bell.** ***Merc. Nux v. Phyt.**] When swallowing, sensation as of a *splinter* in throat, [**Arg. n. Nit. ac.**] *Roughness and scraping in throat, [**Am. c. Ars.**] *Quinsy, with impending suppuration, [**Merc. Mur. ac. Sil.**] Stitches in the throat, extending to the ear when swallowing.

**STOMACH and ABDOMEN.** *Longing for acids, wine and strong-tasting food, [**Bry. Chin. Nux.**—For *bitter* things, **Dig. Nat. m.**—For *chalk, lime,* etc., ***Nit. ac. Nux.**—For *fat* food, **Nit. ac.**—*Milk,* ***Merc. Nux.**—*Salt* food, ***Calc. c. Carb. v.**—*Sweet* things, **Ipe. Lyc.**—For refreshing, juicy things, ***Phos. ac. Verat.**] *Aversion to fat* food, [***Hep. Pet.** ***Puls.**—To bread, coffee, **Lyc.** ***Nux.**—To *meat, milk,* **Ign. Sep. Sulph.**—To *sweet* things, **Caust.** ***Graph. Nit. ac.**] *Frequent eructations, without taste or smell, [putrid, as from bad eggs, ***Arn.** ***Merc. Sep. Sulph.**—*Tasting of ingesta,* ***Chin. Con.** ***Puls.**—Of garlic, **Mosch.**] *Distention of stomach,* compelling one to loosen the clothing, [**Chin.** ***Lyc.** ***Nux.**] Burning in stomach, [***Ars.** ***Nux. Puls.**] Heaviness and pressure in stomach after a slight meal, [as from a stone, **Ars. Cham. Nux v.**] Stitches in region of liver when walking, coughing, breathing, or touching it, [**Bry. Merc. Nux v.**] Swelling and suppuration of inguinal glands, [**Merc. Nit. ac.**]

**STOOLS.** *Painless diarrhœa;* stools light-yellow, *undigested; whitish, smelling sour,* [**Calc. c.**—See **Ferr. Phos. Phos. ac. Podo.**] Clay-colored stool, [black, **Lept. Verat.**—Changeable, **Puls. Sulph.**] Protrusion of varices.

**URINARY O'S.** *Sharp, burning urine corroding the prepuce. Burning in urethra during micturition, [see **Canth.**] *Ulceration in kidneys, [**Mur. ac. Phos. Sil.**] Urine dark-red, hot; bloody. Inflammation of orifice of urethra, with mucous discharge, [see **Cann. s.**]

**SEXUAL O'S.** *Men.* Ulcers like chancres on prepuce, [with a cheesy bottom, **Merc.**] *Women.* Menses delayed and too scanty, [too late, pale and scant, **Graph. Puls. Sulph.**] Between menstrual periods discharge of blood.

**RESPIRATORY O'S.** Hoarseness, with loss of voice, [see **Phos.**] *Dry, hoarse cough,* [***Bell. Merc. Nux.** ***Phos.**] *Cough excited whenever any part of body gets cold, [**Rhus**], or from eating anything cold, [relieved by eating or drinking, **Spong.**] **Croup,* with loose, rattling cough, worse in morning, [*dry, barking, wheezing cough,* with rattling breathing,

**Brom.** ***Spong.**—*Crowing* inspiration, expiration almost impossible, ***Chlorine.**] Rattling, croaking cough; suffocative attacks, has to rise up and bend head backwards, [see **Acon.**] *Anxious, wheezing breathing,* [***Spong.**] *Palpitation of heart.*

**EXTREMITIES.** *In early stage of *whitlow,* when pain is violent and throbbing, [**Merc. Sil.**] Roughness of hands, with a dry, grating skin. Swelling and suppuration of axillary glands, [**Sil.**] Coxagra, with throbbing pain and disposition to suppurate, [after suppuration, **Calc. Phos. Merc.**—Caries and suppuration of bones, **Asa. Sil.**] Swelling of ankles and feet.

**FEVER.** Chilliness and heat alternating, with photophobia. Great chilliness in open air. *Intermittent fever;* first *chill,* 8 P.M., then thirst, and, an hour later, fever, with interrupted sleep, [*chill* and *heat* simultaneous, **Ars.**] *Itching, stinging nettle-rash before and during chill, [itching, stinging nettle-rash during fever, **Ign.**] Cold, clammy, offensive perspiration.

**SKIN.** *Unhealthy skin; every little injury suppurates, [**Calc. c.** ***Graph. Sil.**—Slight injuries bleed much, **Phos.**] Chapped skin, with deep cracks on hands and feet. *Ulcers, with bloody suppuration, smelling like old cheese, [gangrenous ulcers having a *putrid* smell, **Ars. Lach.**—Ulcer feels as if burnt; discharges a putrid fluid, **Sec. c.**] Ulcers very sensitive to contact, *burning, stinging,* easily bleeding, [see **Ars.**] *Jaundice,* with blood-red urine.

**CHARACT. PECULIARITIES.** *In diseases where suppuration is inevitable, [**Mur. ac.** ***Sil.**] Sweats day and night, without relief, [**Merc.**] Cannot bear to be *uncovered;* wants to be wrapped up warmly, [*skin cold,* but wants to be *uncovered,* **Camph. Sec.**] *Sticking* or *pricking* in affected part. *Worse* lying on painful side, [**Ars. Iod. Nux m.**—*Better,* ***Bry. Calc. c. Puls.**] *Better after eating,* (stomach symptoms,) [worse, **Ars. Nux.**]

## HYDRASTIS CANADENSIS.

**MIND.** *Forgetful,* [**Bell. Calc. Graph. Rhus.**] Cannot remember what he is reading or talking about. Irritable; disposed to be spiteful, [**Nux v.**]

**HEAD.** Feeling as if intoxicated, [see **Gel.**] **Dull frontal headache* over eyes, better from pressing with hand. Headache of a nervous, gastric character. *Eczema on margin of hair in front,* worse coming from cold into warm room; oozes after washing.

**NOSE.** Coryza watery, excoriating, [**Ars. Arum t.**] Sneezing, with fulness over eyes, dull frontal headache. The air feels cold in nose. Thick, tenacious secretion from posterior nares, [*dropping* back into pharynx, **Ferr. Kali b.**] Ozena, with bloody, purulent discharge.

**MOUTH.** *Peppery taste,* [see **Lach.**] Tongue coated white, or with a yellow stripe. Tongue swollen, shows *imprint of teeth,* [**Ars. Merc.**] Tongue feels as if *scalded,* [**Colo.** ***Verat. v.**]

*Stomatitis* after mercury or chlorate of potash, also in *nursing women*, or *weakly children*.

**THROAT.** *Hawking yellow, tenacious mucus from posterior nares, [see **Arg. n.**] Ulcers in throat.

**STOMACH.** Eructations of sour fluid, [see **Nux.**] Vomits all he eats except milk and water. *Dull, aching pain in stomach, which causes a weak, faintish "goneness." Chronic gastric catarrh. Cutting in lower abdomen, extending to testicles.

**STOOL.** Diarrhœa, stools light-colored, acrid, greenish. *Constipation, stool lumpy, covered with mucus, [see **Opi.**] *Fistula ani.* Bleeding piles, *exhausting*.

**URINE.** Dull aching in region of kidneys. Catarrh of bladder, with thick, ropy sediment in urine.

**SEXUAL O'S.** *Gonorrhœa*, second stage, thick, yellow discharge; painless. *Leucorrhœa*, tenacious, ropy, thick, yellow. *Pruritus* vulvæ, with profuse leucorrhœa. Prolapsus uteri, with ulceration of cervix and vagina, [see **Arg. n.**]

**LUNGS.** Dry, harsh cough, from tickling in larynx. Rawness, soreness and burning in chest. *Bronchitis* of old exhausted people, thick, yellow, tenacious, stringy sputa, [**Kali b.**]

**FEVER.** Chill morning or evening. Chilliness, especially in back or thighs, with aching. *Heat in flushes.* *Slow pulse, [**Opi.**] Gastric, bilious or typhoid forms of fever, with gastric disturbance.

**CHARACT. PECULIARITIES.** Adapted to old people, with debility, [see **Opi.**] *Frequent sudden attacks of fainty spells, with cold sweat all over. *Faintness, "goneness" in stomach. *Left side* most affected.

## HYOSCYAMUS NIGER.

**MIND.** **Mental derangement*, with muttering. *Fear of being *poisoned*. *Very talkative*, [talks continually, **Cicu. Lach.** ***Stram.**] *Delirium* without consciousness; does not know his own family. *Muttering, with picking at bed-clothes, [during sleep, **Opi.**—Grasping at flocks, **Bell. Bry. Phos. ac.**] Delirium, with jerking of limbs, wild, staring look, or closed eyes, [silent delirium with open eyes, **Opi. Stram.**] *Lascivious furor, without modesty, [**Canth. Verat.**] Involuntary loud laughter, with silly actions and trembling, [**Croc.**—Weeps and laughs alternately, **Aur. Bell.**] Aversion to light and company, [desire for, ***Stram.**] *Loss of memory. Complete stupefaction*, [**Opi.**]

**HEAD.** Vertigo, with stupefaction, [**Coni. Opi. Puls.**] *Congestion* to the head, with delirium, unconsciousness, yet answering all questions properly. *Congestion to the head, with red, sparkling eyes and purple-red face. *Inflammation of brain*, with tingling, and violent pulsations in head like waves, [violent *pulsations of carotids* and *throbbing headache*,

**Bell. Glon.**] The brain feels as if it were loose, [**Bry. Nat. sul. Nux m.**] Hydrocephalus, with stupor and sensation of swashing in head, hands closed, with *clinched thumbs*, [see **Hell.**]

**EYES.** Red, sparkling, staring eyes, [**Bell.**] Spasmodic closing of lids; inability to keep them open, [see **Gel.**] *Pupils dilated*, [***Bell. Opi.**—*Contracted*, **Cicu. Phos.**] *Objects appear red, *too large*, or double.

**MOUTH and THROAT.** Foam at mouth, [bloody, **Stram.**] Lips look like scorched leather, [dry, parched and cracked, **Bry. Stram.**] *Clean, parched, dry tongue*, [red and cracked, **Bell. Rhus.**] *Constriction of throat, with inability to swallow, especially fluids, [**Bell. Laur. Stram.**—Sensation of *expansion* of throat, **Hypericum.**]

**STOMACH.** *Dread of drink, [**Bell. Canth.**] Great thirst, but drinks very little, [drinks little and often, **Apis. Ars. Chin.**] *Eating produces vomiting*, [vomits after *eating or drinking*, **Ars. Ipe. Verat.**—Comp. **Ipe.**] *Vomiting of blood and and bloody mucus. Colic relieved by vomiting, [relieved by eating, **Hepar.**]

**STOOL.** *Painless diarrhœa;* stools, yellow, watery, [**Chin. Hep.**] Involuntary stools in bed, without being conscious of it, [**Carb. v. Rhus. Sec.**] *Diarrhœa during typhoid fever, and during lying-in.

**URINE.** *Involuntary micturition*, as from paralysis of bladder, [**Ars. Bell. *Puls.**] *Suppression* of urine.

**RESPIRATORY O'S.** Dry *spasmodic* cough, [old persons,] with tickling in throat; worse at night, when at rest, during sleep, in cold air, after eating and drinking, [better by eating or drinking, **Spong.**] *The cough is relieved by sitting up, [**Puls.**—Worse from sitting up, **Kali c. *Zinc.**—Better by a swallow of water, **Cup. Caust.**] Violent, spasmodic cough, with expectoration during day of saltish-tasting mucus, or bright-red blood, mixed with clots. Slow, rattling breathing.

**SLEEP.** *Deep sleep*, with convulsions, [with stertorous breathing, ***Opi.**] Starting from sleep, [when closing the eyes, **Bell.**] *Nightly sleeplessness*, [see **Opi.**]

**FEVER.** Pulse accelerated, full, hard. Chilliness over whole body, with hot face and cold hands. In evening, great heat over whole body. *Typhoid fever, with low, muttering delirium; *subsultus tendinum; picking at bed-clothes;* involuntary discharges of fæces and urine, and *desire to escape*, [see **Opi.**] *After a correct answer, relapses into delirium and unconsciousness, [see **Arn.**] Debilitating perspiration during sleep, [**Chin. Merc.**]

**CHARACT. PECULIARITIES.** Adapted to *hysterical subjects* and to drunkards, [***Nux v. Stram.**] Things look too *large*, [too *small*, **Plat. Stram.**] *Spasms, with twitching and jerking of every muscle of body, eyes, eyelids and face. Epileptic attacks, ending in deep, heavy sleep. *Spasmodic, dry cough, always worse when lying down, relieved by sitting up, [**Puls.**] ***Desire to uncover and remain naked, [skin cold as ice, yet he must be uncovered, ***Camph.** ***Sec.**] *Subsultus tendinum.* Bad effects from jealousy and unhappy love. *Worse* in evening; after eating and drinking, [see **Ars.**] *Better* from stooping [head, and breathing.]

## IGNATIA AMARA.

**MIND.** *Full of suppressed grief, [**Phos. ac. Puls.**—Gay and cheerful, **Croc. Lach.**] *Great indifference to everything,* [***Phos. ac. Lach. Merc.**] Avoids talking, [**Con. Bell. Phos. ac.**—*Wants to talk continually, **Stram.**] Changeable disposition, jesting, laughing and crying, [sings involuntarily and then laughs, **Croc.**]

**HEAD.** Sensation of hollowness in head, [see **Opi.**] Heaviness of head, [*lightness,* ***Stram.**] *Headache, increased by stooping,* [relieved by stooping, **Hyos.**] Tearing pain in forehead, relieved by lying on back. *Sensation as if a nail were driven out through side of head, relieved by lying on it, [see **Nux v.**] *Cramp-like* pain over root of nose, [*boring pain* in *upper bones* of orbit, **Bell. Hep.**] *Beating* headache in occiput; worse from smoking or smelling tobacco-smoke, [relieved by smoking, **Diad. ar.**]

**EYES.** Sensation as if grains of sand were under upper lids, [**Carb. v. Caust. Euph.**—Smarting as from salt, **Nux v.**] *Cannot bear the glare of light, *[aversion to or desire for light, **Acon. Bell.**] Flickering zigzags before the eyes, [**Nat. m.**]

**MOUTH and THROAT.** Boring pain in front teeth; worse after drinking coffee or smoking, [see **Nux v.**] *Toothache, as if the tooth were *crushed* in pieces, [as if burst, **Sabi.**] *Increased secretion* of saliva; foam at mouth. Stitches in throat when *not* swallowing, [when *swallowing,* **Hep.**] Stitches in throat, extending to ear, [**Hepar.**] Sensation as of a lump in throat, when *not swallowing,* [**Cham. Nux v.**—When swallowing, **Bell. Hepar. Merc.**]

**STOMACH.** Taste flat, like chalk, [**Nux m.**] Food has no taste, [all food tastes like straw, ***Stram.**] *Aversion to warm food, meat and tobacco,* [see **Hep.**] Gulping up of a *bitter* fluid, [**Bry. Nux v. Puls.**—*Sour* eructations, **Nit. ac. Phos. Sulph. ac.**—Of sweetish water, **Merc. Plumb.**] *Weak, empty feeling at pit of stomach, not relieved by eating, [**Mur. ac.** ***Sep.**—*Gone feeling* in stomach, ***Hydras.**—*Sudden feeling of fulness after taking a small quantity of food, **Chin.** ***Lyc. Nux. Phos. Sulph.**—Feels empty after eating, **Sang. Sars.**] Spasmodic pains in stomach. *Fine, stinging pains,* like pins sticking in stomach, [**Rhus.**] Throbbing in abdomen, [**Aloe. Sang.**]

**STOOL.** Difficult stool, causing *prolapsus ani,* [see **Podo.**] *After stool, a violent stabbing stitch from anus upwards into rectum, [**Mez.**] Bleeding after and during stool. *Hemorrhoids; the tumors prolapse with every stool; they are sore, as if excoriated; pain and bleeding worse when the stool is loose.

**SEXUAL O'S.** *Menses scanty, black, of putrid odor, [**Puls.**—Delayed, *scanty, pale*, **Graph.**] During menses, great languor, even to fainting, with spasmodic pains in stomach and abdomen, [**Cham. Cocc .Nux v.**] *Uterine cramps, with cutting stitches. [**Coco.**]

**RESPIRATORY O'S.** Constrictive sensation in throat, exciting cough, as from vapor of sulphur, [**Ars. Chin.**] *Dry, spasmodic* cough, day and night, with fluent coryza. Stitches in left side, [**Phos.**—In the right side, **Bell.**] *Oppression of chest at night:* *Palpitation of and stitches in heart, [**Dig. Spig.**]

**EXTREMITIES.** Pain in shoulder-joint, as if dislocated, on moving arm, [**Bry. Ruta.**] When rising, stiffness in knees and tarsal bones. Cracking in knees when moving them, [**Coni.**—Cracking in all the joints, **Kali b.**] Heaviness of feet.

**SLEEP.** *Restless sleep*, with nightmare, [**Puls. Sulph.**] Moaning and groaning while asleep. Sudden startings of limbs when falling asleep.

**FEVER.** Chill relieved by external heat, [**Ars. Kali c.**—Not relieved by external heat, **Bell. Phos. Nux.**] External coldness, with internal heat, and *vice versa*. *Intermittent* fever. During fever, violent itching; nettle-rash over whole body. Burning heat of face, only on one side, [see **Cham.**]

**CHARACT. PECULIARITIES.** Adapted to *excitable, sensitive, hysterical* individuals. *Convulsive twitchings, especially after fright or grief, [**Gel. Opi.**] *Hysterical spasms. Pains are *relieved* by a change of position, [***Rhus.**] Pains as from a sprain, [***Arn. Bry.** ***Ruta.**]

## IPECACUANHA.

**HEAD.** Vertigo, when walking and when turning round, [*when turning over in bed, **Coni.**] *Headache, as if bruised all through bones of head, and down into root of tongue, with *nausea and vomiting*. *One-sided headache, with nausea and vomiting*, [see **Kali c.**]

**FACE.** Pale face, with blue margins around the eyes, [**Ars. Chin. Cina.**—*Yellow* margins, **Spig.**]

**MOUTH and THROAT.** Flat taste, with *white, thickly-coated* tongue, [**Ant. c. Nux v.**—Dirty-yellow or black tongue, **Chin. Merc.**] Spasmodic, constrictive sensation in throat, [***Bell.** ***Hyos.**]

**STOMACH.** Aversion to food; craves dainties and sweet things, [see **Hepar.**] *Constant and continual nausea*, [**Phos.** ***Tart. e.** ***Verat.**] Vomiting the ingesta, [***Bry.** ***Nux. Puls.**] Vomiting bilious bitter fluids, [**Cham. Merc. Phos. Verat.**—A *sweetish* fluid, **Iris. Kreo.**—A *sour* mucus, **Nux.** ***Phos.** ***Puls. Sulph.**] Vomiting green, jelly-like mucus, [**Merc. sub.**

**Verat.**—A pinkish, glairy fluid, **Kali b.**—A watery, albuminous substance, **Jatro. c.**] Vomiting blood, [**Bry. Ham. Hyos. Nux.**] Vomiting black, pitch-like substance, [***Ars. Sec.** ***Verat.**—Fæces and urine, ***Opi. Plumb.**] Vomiting when stooping, [**Alum. Rhus t.**—From motion of a carriage, boat, etc., **Ars.** ***Cocc. Pet.**—After eating, ***Ars. Bry. Nux. Puls.**—After drinking, ***Ars.** ***Bry. Crot. t.** ***Verat.**] Great sense of emptiness and relaxation in stomach, [**Ign. Mur. ac. Sep.**—Great fulness, ***Chin.** ***Lyc. Nux. Phos.**] *Horrible pain and sick feeling in stomach. Cutting, pinching around umbilicus, as if grasped with a hand; worse from motion, [see **Bell.**]

**STOOL.** *Diarrhœa;* *stools as if fermented, [**Rheum. Saba.**—Like *yeast*, **Arn.**] *Stools green as grass,* [dark-green mucus, **Merc.**—Green, slimy, like scum on a frog-pond, ***Mag. car.**] Dysenteric stools, with tenesmus. Bloody stools, with cutting, burning at anus, [see **Merc.**]

**URINE.** *Bloody urine, [**Cact.** ***Millef. Nit. ac.**] *Turbid* urine, with brick-dust sediment, [**Bell. Phos.**—*Reddish* urine, with brick-dust sediment, **Nux v.**—*Dark* urine, with brick-dust sediment, **Chin.**]

**SEXUAL O'S.** Menstruation too early and too profuse, [**Bell. Calc. c. Sabi.**] **Metrorrhagia;* blood bright-red, *profuse*, clotted, with oppressed breathing.

**RESPIRATORY O'S.** *Rattling in bronchial tubes when breathing. *The chest *seems full of phlegm*, but does not yield to coughing [***Tart. e.**] *Suffocative cough, occasioned by a contractive tickling in throat, sometimes vomiting phlegm, [vomiting large quantities of mucus, ***Tart. em.**] *Suffocation threatens from constriction in throat and chest, [asthma.] *Suffocative cough;* child becomes quite stiff and blue in face, [**Coral r.**] *Hæmoptysis from slightest exertion, [better from walking *slowly* about, ***Ferr.**]

**FEVER.** Chilliness, but is unable to bear the least heat, [better from external heat, **Ars.** ***Ign. Kali c.**] About 4 P. M. *sudden attack of heat; no thirst.* *Intermittents, where *gastric symptoms predominate;* backache, short chill, long fever; mostly heat, with thirst, headache, nausea, cough and sweat last. *External coldness and internal heat,* [see **Ars.**]

**CHARACT. PECULIARITIES.** Great weakness and aversion to all food. **Nausea and vomiting,* with almost all ailments, [**Tart. e. Verat.**] Hemorrhages from all orifices of the body. [**Crotal. Erig. Ham.**—After great depletion, **Ars.** ***Chin.**]

## KALI BICHROMICUM.

**HEAD.** Sudden, transient attacks of vertigo, [when rising, stooping, looking up, **Podo.** ***Puls.**—When riding in carriage, **Cocc. Hepar.**—When lying down, or turning over in bed, ***Con.**—When raising head, **Chin.**—When *ascending* a height, **Calc. c.**—When *descending*, **Ferr.**] *Throbbing* headache at angles of forehead, with dimness of sight. ***Frontal headache,***

mostly over *left* eye, [over *right* eye, with *nausea and vomiting*, **Sang.**] *The pain is of a dull, heavy, throbbing character, mostly in forehead; worse after eating. Headache from suppressed coryza, [**Chin. Nux v.**] Pressure on vertex, as from a weight, [**Aloe. Cann. s. Caot. g.**—On forehead, **Acon. Bell. Nux v. Sulph.**]

**EYES.** Great heaviness of eyelids on waking, [see **Gel.**] Eyelids burning, inflamed, much swollen; rash on adjacent parts. Œdematous swelling of eyelids, [see **Kali c.**]

**EARS.** Violent stitches in *left* ear, extending to roof of mouth, [in *right* ear, **Nit. ac.**] Discharge of thick, yellow, fetid pus from ears, after scarlet fever, [**Bell.**—After measles, **Puls.**—After suppressed crusta lactea, **Sulph.**]

**NOSE.** *Great dryness* of nose, [**Graph. Nit. ac.**—Nostrils ulcerated, scabby, **Calc. c. Nit. ac. Sil.**] *Green, fetid discharge from nose*, [**Graph. *Merc. *Puls. Rhus.**—Yellow, fetid discharge, **Aur. m. Puls.**] *Discharge of hard, elastic plugs, [**Alum Sep. Sil. Thuy.**] Caries of bones of nose, [**Aur.**] Fetid smell from nose, [**Calc. c. Merc. Nit. ac.**] *Ropy, tough discharge from posterior nares.*

**MOUTH and THROAT.** Tongue coated with *thick, yellowish-brown fur*, like felt, [*thick, dirty-yellow*, ***Merc. iod.**] Tongue dry, smooth, red, and cracked, [***Bell. *Rhus.**—Dry, hard, coated black, **Merc.**] Soft palate, reddened; uvula relaxed, with sensation of a plug in throat, [see **Hepar.**] *Pseudo-membranous deposit on fauces, tonsils, soft palate, and respiratory mucous surfaces, pearly in appearance and fibrinous in character, [similar deposit, more limited in extent, easily detached, and slow to reorganize, ***Merc. iod.**—*Dark-colored pseudo-membrane*, ***Phyto.**—*Dirty-gray* color, **Apis.**] Ulceration of uvula and tonsils, [**Apis. Bell. *Merc. Mur. ac.**] Burning in pharynx, extending to stomach. *Discharge from mouth and throat *tough and stringy.*

**STOMACH and ABDOMEN.** Desire for beer, acids, and sour things, [see **Hepar.**] *Vomiting* undigested food, bitter bile; glairy, pinkish fluid, or blood, [see ***Ipec.**] **After eating*, the food lies in stomach like a heavy load, [***Ars. Bry. Merc. *Nux v. Sep.**] Swelling of stomach, with fulness; cannot bear tight clothes, [**Lyc. Nux v.**] Dull, heavy *pressure* or *stitches* in region of liver. Cutting pain in abdomen, soon after eating. *Chronic intestinal ulceration, [**Merc.**]

**STOOL.** Constipation, stools dry, knotty, with burning at anus, [**Nat. m. Verat.**] stools slate-colored, bloody. *Morning diarrhœa*; wakes with urgent pressure to stool, [**Nux v. *Sulph.**] Stools *watery*, gushing out, followed by tenesmus. *Bloody, jelly-like* stools. Sensation of a plug in the anus, [of a *weight*, **Sep.**]

**SEXUAL O'S.** Menses *too soon*, with vertigo, nausea, and headache. *Yellow, ropy leucorrhœa, with itching, burning in the parts. Rawness, *soreness* in vagina.

**RESPIRATORY O'S.** Hoarseness in *evening*, [**Calc. c. Carb.**

v. **Lach**.—In *morning*, **Caust. Phos.**] **True membranous croup*, [**Brom. Iodi.**] Tickling in larynx; every inhalation causes cough. Cough in morning, with viscid expectoration, and stitches in chest, [see **Bry.**] *Violent, rattling cough, with expectoration of *tough*, *stringy* mucus, [**Phos. Staph.**] Cough, with pain in sternum, extending back between shoulders. Pricking pain in region of heart.

**EXTREMITIES**. *Stitches* at lower angle of *left scapula*, [constant pain under lower inner angle of *right scapula*, ***Chelid.**] Rheumatic pains in joints, especially wrists, [as if dislocated, **Bry. Ruta.**] Cracking of all the joints from least motion. Heaviness of legs, [*numbness*, **Nux v. Sil.**]

**FEVER**. Great inclination to yawn and stretch. *Chilliness*, with vertigo and nausea, then *heat*, with coldness and shooting pains in temples; no thirst. Attacks of chilliness extending from feet upwards; wants to be in a warm place, [***Ars. Hep. Rhus.**] Heat alternating with general perspiration. Fever in first part of night.

**SKIN**. Hot, dry, red skin, [see **Bell.**] Solid eruption, like measles, [see **Puls.**] *Pustular eruptions, resembling smallpox. Suppurating tetter, [**Calc. c. Merc.**]

**CHARACT. PECULIARITIES**. Especially adapted to fat, light-haired people, scrofulous and syphilitic diseases, [**Merc.**] *Discharges from nose, mouth, throat, stomach, vagina, etc., of a *tough*, *stringy* mucus. Daily headache in morning, at same hour, [**Nux v. Sulph.**] Pains which shift quickly from one part to another, [**Bell.** ***Puls.**] Symptoms appear and disappear suddenly, [***Bell.**]

## KALI CARBONICUM.

**HEAD**. Headache when riding in carriage, [**Bell.** ***Cocc.**] *One-sided headache, with nausea, [**Colo. Coni. Ipe.**—As if brain would burst, **Puls.**] *Aching in back part* of head, [in fore part, **Bell. Bry. Puls.** —In top, **Hep. Lach.**] Stitches in temples. *Throbbing* pain in *forehead*, [**Bell. Con. Graph.**—In *top of head*, **Cap. Kreo. Nat. c. Stam.**—In back of head, **Calc. c. Sep.**—In *temples*, **Acon. Bell. Nit. ac. Stan.**—In *whole head*, **Lach. Puls.**] *Liability to take cold in head, [**Bell. Sil.**] Great dryness of hair, [greasiness of, **Bry.**]

**EYES**. Redness of the whites, [blood-red, **Thuy.**] Stitches in eyes, [**Bry.**] Agglutination of lids in morning. Spots, gauze, and black points before the eyes, [**Cocc. Caust. Dig.**] *Swelling over *upper* eyelids, like little bags, [under the *lower* lids, **Apis.**] Eyes sensitive to daylight.

**EARS**. Stitches in both ears, [**Con. Nit. ac.**] *Cracking in ears, [when masticating, **Graph.**] Singing, whizzing, and roaring in the ears, [see **Chin.**] Hardness of hearing. *Hard swelling of parotid gland.

**NOSE**. *Sore, scurfy nostrils*, for a long time. Ulcerated nostrils; bloody nasal mucus, [comp. **Kali b.**]

**STOMACH and ABDOMEN.** Desire for acids or sugar, [see **Hepar.**] Milk and warm food disagree, [**Puls. Sep.**] Sour eructations after a meal, [**Bry. Calc. c. Phos.**—*Bitter*, **Bell. Chin. Nux v.**—Tasting like garlic, **Mosch.**] *Nausea*, as if he would faint, subsiding when lying down. *Sour* vomiting of food, [**Nux v. Phos.**—Vomiting an *exceedingly* sour fluid, ***Iris v.**] Sensation in stomach as if cut to pieces, [as if torn to pieces, ***Ars.**] *Throbbing* in stomach, [**Nux v. *Puls.**] *Stitches in region of liver; also burning pain, [see **Bry.**] Inactivity and coldness in abdomen, [**Ars. Phos. Sep.**]

**STOOL and ANUS.** **Constipation*, with distress and colicky, stitching pains an hour or two before stool. *Large, difficult stool*, [see **Nux v.**] Passing of *white mucus* before and during stool. Itching and burning of the anus. *Large, painful varices*, [**Mur. ac.**]

**SEXUAL O'S.** *Deficient sexual* instinct, [*increased sexual desire*, **Canth. Phos.**] *Menses* too late, pale, and scanty, [**Dulc. Hep. Nat. m. Puls. Sulph.**] Menses too early and too profuse, [***Bell. *Calc. c. Nux v. Phos. Sabi.**] Yellowish leucorrhœa, with pain in small of the back, [**Alum. Sulph.**—Yellow, ropy, **Kali b.**]

**RESPIRATORY O'S.** *Hoarseness and loss of voice*, [see **Phos.**] Cough from titillation in throat, [**Bell. Chin. Nux v. Phos.**] *Dry, hard cough, worse about 3 A.M., with sticking pains in left side. Stitches in right chest through to back, when taking an inspiration, [see **Bry.**] Violent palpitation of heart, with dulness of head and nausea. *Burning* in region of heart, [*coldness*, **Nat. m.**] Crampy pain in region of heart.

**BACK.** Drawing pain in small of back. *Stiffness and paralytic feeling in back, [in nape of *neck*, **Sulph.**] *Stitches* in region of both kidneys. Stiffness in nape of neck, [**Bell. Phos. Sep.**] *Swelling of cervical glands, [**Caust. Merc. Sil.**]

**EXTREMITIES.** Tearing pain in arm, from shoulder to wrist-joint, [**Rhus. t.**—In shoulder-joint, **Bry. Sulph.**] Lacerating in wrist-joints. Nightly rheumatic pains in legs of a *tearing character*. *Jerking up of limbs, much frightened when feet are touched. Heaviness and stiffness of feet.

**FEVER.** Pulse variable. Chilliness mostly in morning, [increased towards evening, **Puls.**] Chill frequently *after* pains, [*with* the pain, **Ars. Merc. *Puls.**] Chilliness in evening, relieved by warm stove, [**Ars. *Ign.**—Chilliness increased near warm stove, **Ipec.**] Internal heat with external coldness, [see **Ars.**]

**CHARACT. PECULIARITIES.** **Stitching, darting pains, worse* during rest, [pains as if sprained, *worse during rest*, **Rhus.** —*Stitching, darting pains, *better during rest*, **Bry.**] Intense thirst, morning, noon, and night. *Dropsical affections, and paralysis of old people. Great aversion to being alone, [**Ars. Lyc.**—Wishes to be alone, **Nux v.**] *Worse* in cold air, or from being cold.

# LACHESIS TRIGONOCEPHALUS.

**MIND.** *Great disposition to feel sad,* [**Nit. ac. Puls. Sep.**] Indolence of mind, [indisposed to work, **Con. Nit. ac. Phos.**] Excessive moaning and complaining of one's pains. Inability to think, [**Gel.**]

**HEAD.** Giddiness, with headache. *Dull pain* in vertex, [see **Kali c.**] *Heaviness* of head, [**Bell. Calc. c. Nux v. Puls. Sulph.**—*Lightness of,* ***Stram.**—Sensation of emptiness in head, **Cocc. Puls.**] **Beating* headache, most violent over eyes, [*beating* in middle of brain, **Calc. c.**—In the occiput, **Sep.**] Headache, mostly in forehead, with nausea and chilliness, [**Puls.**]

**MOUTH and THROAT.** *Burning* in mouth, as from pepper, [**Hydras.**] Tongue *dry, red, cracked at tip.* Great dryness of mouth, feeling sore. **Anterior half* of tongue red, smooth, and shining. *Great difficulty in protruding the trembling tongue, [**Ars. Bell.**] Cracks and large papillæ on tongue, [*vesicles* on tongue burning, smarting when eating, **Nat. m. Hell.**] Inflammation of tongue, [***Bell. Merc.**] Inflammation of tonsils, with disposition to suppurate, [see **Hep.**] *Ulcers* in throat, and on inflamed tonsils. * Diseases of throat that begin on *left* side, [begin on *right* side, **Gel.** ***Lyc. Podo.**] *Malignant diphtheria,* [see **Kali b.**] *Painful deglutition; fluids regurgitate through nose, [***Bell. Merc.**] *Cannot bear anything to *touch throat,* it is so sensitive and causes suffocation, [**Apis.**]

**STOMACH and ABDOMEN.** Bitter taste, [everything tastes bitter, **Bry. Chin. Colo. Puls.**] *Regurgitation of food after eating, [**Puls. Phos.**] Eructations of sour water after eating, [see **Nux**]. *Vomiting* the ingesta, [see **Ipec.**] Vomiting with diarrhœa, [**Ars. Verat.**] *Gnawing* pressure in stomach, relieved by eating. *Burning in abdomen,* [**Ars. Phos. Sep.**—*Coldness in,* **Calc. c. Kreo. Phos.**]

**STOOL.** *Chronic constipation;* hard stools, resembling sheep-dung, [**Chel. Plum. Ruta.**] *Chronic diarrhœa,* mostly in evening or at night. Alternate diarrhœa and constipation. Discharge of blood and pus from anus, *very offensive.*

**URINARY O'S.** Stitches in region of kidneys, [**Kali c.**] *Dull pain* in bladder. Frequent micturition, with copious emissions of foaming urine of a dark color. *Yellow urine, like saffron. *Dark and turbid urine.* *Sensation of a *ball* in bladder, [of a *worm,* ***Bell.**]

**SEXUAL O'S.** *Especially suited to women at climacteric period, with frequent uterine hemorrhages, [**Puls. Sep.**] *Menses at regular time, but too short and feeble, [irregular, never at right time, **Nux v. Nux m.** ***Sep.**] Before menses, vertigo and headache. *Cannot bear the *least pressure* in uterine region. **Left* ovary swollen, with pressing, stitching pains, [see **Apis.** ***Bell.**]

**RESPIRATORY O'S.** *Hoarseness,* with feeble voice. Cough, occasioned by ulcers in throat. *Can bear nothing to touch the neck, [**Apis.**] *Slight pressure on throat produces violent cough. *Cough worse after sleeping, [**Apis.**] Bloody expectoration, with frothy mucus. *Oppression of chest*, accompanied by cough. *Stitches in left chest, with difficult breathing; worse when coughing or breathing, [see **Bry.**] Burning in chest, [*coldness*, **Ars.**] *Palpitation of heart.* Irregularity of beats of heart, [**Kali c.**]

**BACK.** Pains in back, with constipation, or palpitation of heart and dyspnœa. **Great* painfulness and sensitiveness of neck to contact, [stiffness in nape of neck, **Kali c. Phos. Sep.**]

**EXTREMITIES.** Pains in wrist-joints, as if sprained, [***Arn. Gel.**—As if dislocated, **Bry. Ruta.**] Stinging in tips of fingers. *Whitlow, [**Merc.** ***Sill.**—See **Hepar.**] Stinging in knees. Left knee feels as if sprained, [sharp stitches in right knee, **Bry. Calc. c.**] *Gangrenous ulcers on legs*, [see **Ars.**] *Caries of the tibia.*

**FEVER.** Pulse small, weak, and accelerated; intermittent pulse, [**Kali c. Nat. m. Spig.**] Chilliness, with chattering of teeth. Heat, especially in evening, in hands and feet, [in face, with cold hands and feet, **Ruta.**] *Chills at night and flushes of heat by day. *Intermittent fever*, the disease returns every spring, or after being suppressed the previous fall by quinine. *Typhoid fever*, with stupor, muttering, sunken countenance, dropping of lower jaw, dry, red, or black tongue, cracked at tip and trembles. Perspiration yellow, cold, bloody, [**Lyc.**]

**SKIN.** Color of skin bluish red, or *yellow*, [**Chin. Hepar.** —*Dirty* yellow, **Merc.**] *Ulcers* very tender, and burning when touched, with ichorous, fetid discharge, [**Ars. Carb. v.**—*Ulcers* hard on edges, stinging, burning; with proud flesh; turning *black*, thin ichorous pus, ***Ars. Graph.**—Ulcers tingling, pulsating, burning, stitches when touched, **Clem.**—*Black* ulcers, with bloody, fetid discharges, **Ars. Con.**—Ulcers, with tearing, itching pains, burning when touched, **Lyc.**—Ulcers corroding, easily bleeding, **Ars. Merc.**—*Cancerous ulcers*, **Ars. Con. Sulph.**] *Carbuncles*, surrounded by boils and purple spots.

**CHARACT. PECULIARITIES.** *Very unhappy and distressed after sleeping. Can bear nothing tight about waist. *Great sensitiveness of the surface to slight touch or pressure, [see **Apis.**] *Left side most affected, [*right side*, **Lyco.**] Suitable to persons of intemperate habits, [also **Nux v. Opi.**] Bad effects of mercury, china, [**Puls. Sulph.**] *Symptoms all worse after sleep, [**Apis Calc. c. Opi. Verat.**—Better after sleep, **Crot. Phos. Sil.**]

## LYCOPODIUM.

**MIND.** *Melancholy*, [cheerful, **Croc. Lach.**] Weeping mood, with chilliness, [Puls.] *She is afraid to be alone, [**Ars. Bis.**—Wishes to be alone, **Chin. Mag. m. Nux v.**] *Ex-*

*tremely sensitive*, [**Cham. Coff.**] Great indifference, [**Chin. *Phos. ac.**] Vehement, *angry*, headstrong.

**HEAD.** Pressing headache on vertex; worse from 4 to 8 P. M., and *from lying down* or stooping, [pressing pain in the vertex, as if a nail were driven in, **Nux v. *Ign. Thuya.**] *Pain in temples, as if they were screwed towards each other, [**Æthu. Merc.**] Stitches in temples, mostly on right side, [see **Kali c.**] *Tearing* pain in *occiput*, [**Con.**—**Stupefying* pain, ascending from nape of neck, **Dulc.**] *Great falling out of hair.*

**EYES.** *Stitches in eyes*, without any redness, [**Bry. Kali c.**] Smarting in eyes, [as from salt, **Nux v.**] Burning in eyes, [**Cap. Kreo.**—*Coldness*, **Con. Kali c.**] Styes on lids, near internal canthus, [see **Puls.**] Eyes wide open, insensible to light, [**Hyos.**]

**EARS.** Dulness of hearing, [**Graph. Kali c.**—From *suppressed* fever and ague by quinine, **Calc. c.**—From abuse of mercury, **Hepar. Nit. ac.**] Roaring, humming and whizzing in the ears, [see **Chin.**]

**NOSE.** Sense of smell very *acute*, [**Bell. Con. Hep.**—Very *obtuse*, **Alum. Calc. Mez.**] Ulcerated nostrils, [**Aur. Calc. c. Graph. Nit. ac.**] *Fluent* coryza, [**Ars. Lach. Merc.**—*Dry* coryza, **Nit. ac. Nux v. Sep.**—Green discharge, **Phos. Puls.**—Purulent, **Calc. c. Sulph.**] **Fan-like* motion of alæ nasi. [**Phos.**]

**FACE.** *Grayish-yellow color of face, with blue circles around eyes, [**Ars. Chin.**] *Dropping of lower jaw, in typhoid fever, [**Lach. Opi.**] *Itching, scaly herpes* in face and corners of mouth.

**MOUTH and THROAT.** Teeth excessively painful to touch. Toothache, with swelling of cheeks, *relieved* by warm applications, [*worse* from warm, **Bry.**—Cold water relieves, **Puls.**] Dryness of mouth and tongue *without thirst* [*with thirst*, **Nat. m. Nit. ac. Rhus.**—Dryness of throat, *without* thirst, **Mur. ac. Nux m.**—*With* thirst, **Pet. Phos.**] *Tongue dry; becomes *black* and cracked, [***Ars. Merc. Verat.**—Red and cracked, ***Bell. Rhus. t.**—*Clean*, parched, **Hyos.**] Inflammation of throat, with stitches on swallowing, [**Hep.**] Swelling and suppuration of tonsils, [**Hep. Merc.**] *Ulceration of tonsils, beginning on *right* side, [**Bell. Podo.**—Beginning on *left* side, ***Lach.**]

**STOMACH and ABDOMEN.** *Excessive hunger, [soon *after eating*, **Cina. Merc.**] Aversion to bread, etc., [see **Hepar.**] Desire for sweet things, [**Ipe. Lyc.**—Aversion to sweets, **Caust.**—See **Hepar.**] Food tastes *sour*, [**Nux v. Puls.**] *Sour* eructations, [see **Nux v.**] *Great weakness of digestion, [**Carb. v. Chin.**] After eating, pressure in stomach, with bitter taste in mouth. *Immediately after a light meal, abdomen is bloated, full, [***Chin. Nux v. Phos.**—Feels empty after eating, **Sang. Sars.**] **Constant* sense of *fermentation in abdomen*, like yeast working, [**Angus. Chin. Phos.**] *Much

> from eructa.

rumbling, particularly in left hypochondria, [sensation of something alive in abdomen, ***Croc.**] *Incarcerated flatulence,* [**Carb. v. Chin.**]

**STOOL.** *Constipation, *stool passed with great difficulty.* Scanty stool, with sensation as if much remained behind.

**URINARY O'S.** *Dark and scanty urine,* [**Bell. Nit. ac.**] **Red, sandy* sediment in urine, [**Caot. g. Phos. Sep. Sil.**—Yellow, sandy sediment, **Am. c. Sil.**—Brick dust-like sediment, **Chin. Nat. m. Phos. Puls.**—*Clay-like,* **Am. m.**—*Jelly-like,* **Berb. Puls.**—*White,* **Calc. c. Sep.**] *Before passing urine, child screams with pain.

**SEXUAL O'S.** *Diminished sexual desire;* penis small, cold, relaxed, [**Arg. n. Hep. Mag. c.**—**Increased* desire, ***Canth. Nux v. Phos.**] *Menses too soon and too profuse, [***Calc. c. Bell. Bry.**] Suppression of menses, also from fright, [**Acon. Opi.**] Chronic dryness of vagina, [**Bell.**] *Discharge of wind from vagina, [**Bromi.**—From *bladder,* **Sars.**] *Profuse leucorrhœa, with cutting pains across right side to left; discharge like milk, or bloody.

**RESPIRATORY O'S.** Dry cough, with wheezing. *Cough, with *gray salt expectoration,* [*green,* tasting *sweet,* ***Stan.**] Cough, with bloody expectoration, [**Merc.**] *Pulmonary phthisis,* with cough and expectoration of large quantities of pus. Stitches in left side of chest, [**Bry. Kali c.**] The least exertion causes shortness of breath. *Oppressed breathing, with *fan-like motions alæ nasi,* [**Phos.**] *Cough worse from 4 to 6 P. M. Typhoid and neglected pneumonia, [**Sulph.**]

**BACK.** Swelling of cervical glands, [**Caust. Merc. Sili.**] Painful stiffness of neck, [**Kali c.**] Drawing pain in small of back, [as if sprained, **Arn. Calc. c.**] Burning between the scapulæ, [coldness, **Am. m.**]

**EXTREMITIES.** Redness, inflammation and swelling of joints of fingers. *Great dryness of skin of hands. Pain as if sprained in hip, [**Mez.**—Feels as if dislocated, **Caust. Bry.**—*Pulsating* pain in hip-joint, the beginning of suppuration, **Merc. Hep.**] *Inflammation of end of bones. *Cold feet constantly,* [as if they had on damp stockings, ***Calc. c.**] One foot cold, other hot, [see **Dig.**] *Old ulcers on legs, tearing, itching and burning at night, [**Ars.**]

**SLEEP.** *Drowsiness during day, and sleepless at night, [**Merc. *Phos. ac. Sulph.**—Sleepy, but cannot sleep, ***Bell. Opi.**] Starting when falling asleep, [**Bell. Bry.**] *Palpitation,* cannot lie on left side.

**FEVER.** Sensation as if circulation stood still. Chilliness from 4 to 8 P. M., with sensation of numbness in hands and feet, [fingers *feel as if dead,* ***Sep.**] *One-sided* chilliness, mostly on left. **Intermittent fever;* paroxysm at 4 P. M., terminating at 8 P. M., [see **Rhus.**] Shaking chill and great coldness, as if lying in ice, followed by perspiration and violent thirst, without previous heat. *Sweat smelling like onions.*

**SKIN.** Itching of skin, as if caused by fleas, [**Nico.**] *Humid suppurating herpes*, [**Kali b.**] Full of deep cracks, and covered with thick crusts. Fistulous ulcers, with hard, everted edges, [**Ant. Calc. c. Sil.**] Ulcers, with tearing, itching pains, burning when touched, [see **Lach.**] *Caries*, [**Calc. c. Hep.**] Mercurial ulcers, [**Hepar. Nit. ac.**] *Dry porrigo of children.

**CHARACT. PECULIARITIES.** Adapted to subacute and gradually advancing chronic diseases. *Great emaciation of upper part of body. *Great fear of being left alone, [**Ars. Kali c.**—Wishes to be alone, ***Nux v.**] *Constant sense of satiety, or fulness in abdomen, [see **Sep.**] *Disease always *worse*, 4 P. M., and better in the evening, [*worse* in evening, **Merc. Nit. ac.** ***Puls.**] Patient feels *better* on getting cold, from being uncovered, [**Sec. Verat.**—**Reverse, Ars. Hep.**]

## MAGNESIA CARBONICA.

**MIND.** Sad and indisposed to talk, [wants to talk continually, ***Stram.**] Trembling, anguish, fear, as if some accident would happen.

**HEAD.** Vertigo when kneeling or standing as if everything were turning around. Headache from mental exertion, or when in a crowd. Pulsating sensation in forehead, [see **Bell.**] *Headache increased by stooping and relieved by lying down, [increased by lying down, **Bell. Colo. Lyc.**] Pain on top of head as if hair were pulled.

**EYES.** Burning, stinging in eyes, which are inflamed. *Agglutination of lids in morning, [**Bry. Calc. c. Merc. Sulph.**] *Black motes* before eyes, [**Acon. Merc. Phos.**]

**EARS.** Great sensitiveness to noise, [**Acon.** ***Bell. Bry. Chin.**] Whizzing and ringing in ears, [see **Chin.**]

**NOSE.** *Nosebleed* in the morning, [**Am. c. Nit. ac. Nux.**] *Dry coryza, with obstruction of the nose.

**FACE.** Earthy, sickly complexion, [*pale, death-like*, **Ars. Verat.**] Alternate redness and paleness of the face, [**Bell. Croc. Ign. Puls.**] Boring pain in the malar bone at night, worse during rest.

**MOUTH and THROAT.** Toothache while riding in a carriage, [headache, **Bell.** ***Cocc.**] Toothache during pregnancy, [**Sep.**] Burning vesicles on gums, cheeks, tongue, lips and palate, bleeding easily. *Bloody saliva*, [**Ars. Merc. Nux.**] Burning in throat, with dryness and roughness, as if scraped, [**Ars. Hep. Nux. Phos.**] *Hawking up fetid tubercles color of peas*, [see **Arg. n.**]

**STOMACH and ABDOMEN.** Bitter or sour taste in mouth, [sweet, **Merc. Mur. ac.**] Desire for fruit and acid things, [***Phos. ac. Verat.**] Sour eructations. Eructations, tasting of ingesta, [**Calc. c. Chin.** ***Puls.**] Vomiting bitter water. *Contractive pain in stomach. Stitches and sensation of hardness in region of the liver. *Contractive, pinching* pain in right iliac region. *Great heaviness* in abdomen.

**STOOLS.** ******Green, watery, frothy stools, like the scum on a frog-pond,* [*like chopped spinach,* ***Acon.**—Like *chopped eggs and spinach,* ***Cham.**] *Bloody mucous stools.* Sour-smelling stools of children, [**Hep. *Rheum. Sulph.**] *Before stool,* cutting, pinching in abdomen. *During* and *after* stool *tenesmus.*

**SEXUAL O'S.** Pressing towards pelvis, as if menses would come on. Menses too late or suppressed. *Menstrual blood thick, dark, like pitch, [**Nux. Sang.**—Black, clotted and offensive, **Ign. *Mag. m. Plat. Stram.**] *During* menses, great debility, chilliness, headache, pale face, and pain in small of back.

**RESPIRATORY O'S.** Spasmodic cough during night, with pain in chest. Oppression of chest, with a sensation of constriction, [**Acon. Ars. Nux v. *Phos. Puls.**] Soreness in chest as if bruised during motion.

**BACK.** Stiffness in neck, [**Bell. Bry. Nit. ac. Rhus. Sulph.**] Pain in small of back, as if broken.

**EXTREMITIES.** *Pain as from a sprain in right shoulder, when moving arm. Rheumatism of shoulder, pain prevents least motion of arm. Spreading blisters on fingers. *The lower,* especially knees, are very painful. Painful swelling in bend of knees. Heavy, weary feeling in feet, [***Bell. Lach. Nat. m.**]

**SLEEP.** *Sleeplessness at night from oppression in abdomen, [from itching of head, face, and shoulders, **Gels.**—From *palpitation* of heart, **Cro. t.**]

**FEVER.** Pulse accelerated only during night. Chilliness with external coldness in evening. Chill running down back, [see **Cap.**] Heat after evening chill, and perspiration with thirst from midnight till morning.

**SKIN.** *Vesicles and pimples,* sometimes itching violently, [**Rhus t.**] *Small, red elevated herpes,* scaling off.

**CHARACT. PECULIARITIES.** Epileptic attacks, falls down suddenly with consciousness, [without consciousness, **Lyc.**] Painfulness of whole body. Feels tired, especially in feet. Most symptoms come on at night and while at rest. Better while moving about.

## MERCURIUS.

**MIND.** *Great restlessness.* Anxiety, with fear of losing one's mind. Indifference to everything, [***Phos. ac.**] Continuous moaning, [**Lach.**] Suspicious, distrustful. *Great weakness of memory* Hurried speech, [talks all the time, **Cicu. *Stram.**] Craziness, absurd talking.

**HEAD.** Vertigo, when *lying on back,* things turning black before the eyes, [vertigo when lying down, or turning over in bed, ***Con.**—When sitting up in bed, **Cocc.**] Compressive headache, head feels as if in a vise, [**Nat. m. Puls.**—Sensation as if skull *were open,* **Carb. a.**—As if skull *would* split, **Bell. Bry.**] Head feels as if it would burst with fulness, [**Acon.**

***Bell. Bry. Sulph.**—Sensation of emptiness in head, **Cocc. *Oxal. ac. Sep.**] *Stitches through whole head. *Open fontanels*, with dirty color of face, sour-smelling night-sweat, [***Calc. c. *Sil. Sulph.**] *Stinging, burning, fetid eruptions on hairy scalp, [**Graph. Hep. s. Lyc.**]

**EYES.** *Scrofulous ophthalmia; lids swollen, edges ulcerated and scabby, [**Bell. Calc. c. Phos.**] *Ulceration* of margins of lids, [**Euph. Nat. m. Sulph.**] Inflammation, with redness of whites, [**Bell. Puls. Rhus t.**] *Pustules on conjunctiva. *Ulcers on cornea, [**Ars. Calc. c. *Sil. *Sulph.**]

**EARS.** *Sticking* pains in ears, [*shooting* pains, **Puls.**—*Stitching, tearing* pains, ***Cham. Chin.**—*Pulsations* in ears, **Hep. Phos. *Rhus. Sil.**—*Stinging*, **Bell. Nux m.**—*Cracking*, **Baryt. Kali c. Nit. ac.**] *Buzzing, roaring*, [**Caust. Con. Croc.**] *Discharge of pus* from ears, [**Nit. ac. *Puls. Sulph.**—*Bloody* pus, **Graph. Pet. *Rhus.**]

**NOSE.** Greenish, fetid pus from the nose, [**Puls. Rhus t.** —See **Kali b.**] Swelling of nasal bones. **Profuse fluent coryza*, with much sneezing, [**Euphr. Gel. Kali c.**—Coryza, with *acrid, corroding* discharge, **Ars. *Arum. t. Lyc.**—*Dry, coryza*, **Dulc. Nit. ac. Nux v. Sep.**—*Dry* at night, fluent during day, ***Nux v.**]

**FACE.** Pale, yellow, earthy color of face, [**Ars. Puls.**—*Greenish* color, **Ars. Carb. v.**—Yellow saddle across nose, ***Sep.**] *Crusta lactea*, [with thick crusts and fetid, bloody ichor, **Rhus t.**] *Ulcerated corners of mouth, [**Bell. Graph.**] *Syphilitic* pustules on face.

**MOUTH and THROAT.** *Bitter, sour, putrid, or sweet taste, [see **Puls.**] Dry, rough, black lips, painful to touch. **Ulcerated gums;* they recede from teeth and bleed when touched. *Very fetid breath*, [**Nux v.**] *Grayish ulcers on inner surface of lips, cheeks, gums, tongue, palate, [*fetid ulcers* in mouth and fauces, ***Kali c. Nit. ac. Nux. v.**] Tongue coated with a dirty-yellow fur. *Dry, hard, blackish tongue, [***Ars. Lach.**] The tongue *feels as if burnt*, [**Colo. Verat. v.**] **Ptyalism*, the saliva often fetid and tenacious, [**Bell. Lach. Sul. ac.**—Ptyalism from abuse of mercury, **Hep. Nit. ac. Sulph.**] **Bloody saliva*, [**Ars. Hyos. *Nux v. Rhus.**] *Complete loss of speech* and voice, [***Bell. Con. Laur.**] Catarrhal sore throat; stitches when swallowing. Fluids return through nose when being swallowed, [***Bell. Lach.**] *Ulcerated tonsils*, with sharp, stinging pains, [***Bell. Lach. Nit. ac.**] *Burning* in throat, as from *hot vapor ascending*, [as of something *cold* ascending, **Caust.**—As of a ball rising, **Asaf. Kalmia. Lach. Mosch.**]

**STOMACH and ABDOMEN.** Hunger soon after eating, [**Cicu. Phos. *Staph.**—Sensation of emptiness after eating, **Sang. Sars.**—Great fulness after eating. **Chin. *Lyc. *Nux m.**] Rising of air, or acrid, putrid eructations. *Complete loss of appetite, [**Chin. Rhus t.**—Canine hunger, **Lyc. Sulph.**] *Great weakness of digestion*, with continuous hunger. *After a meal food weighs like a stone in stomach, [***Ars.** **Bry.** ***Nux v.**] *Region of stomach sensitive to touch, [**Bry.** **Lach.** **Nux v.**] *Hepatitis, with stinging pains and great soreness in region of liver to contact, [**Bell.** **Bry.**] *Induration of liver*, [**Chin.**] *Stabbing, pinching pains in abdomen, with chilliness, [pains mostly accompanied by chilliness, **Ars.** **Bell.** **Sep.** ***Puls.**] *Syphilitic and scrofulous buboes*, [**Nit. ac.** **Thuya.**]

**STOOL.** *Diarrhœa:* *stools *dark-green*, *frothy*, or yellowish like sulphur, preceded by chilliness, [see **Dig.**] *Tenesmus during and after* stool, [**Bell.** **Cap.** **Colch.** **Mag. c.**] **Dysentery;* stools *bloody mucus*, [***Cap.** **Canth.** **Colo.** ***Nux v.**] *Dark-green mucus; whitish-gray mucus*, [*white, slimy stools*, **Cham.** **Colch.** **Sulph.**] *The discharges are accompanied by chilliness, sick stomach, cutting colic, *violent tenesmus during and after stool.* Black, pitch-like stools, [***Ars.** **Chin.** ***Verat.**—*White* stools, **Calc. c.** **Dig.** ***Phos. ac.**—*Jelly-like, mucous stools*, but little pain, worse at night or in morning, ***Colch.** **Hell.** ***Podo.**]

**URINARY O'S.** Urine dark-red, soon becoming *turbid and fetid.* *Dark-red urine, as if mixed with blood, [dark like coffee, **Nat. m.** **Tereb.**] *Urine smells sour*, [strong like *horse* urine, **Ben. ac.** ***Nit. ac.**—Like *cat's* urine, **Viol. try.**] Burning in urethra, [during micturition, **Cap.** **Caust.**—After micturition, ***Canth.** **Nit. ac.**] *Gonorrhœa; thick *greenish* or *yellow* discharge, [**Thuya.**—*Purulent* discharge, **Agn. c.** **Cap.** —Soreness of urethra, with *bloody* discharge, **Canth.**]

**SEXUAL O'S.** Painful inflammation and swelling of glans and prepuce. *Chancre ulcers on prepuce and glans, [the chancre assumes a phagedenic appearance, and secretes a thin, ichorous pus, ***Merc. cor.**—*Indurated* chancres, old, obstinate cases, **Merc. pre. rub.** **Merc. v.** **Cinna.**—Old cases after abuse of mercury, ***Kali iod.** **Nit. ac.**—*Cauliflower-like excrescence* on glans and prepuce, ***Thuya.**] Suppression of menses. **Prolapsus of vagina*, with sensation of great rawness, [**Ocimum c.** ***Sep.** **Stann.**—Prolapsus uteri, **Calc. c.** **Con.** ***Nux v.** **Sep.**]

**RESPIRATORY O'S.** **Catarrh with chilliness*, fluent coryza, hoarseness, sore throat, cough, dread of open air. **Dry*, fatiguing cough; pain in chest and small of back, [**Cham.** ***Nux v.** **Phos.**] **Whooping cough.* *Shortness of breath* when walking or going up-stairs, [**Ars.** **Calc. c.**] *Pneumonia*, with bilious symptoms. Stitches in *right* chest through from the shoulder-blade, [stitches in *left* chest, **Lach.** **Lyco.**] Burning in chest, extending to throat, [**Cocc.**—Sensation of coldness in chest, **Ars.** **Sulph.**]

**BACK.** *Bruised pain* in small of back, especially when sitting, [when touching the part, **Graph.**] *Swelling of the cervical glands, with painful closing of jaws, [**Caust.** **Kali c.**]

**EXTREMITIES.** **Lacerating* in shoulder-joint, humeri and wrist-joint, particularly at night, and when moving the parts. *Itch-like eruption on hands. *Cold, clammy sweats on thighs and legs at night. *Coxalgia;* pulsating pain, suppuration beginning, [***Hep. Mur. ac. *Sil. Staph.**] Dropsical swelling of feet and legs, [**Apis. Ars. Colch.**]

**SLEEP.** *Great inclination to sleep in daytime, [**Puls. Sulph.**—Especially after meals, **Bry. Nux. *Phos.**] *Wakeful until* 3 A. M., [**Am. c.**—Cannot sleep after 3 A. M., **Calc. c. Nux.**] *Sleepless at night.*

**FEVER.** *Accelerated pulse,* at times slow and trembling. *Chills, especially in evening,* [**Bell. *Puls.**] *Paroxysms of fever, especially at night, with thirst. *Profuse, debilitating *night-sweats,* [**Chin. Phos. *Sil.**—Copious *morning sweat,* after waking, **Puls. Sulph.**]

**SKIN.** Itching eruptions, burning after scratching, [**Cro. t. Rhus. Staph.**—*Sore* after scratching, **Sulph.**] **Itch,* bleeding easily, [see **Sulph.**] *Ulcers and eruptions, having a *raw appearance,* [like *raw flesh,* ***Nit. ac.**] *Syphilitic ulcers and herpes. *Watery vesicles and blotches; turn yellow and maturate.

**CHARACT. PECULIARITIES.** *Affects especially the glandular system, [**Hep. Iodi. Kali b.**] The parts are much swollen, with a raw, sore feeling. *Profuse perspiration with most complaints, but does not relieve, [better after perspiring, **Verat.**] All symptoms are *worse at night,* and in damp, rainy weather, [**Dulc. Rhus.**]

## MERCURIUS CORROSIVUS.

**MIND.** *Anxiety, preventing sleep.* Stares at persons who talk to him, and does not understand them.

**HEAD.** Vertigo, with coldness, cold perspiration; [with *chilliness,* ***Puls.**] Vertigo, with dizziness when stooping. Violent temporal headache. Head feels heavy, [**Calc. c. Phos. ac. Sulph.**—Feels *light,* **Stram.**] Swelling of head and neck.

**EYES.** Pupils contracted, insensible, [**Ars. Cicu. Laur.**—Pupils *dilated,* **Acon. *Opi. *Stram.**] Ophthalmia, with deep ulcers on the cornea, discharge ichorous, making surrounding parts sore. Iritis, especially of *syphilitic* origin. Eyelids swollen, red, excoriated; *edges covered with thick crusts or pustules, [see **Sulph.**]

**EARS.** Inflammation, with stitches in ears, [**Bell. Merc.**] Discharge of fetid pus from the ear, [see **Rhus.**]

**NOSE.** Ozæna, discharge from nose like glue, drying up in posterior nares; perforation of the septum, [see page 62.]

**MOUTH.** *Sensation as if mouth was *scalded,* [**Jatro. Mag. m. Sep.**—As if tongue was scalded, **Colo. Hydras. *Verat. v.**] Gums swollen, covered with false membrane; gangrenous; bleed freely, [see **Ars.**] Tongue coated with thick white mucus, or dry and red. Papillæ elevated, strawberry-like, [**Bell.**] Ulcers in the mouth, throat and gums, with fetid breath, [**Nit. ac. Nux.**] Burning in mouth extending to stomach.

**THROAT.** Uvula swollen, elongated, dark red. *Throat intensely inflamed, [**Bell. Merc. Phyto.**], swallowing causing suffocation. *Tonsils swollen and covered with ulcers, [**Lach. *Merc. Nit. ac.**] Pricking in throat as from needles.

**STOMACH.** Vomiting albuminous matter, [**Jatro.**] Vomiting tough or stringy mucus. *Vomiting blood, [**Ars. Ipe. Phos.**] Vomiting a substance like *coffee-grounds*, [**Ars. Con. Phos. Verat.**] *Burning in the stomach, extending up to the mouth. *Bloated abdomen, painful to touch.*

**STOOLS,** etc. *Diarrhœa*, yellow, green, bilious, bloody stools; with *tenesmus* and severe cutting, colicky pains. *Dysentery*, *painful bloody discharges, with vomiting; tenesmus during and after stool; worse after midnight. Autumnal dysentery, [***Acon. Colch.**] *Burning* and *tenesmus* of rectum and *bladder* after stool.

**URINE.** Scanty, brown, with brick-dust sediment, [**Chin. Phos. Puls.**] *Tenesmus vesicæ; urine scanty, hot, bloody,* or *suppressed*, [see **Canth.**] The urine passed only in drops, with great pain. *Albumen* in the urine, [**Apis. Berb. Helon.**] *Filaments*, flocks, or dark flesh-like pieces of mucus in urine, [**Apis, Canth. Kalmia.**]

**SEXUAL O'S.** *Men.* Gonorrhœa greenish, worse at night burning smarting urination. Violent erections during sleep. Buboes, [see **Merc.**] *Women.* Leucorrhœa, pale yellow, of a disgustingly *sweetish smell*, [odor of menses, **Caust.**]

**CHEST.** *Hollow, fatiguing dry cough. *Cough with bloody expectoration*, [**Bell. Merc. Nitrum.**] Hæmoptysis, followed by pulmonary phthisis, attended with hectic fever. *Pulmonary tubercles.* Great dyspnœa.

**FEVER.** Pulse small, weak, intermitting, [see **Dig.**] Chilliness from the least movement, [**Merc. Nux. Rhus. Podo.**] Generally with colic. Burning and stinging heat in the skin. Night-sweat, [**Chin. *Merc. Phos.**] Cold perspiration, often only on forehead, [see **Verat.**]

## NATRUM MURIATICUM.

**MIND.** *Dejection of spirits*, [gay and cheerful, **Croc. Lach.**] Out of humor; gets angry at trifles, [***Bry. *Cham.**] *Great tendency to start, [**Con. Ign.**]

**HEAD.** Vertigo when rising from bed, [see **Kali b.**] Sensation of *emptiness* in head, [**Cocc. Coral. r. Sep.**—*Great fulness*, ***Acon. *Bell. Sulph.**] Pressing headache from both sides, as if head were in a vise, [**Æthu. *Merc. Puls.**—*Pressing on the vertex*, as from a weight, **Aloe. Cact. Can. s. Kali b.**] Beating in forehead, with nausea and vomiting; worse in morning, and better when lying down, [*worse* about 3 P.M., and when lying down, ***Bell.**] *Awakens every morning with a violent, bursting headache. [**Sulph.**] *Burning* on vertex, [see **Sulph.**] *Periodical* headaches during menses.

**EYES.** *Excessively sore, red, disgusting eyelids. *Thin, watery, excoriating discharge from eyes after abuse of *nitrate of silver*. Fiery, zigzag appearance around things, [see **Ign.**] Gauze before the eyes, [**Caust. Phos. Sulph.**] *Letters run together when reading*, [**Chin. Coco.**] Long-sighted, [**Calc. c. Pet.**—Short-sighted, **Nit. ac.**]

**EARS.** *Otalgia*, with stitches in the ears, [**Cham. Chin.**] Singing or tingling in the ears. Ringing, humming, or buzzing in the ears, [see **Chin.**]

**NOSE.** Boring pain in nasal bones. *Excessive fluent coryza, with loss of smell and taste, [see **Puls.**] *Scabs* and scurf in nose. Posterior nares dry.

**MOUTH AND THROAT.** *Lips dry, cracked; upper lip swollen, [see **Bry.**] *Heaviness of tongue, with difficult speech, [**Mur. ac. Nux v.**] *Vesicles* on the tongue, [**Mur. ac.**] *White coated, or *map tongue*, [**Tarax.**] *Sore throat;* it feels as if a *plug* had lodged in it, [see **Hepar.**]

**STOMACH AND ABDOMEN.** *Sour taste.* Longing for bitter food and drink, [see **Hepar.**] *Sour regurgitation of food, [**Lach. Phos.**—Regurgitation of a sweetest water, **Merc. Plumb.**] *Great aversion to bread, [**Lyc. Nux v.**—Bread tastes bitter, **Chin.**] *Craves salt, [**Calc. c.**—Food tastes too salt, **Carb. v. Sep.**] Soreness in pit of stomach when pressing on it, [**Bry. Merc. Sulph.**] *She always has heartburn after eating, [**Calc. c. Croc.**] Vomiting, first food, later bile, [first bile, later food, **Bry.**] *Stitches in region of liver, [see **Bry.**] Fermentation in abdomen, [like a pot of yeast working, ***Lyco. Phos.**—After eating fruit, **Chin.**]

**STOOL.** *Constipation;* stools hard, dry, *crumbling*, very difficult to discharge, [**Am. m. Mag. m.**—Stools *tough*, shining like grease, ***Caust.**] *Diarrhœa;* stools *thin*, watery, with colic. **Excoriating* diarrhœa, like water, only in *daytime*, [***Pet.**] *Burning in rectum* during and after stool, [**Ars. Canth. Iris v.**]

**URINARY O'S.** Pale urine, with brick-dust sediment, [**Puls.**—Dark-brown, with white sediment, **Calc. c. Sep.**—Urine white, like milk, **Con. Phos. ac.**—Turning white after standing, ***Cina.**] *Brown, black* urine, [***Colch. Tereb.**] Red sand in urine, [see ***Lyco.**] *Severe cutting pains in urethra after micturition. *Involuntary* micturition when coughing.

**SEXUAL O'S.** *The menses delay, and grow more and more scanty, [see **Puls.**] * *Very sad and gloomy during menses*, with palpitation of heart and morning headache. *Pressing, bearing down* in genitals, must sit down to prevent prolapsus, [***Bell. *Nit. ac. Plat. *Sep.**] *Leucorrhœa, acrid, greenish*, especially when walking, [**Bovista.**]

**RESPIRATORY O'S.** *Cough after going to bed, spasmodic, suffocating, expectoration mostly in morning, [dry cough at night, going off when sitting up, ***Hyos. Phos.**] Tensive pains in muscles of right chest. Stitches in chest during a deep inspiration, or when coughing, [**Bry. Lyc. Puls.**] *Palpitation of heart from slightest motion, [**Dig.**

**Iod.**] Irregular, intermitting beats of heart, [**Kali c. Lach. Sep.**—see **Dig.**]

**BACK.** Pain in small of back, as if bruised. Painful stiffness of neck, [**Bell. Bry.**] The pain in back is relieved by lying on something hard, [***Rhus t.**]

**EXTREMITIES.** Languor, heaviness of arms, [**Caust.**] Sensation of lameness, and as if sprained in shoulder-joint, [**Nux v.**—*Lacerating* in shoulder-joint, **Sulph.**] Pain in hip, as if sprained, [as if dislocated, **Bry. Ruta.**] *Great heaviness of legs and feet. Swelling of feet, [***Ars. *Chin.**]

**SLEEP.** Sleepiness during day, wakeful at night, [**Merc. *Sulph.**] Sleep full of fanciful ravings. Talks while asleep, and is very restless, [**Sep. *Sulph.**]

**FEVER.** Pulse very irregular, especially when lying on left side. Constant chilliness, and want of animal heat, [**Ledum.**] *Intermittent fever.* Chilliness, with great thirst; afterwards fever, with violent thirst and excessive headache; at last profuse perspiration. *The chill occurs about 10 A.M., commencing mostly at feet, [**Petro.**—Chill at 7 A.M., **Eup. per.**—At 11 A.M. or 11 P.M., **Cactus.**—Every day at 3 P.M., **Angus.**—At 4 P.M., **Lyc. Puls.**] *Inveterate, or badly treated cases of fever and ague, especially after abuse of quinine, [**Puls.**]

**SKIN.** Rash over whole body, with stinging in skin. *Nettle-rash after violent exercise, [after taking cold, ***Dulc.**—After getting wet, **Rhus t.**—After suppressed itch, **Psorin.**—During menses, **Kali c.**]

**CHARACT. PECULIARITIES.** *Losing of flesh while living well, [**Calc. c. Iodi.**—*Young people who incline to grow fat, **Calc. c.**] Pulsation in whole body from least exertion. Bad effects from loss of animal fluids, [**Calc. c. Chin. Phos. ac.**] Great liability to take cold. Most complaints are aggravated at 10 A.M., appear or grow worse while lying down, and are relieved by sitting up; also *better* from lying on right side, [*better* lying on painful side, **Bry. Ign. Puls.**]

## NITRIC ACID.

**MIND.** Sad, desponding, [**Nat. m. *Puls. Rhus t.**—Gay, cheerful, **Croc. Lach. Oxal. ac.**] Anxiety, with fear of death. [***Ars. Nux v.**—Predicts the day he will die, ***Acon.**] Excessively nervous, [**Canth.**] *Indisposed to work*, [**Con. Phos.**—Indisposed to talk, **Dig. Phos. ac. Stan.**]

**HEAD.** Headache in the morning on waking, [**Calc. c. Nat. m. *Sulph.**] Headache, as if head were surrounded with a tight bandage, [**Merc. Ther.**—Headache relieved by tight bandaging, **Arg. n. *Puls.**] *Stitches* in temples, particularly right, [**Kali c. Lyc.**—Vide **Caust.**] **Throbbing* pain in temples, [***Acon. *Bell.**]

**EYES.** Stitches in eyes, [**Bry. Kali c. Lyc.**] Smarting sensation in eyes, [as from *salt*, **Nux v.**—As from *sand*, **Caust.**

**Euph.**] Paralysis of upper lids, [see **Gel.**] Black spots before the eyes, [**Carb. v. Merc.**] Double vision, [**Hyos.**] Short-sightedness, [long-sighted, **Nat. m. Calc. c. Pet.**] Fistula lachrymalis, [ ***Pet. Puls.**]

**EARS.** *Stitches* in right ear, [see **Kali c.**] **Hardness of hearing*, especially from induration of tonsils, after abuse of mercury, [from abuse of quinine, **Puls.**] *Roaring, throbbing, cracking*, in ears, [see **Chin.**]

**NOSE.** Soreness, burning, and scurf in nose. *Fetid, yellow* discharge from nose, [**Aur. m. Puls.**—*Green, fetid* discharge. **Graph. Kali b.** ***Merc. Puls.**—See **Kali b.**] *Violent fluent* coryza, with pain in limbs, [**Ars. Merc. Pet.** —*Dry coryza*, **Dulc.** ***Nux v.** ***Sep.**] *Fetid smell from nose.

**FACE.** Dark yellow, almost brown, complexion. *Black pores in face, [**Dig. Sabi.**] *Small pimples on face.* Drawing pain in cheek-bones. Swelling of submaxiliary glands.

**MOUTH.** *Throbbing toothache, mostly at night in bed, [**Mur. ac. Sep.**] Gums white, swollen, bleeding, [**Nux v.**] Great dryness in mouth, with thirst, [*without* thirst, **Bell.** ***Nux m.**] *Mercurial* and *syphilitic* ulcers in mouth and fauces, with pricking pain, [see **Merc.**] *Mouth full of fetid ulcers; bloody saliva; putrid-smelling breath [ ***Nux v.**]

**STOMACH and ABDOMEN.** *Bitter taste, particularly after eating, [**Ars. Bry. Puls.**—Food tastes *sour*, **Nux v. Puls.**] Longing for fat, herring, chalk, lime, earth, [see **Hepar.**] *Great thirst continually. *Sour eructations*, [**Bry. Calc. c. Kali c. Phos.**] *Much nausea and gastric trouble, relieved by moving about or riding in a carriage, [see **Cocc.**] Stitches in region of liver. Cutting pain in abdomen, in morning in bed, and after rising. *Swelling and suppuration of inguinal glands, [**Merc. Thuya.**]

**STOOL and ANUS.** *Hard, difficult, and scanty stool, [**Alum. Lyc. Ruta.**—Large, hard, difficult stools, crumbing as they pass, **Am. mur. Mag. m.**] *Diarrhœa;* stools putrid or mucous, fetid or undigested. *Dysentery*, with bloody stools and tenesmus, [see **Merc.**] *Hemorrhage from bowels in typhoid fever, [*discharges of black, decomposed blood, **Phos.**—*Involuntary* and *cadaverous smelling.* ***Ars.** ***Carb. v.**] *Old hemorrhoidal tumors, secreting much slime, and bleeding profusely after stool. *Fissures of anus*, [see **Carb. v.**]

**URINARY O'S.** Discharge of dark-brown, badly-smelling, urine. *The urine has an intolerably strong smell, like that of horses, [**Chin. s.**—Dark-colored and heavy, with an *exceedingly strong smell*, ***Ben. ac.**—Smells, like *cat's* urine, **Viola t.** —Like *violets*, **Nux m. Tereb.**—Like ammonia, **Asaf. Iodi.**—Smells sour, **Ambr. Merc.**—Thick, purulent urine, smelling like *musk*, **Ocim. can.**—Smelling like *onions*, **Gum g.**] *Active hæmaturia; urging after micturition, with shuddering along the spine.

**SEXUAL O'S.** Chancre-like ulcers on prepuce and on corona glandis, with pricking, stinging pains, [see **Merc.**]

*Secondary syphilis, *after abuse of mercury.* Uclers in vagina, burning, and itching, [painless, ***Sulph.**] *Menses too early and too profuse, [see **Puls.**] *Pressing down in genitals as if everything would protrude, [***Bell. Nat. m. Sep.**] Pain in the small of the back, through the hips, and down the thigh. **Leucorrhœa*, cherry-brown color, fetid, [**Am. m. Chin.**—Green, corrosive, **Bovis. Merc. Sep.**—White, like milk, **Con. Puls.**] *Tumors in mammæ, [**Carbo a.** ***Con.** ***Phyto.**]

**RESPIRATORY O'S.** **Dry, barking* cough in evening after lying down, [see **Hepar.**] Violent, shaking, barking cough, with expectoration of blood mixed with clots, or of yellow, acrid pus, tasting bitter, sour or salt. *Shortness of breath*, palpitation of the heart, and anguish when going up-stairs, [**Ars.** ***Calc. c. Merc.**] Atrophy of mammæ, [***Iodi.**—*Swelling and induration* of, **Bell. Con. Graph.**]

**FEVER.** Pulse very irregular. *Afternoon fever*, heat, and chilliness. Heat, with perspiration and debility after eating. *Intermittent fever;* chilliness in afternoon; then heat over whole body; afterwards perspiration; no thirst in either stage, [see **Puls.**] Perspiration offensive, smelling like urine, [**Colc.**—Like sulphur, **Phos.**—*Putrid*, **Staph.**—*Sour*, **Merc.**]

**SKIN.** *Easily-bleeding ulcers; look like raw flesh, [**Merc.**] Ulcers, with boody, ichorous matter, [see **Lach.**] *Mercurial ulcers and caries, [**Aur. Sulph.**] Black pores on skin, [**Sulph.**]

**CHARACT. PECULIARITIES.** *Acts especially on mucous outlets, as rectum, anus, vagina, mouth. *Adapted to diseases depending upon presence of some virulent poison, as syphilitic, mercurial, and scrofulous miasm. Especially suited to lean persons with dark complexion, black hair and eyes, [lean persons who walk stooping, ***Sulph.**] Great debility, with heaviness and trembling of limbs. Symptoms *worse* in evening and at night; *better* from riding in a carriage, [reverse, **Cocc.**]

## NUX VOMICA.

**MIND.**—*Hypochondriac mood*, [**Bell. Calc. c. Puls.**—Cheerful mood, **Angus. Cann. Croc.**] *Noise, talk, strong odors, and bright light are intolerable. *Very irritable, and wishes to be alone, [**Chin. Mag. m.**—Fear of being alone, **Ars. Kali c. Lach.**] *Disposed to quarrel and feel vexed, **Bry. Cham. Lyc.**] He makes mistakes in speaking, and gives wrong, absurd answers, [see **Gel.**] *Insane desire to kill even his *best friends.* *Mental derangement, in case of drunkards, [*delirium tremens.*] Muttering delirium, [**Hyos. Mur. ac. Rhus.**] *Ailments from intoxication and nightly revelling. Time passes too *slow*, [**Arg. n. Pall.**—Too *fast* **Cocc. Ther. cur.**] Aversion to all kinds of labor, [**Nit. ac. Phos.**—Aversion to talk, **Dig. Phos. ac.**]

**HEAD.** *Vertigo, with obscuration of sight, and whizzing

in ears. *Head feels much too large, [**Arg. n. Glon. Lactu.** —*Too small*, **Coff.**—As if it became elongated, **Hyp. per.**] *Headache*, feels as if head would split, with sour vomiting, [**Bry. Sars.**—*Gastric sick headache*, with vomiting of sweetish water ***Iris.**] Sick headache from wine, coffee, close mental application, sedentary habits. *Pressing pain on vertex, as if a nail were driven into it, [**Ign.**—Semi-lateral pains, as if a nail were driven into side of head, **Coff.**] Head symptoms *worse* in morning; in cold air; from mental exertion, and when lying down, [see **Bell.**]

**EYES.** *Pressure on upper lids*, especially in morning. *Painless spots, like extravasated blood in sclerotica. Oozing of blood from eyes, [**Bell. Carb. v. Cham.**] Burning and smarting in eyes as from salt, [see **Nat. m.**] *Streaks*, like lightning, before eyes, [*flickering zigzags*, **Ign. Nat. m.**] *Intolerance of light of day*, [of candle-light, **Borax. Hepar. Phos.**]

**EARS.** Otalgia, with tearing, stinging pains, [see **Cham.**] Tingling, hissing in ears. *Ringing in ears, [see **Chin.**] *Roaring in ears*, early in morning, [**Bell. Lyc. Nit. ac.**]

**NOSE.** **Fluent coryza* during day, and *dry coryza* at night, [see **Merc.**] *First stage of ordinary catarrh*, with oppressive dulness in head.

**FACE.** Pale, yellowish complexion, [**Merc.**—Gray-yellow, **Carb. v.**—Pale face, pointed nose, sunken eyes, with blue margins, ***Ars. Chin.**] Redness and heat of one cheek, and paleness of the other, [**Acon.** ***Cham.**]

**MOUTH and THROAT.** Tearing toothache, renewed by cold drink, relieved by warmth, [*better* from *cold* things, and *worse* from *warm*, ***Bry. Coff. Puls.**] Gums swollen, white, putrid, bleeding, [**Nit. ac.**] *Bloody saliva*, [**Ars. Hyos. Merc. Rhus.**—See **Merc.**] **Stomacace;* fetid ulcers in mouth and fauces, [***Kali chlo. Nit. ac.**] Tongue black and cracked, with bright-red edges. The tongue *feels heavy*, [**Coloh.** ***Mur. ac. Nat. m.**] *Sore throat; when swallowing, feels as if it were raw. Burning in throat up to mouth, [*coldness* in throat, **Carb. v. Laur. Verat.**] Feeling as of a plug in throat, [**Hepar. Ign.**—As of splinters in the throat, **Arg. n.** ***Hepar.** ***Nit. ac.**] Throat feels constricted, [**Nat. m. Hyos.**] *Catarrhal* sore throat.

**STOMACH and ABDOMEN.** *Hunger, with aversion to food.* Longing for brandy and chalk, [see **Hepar.**] *Putrid* or bitter taste early in morning, [**Merc. Puls.**—*Bitter or sour* taste after a meal, **Lyc. Puls.**] *Bitter, sour eructations, [**Nit. ac.** ***Phos. Sul. ac.**] *Gulping up a bitter fluid, [**Bry. Ign. Puls.** — A sweetish water, **Merc. Plumb.**] *Nausea after a meal*, [**Ars.** ***Bry. Puls.**—After drinking, **Puls. Rhus.**] Vomiting food, sour-smelling mucus, dark-clotted blood, [see ***Ipe.**] *Vomiting of pregnant females, [**Con.** ***Kreo.** ***Euphor. Verat.**] *Region of stomach very sensitive to pressure*, [**Ars. Bry.** ***Merc.** ***Phos.**] **Cannot bear clothing tight* about waist, [**Chin. Hep.** ***Lyc.**] *Sensation of great fulness after eating a small quantity of food, [ *Chin. Lyc. *Nux m. —Feeling of *emptiness* after eating, **Sang. Sars.**—Sensation as if the stomach hung down relaxed, **Arg. n.** ***Staph.**] *Pressure in the stomach, as from a stone, especially after eating, [**Ars. Bry. Merc. Puls.**] **Constrictive, cramp-like pain in stomach*, [see ***Colo.**] Throbbing in stomach, [**Iod.** ***Puls. Rhus. Sep.**] *Burning in stomach, [see **Ars.**] *Throbbing in region of liver.* *Cutting or pinching pain in abdomen, with desire to vomit. *Incarcerated hernia*, [**Opi.** ***Tabac.**] * *Umbilical hernia of infants.*

**STOOL.** * *Habitual constipation* of large, difficult fæces, *with frequent, and often ineffectual, attempts at stool*, [**Bry. Con. Lyc.**—*Small*, hard stools, with ineffectual efforts, **Lyc. Sulph.** —*Too large in size, *hard, and dry*, **Bry.**—See **Lyc.**] Dysentery, with cutting at the navel, *pressing on rectum; stools, bloody mucus with fæces*, [liquid, fæcal, mingled with hard lumps, **Con. Lyc.**] *Pitch-like* stools, with blood, [**Merc.** ***Lep.**—*Black, putrid stools*, **Ars. Chin.**] *Painful hæmorrhoids, blind or flowing.

**URINARY O'S.** *Renal colic*, pain extending to genitals and leg. Painful and almost ineffectual urging to urinate, [**Cann. Puls.**] *Urging to urinate, passing only a few drops of red, bloody, burning urine, [**Cann. Canth.**] *Bloody urine, [**Ipec. Millef. Tereb.**]

**SEXUAL O'S.** Constrictive pain in testicles. *Menses* too early and too profuse, with dark, black blood, [**Bry.** ***Cal. phos. Cimic.**—Too late, pale, and scant, **Graph.** ***Puls. Sulph.** —See **Puls.**] *Menses irregular, never at the right time, [**Iod.** ***Nux m. Ruta.** ***Sep.**] *Dysmenorrhœa*, [***Cimi.**] *Fetid leucorrhœa*, tinging linen yellow, with uterine pains, [see **Nit. ac.**] *False and inefficient labor-pains, with frequent desire to urinate and go to stool. *Prolapsus uteri from overlifting, straining*, [**Rhus.**—Prolapsus vagina, ***Merc.** ***Sep.**]

**RESPIRATORY O'S.** *First stage* of ordinary bronchial catarrh, with *dry coryza.* *Dry cough, with a sense of constriction around waist. The cough is worse after midnight and in morning, from exertion, when lying on back, from eating and drinking, [see **Spong.**] Painful pulsative shocks in direction of heart, [**Cann. Con.**] *Palpitation of heart, with inclination to vomit and heaviness in chest, [see ***Dig.**] Pressure on outer parts of chest, as from a load.

**BACK.** Drawing pain in nape of neck, [**Chin. Puls.**] Bruised pain between scapulæ, [aching under outer edge of left scapulæ, **Bell.**—*Constant pain under inferior angle of right scapula, **Chel.**] *Bruised pain in back*, worse 3 or 4 A.M. Spine affected by *sexual excesses.*

**EXTREMITIES.** *Upper.* Sudden loss of strength in arms, early in morning. Paralysis of arm, with tumult and shocks in it, as if blood would start out of vessels. The hands go to sleep and feel dead. *Lower.* *Numbness and paralysis of lower limbs, [**Lyc. Plum.**—Paralytic heaviness, **Stan. Sulph.**] Numbness and deadness of lower legs. Cracking in knee-joint during motion, [**Coco. Con.**—Buzzing sensation in lower limbs, **Kreo.**]

**SLEEP.** *Cannot sleep after 3 A.M., ideas crowd upon the mind so, [**Calc. c. Sep.**—Cannot sleep before 3 A.M., **Am. c. Merc.**] Great drowsiness during the day and after meals, [**Bry.** ***Phos.**] Night seems long.

**FEVER.** *Chilliness*, not relieved by external heat, [**Bell. Phos.**—Heat relieves, **Ars.** ***Ign. Kali c.**] Chilliness, with shuddering, in evening and at night; worse from movement and after drinking, [see **Ars.**] Coldness of whole body, with blue skin and finger-nails. Fever and ague, with much gastric disturbance, [**Ipe. Puls.**] Great heat, and yet wants to be covered, [**Hepar.**—Wants to be uncovered, **Hyos. Sec.**] Afternoon or evening fever, [**Chin. Phos. Puls.**] *Sweat* after midnight.

**CHARACT. PECULIARITIES.** Suitable to thin, slender persons, [*lean persons with dark complexion, black hair and eyes*, **Nit. ac.**—Tall, slender, fair skin, nervous temperament, **Phos.** —Thin, scrawny, with shrivelled skin, **Sec.**] *Shocks and jerks through whole body, [pulsations through whole body, **Puls.** ***Zinc.**—Buzzing through whole body, **Opi.**] *Heaviness* of body, [*lightness*, **Sep. Thuya.**—Feels too tall, ***Stram.**] *Bad effects from coffee, tobacco, spirituous liquors, sedentary habits, loss of sleep. *Aggravation* in morning, after eating, from touch; *strong pressure* relieves, **Nat. c.**]

## OPIUM.

**MIND.** *Fearfulness* and tendency to start, [**Ign. Kali c. Nat. m.**] Stupid indifference to pain and pleasure, [*insensibility to mental impressions, **Stram.**] *Thinks she is not at home, [see **Bry.**] *Delirious talking; eyes wide open, face red and puffed up, [unconscious delirium, with closed eyes, **Hyos.**] *Complete loss of consciousness*, [**Bell. Laur.**] **Complete loss of memory*, [see **Hydras.**] **Dilirium tremens*, with dulness of sense, stupor, and loud snoring, [with clonic spasms, unconsciousness, and *aversion* to light and company, **Hyos.**—With *consciousness* and *desire for light and company*, **Stram.**] *Apoplexy, with loss of consciousness, red, bloated face; half-closed eyes, dilated, insensible pupils; foam at the mouth, loud snoring.

**HEAD.** Dulness and stupefaction of head as from drunkenness, [**Gel.**] *Vertigo* when rising, has to lie down. Sensation of *tightness* in head, [*of looseness*, **Nat. sul. Nux m.**—Brain feels as if it fell forward when stooping **Dig.**—As if it fell to left side, **Nat. s.**—*Feeling of hollowness* in head, **Carol. ru. Ign.**] Throbbing of arteries of the head, [**Hyos. Stan.**—* *Of the neck*, **Bell.**] *Great *heaviness* of head, [**Calc. c. Phos. ac. Sulph.**—*Ligthness* of, **Stram.**]

**EYES.** Eyes half open and turned upwards, [heaviness of

lids, cannot keep them open, ***Gel. Rhus. Sep.**] ***Pupils dilated and insensible to light, [*contracted*, **Ciou. Phos.**]

**FACE.** *Dark-red, bloated, swollen face, [**Bell. Hyos.**] Spasmodic movements of facial muscles. Veins of face distended. *Hanging down of lower jaw, [**Lach. Lyc.**—*Lock-jaw*, **Ciou. Hyos.**] Corner of mouth-twitch.

**STOMACH.** Vomiting, with violent colic and convulsions. *Vomiting blood*, [see **Ipec.**] *Vomiting fæces and urine, [**Plumb.**] *Lead-colic*, [***Nux v.**] *Incarcerated hernia*, [**Nux v.**] *Ileus, with retention of stool.

**STOOL.** *Constipation; stools composed of *round, hard, black balls*, [**Thuya.**—Hard, white, like chalk, **Pallad.**—Light-colored, lumpy, **Collin.**—Stools like *sheep's dung*, **Chel. Plumb. Ruta. Verbas.**—Stools long, narrow, hard like a *dog's*, **Caust.** ***Phos. Prun. spin.**—Too large, hard, and difficult, ***Bry. Kali c.** ***Nux v. Verat.**] *Involuntary stools after fright. **Cholera infantum* with stupor.

**RESPIRATORY O'S.** Difficult, intermitting breathing, as from paralysis of lungs, [**Lyc. Tart. e.**] *Deep snoring, breathing, with open mouth, [deep, like a sigh, **Cap.**—Unequal, quick, and moaning, **Bell.**]

**SLEEP.** *Very sleepy, but cannot go to sleep, [***Bell. Ferr.**] **Great drowsiness* and inclination to sleep, [**Camph. Hep.** ***Phos. Sec.**—Very *wakeful*, ***Coff. Colo.**] *Coma vigil*, [***Hyos. Hydro. ac. Verat.**] *Stupefying sleep, with *eyes half open and loud snoring*, [**Stram.**—Screams out during sleep, **Bell. Cham. Stram.**] During sleep, *picking at the bedclothes*, [**Hyos. Mur. ac.**—Grasping at flocks, **Ars. Zinc.**]

**FEVER.** *Pulse *full and slow*, with difficult snoring, breathing, [pulse *thread-like, weak*, slow, **Verat.**] *Intermittent fever;* shaking chill, falls asleep in cold stage, no thirst; during hot stage, *thirst*; with copious perspiration. *Typhoid fever with *sopor;* snoring with mouth open, twitching of limbs, and perspiration on hot body.

**CHARACT. PECULIARITIES.** Suitable to children and old people, [**Mill.**] *All complaints, with great sopor. *Buzzing* through whole body. **After a fright* with fear, convulsions, *Screaming before and during spasm*, [comes out of spasm happy, **Sulph.**] *After fright; the fear seems to remain, [***Acon.**] Bad effects from fright, [**Hyos. Verat.**—From grief, ***Ign. Phos. ac.**] *Bed feels so *hot*, cannot lie on it, [feels too *hard*, ***Arn. Bapt.**] Patient *worse* while perspiring, during and after sleep, [worse after sleep, **Apis.** ***Lach. Verat.**—Better after sleeping, **Cro. t. Phos. Sil.**]

## PHOSPHORUS.

**MIND.** *Great lowness of spirits*, [**Plat. Puls. Rumex.**—Hilarity of, **Croc. Lach. Sabi.**] *Fearfulness, as if something were creeping out of every corner, [fear of ghosts, **Acon.**] *Great tendency to start, [**Kali c. Nat. m.**] Indisposed *to work*, [**Con. Nit. ac. Nux.**—Indisposed *to talk*, **Dig. Phos. ac. Stan.**] Loss of memory, [**Merc. Nat. m. *Opi.**]

**HEAD.** Vertigo when rising from bed in the morning, or from a seat, [see **Kali b.**] Dull, stupefying headache, worse in morning and when stooping; better when lying down and in cold air, [worse lying down and in cold air, **Bell. Nux.**] Congestion to head, with burning, stinging, pulsating pains. Burning in forehead, [**Stan.**—On vertex, **Graph. *Sulph.**] Sensation of *emptiness in head*, with vertigo, [**Carol. r. Ign. Oxal. ac.**—Great fulness, ***Acon. Bell. Bry.**] *Humming* and roaring in head.

**EYES.** *Ophthalmia, with burning, itching, and pressure as from sand in eyes. *Scrofulous ophthalmia*, [see **Merc.**] Agglutination of lids in morning, with secretion of gum during day, [**Caust. Kali c.**] *Frequent attacks of sudden blindness, [***Caust. Merc. Sil.**] Black spots passing before eyes, [**Carb. v. *Merc. *Nit. ac.**—As of insects, **Caust.**]

**EARS.** Throbbing in ears, [**Calc. c. Hep. Nat. m.**] *Loud whizzing before ears, [ringing, whizzing, **Ledum. Lyc.**] Hardness of hearing, as if a foreign body were in the ear, [see **Puls.**] Polypi in the ears.

**NOSE.** **Frequent bleeding of nose*, in morning, [**Am. c. Bry.**—At night; during stool, or from exertion, **Rhus.**—*Epistaxis instead of the menses*, ***Bry. Puls.**—After suppressed bleeding piles, **Nux.**] *Polypi nasi bleeding easily.

**FACE.** *Pale, sickly complexion. *Hippocratic countenance*, [***Ars. Carb. v. Verat.**] *Tearing pains in facial bones, as if parts would be torn out. *Circumscribed* redness of face, [**Calc. c. Sang. Sulph.**] Bloated lips.

**MOUTH and THROAT.** *Toothache*, with swelling of cheeks, [**Arn. Cham. Sep.**] Toothache from washing, [**Nux m.**] *Dry tongue; coated with white mucus. *Nursing sore mouth. *Burning* in œsophagus, [***Ars. Canth. Merc.**—*Coldness* in, **Carb. v. Verat.**] *Dryness in pharynx and fauces*, day and night, Spasmodic constriction of the throat, [**Bell. Hyos. Laur.**] *Hawking up mucus in morning, [**Lach. Nat. m.**—See **Arg. n.**]

**STOMACH and ABDOMEN.** **Thirst for very cold drinks.* Hunger soon after eating, [**Cicu. Merc. Staph.**—Stomach feels empty after eating, **Sang. Sars.**] Sour taste after eating, [**Lyc. Puls.**—All food or drink tastes bitter, ***Bry. Colo.**—Tastes sour, **Nux v. Puls.**] *Sour eructations after every meal, [**Bry. Calc. c. Kali c.**—Bitter eructations after a meal, **Bell. Chin. Nux v.**] *Belching large quantities of wind after eating, [***Arg. n. *Iodi. Hepar.**] *Sour* regurgitation of food, [**Nat. m. Nux v. Sulph.**—*Bitter* regurgitation, **Bry. Merc. Pet.**] *Vomiting bile or a sour substance, [***Ipe. Nux v.**] Vomiting what has been drunk, soon as it becomes warm in stomach. *Region of stomach painful to touch*, or when walking, [**Ars. Bry. Merc.**] *Inflammation of stomach*, with *burning* extending to throat and bowels, [**Ars. Canth. Merc.**] *Feeling of coldness* in abdomen, [**Ars. Pet. Sec. Sep.**—*Burning* in, **Canth. Lach. Sep. Sil.**] *Sharp, cutting pains in bowels.

**STOOL.** *Stools, *long, narrow, hard, like a dog's;* difficult to expel, [**Caust. Prun. spi.**—*Stools like *sheep's* dung, **Chel. Plumb. Ruta. Verbas.**] Alternate constipation and diarrhœa, [see **Ant. c.**] *Painless,* debilitating diarrhœa; worse in morning, [**Apis. *Podo. Sulph.**] Stools of *green mucus;* *white, watery, with *little grains like sago,* [green, like scum on frog-pond, ***Mag. c.**] *Stools* undigested, [***Chin. Ferr. Phos. ac. Podo.**] Bloody stools, [**Cap. Colch. Colo. *Merc.**] *Involuntary stools, *anus remaining open,* [**Apis.**—Anus as if *constricted,* **Nux.**]

**URINE.** Brown urine, with sediment of red sand, [***Lyc.**] *Hæmaturia.* The urine *deposits a brick-dust* sediment, [**Chin. Nat. m. Puls.**—Urine dark-brown, with *white sediment,* **Calc. c. Sep.**] Profuse, pale, watery.

**SEXUAL O'S.** *Male.* *Irresistible desire for an embrace, [**Calc. c. Canth. Nux v.**—Diminished sexual desire, **Arg. n. Hepar. Lyc. Mag. c.**] Stitches through pelvis, from vagina to uterus. **Menses* too *early* and scanty, [**Con. Nat. m. Sil.**—Too *late* and too scanty, **Grap. Hepar. *Puls.**—Too *early and too profuse,* ***Bell. *Calc. c. Nit. ac. Sabi.**] *Profuse, smarting, corrosive* leucorrhœa, [**Con. Kreo. Puls.**]

**RESPIRATORY O'S.** *Hoarseness* in *morning,* [**Carb. v. *Caust. *Iodi. Sulph.**—In *evening,* **Calc. c. Kali b. Lach.**] *Complete loss of voice, [**Bell. Bapt. Merc. Sulph.**] *Violent catarrh, with hoarseness, [**Cham. Merc. Nux v.**] *Cannot talk, the larynx so painful, [**Bell. Dros.**] *Cough from tickling in throat;* worse from cold air; reading aloud; talking, laughing, eating or drinking, [**Chin. Dros.**—See **Spong.**] *Cough, with *pale-red, rust-colored,* or bloody, frothy expectoration, [***Bry. Rhus. Sang.**—Dirty, slate-colored, **Kali b.**—**Gray,* saltish, **Bary. c. Lyc.**—*Green,* **Lyc. Phos. Puls.**—Jelly-like, with specks of blood, **Laur.**—*Green,* with sweet taste, **Stan. Sulph.**—*Salt, fetid,* purulent, **Kali b. Nit. ac. Sep.**—*Transparent,* tenacious, **Ferr. *Kali b.**—*Yellow,* **Ign. Phos. ac. Puls. *Stan.**] **Tightness across chest,* with a dry, tight cough, [**Puls.**] **Pneumonia,* (left side,) *with sharp stitches in chest; rust-colored sputa; respiration oppressed, quick, anxious;* better lying on *right* side, [**Apis.**] *Heaviness and fulness* in chest, [**Calc. c. Puls. *Sep.**—*Emptiness,* **Cocc. Crot. Zinc.**]

**BACK.** Pain in back, as if broken, [**Graph. Mag. c.**—As if it would break, **Kreo. Kalm.**] Burning in back, [**Ars.**—Between scapulæ, **Bry. Lyc.**—*Coldness* between shoulders, **Am. m.**] *Rachitis.*

**EXTREMITIES.** *Stitches* in elbow and shoulder-joints. Cramp in hands. Heaviness of lower limbs. Numbness of thighs and toes. *Burning of feet, [**Calc. c. Sulph.**]

**SLEEP.** *Very sleepy after meals, especially after dinner, [**Bry. Lyc. Nux v.**] *Great drowsiness;* coma vigil, [see **Opi.**] *Somnambulism.*

**FEVER.** *Pulse quick and full*, or small and weak. Chilliness, generally in evening, not relieved by heat of stove, [**Bell. Nux v.**] Absence of thirst, and aversion to being uncovered. *Febrile heat* and sweat at night. *Typhoid fever, with soporous condition, dry, black lips and tongue, open mouth, [see **Lyc.**] *Hectic fever* *Nightsweats.

**SKIN.** Burning itching of whole body, [**Kali c.**] *Dry herpes*, [**Calc. c. Kali c. Sulph.**—*Humid tetters*, **Kreo. *Ledum. Kali c. Merc.**—Eruptions oozing a sticky fluid, ***Graph.**—Oozing a watery fluid, **Dulc.**]

**CHARACT. PECULIARITIES.** Especially suitable to *tall, slender persons*, with fair skin, blonde, or red hair, [fat, light-haired persons, **Kali b.**] *Weakness from loss of animal fluids, [***Chin. Calc. c. Phos. ac.**] *Great nervous debility*, trembling, [**Cocc. Plat. Stram. Valer.**] Great emaciation, [**Ars. Bary. c. Lyc.**—*Children and young persons who incline to *grow fat*, **Calc. c.**] *Slight wounds bleed much, [**Lach.**] *Worse*, in evening, from light, [better from light, **Stram.**] *Better*, in *dark*, [**Con. Sang.**—Afraid in *dark*, **Caust.**] Better lying on *right* side, [**Apis.**] Better after sleeping, [*worse*, **Apis. *Lach. Opi. Verat.**]

## PHOSPHORIC ACID.

**MIND.** **Perfect indifference* [**Chin. Lyc. Merc. Sep.**] *Not disposed to talk, [***Bell. Con. Ign. Nit. ac.**—Hurried speech, **Lach. Merc. Stram.**] *Silent sadness*, [***Ign. Puls.**] Low-spirited and anxious about the future, [**Lyc. Nat. m. Nit. ac.** *Delirium, drowsiness, and stupor.

**HEAD.** Sensation of intoxication, with buzzing in head, [see **Gel.**] *Dreadful pain on top of head, as if brain were crushed, after long-continued grief. *Great heaviness of the head*, [**Calc. c. Nat. m. Rhus t. Sulph.**—Sensation of lightness, **Hipp. Stram,**] Headache, compelling one to lie down; *worse from the least shaking or noise*, [**Bell.** [**Kali b.**] Buzzing in head.

**EYES.** Inflammation of eyes, and stye on the upper lids, [**Lyc. Puls.**—Styes on lower lids, **Rhus.**] *The eyes are dazzled by looking at bright things.* Coldness of internal surface of eyelids, [**Alum. Kali c.**]

**EARS.** Ringing in ears, [see **Chin.**] Roaring, humming in ears, [**Bell. Lyc. Nit. ac.**] Intolerance of noise and conversation, [**Acon. Ars.**—Intolerance of music, **Lyc. Phos. Sulph.**]

**MOUTH.** Burning pain in front teeth at night; worse from hot or cold things. The *gums stand off from the teeth, are sore, and bleed when being rubbed*, [**Carb. v. Merc. Nit. ac. Nux v.** —*Scorbutic* gums, **Am. c. Kreo. Mur. ac.**] *Clammy, sticky mucus in mouth and on tongue, [**Merc. Nux m. Puls.**—*Dry, blackish tongue, **Ars. Lach. Lyc. Merc.**—See **Lyc.**] *Dryness* of *tongue* and *throat, without thirst*, [**Bell. *Nux m.**—With thirst, **Nit. ac. Phos.**]

**STOMACH and ABDOMEN.** Nausea, as if in the palate. ***Desire** for something refreshing or juicy, [**Verat.**—See **Hepar.**] *Bread tastes bitter, [all food and drink taste bitter, ***Bry. Colo. Puls.**] Pressure in stomach, as from a load, with drowsiness, [**Ars. Bry. Nux v. Sep.**] *Sensation as if the stomach were balanced up and down, [as if hanging down, relaxed, **Arg. n.** ***Staph.**—Sensation of a worm in stomach, **Croc. Lach.**] *Feeling of heaviness in region of liver,* [see **Podo.**] Crampy pain in abdomen.

**STOOL.** *Diarrhœa, preceding epidemic cholera, [**Phos. Sec. Verat.**] *Copious, *watery-whitish* stools; painless, [**Ben. ac. Cast. Phos. Podo.**—Stools *black,* **Camp. Chin.** ***Lep.** ***Verat.**] *Diarrhœa not debilitating,* [*reverse,* ***Ars. Chin. Sec.** ***Verat.**]

**URINARY O'S.** Urine like milk, mixed with jelly-like, bloody pieces, with pain in kidneys, [urine turns *milky* after standing, **Cina.**—Like curdled milk, with brick-dust sediment, **Phos.**—*Transparent, jelly-like, or reddish, with mealy sediment, **Berb. v.**] *Passes large quantities of colorless urine at night, [***Cham.**] *Diabetes mellitus,* [**Arg. n. Bovis. Trill.**]

**SEXUAL O'S.** Itching, stinging in glans penis. *Gnawing in testicles,* [**Plat.**—*Constrictive* pain in, **Nux v.**] **Seminal emissions,* especially after onanism, [**Chin.** ***Gel. Phos.**] *Too early and too long-continued menstruation, with *pain in liver.* *Uterine ulcers; has a copious, putrid, bloody discharge, with itching, corroding pain, [**Hepar. Sec. Zinc.**]

**RESPIRATORY O'S.** *Hoarseness and roughness* of throat, [**Carbo a. Phos.**—*Soreness and rawness in throat, **Æscul. Iris.**] Cough from tickling in throat and pit of stomach, with expectoration only in morning, [***Mag. c. Nux v. Puls. Sep.**—Expectoration only *at night,* ***Caust. Staph. Tart.**—Expectoration only *in evening,* **Dig.**] Cough, with purulent, *offensive expectoration,* [**Ars. Calc. c. Stan. Sulph.**—*Hoarse, barking cough,* **Bell. Dros. Nit ac.** ***Rumex.** ***Verbas.**]

**SLEEP.** *Great drowsiness* in daytime; sleeplessness at night, [**Lyc. Merc.** ***Sulph.**—*Sleepy, but cannot go to sleep, **Bell.** ***Opi.**] Anxious dreams.

**FEVER.** Pulse irregular, frequently intermitting, [**Kali c. Lach. Nat. m. Spig.**] Chills, with shuddering *in evening,* followed by exhausting sweat. *Typhoid fever. Intermittent fever.* —Shaking chills over whole body; the fingers being cold as ice, without any thirst, followed by heat without thirst, or by excessive heat, depriving one almost of consciousness. *Profuse morning sweats, [**Chin. Sulph. ac.**—Debilitating night-sweats, **Calc. c.** ***Merc. Sil. Stan.**]

**SKIN.** *Scarlet-like* exanthems, [**Am. c. Bell.**—Black, pock-shaped exanthems, **Ars. Rhus.**] Rash over whole body, more burning than itching. *Ulcers, itching,* inveterate or flat, with dirty pus, [see **Merc.**]

**CHARACT. PECULIARITIES.** Affects especially the *nerv-*

*ous system,* [Cocc. Plat. *Valeri.—Affects *glandular system,* Hepar. Iodi. Kali b. Merc.] *Children with pale, sickly look; *painless diarrhœa,* and tottering gait. Children and young persons who grow *too fast,* [grow too *fat,* Calc. c.—Those who incline to grow thin, Ars. Bary. c. Phos.] *Weakness from loss of animal fluids, [Calc. c. *Chin. *Phos.] *Bad effects from grief, chagrin, unhappy love,* [Gel. *Ign.] *Pain in periosteum, as if scraped, [Rhus.] Pains *worse during rest;* and better from motion, [Dulc. Kali c. Rhod. *Rhus.—*Better* during rest, worse from motion, Acon. *Bry. Hep. Merc.]

## PHYTOLACCA DECANDRA.

**MIND.** Entire *indifference* to life, [Chin. Merc. Phos. ac.] Melancholy, is sure he will die, [see Acon.]

**HEAD.** Vertigo and dimness of vision, with danger of falling. Pain in back of head and neck. One-sided headache, [see Puls.] *Dull, heavy headache in forehead.* *Sick-headache, worse in forehead, with backache and bearing down, comes every *week,* [comes every *three or four days,* Aur.—Every two weeks, Sulph.] *Shooting pain from left eye to vertex.*

**EYES.** *Burning, smarting in eyes, with profuse lachrymation, [Euph.] Feeling of sand in eyes, [see Nux.]

**NOSE.** Thin watery discharge from nostrils, nose becomes stuffed. Flow of mucus from one nostril while the other is stopped.

**FACE.** *Hippocratic face,* [*Ars. Carb. v. Verat.] *Chin drawn closely to sternum, by contraction of muscles, in tetanus. *Lips everted and firm. Glands of neck swollen.

**MOUTH.** *Metallic* taste, [Arg. n. Merc. Plumb.] Back part of tongue feels as if burnt, [see Verat.] Tongue fiery red at tip, tender and smarting. Profuse saliva, sometimes yellowish, thick, ropy.

**THROAT.** *Sore throat,* right side. Fauces dark, bluish-red, worse on swallowing, [see Bell.] *Throat feels as if a red-hot ball was lodged in fauces, [as if a *splinter* was, Arg. n. Hepar. Nit. ac.] Diphtheric inflammation and ulceration of throat. *Fauces, tonsils and pharynx covered with dark-colored pseudo-membrane. Cannot drink hot fluids, [Lach.] Mucus hangs down in strings from posterior nares, and is hawked up with difficulty, [see Arg. n.].

**STOMACH.** Eructations of flatus and sour fluid. Vomiting ingesta, bile, blood, and slime, with intense pain. Bruised and sore feeling in pit of stomach. Soreness and pain in right hypochondrium.

**STOOL.** *Thin, dark-brown stools, [Scilla.] Stools of mucus and blood, like scrapings off intestines, [*Canth. Colch. Colo.] Bleeding piles. Fissured rectum.

**URINE.** *Dull pain and soreness* in region of kidneys,

[burning, stinging, ***Canth.**] Uneasiness down ureters, [*dragging, shooting* pains, **Cann. s.**] Urine *albuminous*, [**Apis.** ***Berb.** ***Helon. Terb.**] *Urine dark-red, stains vessel mahogany color, [*clay color*, ***Sep.**]

**SEXUAL O'S.** Gonorrhœa and gleet, [**Cann. Gel. Merc.**] *Syphilis, chancres, ulcerated throat; ulcers on genitals.* Menses too frequent and too copious, [see **Puls.**] *Inflammation, swelling and suppurations of breasts. Mammary gland full of hard, painful nodosities, [**Con. Nit. ac.**]

**LARYNX.** *Hoarseness*, with loss of voice, [see **Phos.**] Burning in larynx and trachea, with sensation of constriction. *Dry, hacking cough, with hawking. Cough excited by *tickling in larynx*, or dryness in pharynx, worse at night soon as he lies down, [see **Puls.**]

**CHEST.** Aching pains in chest and side, with cough. Pain through mid-sternum, with cough. Shocks of pain in cardiac region. *Angina pectoris, pain goes into right arm, [with *numbness* of left arm, **Rhus.**]

**BACK.** Neck stiff, tonsils swollen. Glands on right side of neck *hard*. *Rheumatism in lumbar muscles, aching pain day and night.

**UPPER LIMBS.** Both scapulæ ache continually. Shooting pains in right shoulder-joint, with stiffness and inability to raise the arm. *Finger-joints swollen, hard, shining. Lame feeling in arms.

**LOWER LIMBS.** Sharp cutting pains in hip, drawing; leg drawn up, cannot touch floor. *Rheumatism of left knee, hamstrings feel shortened. Chronic rheumatism of left hip. Ulcers on the legs.

**SKIN.** Barber's itch, local application of tincture. *Ringworm*, [**Lith. c. Sep. Tellu.**] Black-looking, tettery, suppurative eruption. Ulcers, with an appearance as if punched out, [see **Sili.**] Scarlatina, with angina.

**CHARACT. PECULIARITIES.** Adapted to persons of a *rheumatic diathesis* [**Bry. Cimi. Rhus.**] Syphilitic rheumatism. Pains, pressing, shooting and sore. Erratic pains, [***Lac can.** ***Puls.**] Glands inflamed, swollen. Hastens suppuration in abscesses, [**Lach. Merc.** ***Sili.**]

## PODOPHYLLUM.

**MIND.** Depression of spirits, [**Bovis. Chel. Iris.**] Imagines he is going to die, [**Acon. Ars. Nux. Phyto. Sec.—Is very cheerful, Cocc. Lach.**]

**HEAD.** *Vertigo, with tendency to fall forward.* Morning headache, with flushed face, [see **Nux v. Sulph.**] Headache, alternating with diarrhœa. *Rolling of head during difficult dentition, [boring head into pillow, **Apis.** ***Bell. Hell.—Jerking head up from pillow,** ***Stram.**]

**MOUTH and THROAT.** Tongue furred white, with *foul*

*taste*, [Ant. Nux. Sep.] Dryness of mouth and tongue in morning, [Mag. c. Puls. Spig.] Grinding of teeth at night, [Cicu. *Cina. Seo. Stram.] *Sore throat, beginning on right side and going to left, [see *Lach.] *Rattling of mucus* in throat. Dryness of throat. *Goitre*, [Calc. c. *Iod. *Spong.]

**STOMACH and ABDOMEN.** Regurgitation of food, [see *Phos.] Vomiting food, with putrid taste and odor. *Waterbrash, [Ars. *Nux. Phos.] *Belching of hot flatus, very sour. Gagging, or empty retching* **Fulness** and pain in region of liver, [Acon. Berb. Eup. per.—*Constant dull pain* in region of gall-bladder, Bapt. *Lept. *Phyto.—*Burning pain* in region of liver, Kali c. Merc.—Drawing, burning, stinging pain, Bry. Calc. c.—*Induration* of liver, Ars. Bell. Chin. *Merc. *Sil.]

**STOOL and ANUS.** *Chronic diarrhœa*, worse in morning, [Kali b. Nat. s. Phos. Sulph.—Worse at night, *Ars. Chin. *Puls. Verat.] **Greenish, watery stools*, [Dulc. Grat. *Mag. c. Puls.—*White, watery*, Benz. ac. *Castor. Phos. *Phos. ac.—*Black, watery*, Ars. Kali b. Verat.—*Yellowish, watery*, Apis. Chin. Crot. t. Dulc. Hyos.] *Profuse stools, gushing out like a torrent, [*Jatro. *Thuya.] *Frequent chalk-like stools*, very offensive, with gagging and great thirst in children, [see *Calc. c. Copa.] *Dark, yellow, mucous stools, smelling like carrion. *Jelly-like*, mucous stools, [Aloe. *Colch. *Hell.] *Painless, undigested stools*, [Ars. *Chin. *Ferr. Hyos. Phos. ac.—Painless, morning diarrhœa, Rumex c. *Sulph.] *White, slimy, mucous stools.* **During and after* stool, *prolapsus ani*, [Merc.—*During* stool, Gum. g. Ign. *Ruta. Sep.] Diarrhœa worse after eating or drinking.

**URINE.** Diminished secretion of urine, [Kreo.] *Suppression* of urine, [Hell. Laur.—Suppression in fever, Cact.]

**GENITALS.** *Suppression of menses in young girls, [see Puls.] *Leucorrhœa;* discharge of thick, transparent mucus, with bearing down in genitals and constipation. *Prolapsus uteri, [Calc. c. *Coni. Nux v. *Sep.—Prolapsus of vagina, with a sensation of great rawness, *Merc. Sep. Stan.] *Numb, aching pain in left ovarian region, [see Lach.]

**CHARACT. PECULIARITIES.** Symptoms generally worse in morning, especially those of abdomen. *Painless cholera morbus. *Violent cramp in feet, calves, and thighs, [with painless, watery stools.] Sudden shocks of jerking pain.

## PULSATILLA.

**MIND.** *Melancholy, with weeping, sadness*, [Lyc. Plat. Phos.—Gayety, cheerfulness, Croc. *Lach.] Disposed to weep or laugh, [Berb. Calc. c. Staph. Sulph.] *Anguish in region of heart, even to a desire for suicide. *Hypochondriac peevishness.* *He is disgusted with everything, [Calc. c.—Indifferent to everything, Ign. *Phos. ac. Phyto.]

**HEAD.** Vertigo, as if intoxicated, [Bry. Can. s. Croc. *Gel.] *Vertigo, when rising from a sitting posture, with chilliness. *Vertigo, when stooping, lifting up the eyes, after eat-*

*ing*, [see **Kali b.**] Confusion of head, with pain, as after intoxication or watching. Sensation of *emptiness* in head, with great indifference, [***Coco. Coral. r. Ign.** ***Oxal. ac.**—Great fulness in head, **Acon.** ***Bell. Bry.** ***Merc.**] *Beating pain in head; worse in evening, from stooping, mental exertion, in a warm room. *Hemicrania, as if brain would burst. *Headache relieved by compression, [**Apis. Arg. n.**] **Headache* from overloading stomach, *or after eating fat food*, [***Ant. Ipe.** ***Iris.** ***Nux.**—Headache from abuse of *coffee*, **Cham. Ign.** ***Nux.**—From abuse of *spirituous liquors*, **Carb. v. Coff.** ***Nux. Puls.**—From *excessive study*, **Calc. c. Nux. Sulph.**—From *moral emotions, grief*, etc., ***Ign. Phos. ac. Staph.**] *Headache, worse in evening, after lying down; better in open air and from compression, [**Apis.**]

**EYES.** *Inflammation of margins of lids, with swelling, [*ulceration* of margin of lids, **Euph.** ***Merc. Sulph.**] Pressure in eyes as from sand. [**Caust. Chin. Euph. Sulph.**—Burning, smarting, as from salt, **Nux v.**] **Styes*, especially on *upper lids*, [**Phos. ac. Lyc.**—On *lower lids*, **Rhus t.**]

**EARS.** *Otalgia, with *darting*, tearing pains, [see ***Merc.**] *Stinging* in ears. *Hardness of hearing*, as if ears were stopped, [**Calc. c. Caust. Sil. Sulph.**] **Discharge of pus* from ears, especially after measles, [**Bell. Merc. Sulph.**] Humming and tingling in the ears.

**NOSE.** **Bleeding* of nose, with dry coryza, [see **Bell.** ***Phos.**] *Green, fetid* discharge from nose, [**Merc. Rhus.**—*Fetid, yellow* discharge, **Coni. Graph.** ***Nit. ac.**] *Coryza, with loss of taste and smell*, [**Nat. m.** ***Mag. m.**]

**FACE.** *Yellowish* complexion, [**Ars. Caust. Merc.**—*Greenish* color of face, **Ars. Carb. v.**] Alternate redness and paleness of the face, [***Bell. Croc. Ign.**]

**MOUTH and THROAT.** *Toothache*, with *otalgia, one-sided headache, and chilliness.* *The toothache comes on every time he eats or takes anything warm in mouth, relieved momentarily by cold water, [**Bry.**] *Tongue coated yellow or white, and covered with tough mucus, [**Merc. Nux m. Phos. ac.**] * Sore throat; it feels too narrow or as if closed up when swallowing. Back part of throat feels sore and raw.

**STOMACH and ABDOMEN.** *Putrid taste in mouth, with inclination to vomit, [**Arn. Bry.** ***Merc. Nux v.**] *Absence of thirst, [***Bell. Ipe. Sep.**] *Every kind of nourishment tastes bitter*, [***Bry Chin. Colo.**—All food tastes *sour*, **Lyc. Nux v.**—All food tastes too *salt*, **Ars. Bell. Chin. Sulph.**] *Eructations tasting of ingesta, [**Ant. Calc. c. Chin. Con.**—Tasting like bad eggs. **Arn. Mur. ac. Sep. Sulph.**—Without taste or smell, **Hepar. Staph.**] Gulping up *bitter fluid*, [**Bry. Ign. Nux v. Phos.**—*Sourish fluid*, **Dig. Hydras. Lach. Nat. s.**—*Sweetish fluid*, **Nat. c. Plum. Stan.**] Vomiting after every meal, [***Ars. Ferr. Iris. Nux v.**] *Vomiting mucus. *Morning sickness*, [**Con. Cyclamen. Ipe. Phos.**] **Disordered stomach from eating fat, rich food*, [***Ant. Ipe. Nux v.**] Pain in stomach after eating, [*Ars. Ferr. *Nux. Sulph.] Perceptible *pulsations* in pit of stomach, [Iod. Rhus. Sep. Tart.] Distension of abdomen after every meal. *Enteritis, with painful sensitiveness of abdominal walls.* **Colic, with chilliness* and rumbling in abdomen, especially in evening.

**STOOL and ANUS.** *Nightly diarrhœa; *stools watery or green like bile* preceded by rumbling and colic. *Frequent loose stools mixed with mucus,* [*Ars. Bell. *Cham.] **Diarrhœa* from eating *fruit,* [Ars. *Chin. Cist. Colo.—From eating *pears,* Verat. a.—From eating *onions,* Thuya.—From eating *oysters,* *Brom. Lyc.—From eating *veal,* Kali n.—After taking cold, *Acon. Bry. Cham. *Dulc.—After taking *cold drinks,* *Ars. Bry. Nux m. *Puls.—After cold food, ice-cream, *Ars. *Puls. —After drinking *impure water,* *Camph. Zing.—After drinking *milk,* *Calc. c. Nat. c. *Nico. Sulph.] **Dysenteric* diarrhœa, stools nothing but mucus and blood, with chilliness during stool, [Ipe. *Merc. Sulph.—See Merc.]

**URINARY O'S.** *Incontinence of urine* [Bell. Gel. *Euph. pur. *Kreo.] *Frequent desire to urinate, with drawing in abdomen. *Colorless, watery urine, with jelly-like sediment,* [Berb.— *Milky urine, with bloody, jelly-like lumps, Phos. ac.] *Hæmaturia,* with purulent sediment and pain in kidneys, [*Ars. Cann. Canth. *Phos.] Gonorrhœal discharge resembling semen, [see Phyto.]

**SEXUAL O'S.** *Menses *too late* and too scanty, and of too short duration, with cramps in abdomen, [Con. *Dulc. Phos. *Sulph.—*Too early* and too *scanty,* Con. Nat. m. *Phos. Sil.—Too early and too *profuse,* *Am. c. Bell. *Calc. c. *Plat.— Too *late* and too *profuse,* Caust. Iod.] **Suppression of menses,* especially from cold, [*Dulc. *Merc. *Podo. *Sulph.—From *fright,* *Acon. Lyc.—*Vicarious menstruation,* (spitting blood), Ars. *Phos. Puls.—*Epistaxis,* when menses should appear, Bell. *Bry. Puls.—*Discharge of white water instead of the menses, Sil.] *Delayed and difficult first menstruations, [Kali c. Nat. m. Sulph.—*Climacteric disorders,* *Lach. Sang. *Sep.—Menses irregular, *never at right time,* Iodi. *Nux m. Nux v. Ruta.] Menstrual blood, *black and clotted,* putrid, [Ign. *Mag. m. Plat. Stram.—Thick, *black like pitch,* *Mag. c. Nux v. Sang.] **Menstrual colic,* pains so violent she tosses in every direction, with cries and tears; blood thick and dark, [*Caul. Cham. *Cimi. Nux v.] Irregular labor-pains, [Bell. Caul. *Nux.] **Malposition of fœtus.* Thin, acrid, or or milky leucorrhœa.

**RESPIRATORY O'S.** Hoarseness, which does not permit one to speak a loud word, [Bell. *Kali c. Merc. *Phos.— Hoarseness in the morning, with intolerable tickling in the throat, [*Iodi. Sep.] Scraping and dryness in throat, [Nit. ac. Nux v.] *Dry cough at night, when lying down, going off when sitting up, [*Hyos. Sang.—Worse from sitting up, Kali c. *Zinc.—*Worse* lying on *back,* Am. m. Nux v. Phos.—On *left side,* Ipe. Merc. Phos.—On *right side,* Am. m. Stan.] *Cough, with easy expectoration of yellow mucus, especially in morning, [**Calc. c. Phos. ac. Stan. Sulph.**—*Dry, barking cough*, **Bell. Nit. ac. *Rumex. *Spong.**] Cough, with expectoration of *black coagulated blood*, [**Am. Collin. *Nit. ac.**] *Stitches in side and chest*, [***Acon. Bell. *Bry. *Kali c.**] *Sensation of tightness or constriction across chest, [**Bell. Nux. *Phos. Stan.**] Dyspnœa, especially when lying on back. Burning in region of heart, [**Opi.**]

**SLEEP.** *Drowsiness in day-time*, [**Merc. Nux. *Phos.**] *Sleep at night is prevented by ideas crowding upon one, [see **Nux v.**] *Restless sleep*, with tossing about; frequent waking. *Sleep full of frightful dreams, [***Bell. Nit. ac. Phos.**]

**FEVER.** *Continuous internal chilliness, even in warm room. Increased chilliness towards evening, [**Ars. Bell. Phos. Rhus.**] *Intermittent fever; long chill, little heat, no thirst. Sometimes thirst before chill or heat, seldom in hot stage. Ague, with much gastric disturbance, [**Ant. *Ipe. Nux.**]

**SKIN.** **Measles*, and their secondary ailments, [**Bell.**] Eruptions, like *chicken-pox*, from eating *pork, fat things*. Erysipelas, with swelling, hardness, burning heat, stinging when touched or moving parts, [see **Bell.**]

**CHARACT. PECULIARITIES.** *Pulsations* through whole body [in *back*, **Bary. c. Thuya.**] *Adapted to females, or persons of a mild, tearful disposition, [**Bell. *Sep.**] *The pains are accompanied with chilliness*, [**Ars. *Bell. Sep. Ign.**—Chilliness *after* pains, **Kali c.**] *Erratic pains, rapidly shifting from one part to another, [**Bell. *Kali b. *Lac can.**] Burning, stinging pains, [***Apis. Merc.**] *Aggravation* in *evening; in twilight*, [**Bry Iris. Merc. Phos.**—In *morning*, **Nux Rhus. Sang.**] *Worse* when lying on *left side*, [**Acon. Cact. Phos.**—*Better* on left side, **Pallad.**—*Worse* on *painful side*, **Ars. Hepar. Iodi. Nux m. Sil.**—*Better* on *painful side*, ***Bry. Calc. c. Ign.**] *Better in open air, or in a *cold room*, [**Croc. Sec. Verat.**—Better from heat, or in warm room, ***Ars. Hepar. Kali b. Rhus.**]

## RHUS TOXICODENDRON.

**MIND.** Restlessness, with continual change of position, [***Ars.**] Great anxiety towards evening. Fear that he will die, [***Ars. Bry. Nux. Sec.**—*Predicts the day*, ***Acon.**—Desires death, ***Aur. Kreo. Sil.**] Inclination to weep, especially in evening, with desire to be alone, [**Lyc. Nux.**—With dread of solitude, **Sep.**] *Desire to commit suicide*, [***Aur. Hepar. *Nux. Puls.**] *Delirium, with stupefaction of mind.*

**HEAD.** Giddiness, as if intoxicated when rising from bed, [see **Gel.**] *Fulness and heaviness* of head, especially in forehead, [**Acon. *Bell. Bry. *Merc.**] When stooping, sensation as if a weight fell forward in forehead, [**Dig.**] *When walking, sensation as if brain were loose, [**Cicu. Mur. ac. Nat. s. Nux m.**] *Stinging headache, extending to ears. *Humid sup-*

*purating eruptions on head,* forming heavy crusts, eating off hair, offensive smell and itching, worse at night, [**Calc. c. Graph. Lyc. *Staph.**]

**EYES.** Inflammation of lids, with agglutination in morning, [see **Caust. Dig. *Phos.**] *Erysipelatous swelling of eyes and adjacent parts. *Incipient amaurosis.*

**EARS.** *Otalgia,* with painful beating in ear at night, [see **Puls.**] Discharge of *bloody pus,* with hardness of hearing, [**Graph. *Merc. Pet.**—Of *yellow, fetid pus,* **Hepar. *Kali b. *Merc. *Puls.**] Parotitis, also *after scalet fever.*

**NOSE.** *Bleeding of nose at night. Green, fetid discharge from nose, [**Graph. Kali b. Merc. Puls.**]

**FACE.** * *Vesicular erysipelas of face,* with burning, tingling, stinging, [***Cist. c. Euphor.**—*Vesicular* erysipelas, with pricking in parts, **Hepar.**—*Vesicular eruptions, discharging a sticky, glutinous fluid, **Graph.**—*Œdematous swelling, with *burning, stinging pains,* **Apis.**—See **Bell.**] *Crusta lactea, with thick ceusts* and secretion of a fetid, bloody ichor, [**Lyc. Merc. *Staph.**]

**MOUTH and THROAT.** Dry mouth, with much thirst, [**Nat. m. Nit. ac.**—*Without thirst,* **Bell. Lyc. *Nux m.**] *Tongue, with red tip, in shape of a triangle. *Tongue dry, red, and cracked. Throat sore, as from an internal swelling, stinging when swallowing.

**STOMACH and ABDOMEN.** *Complete loss of appetite for any kind of food,* [***Chin. Hep. *Merc. Puls.**—*Ravenous* appetite, **Bry. *Nux v. Pet. *Verat.**] Food tastes *bitter,* especially bread, [see **Merc.**] *Sudden vomiting when eating. Pressure* in stomach, as from a stone, [***Ars. Bry. Merc. Nux.**] *Violent throbbing in stomach, [**Nux. *Puls.**] *Colic, compelling one to walk bent,* [to *bend double,* ***Colo.**] *Cramp-like* drawing in umbilical region.

**STOOL.** *Thin, red, mucus,* [***Canth. Graph. Sulph.**—*Thin, yellow, mucus,* ***Apis. Cham. *Sul. ac.**] *Jelly-like mucous* stools, [**Colch. Kali b.**—See **Podo.**] *Bloody* stools, [**Cap. Colch. Colo. Phos.**] *Before* stool, urging, cutting colic. *During* stool, cutting colic, nausea. *After* stool, *remission of pains.* Also *frothy, painless stools.*

**URINE.** Dysuria, with discharges of drops of bloody urine, [**Cann. Nux v.**] *Urine, with snow-white sediment, [**Cap. Colch.**—Brick-dust-like sediment, **Nat. m. *Phos. Puls.**—*Red, sandy sediment,* ***Lyc.**] Incontinence of urine, [see **Puls.**]

**SEXUAL O'S.** *Derangement of uterine functions, from being drenched in rain, [from taking cold, ***Dulc. Merc. Podo. *Puls.**] Metrorrhagia, with labor-like pains; blood clotted, [**Bell. Cham. Cimi.**] *Vitiated and diminished lochia, with shootings upwards in vagina, with a bursting sensation in head, [**Bry.**] *Abortion from a strain or overlifting, also *prolapsus uteri.*

**RESPIRATORY O'S.** *Hoarseness from overstraining voice.* Roughness of throat, inducing a short and hacking cough.

*Short, dry, tickling cough, especially in evening and before midnight, [after midnight and in morning, **Hyos. Nux v.**] *Terrible cough, which seems as if it would tear something out of chest. *Putting hand out of bed brings on cough, [see **Hepar.**] Cough excited from tickling under sternum, [**Rhus r. Rumex. Plat.**] Cough in evening, with vomiting the ingesta, [**Carb. v. Dros. Ferr.**] Cough, with *stitches in chest*, [**Acon.** ***Bry. Kali c.** ***Puls.**—With stitches over eye and splitting headache, **Phos.**] *Stitches* in chest and sides, *worse at rest*, [*better* at rest, ***Bry. Puls.**] Sensation of weakness and trembling of heart, [**Bell. Nit. ac. Nux m. Spig.**] Violent palpitation when sitting still, [***Aspar. Phos. Spig.**—When lying down, **Nux v. Oxal. ac.**—On the left side, **Cact.** ***Nat. c. Nat. m.**]

**BACK.** Pain in small of back, as if bruised, relieved by lying on something hard, or by motion, [**Rhod. Ruta.**] *Pain between shoulders when swallowing. Creeping coldness in back.

**EXTREMITIES.** Tearing, burning in shoulder, with lameness of arm. Paralysis of arm, with coldness and insensibility. *Tearing in all the joints of the fingers. Coxalgia;* pain, as if sprained. *Rheumatism, with drawing, tearing pains, caused by damp weather, bathing, or straining, [**Rhod. Ruta.**] *Sciatica*, worse at night.

**SLEEP.** *Sleeplessness, especially before midnight, [**Bry. Graph. Phos.**—Sleeplessness after midnight, ***Ars. Rhod.**—See **Nux v.**] *Heavy sleep*, as from stupor.

**FEVER.** Pulse slow and irregular, [**Dig. Merc. Mur. ac.**] The *chilliness*, with paroxysms of pain and other symptoms, mostly occurs in evening, [**Ars. Bell.** ***Puls.**] **Typhoid fever;* tongue dry and brown; sordes on teeth; bowels loose; great weakness; powerlessness of lower limbs, can hardly draw them up; *great restlessness after midnight, has to move often to get relief. Intermittent fever.* Paroxysms 7 P. M., [**Eup. per. Gel.**—See **Nat. m.**] Chilliness, as if cold water were poured over him, followed by heat and inclination to stretch the limbs; sweat towards morning.

**SKIN.** **Burning, itching eruptions*, with swelling of parts, and *small, yellowish vesicles*, which run together and become moist. *Erysipelas, with more burning than itching, and exudation of serous fluid, forming blisters*, [**Canth. Cro. tig.**—*Eruptions oozing a *sticky fluid*, **Graph.**—Oozing a watery fluid, **Canth. Dulc.**] Confluent vesicles containing a milky or watery fluid. *Herpes*, alternating with pains in chest and dysenteric stools. *Nettle-rash*, with burning itching, [**Dulc.**—*Stinging, burning, **Apis.** ***Urtica.**] *Glandular* swellings.

**CHARACT. PECULIARITIES.** *Pain in bones, as if scraped. [**Phos. ac.**] *The pains are *worse* at night, particularly after midnight, [***Ars. Bell. Calc. c. Sulph.**—Worse before midnight, **Phos. Saba.**] *Pains *worse during rest*, and on *beginning to move*, **Con. Lyc. Sep. Sulph.**—*Better while at rest,*

**Acon. *Bry. Merc.**] Aggravation from a change of weather; in wet, damp weather, [***Dulc. Ruta.**] *Better* from moving affected parts; from stretching out limbs, [from drawing up limbs, **Sep.**] From warmth in general.

## SEPIA.

**MIND.** *Sadness and weeping,* [**Lyc. Plat. Phos. *Puls.**—Merry, cheerful, **Croc. Lach. Oxal. ac.**] *Indifference, even to one's own family, [**Chin. Lyc. Merc. *Phos. ac.**] *Weakness of memory,* and inability to think, [**Colch. Pet. Nit. ac.**]

**HEAD.** *Vertigo only when walking in open air,* [see **Kali b.**] *Violent *beating* headache, in evening mostly in temples, [**Ars. *Bell. *Puls. *Sulph.**] Headache, as if head would burst, [**Bell. Bry.**] *Dull, aching pain over orbits,* as if the eyes would fall out. *Paroxysms of hemicrania, with nausea and vomiting. Sensation of *coldness* on vertex, [***Verat. a.**—Coldness in *back part* of head, **Dulc. Phos.**—*Heat* on vertex, **Graph. *Sulph.**]

**EYES.** *Pain in eyelids when waking,* as if *too heavy,* [see **Gel.**] Black spots or sparks before the eyes, [streaks like lightning, **Nux v.**] *Swelling of eyes, with headache.

**EARS.** *Herpes* on lobule, and behind ear, with itching. Discharge of thin pus from ear, [thick, *yellow, fetid pus,* ***Kali b. *Merc. *Puls.**] Whizzing and roaring in ears, [**Bell. Lyc. Nit. ac.**—See **Chin.**]

**NOSE.** *Swollen, inflamed nose, with sore, ulcerated nostrils, [***Alum. Lyc. *Nit. ac. Sulph.**] Bleeding of nose, [see **Phos.**] **Dry coryza,* with obstruction of nose, [***Bry. Nit. ac. *Nux v. Phos.**—*Profuse, fluent coryza,* ***Allium c. *Euph. Merc. Sang.**] *Discharge of yellow-green plugs* from nose. [See page 62.]

**FACE.** *Yellowness of face, particularly across nose, *like a saddle,* [herpes across the nose, **Sulph.**—*Yellow blotches* on the face, **Ferr.**—On forehead, **Nat. c.**]

**MOUTH and THROAT.** *Toothache during pregnancy, [**Bell. *Nux m. *Puls. Staph.**—During *lactation,* **Chin.**—During *menstruation,* **Calc. c. Carb. v. Cham.**] *Drawing* or *beating toothache,* extending to ear; pain worse from taking hot or cold things in mouth. *White-coated tongue, feeling as if burnt, [**Colc. *Verat. v.**] *Stinging sore throat,* [***Apis. Bell.**]

**STOMACH and ABDOMEN.** Aversion to all food; *everything tastes too salty,* [**Carb. v. *Chin.**—Not salty enough, **Ars. Thuya.**—Craves salt, **Calc. c.**—See **Hepar.**] *Bitter* or *sour eructations,* [**Nit. ac. *Nux. Phos.**] *Nausea and vomiting during pregnancy, [**Con. Kreo. *Nux. Verat. a.**] *Pressure in stomach,* as from a stone, after eating, [see **Nux v.**] *Painful sense of *emptiness* in pit of stomach, not relieved by eating, [***Ign. Mur. ac. Pet.**—Feels full up to throat after eating but little, ***Chin. *Lyc.**—Feels *empty after eating,* **Sang. Sars.**] *Burning* in abdomen, [***Ars. Phos. Sec.**—Coldness, ***Ars. Calc. c. Laur. *Pet.**]

**STOOL and ANUS.** *Hard, difficult stools, with a sense of *weight in anus;* not relieved by evacuation, [**Cact.**—*The rectum feels as if stopped up, **Anacar.**] *Constipation during pregnancy,* [**Alum. Bry. Lyc.** ***Nux.**—*Lying-in* females, **Ant. Bry. Nux. Plat.**—Diarrhœa *during pregnancy,* **Ant. Dulc. Hyos. Phos.**] *Diarrhœa,* stools green, smelling sour. Prolapsus ani, [***Podo.**]

**URINARY O'S.** *Fetid urine, depositing a *clay-colored sediment, which adheres to chamber,* [dark-red urine, staining chamber color mahogany, **Phyto.**] Turbid urine, with sediment of red sand, [see ***Lyc.**] *Blood-red urine.* *Wetting bed, particularly in *first sleep.*

**SEXUAL O'S.** *Pressing in uterus, as if everything would protrude, [***Bell. Nat. m.** ***Nit. ac.**] **Prolapsus uteri and vagina,* with burning pain in small of the back, [see **Merc.**] *Burning, shooting pains in neck of the uterus, [burning, sore, aching pain, ***Con.**] Menses *too early* and too scanty, [*too late* and too scanty, ***Dulc. Phos.** ***Puls.** ***Sulph.**—See **Puls.**] **Climacteric disorders,* [***Lach. Sang.**] *Leucorrhœa,* with *itching* in vagina; discharge *yellowish* or watery. Leucorrhœa, *like milk,* only in daytime, [*only at night, of bluish-white mucus, **Amb. g.**] *Profuse,* watery, offensive leucorrhœa.

**RESPIRATORY O'S.** Hoarseness, with dry cough, from tickling in throat. *Cough in morning, with profuse expectoration, *tasting very salty,* [**Amb. g. Mag. c.** ***Phos.**—Cough, with profuse expectoration, *tasting sweet,* ***Stann. Zinc.**—Expectoration tasting *putrid,* ***Carb. v. Con.** ***Puls.**] *Pressure on upper part of sternum, as from a weight, [**Nux m. Phos. Sulph.**] *Feeling of heaviness in chest,* [**Kreo. Lach.** ***Sulph.**—Of *lightness,* **Stann.**—Of *fulness* in the chest, **Calc. c.** ***Phos. Puls.**—Of *emptiness,* **Cocc. Cro. tig.**—Of *rawness* in the chest, **Anacar. Psor. Staph.**]

**BACK.** *Great weakness* in small of back, [**constant aching,* affecting sacrum and hips, **Æsculus.**] Beating in small of back, [**Bary. c. Thuya.**] Stiffness in nape of neck, [**Bell. Kali c.** ***Phos.**] Coldness between shoulders, [*burning,* **Bry.** ***Lyc.**]

**ARMS.** Violent pain in shoulder-joint, as if dislocated, [**Bry. Ruta.**] Pain in upper arm, as if bruised, [**Arn. Gel.**] *Heat in hands,* [heat of one, coldness of the other, **Chin. Dig. Ipe. Puls.**] *Panaritium,* beating pains.

**LEGS.** *Heaviness of the legs.* *Icy coldness of feet, [**Graph.** ***Phos.** ***Verat.**—As if they had on *cold, damp stockings,* ***Calc. c.**—Burning and heat of soles, **Calc. c.** ***Phos. ac.** ***Sulph.**] *Profuse sweat on feet,* [**Bary c. Lach. Phos. ac.**—Very fetid, **Carb. v. Nit. ac.** ***Sil.**] Swelling of feet, [***Apis. Ars.** ***Kali c. Merc.**] Cramp in calves at night, in bed, [***Colo. Rhus. Sulph.** ***Verat.**]

**SLEEP.** *Drowsiness* in daytime, *wide awake* at night, [see **Phos. ac.**] *Loud talking during sleep,* [**Nat. m.** ***Sulph.**] **Jerking* of limbs at night, *fidgety feeling* in feet, [**Sticta. Taran.** ***Zinc.**—*Jerking* of whole body during sleep, **Puls. Sulph.**

*Zinc.] *He awakens with a shriek and start,* [Coff. *Merc. Sulph.—*Awakens with a *shrinking look,* Stram.]

**FEVER.** *Intermittent fever,* with thirst during chill; pain in limbs; hands and feet icy cold. **The fingers feel as if dead.* Chill followed by violent heat, and inability to collect one's senses, after which profuse sweating. **Frequent flushes of heat,* especially in afternoon and evening, [*Lyc. Puls. *Sulph.] Profuse night-sweat, [Chin. *Merc. *Sil. Stan.—*Morning* sweat after waking, Nux v. Puls. Sulph.] *Sweat* from least motion.

**SKIN.** Dry itch, and itch-like eruptions, [*Merc. Staph.] *Humid herpes,* with itching and burning, [see Graph.] **Ringworm,* [over whole body, Tellur.—Herpes, in yellow rings, or suppurating, Nat. car.]

**CHARACT. PECULIARITIES.** *Suitable in mild, easy dispositions, and females,* [*Puls.] *Climacteric disorders,* [Lach. Sang.] *Disease in women, with sudden prostration and *sinking faintness.* Pains with shuddering, [Ars. Bell. *Puls.] Want of natural heat, [Ledum.] *Worse* in afternoon and evening; when at rest, [see Rhus t.] *Better* from the application of warmth; from violent exercise.

## SILICEA.

**MIND.** *Yielding mind, faint-hearted, anxious mood. *Gloomy, feels if she would die.* *Great tendency to start, [Kali c. Nat. m. Opi. *Phos.] *Difficulty of thinking,* [*Gel. Lach.] *Child cries if spoken to, [see Cham.]

**HEAD.** *Feels as if intoxicated,* [Gel. Cann. s. *Nux.] *Vertigo* as if one would fall forward; worse when stooping, riding, or raising eyes. *Headache from nape of neck to vertex, pain, throbbing.* Pulsating pain, most violent in forehead and vertex, with chilliness, [see Puls.] Sensation of a heavy weight pressing in forehead, [Aloe. Cact. Kali b. *Nux v.—*As if brain were pressing out through forehead, Acon.] *Sensation* as if *everything in head were alive,* [Pet.—Of a *lump* in brain, Con.—Of *numbness* in brain, Graph. *Mag. m. Plat.] *Large head, with open fontanels, [*Calc. c. Merc. Sulph.] *Itching, humid porrigo* on scalp, [Graph. Hep. *Lyc. Sulph.] *Profuse sweating on head, in evening, [*Calc. c. Merc.]

**EYES.** Smarting or burning in eyes, [as from salt, Nux v.] *Agglutination at night,* with smarting of lids. *The eyes are dazzled by light. Black spots and fiery sparks before the eyes, [see Nux.] *Ulceration* of *cornea.*

**EARS.** Stoppage of ears, which open at times with a loud report, [as of a gun, Graph.—Cracking in the ears when chewing, Cal. c. Graph.] *Otitis* interna.

**NOSE.** Ulcers in nose, [see Sep.] *Loss of smell,* [Kali b. Sep.] Stoppage of nose from hardened mucus. *Long lasting itching of the tip of the nose. *Ulcers* in nose.

**MOUTH and THROAT.** *Toothache when eating warm

food, or from breathing cold air through mouth, [**Calc. c** ***Merc. Sulph.**—Pains relieved by ice-cold water, **Bry. Coff.** ***Puls.**—By external heat, **Rhus.**] Sensation as of a hair on *front part of tongue*, [on *back part*, **Kali b. Nat. m.**—In *nose*, **Hydras.**—In *throat*, **Kali b.**] Stinging sore throat, only when swallowing, [see **Apis.**]

**STOMACH and ABDOMEN.** *Bitter taste in morning, [*putrid* taste, **Arn. Bry.** ***Merc.** ***Puls.**—Bitter taste after eating, **Ars.** ***Nit. ac. Puls.**—Sour taste after eating, **Lyc. Phos.**] *Water tastes badly; vomits after drinking, [see **Ars.**] *Hungry, but cannot eat, the food is so nauseous, [hunger, with aversion to food, **Nux v.**] *Burning* in pit of stomach, [***Ars. Canth.** ***Nux v. Phos.**—*Coldness*, **Colch. Sulph.**] *Burning in bowels*, [see **Ars.**] Much *rumbling* in bowels.

**STOOL.** *Constipation before and during menstruation; stools in hard lumps, [constipation before and diarrhœa after menstruation, **Graph.**] **Hard*, difficult stools; *they recede after having been partially expelled*, [*large, hard stools, with a sensation as if anus were closed or too *narrow*, **Nux v.**—*The rectum feels as if stopped up, **Anacar.**—See **Nux.**] Ascarides with the stool.

**URINE.** Urging to urinate, with scanty discharge. *Red or yellow sand* in the urine, [see ***Lyc.**]

**SEXUAL O'S.** *Male.* Redness of prepuce near the corona, as if excoriated with itching. [see ***Merc.**] *Weak and almost extinguished sexual desire, [**Arg. n. Hepar. Lyc. Mag. c.**] *Women.* *Increased menses, with icy coldness over whole body. Discharge of pure blood from uterus, *when babe nurses.* *Discharge of white water instead of menses, [see **Puls.**] *Menses irregular.*

**RESPIRATORY O'S.** *Continual cough, with discharge of transparent mucus, [**Ferr. Chin.**] *Dry, hacking cough, with soreness of chest*, [**Ars.** ***Caust. Nux m. Sep.** ***Staph.**—Cough, with stitches in chest, ***Bry. Bell.** ***Puls. Sulph.**]

**BACK.** *Spinal curvature*, painful to touch, [***Calc. c. Puls. Sulph.**] Swelling and suppuration of cervical glands.

**EXTREMITIES.** *Frequent panaritia*, also with proud flesh, or even where caries have set in, [***Hepar. Merc.**—In early stage, pain, *burning, stinging*, ***Apis.**] *Ulcers* on lower leg, [*Gangrenous*, **Lach.**—*Old ulcers, with burning and lacerating pains*, ***Ars. Lyc.**] **Fetid sweating of feet*, [***Bary. c. Nit. ac.** ***Plumb.**] Cold legs and feet.

**FEVER.** *Hectic fever*, particularly during a long suppuration, [***Calc. c. Hep. Phos.** ***Sulph.**] *Worm fever.* *Profuse, general night-sweat, [see **Merc.**]

**SKIN.** Lymphatic swellings, with suppuration. *Ulcers with *proud flesh* and putrid, acrid ichor, [***Ars. Kreo. Hep.** ***Sulph.**—Ulcers, with elevated, bluish edges, thin, fetid pus, **Asaph. Kreo.**—*Old, foul, flat ulcers*, with ichorous discharge, ***Lach. Puls. Sang.**—Indolent ulcers, *destitute of any organized reaction*, much burning at night, very fetid discharge, ***Carb.**

v. **Lach.**—Readily bleeding ulcers, *burning like fire*, ***Ars. Cap.**] **Fistulous ulcers*, with fetid, yellow discharge, [**Ant. Calc. c.** ***Kali hyd.**] The skin heals badly.

**CHARACT. PECULIARITIES.** **Silicea** has great control over suppurative process, *maturing abscesses* when desired, [***Hep. Mur. ac. Phyto.**] *Want of vital heat, [***Ledum. Sep.**] *Feels better with head covered up. *Ailments following vaccination*, [**Thuya.**] Symptoms *worse* at night and during full moon. *Better* in warm room, and from being wrapped up warmly.

## SPIGELIA.

**HEAD.** Vertigo, when looking downwards, [when looking upwards, **Puls.**—See **Kali b.**] Pressing headache in ~~right~~ temple, worse from least motion, stooping, or noise; better from rest and lying with head high. Sensation of *swashing* in brain when walking, [**Hep. Hyos. Nux v.**—Of *looseness*, **Cicu. Graph. Mur. ac. Rhus.**] Burning in *temples*, [in *vertex*, **Graph. Nat. m.** ***Sulph.**—*Coldness*, **Calc. c. Sep.** ***Verat.**—*Coldness* in back part of brain, **Dulc.** ***Phos.**]

**CHEST.** Shortness of breath, especially when talking, with redness of cheeks and lips. *Dyspnœa and suffocating attacks on moving and raising the arms. *Can lie only on right side*, [worse on *left* side, **Acon. Cact. Phos.**] *Stitches* about heart, worse from least movement, [**Bry.**—See **Dig.**] *Violent (visible and audible) palpitation of heart, [**Sulph. Tart. Thuya.** ***Verat.**] *Worse when bending forward*, [worse *lying down*, ***Ars.**] *Rubbing, bellows* sounds of heart, [**Spong.**—Trembling, fluttering, **Lithium.**—Wave-like beating of heart, **Viola.**] Palpitation caused by worms.

**STOMACH.** *Ravenous hunger*, with nausea and thirst, [*hungry, but cannot eat, the food is so nauseous, **Sil.**—Hunger, with aversion to food, ***Nux v.**] Nausea in morning, as if something were rising in throat from the stomach. *Worm colic*, [***Cina.**—Wants to press abdomen against something hard, **Stan.**]

**STOOL.** Frequent, inefficient urging to stool, [**Anac. Caust. Lyc.** ***Nux.**] Discharge of fæces with worms, [**Cina. Ign. Merc.** ***Sulph.**] Itching and crawling in rectum, [**Ign. Mez. Tereb.**] *Ascarides*, with itching of anus.

**CHARACT. PECULIARITIES.** Adapted to anæmic and debilitated subjects, and to scrofulous children afflicted with worms. Symptoms worse from the least movement, [**Acon.** ***Bry. Merc.**—See **Rhus.**] *Attacks periodical.* Worse from noise, [***Bell. Nux.**]

## STRAMONIUM.

**MIND.** *Desires light and company, [***Bis.**—Aversion to, **Hyos.**] *Disposed to talk continually, [**Cicu. Lach.**—Indisposed to talk, **Dig.** ***Phos. ac.** ***Verat.**] *Imagines all sorts of things; that she is double, lying crosswise, etc., [thinks another person is in bed with him, **Petro.**—Thinks he is *dead*, and they are preparing to bury him, **Lach.**—Thinks his limbs are made of *glass*, and will break, **Thuya.**—Thinks she is pregnant, or will soon be delivered, **Verat.**—Thinks he is a young child, **Cicu.**—Head feels as if *scattered about*, ***Bapt.**] *Loquacious delirium, with desire to escape, [**Bell. Opi. Rhus.**—Delirium, strange fancies, and *desire to go home*, ***Bry.**] *Insane; he gesticulates, dances, sings and laughs. *Indomitable rage, and desire to bite*, [see **Bell.**]

**HEAD.** Staggering vertigo, [see **Kali b.**] Stupefaction, with vanishing of sight, hearing and loss of consciousness, [**Hyos.** ***Opi.**] Congestion to the head, with pulsation in the vertex, [with throbbing of arteries of head and neck, ***Bell. Hyos.**] Sensation of lightness in head, [**Hipp.**—Of *heaviness*, **Calc. c. Nat. m. Phos. ac. Rhus.**—Of *fulness*, **Acon.** ***Bell. Bry.** ***Merc.**—Of *emptiness*, **Carol. r. Ign. Opi. Oxal. ac.**] *Jerking head up from pillow, and letting it drop back. *Hydrocephalus*, with convulsive motions of head, [with sudden, shrill cries, boring head into pillow, **Apis. Hell. Hyos.**—With automatic motion of one arm and leg, **Apoc.** ***Hell.**] *Rheumatic headache.*

**EYES.** *Dilatation of the pupils, with staring eyes, [***Bell. Hyos. Laur. Opi.**—Pupils contracted, **Ars. Cicu. Chel. Phos.**] *Eyes sparkling. *Dim-sightedness.*

**MOUTH and THROAT.** Grinding of teeth, [**Ars. Cicu. Verat.**—When *sleeping*, **Cina. Podo.**—With foam at mouth, ***Bell. Hell. Hyos.**] *Fear of water and aversion to all fluids, [***Bell. Canth.** ***Hyos.**] Bloody foam from mouth, [**Ars. Sec.**] Difficult deglutition from dryness and spasmodic constriction of throat, [**Ars.** ***Bell.** ***Hyos. Laur.**]

**STOMACH.** *All food tastes like *straw*, [tastes *bitter*, ***Bry. Colo. Puls.**—Tastes *salt*, **Carb. v. Chin. Sep.**—Craves *salt food*, **Calc. c. Carb. v.** ***Sep.**—See **Hepar.**] Vomiting sour mucus or green bile. Pain in abdomen, as if the navel were *pulled out*, [drawn in, as from a string. ***Plumb.**] Colic, with cold shivers.

**SLEEP.** *Sleepy, but cannot sleep*, [***Bell. Lach. Opi.**] He lies on his back, with open, staring eyes, [see **Opi.**] *He awakens with a shrinking look, as if he had been frigthened.

**CHARACT. PECULIARITIES.** Painlessness with most ailments. *Convulsions, with consciousness*, [*without consciousness*, **Bell. Cicu. Cup. Hyos.**] *Bright light or contact renews the spasms, [**Bell.**] St. Vitus' dance, [**Cup. Hyos.**—Especially in girls, **Bell.**—Especially boys, ***Nux v.**] Stiffness of whole body, [**Cicu. Cup. Opi.**] Extreme degree of nervous erethism. *He feels too tall. Aggravation;* after sleeping, [**Apis.** ***Lach. Opi.**] From looking at *glistening objects*, or being touched, [**Bell.**] *Better* from bright light, [better in the *dark*, [**Con. Phos. Sang.**]

## SULPHUR.

**MIND.** *Low-spirited, out of humor, inclines to weep, [see **Puls.**] Dulness, difficulty of thinking, [**Hell.** ***Laur. Spig.**] Misplaces, or cannot find right words when he speaks, [**Graph.**] *Extremely forgetful*, [**Croc. Lach. Thuya.**]

**HEAD.** Vertigo when sitting, [when *rising*, ***Puls.**] *Heaviness and fulness* in forehead, [**Calc. c. Nat. m. Phos. ac. Rhus.**] Sensation of hollowness in head, [**Coral. r. Ign. Opi. Oxal. ac.**] **Constant heat on top of head*, [**Graph. Nat. m.**—*Coldness*, **Sep.** ***Verat.**—On the right side of head, **Calc. c.**—On occiput, **Dulc. Phos.**] Pressure in temples, and tightness in brain, [pressure on vertex, as from a weight, **Aloe. Cact. Cann. s. Kali b.**] *Beating headache, worse in morning, from motion, when stooping, and in open air. *Sick-headache every week or every two weeks*, [**Phyto.**] *Fontanels close too late, [***Calc. c. Merc.** ***Sil.**] *Tinea capitis*, dry form, [see **Rhus.**]

**EYES.** *Burning* in eyes, [**Ars. Bell. Caust. Phos.**—*Coldness* of lids, **Con. Kali c. Lyc.**] *Ulceration* of margins of lids, [***Euph. Merc. Nat. m.**] Specks or ulcers on cornea, [**Lach. Merc. Sil.**] *Intolerance of sun's light, [***Bell. Con. Ign. Puls.**] *Black motes* before the eyes, [**Kali c. Merc. Pet.**—Like a swarm of insects, **Caust.**]

**EARS.** *Deafness, with roaring and itching in ears. *Whizzing* or roaring in ears, [see **Chin.**] Wabbling, as if water was in ears, [escape of wind from ears, **Chel. Stram.**]

**NOSE.** Bleeding of nose, [**Bell.** ***Phos.**] *Loss of smell*, [**Caust. Hep. Phos. Sep. Sil.** —*Acuteness* of, **Bell. Coloh.** ***Lyc.**] Dry ulcers or scabs in nose, [**Sep.**] Herpes across the nose, like a saddle, [see **Sep.**]

**MOUTH and THROAT.** Lips dry, burning. Jerks through single teeth. *Swelling of gums, with throbbing pain, [ulcerated gums, **Lyc.** ***Merc. Staph. Sul. ac.**—Readily *bleeding gums*, **Ars. Merc. Nit. ac. Phos.**] Tongue white, with red tip and borders. *Pressure in throat as from a lump, [**Graph.** ***Hep. Ign. Lach. Nux v.**—Sensation as of a *splinter*, **Arg. n. Hep. Nit. ac.**] Sensation of a hair in the throat, [**Ars. Kali b.**]

**STOMACH and ABDOMEN.** *Putrid taste in the morning, [see **Puls.**] Complete loss of appetite, [see **Rhus.**] Food tastes *too salt*, [**Carb. v. Chin. Sep.**—Not salt enough, **Ars. Thuya.**—See **Hep.**] Milk disagrees, [***Puls. Sep.**] *Sour eructations, with great acidity of stomach, [**Cham. Con. Nit. ac. Nux v.** — *Bitter* eructations after a meal, **Bell. Chin.** ***Nux.**] Region of stomach very painful to pressure, [**Bry. Lach.** ***Merc.** ***Nux v.**] *Painful pressure in stomach, as from a weight, [**Ars. Bry.** ***Nux v. Sep.**] *Burning in stomach*, [see ***Ars.**] *Chronic hepatitis*. *Abdomen sensitive to pressure, internal parts feel raw and sore, [***Bell. Nux.**] Movement in abdomen as of something alive, [**Croc.** ***Saba. Thuya.**]

**STOOL and ANUS.** *Constipation*, with frequent unsuccessful desire for stool, [**Anacar. Caust. *Lyc. *Nux v.**] Hard, knotty, insufficient stool, [**Alum. Graph. Iod. Sep.**] *Painless *morning diarrhœa*, has hardly time to get out of bed, [***Rumex.** —Early morning diarrhœa, *with pain*, **Alœ.**—See **Podo.**] Stools *watery; green mucus; undigested; changeable. Before stool*, cutting colic. *After stool*, tenesmus. *Stool, with ascarides, lumbrici, [**Cin. Ign. Merc. Spig.**] *Prolapsus recti* during stool. *Hemorrhoids, oozing or bleeding.

**URINARY O'S.** Frequent micturition, especially at night; urine at times clear, at times saturated with thick sediment. Very fetid urine, [see **Nit ac.**] Burning in urethra during micturition, [see **Canth.**]

**SEXUAL O'S.** Deep ulcers on glans and prepuce, with puffed edges, [see **Merc.**] *Stitches in penis. Troublesome itching of pudendum*, [**Graph. Kreo. *Sep.**] *Burning in vagina, [**Canth. Lyc. Thuya.**—Smarting and rawness, **Kali b.**] *Menstruation too late*, too short, too scant, [**Con. *Dulc. Phos. *Puls.**] Delayed and difficult first menstruation, [see ***Puls.**] *Catamenia thick, black, acrid, making parts sore. *Burning, painful leucorrhœa, making parts sore.

**RESPIRATORY O'S.** Deep, rough voice—*aphonia*, [***Bell. Bap. Merc. Phos.**] *Loose cough*, with soreness and pressure in chest; talking excites cough, [**Dros. Kali b. Puls.**] *Cough, with greenish, purulent expectoration, having a sweetish taste, [***Stann.**—*Gray, salty* taste, ***Lyc. Phos. Sep.**] *Much rattling of mucus in lungs; the cough worse in morning, [see **Tart. e.**] *Heavy feeling* in chest, [**Kreo. Lach. Lyc. *Nux m.**—*Light* feeling, **Stann.**] *Stitches in chest, extending to back, [**Kali c. Merc. Sil.**] Stitches in right chest to scapula, [**Bell. Sep.**] Palpitation of heart, anxious, visible, [see **Spig.**] *Heart feels too large.*

**BACK.** Stiffness in nape of the neck. Drawing pain between scapulæ, [*burning* between, **Ars. Lyc.**—*Coldness* between, **Am. m.**] Curvature of spine, [see **Sil.**] *Sensation as if one vertebra glided over the other.*

**EXTREMITIES.** *Drawing and lacerating in arms and hands. Trembling of hands, [**Agar. Lach. Phos. Stram.**] *Panaritium, [***Hep. Lach. Merc. Sil.**] *Heaviness* in lower limbs, as if paralyzed, [**Bell. Merc. Nux. Rhus.**] Rigidity in bend of knees, [***Bry. Graph. Led. Sep.**—In the hips, **Acon. *Rhus. Staph.**] *Burning in soles, [**Phos. ac. Puls. *Sil.**]

**SLEEP.** *Drowsiness in daytime; sleepless at night, [**Lyc. Merc.**—See **Stram.**] **Talks* loudly while asleep, [**Bell. Nat. m. Sep.**—*Sings* during sleep, **Bell. Croc. Phos. ac.**] *Jerks and twitches* during sleep.

**FEVER.** Thirst even before chilliness, [**Cimex. Eup. per.** —Thirst only during chill, **Calc. c. Cap. Carb. v. *Ign.**—No thirst during paroxysm, ***Puls. Sep.**] *Chill in evening, followed by heat and profuse sweat, [**Ars. Bell. *Rhus t.**] Slight chill at 10 A.M., continues till 3 P.M., [see **Nat. m.**] *Frequent flushes of heat, [***Lyc. Sep. Puls.**] *Copious morning sweat, [see **Merc.**]

**SKIN.** *Dry, husky, scaly skin.* *Unhealthy skin, every little injury suppurates, [**Calc. c. Graph. *Hep. Sil.**] *Psora, with violent itching and tingling; burning after scratching, [**Cro. t. *Merc. Rhus. Staph.**] *Pimply eruptions filled with pus. *Dry herpes,* scurfy, itching violently, [**Calc. c. Kali c. Phos.**—*Humid* tetter, **Kreo. *Ledum. Kali c. Merc.**] **Excoriation of skin,* especially where it is folded upon itself, [**Cham. *Graph. Lyc. Merc.**] *Old ulcers, with the production of proud flesh, [**Graph. Sang. *Sil.**—Ulcers, which *bleed easily* burn like fire, ***Ars. Carb. v. Kreo. Hep.**—See **Lach.**]

**CHARACT. PECULIARITIES.** *Suitable to lean persons who walk stooping,[thin, scrawny persons, **Arg. nit. *Sec. cor.**—Scrofulous people, with a low, cachectic state, ***Iod.**] Talking fatigues and excites the pains. *Frequent spasmodic jerking in whole body, [**Phos. Puls.**] *Comes out of spasms very happy. *Very weak and faint about 11 A.M., must have something to eat. *Worse* in evening and after midnight, [see **Rhus.**] While at rest, [**Con. Lyc. *Rhus. Sep.**]

## TARTARUS EMETICUS.

**MIND.** Confusion of the head. *Bad humor. Child can't bear to *be touched,* [cries, if spoken to, **Sil.**—Cries if *looked at,* **Ant. c.**] *Great tendency to start.*

**HEAD.** Vertigo on closing the eyes, or when raising head, with flickering before the eyes. Headache, as if a band was compressing the forehead, [headache, *relieved by compression,* **Apis. Arg. n. *Puls.**] Throbbing in right side of forehead. *Trembling of head,* particularly when coughing.

**EYES.** Flickering before the eyes, [**Ign. Nat. m.**—*Streaks,* like lightning before the eyes, **Nux.**] *Dim, swimming eyes. *Rheumatic or arthritic ophthalmia.*

**NOSE.** Sneezing, fluent coryza, with chilliness, loss of taste and smell, [see **Puls.**] Stoppage of nose alternating with fluent coryza.

**FACE.** *Pale, sunken face, or puffed, with coma. *Warm sweat* on forehead from efforts to vomit, [*cold* sweat, **Verat.**] Lips dry, scaly.

**MOUTH.** Violent toothache in morning. *Flat taste, food seems tasteless, [tastes like *straw,* **Stram.**] *Tongue red, in streaks, very red, and dry in centre, [*brown* and dry in centre, **Bapt.**—See **Bell.**] *Aphthae.*

**THROAT.** *Violent sore throat, with painful, dry heat, and redness of the parts. *Much mucus in throat, with short breathing.* Sudden swelling of cervical glands and tonsils. Sensation as if a small leaf obstructed windpipe on hawking.

**STOMACH.** *Violent hiccough,* [**Bell. Hyos. Nux. Puls.**] *Empty or putrid eructations,* [**Arn.**] Continuous anxious nausea, [***Ipe. Lobe.**] *Vomiting large quantities of mucus, [***Ipe.**] *Continuous nausea, vomiting and diarrhœa,* [**Ipe. Verat.**] The vomiting is followed by great prostration, [**Ars.**

**Verat.**] *Pain in epigastrium, as if stomach had been overloaded. *Pulsation in pit of stomach.*

**ABDOMEN.** Abdomen feels as if stuffed full of stones, [as if *intestines were squeezed between stones*, **Colo.**] Violent colic, as if bowels would be cut to pieces, [see **Colo.**]

**STOOL.** Watery diarrhœa, preceded by colic. Stools papescent, slimy, appear like yeast, [see **Arn.**] *Diarrhœa, with vomiting and palpitation of heart.

**URINE.** Dark, brownish-red, turbid urine of strong odor, [see **Nit. ac.**] Deposits of violet-colored sediment.

**LARYNX and TRACHÆ.** Hoarseness in morning, worse on talking. *Much rattling of mucus in trachæ, but little is expectorated, [***Ipe.**] *Rattling of mucus when coughing or breathing. *Catarrhal croup, [**Hepar.**] *Coughing and gaping consecutively. *Cough compels patient to sit up, is loose and rattling, but no expectoration, [see **Bry.**] *Cough, with vomiting food and mucus*, [see **Ipe.**]

**CHEST.** *Difficult respiration, with great rattling of mucus. *Suffocative and oppressed breathing, must sit up to get air. *Chest seems full of phlegm, but does not yield to coughing, [***Ipe.**] *Chest feels as if lined with velvet.* *Pneumonia. *Œdema of the lungs.* *Great præcordial anxiety, with vomiting mucus and bile.

**BACK.** Inclination to unbutton collar of his shirt. Pain in back, as from fatigue. *Violent pain in sacro-lumbar region, the least motion causes retching and cold, clammy sweat.

**LIMBS.** *Trembling of the hands, [**Ars. Caust. Hyos.**] Finger-tips appear dead, dry and hard. Numbness and coldness in legs. Feet go "to sleep" immediately after sitting down. Constant inclination to stretch.

**FEVER.** Pulse full, hard and accelerated. The least exertion accelerates the pulse. Chill, with external coldness, coming on at all times of day, with sleepiness. Feels as if cold water was poured over him. Long-lasting heat, after a short chill, with sleepiness and sweat on forehead.

**SKIN.** Red, itching rash over the body. *Thick eruption like pocks, often pustular, as large as a pea. Violent itching of the skin. Vesicular eruptions.

**CHARACT. PECULIARITIES.** *Trembling of whole body.* Great weakness and lassitude. Children want to be carried, and cry if touched, [see **Cham.**] *Catarrhal inflammation of respiratory organs.

## VERATRUM ALBUM.

**MIND.** Insanity, he wants to cut up everything, [wants to bite, to spit, to strike, and to tear things, ***Bell. Stram.**] Persevering *refusal to talk*, [***Bell. Ign. Nit. ac.** ***Phos. ac.**—Talks continually, **Cicu. Lach.** ***Stram.**]

**HEAD.** *Headache, with nausea and vomiting*, [**Ars. Ipec.**

**Kali b.** ***Nux.**—Gastric sick-headache, ***Iris.** **Puls.**—See **Nux v.**] **Cold perspiration on forehead.* Burning in brain, [**Canth. Hell.**] **Coldness* on vertex, [**Calc. c. Laur. Sep.**—*Burning* on vertex, **Graph. Nat. m. Sulph.**] *Heaviness* of head, [**Calc. c. Opi. Phos. ac. Rhus.**—*Lightness,* **Hipp.** ***Stram.**]

**EYES.** Fixed, watery, sunken, [see **Opi.**] Paralysis of eyelids, [great *heaviness,* cannot keep them open, ***Gel. Rhus. Sep.**] *Double vision.* Blindness at night, [**Bell.**]

**FACE.** *Cold, collapsed face; pinched-up, bluish nose, [pale, death-like face, with distorted features, ***Ars. Canth.**—Distorted, bluish, with mouth wide open, **Hyos.**] *Lockjaw,* [**Bell. Cicu. Hyos.**] Facial neuralgia.

**MOUTH and THROAT.** Grinding of teeth, [see **Stram.**] Tongue red and swollen, or *dry, black, and cracked,* [**Ars. Merc. Lyc.**] Tongue cold, withered, [**Carbo v.** ***Cis. c. Mur. ac.**] Feels as if scalded, [**Colo.** ***Verat. v.**—As if burnt and numb, **Laur.**—Feels *heavy,* **Mur. ac. Nat. m. Nux.**] Spasmodic constriction of throat, [see **Hyos.**] *Roughness* in throat. *Burning* in throat, [***Ars. Bell. Lach. Phos.**—*Coldness,* **Carb. v. Laur.**]

**STOMACH and ABDOMEN.** *Unquenchable thirst, especially for cold drinks, [***Acon.** ***Ars. Jatro. Phos.**] Strong desire for acids and refreshing things, [**Phos. ac.**] *Continuous nausea,* [***Ipe. Phos. Tart. e.**] Vomiting food, acid, bitter, foamy, white, or yellow-green mucus, [see **Ipe.**] *Vomiting black bile and blood,* [***Ars. Hyd. ac. Sec.**] *Vomiting, with diarrhœa and great prostration, [***Ars. Jatro. Tart. e.**] The vomiting is renewed by drinking, or the least motion, [**Zinc.**] Cutting in abdomen, as with knives, [***Colo. Con.**] *Sensation as if bowels were tied in knots, [as if squeezed between stones, ***Colo.**] *Great sinking and empty feeling in abdomen. *Burning* in abdomen, as from hot coals, [***Ars. Phos. Sec.**]

**STOOL.** Constipation, as from inactivity of rectum; stool hard, too large, [**Alum. Kali c. Nux v.**] *Diarrhœa; stools greenish, watery, with flakes,* also *blackish, watery* stools. Before stool, severe pinching colic. *During stool,* paleness, cold sweat on forehead, and vomiting. *After stool, great sinking and empty feeling in abdomen, [see **Ars.**]

**URINE.** *Greenish urine,* [**Ars. Mag. c. Ruta.**—*Blackish,* **Colch. Nat. m.**—White, like milk, **Phos. ac.**] Frequent, but scanty emissions of dark-red urine.

**SEXUAL O'S.** *Dysmenorrhœa, with vomiting and purging, or exhausting diarrhœa, with cold sweat. Suppressed lochia and milk, with delirium.

**RESPIRATORY O'S.** Spasmodic cough, with blue face, suffocation, [**Hyos. Ipe.**] *Deep, hollow cough, as if coming from abdomen, with yellow, tough, bitter, or salt expectoration, only during day, [only at *night,* **Caust. Staph. Tart.**] *Cough, with involuntary urination. [**Caust. Puls.**] Stitches in sides of chest, especially when coughing, [**Bell. Bry. Puls.**] Violent, visible, anxious palpitation of heart, [see **Spig.**]

**FEVER.** Pulse irregular, generally small, thread-like; often imperceptible, [**Ars. Cann. Carb. v.**] *Intermittent fevers;* chill occurs early in morning, or in forenoon, [see **Nat. m.**] Chill, with *external coldness only,* [external heat and internal shuddering, **Ign.**] First, violent chill, afterwards heat, with thirst, then sweat. Blood runs cold through veins, [runs *hot,* **Ars. Rhus.**] *Typhoid fever, with great *prostration; cold sweating;* coma; vomiting, and watery diarrhœa; bluish face; pointed nose; wrinkled skin, [**trembling of hands and coldness of extremities,* **Zinc.**]

**CHARACT. PECULIARITIES.** *Sudden sinking of strength, [**Acon. *Ars. *Camph.**] Attacks of fainting from least exertion. *Excesive weakness.* Shocks in limbs, as from electric sparks, [*shocks through whole body, **Nux v.**] *Violent tonic spsams,* palms of hands and soles of feet drawn inward. After fright, involuntary stools, [***Gel. Opi.**] *Worse* after drinking; after sleep, [**Apis. *Lach. Opi.**—Better after sleeping, **Cro tig. Phos. Sil.**] Better after perspiring, [see **Merc.**]

THE END.

# INDEX.

## REMEDIES.